Nanotechnologies for the Life Sciences
Volume 1

Biofunctionalization of Nanomaterials

Edited by
Challa S. S. R. Kumar

Related Titles

Willner, I., Katz, E. (eds.)

Bioelectronics

From Theory to Applications

492 pages with 241 figures and 4 tables
2005
Hardcover
ISBN 3-527-30690-0

Fecht, H.-J., Werner, M. (eds.)

The Nano-Micro Interface

Bridging the Micro and Nano Worlds

351 pages with 102 figures and 27 tables
2004
Hardcover
ISBN 3-527-30978-0

Baltes, H., Brand, O., Fedder, G. K., Hierold, C., Korvink, J. G., Tabata, O. (eds.)

Enabling Technologies for MEMS and Nanodevices

Advanced Micro and Nanosystems

439 pages with 245 figures and 15 tables
2004
Hardcover
ISBN 3-527-30746-X

Öberg, P. Å., Togawa, T., Spelman, F. A. (eds.)

Sensors in Medicine and Health Care

Sensors Applications Vol. 3

444 pages with 219 figures and 7 tables
2004
Hardcover
ISBN 3-527-29556-9

Niemeyer, C. M., Mirkin, C. A. (eds.)

Nanobiotechnology

Concepts, Applications and Perspectives

491 pages with 193 figures and 9 tables
2004
Hardcover
ISBN 3-527-30658-7

Manners, I.

Synthetic Metal-Containing Polymers

288 pages with 86 figures and 10 tables
2004
Hardcover
ISBN 3-527-29463-5

Caruso, F. (ed.)

Colloids and Colloid Assemblies

Synthesis, Modification, Organization and Utilization of Colloid Particles

621 pages with 273 figures and 8 tables
2004
Hardcover
ISBN 3-527-30660-9

Gómez-Romero, P., Sanchez, C. (eds.)

Functional Hybrid Materials

434 pages with 212 figures and 12 tables
2004
Hardcover
ISBN 3-527-30484-3

Nanotechnologies for the Life Sciences
Volume 1

Biofunctionalization of Nanomaterials

Edited by
Challa S. S. R. Kumar

1st Edition

WILEY-VCH Verlag GmbH & Co. KGaA

The Editor of this Book

Dr. Challa S. S. R. Kumar
The Center for
Advanced Microstructures
and Devices (CAMD)
Louisiana State University
6980 Jefferson Highway
BATON ROUGE, LA 70806
USA

Library of Congress Card No.: applied for
British Library Cataloging-in-Publication Data:
A catalogue record for this book is available from the British Library.
Bibliographic information published by Die Deutsche Bibliothek
Die Deutsche Bibliothek lists this publication in the Deutsche Nationalbibliografie; detailed bibliographic data is available in the Internet at http://dnb.ddb.de.

Printed in the Federal Republic of Germany.
Printed on acid-free paper.

Typesetting Asco Typesetters, Hong Kong
Printing Strauss GmbH, Mörlenbach
Binding J. Schäffer GmbH i. G., Grünstadt

ISBN-13: 978-3-527-31381-5
ISBN-10: 3-527-31381-8

Contents

Nanotechnologies for the Life Sciences Vol. 1
Biofunctionalization of Nanomaterials. Edited by Challa S. S. R. Kumar

ISBN: 3-527-31381-8

Preface

On behalf of a great team of nano researchers who have been part of this exciting project, I am pleased to introduce to the scientific community a comprehensive ten volume series on *Nanotechnologies for the Life Sciences* (*NtLS*), which is going to be a knowledge base of encyclopedic proportions for applications of nanotechnologies in biology, biotechnology and medicine. This is a unique series of books on an important facet of nanotechnology being presented by the nanotechnologists for the nanotechnologists. What you have in your hand is the first volume, *Biofunctionalization of Nanomaterials*, in this exciting series.

The first volume has eleven chapters covering various aspects and techniques for functionalization of different nanomaterials with variety of biomolecules. The book begins with an exciting chapter by *Michael J. Murcia* and *Christoph A. Naumann* from the Indiana University-Purdue University, USA, which provides an overview of developments in *biofunctionalization and biocompatible coating of fluorescent nanoparticles*. There is an explosion of knowledge on carbon nanotubes, long, thin cylinders of carbon, discovered in 1991 by S. Iijima and the focus of their practical applications have been due to their unique physical properties such as optical, electrical, thermal, elastic behavior and so on. However, once it was demonstrated that it is possible to functionalize them with biomolecules, there has been a great interest amongst nanoresearchers to investigate their potential in life sciences. The University of California team of researchers from Riverside, USA, *Elena Bekyarova*, *Robert C. Haddon* and *Vladimir Parpura*, has done a remarkable job in capturing the up-to-date information in their chapter entitled *biofunctionalization of carbon nanotubes*. Metallic and metal oxide nanoparticles are well studied and their extraordinary physical and chemical properties make them useful in variety of applications. Not surprisingly, a great deal of research work was carried out to make them not only biocompatible, but also attach biological molecules in order to extend their applications into the life sciences. Four chapters have been dedicated to capture this information and the authors of these four chapters – 3, 4, 6 and 8 – have done a thorough job in comprehensively providing the information on biofunctionalization aspects of a wide variety of metallic/metal oxide nanoparticles. *Yong Guo* from the Southern Illinois University, Carbondale, USA, dealt with *biofunctionalization of magnetic nanoparticles*. *Ming Zheng* and *Xueying Huang* from DuPont Central Research and Development, USA, described some unique aspects

Nanotechnologies for the Life Sciences Vol. 1
Biofunctionalization of Nanomaterials. Edited by Challa S. S. R. Kumar

ISBN: 3-527-31381-8

of *biofunctionalization of gold nanoparticles*. *Grit Festag*, *Uwe Klenz*, *Thomas Henkel*, *Andrea Csllki* and *Wolfgang Fritzsche* from the Institute for Physical High Technology, Jena, Germany, in a very unique fashion reviewed several approaches towards *biofunctionalization of metallic nanoparticles* for biosensing. In addition to the completely chemical based approach for biofunctionalization, *Raphael Levy* and *Chris Doty* from the University of Liverpool, UK, provided a state-of-the-art review on the use of biomolecules themselves for stabilization of metallic nanomaterials in the chapter entitled *stabilization and biofunctionalization of metallic nanoparticles: the peptide route*.

In addition to metallic nanoparticles, polymeric nanoparticles have been widely investigated for their applications in life sciences primarily in the area of drug delivery. It is again very important for the polymeric nanoparticles to be either biocompatible or biofunctionalized in order to be suitable for life science applications. *Biofunctionalization of phospholipid polymeric nanoparticles* by *Junji Watanabe*, *Jongwon Park*, *Tornomi Ito*, *Madoku Takai*, and *Kazuhiko Ishihara* from the University of Tokyo, Japan, provides information, based on their own research experience, on phospholipid polymeric nanoparticles and their biofunctionalization. The chapter *magnetic core conducting polymer shell nanocomposites for DNA attachment und hybridization* contributed by *Jean-Paul Lellouche* of Bar-llan University, Israel, presents an interesting perspective towards biofunctionalization of magnetic core polymer shell nanomaterials. The researchers from the Northeastern University, Boston, USA, – *Sushama Kommareddy*, *Dinesh B. Shenoy* and *Mansoor M. Amiji* – brought out comprehensive information on *gelatin nanoparticles and their biofunctionalization*.

Amongst all the biomolecules, proteins are unique and their conjugation to nanomaterials provides a very broad base for life science researchers. The research group from Clemson University, USA, led by *Ya-Ping Sun* with *Mohammed J. Meziani* and *Yi Lin* brought out an excellent in-depth analysis of various conjugation approaches to bind proteins to variety of nanomaterials in their chapter entitled *conjugation of nanomaterials with proteins*. In this chapter, they provide an overview of current and emerging approaches in the coupling of metal and semiconductor nanostructures with proteins and their assemblies into different architectures followed by approaches to conjugation of carbon nanotubes with proteins and the mechanistic issues involved with nanotube-protein interactions. The chapter entitled *folate-linked lipid based nunoparticles for tumor-targeted gene therapy* by *Yoshiyuki Hattori* and *Yoshie Maitani*, Institute of Medicinal Chemistry, Japan, contains a review of literature on folate-linked liposomes and nanoparticles, and show the effectiveness of folate-linked lipid-based nanoparticles as a vector for DNA transfection and for suicide gene therapy to treat human nasopharyngeal and prostate tumors.

I am very grateful to all the authors who have shared my enthusiasm and vision by contributing high quality manuscripts, on time, keeping in tune with the original design and theme of not only this particular volume but also the whole series. You will not be having this book in your hand but for their dedication, perseverance and sacrifice. I am thankful to my employer, the Center for Advanced Microstructures and Devices (CAMD), and especially to my superior, Prof. Josef Hormes, Director of CAMD, who has been supporting me in all my creative ventures. Without this backing it would be impossible to make this venture of such magnitude a reality. No words can express the understanding of my wife, Suma, in allowing me to make my office a second home and bearing with my spending innumerable number of hours in front of the computer at home. My little daughter, Saakshi, has been the source of joy and inspiration in bringing forth my intellectual creativity. My families, friends and mentors are integral part of my existence and continue to shape my life and I am indebted to them. While it would be impossible to thank everyone individually in this preface, I must make a special mention of the support from Wiley VCH publishers in general and the publishing editor, Dr. Martin Ottmar, in particular, who has been working closely with me to ensure this project becomes a reality. I am grateful for this support.

I also would like to take this opportunity to provide few glimpses of the rest of the nine volumes in this series. As I write this preface, I am pleased to let you know that the second and the third volumes are in press and will be published shortly after volume one. The second volume, *Biological and Pharmaceutical Nanomaterials*, provides information on variety of nanomaterials from natural sources and also those that are particularly relevant from pharmaceutical stand point of view. As life scientists learn about nanotechnologies, they also need to be familiarized with tools and techniques for characterization and the third volume, *Nanosystem Characterization Tools in the Life Sciences*, brings forth the required information. The rest of the volumes in this series deal in general with sensing, controlled release, devices, engineering, biomimetic approaches that are relevant to life sciences. These volumes are currently under preparation and I hope to present them to you as soon as possible.

As I stop for moment and ponder at the amount of information that the dedicated team of scientists have been compiling for this ten volume series, I can't help but become philosophical. Scientific endeavors by their very nature, while providing answers to several questions, create more and more questions. If one examines the growth of various scientific disciplines one would realize that while we made tremendous progress in scientific achievements, we continue to be puzzled by several unanswered questions in addition to several more new ones popping up every day. In the words of one philosopher, "the measure of our intellectual maturity is our capacity to feel less and less satisfied with our answers to better problems." One could say that the progress in science is directly proportional to the number of unsolved problems. It is pertinent to remember what Einstein said once, "We can't solve problems by using the same kind of thinking we used when we created them." What we need as scientists is lateral thinking. In order for developing lateral thinking one needs to comprehend the existing knowledge and develop the ability to connect seemingly unconnected points in the web of knowledge.

Nanoscience and nanotechnology is beginning to gain respectable place in this web of knowledge that we scientists have been creating. This new scientific discipline is being touted as the greatest revolution in the history of mankind and is anticipated to positively affect every facet of our existence. It is anticipated to improve quality of our life in leaps and bounds. However, Nanotechnology's greatest gift to mankind, in my view, is its ability to promote lateral thinking amongst not only scientists but all those who are associated with this new approach to problem solving. This is what I would like to call "nano vision or nano thinking". It is the ability to think small while thinking big and to connect small and big at the same time." The followers of "nano thinking", so called "nano thinkers", are growing day by day and their presence is beginning to be felt strongly in the field of life sciences. It is my endeavor to be a catalyst in inculcating this new thinking by providing a multi-pronged base of knowledge in nanotechnologies for the life sciences. The ten volume series *NtLS* is anticipated to be the solid foundation for all those who are interested in applying "nano thinking" in life sciences. I am leaving the book in your hands and take your leave sharing a quotation from one of the greatest thinkers from the United States of America, Oliver Wendell Holmes, who said "Man's mind, once stretched by a new idea, never regains its original dimensions." It is my hope that this book series will help in stretching the limits of thinking in all those who come in contact with it.

Challa S. S. R. Kumar

List of Contributors

Mansoor M. Amiji
Department of Pharmaceutical Sciences
School of Pharmacy
Northeastern University
110 Mugar Life Sciences Building
Boston MA 02115
USA

Elena Bekyarova
Departments of Chemistry
Pierce Hall Annex 104
University of California
Riverside, CA 92521-0403
USA

Andrea Csáki
Institute for Physical High Technology
Biotechnical Microsystems Department
P.O.B. 100 239
07702 Jena
Germany

R. Christopher Doty
School of Biological Sciences
Biosciences Building
Crown Street
University of Liverpool
Liverpool L69 7ZB
UK

Grit Festag
Institute for Physical High Technology
Biotechnical Microsystems Department
P.O.B. 100 239
07702 Jena
Germany

Wolfgang Fritzsche
Institute for Physical High Technology
Biotechnical Microsystems Department
P.O.B. 100 239
07702 Jena
Germany

Yong Gao
Department of Chemistry and Biochemistry
Southern Illinois University
1245 Lincoln Drive
Carbondale, IL 62901-4409
USA

Robert C. Haddon
Departments of Chemistry and Chemical &
Environmental Engineering
Center for Nanoscale Science & Engineering
Pierce Hall Annex 203
University of California
Riverside, CA 92521-0403
USA

Yoshiyuki Hattori
Institute of Medicinal Chemistry
Hoshi University
Ebara 2-4-41, Shinagawa-ku
Tokyo 142-8501
Japan

Thomas Henkel
Institute for Physical High Technology
Biotechnical Microsystems Department
P.O.B. 100 239
07702 Jena
Germany

Xueying Huang
Sepax Technologies, Inc.
5 Innovation Way
Newark, Delaware 19711
USA

Kazuhiko Ishihara
Department of Materials Engineering
School of Engineering
The University of Tokyo
7-3-1, Hongo, Bunkyo-ku
Tokyo 113-8656
Japan

Tomomi Ito
Department of Materials Engineering
School of Engineering
The University of Tokyo
7-3-1, Hongo, Bunkyo-ku
Tokyo 113-8656
Japan

Uwe Klenz
Institute for Physical High Technology
Biotechnical Microsystems Department
P.O.B. 100 239
07702 Jena
Germany

Sushma Kommareddy
Department of Pharmaceutical Sciences
School of Pharmacy
Northeastern University
110 Mugar Life Sciences Building
Boston MA 02115
USA

Jean-Paul Lellouche
Department of Chemistry
Bar-Ilan University
Ramat-Gan 52900
Israel

Raphaël Lévy
School of Biological Sciences
Biosciences Building
Crown Street
University of Liverpool
Liverpool L69 7ZB
UK

Yi Lin
Department of Chemistry and Laboratory for Emerging Materials and Technology
Clemson University
Clemson
South Carolina 29634-0973
USA

Yoshie Maitani
Institute of Medicinal Chemistry
Hoshi University
Ebara 2-4-41, Shinagawa-ku
Tokyo 142-8501
Japan

Mohammed J. Meziani
Department of Chemistry and Laboratory for Emerging Materials and Technology
Clemson University
Clemson
South Carolina 29634-0973
USA

Michael J. Murcia
Department of Chemistry and Chemical Biology
Indiana University-Purdue University Indianapolis
402 N. Blackford St.
Indianapolis 46202-3274
USA

Christoph A. Naumann
Department of Chemistry and Chemical Biology
Indiana University-Purdue University Indianapolis
402 N. Blackford St.
Indianapolis 46202-3274
USA

Jongwon Park
Department of Materials Engineering
School of Engineering
The University of Tokyo
7-3-1, Hongo, Bunkyo-ku
Tokyo 113-8656
Japan

Vladimir Parpura
Department of Cell Biology and Neuroscience
1208 Spieth Hall
University of California
Riverside, CA 92521-0403
USA

Dinesh B. Shenoy
Department of Pharmaceutical Sciences
School of Pharmacy
Northeastern University
110 Mugar Life Sciences Building
Boston MA 02115
USA

Ya-Ping Sun
Department of Chemistry and Laboratory for Emerging Materials and Technology
Clemson University
Clemson
South Carolina 29634-0973
USA

Madoka Takai
Department of Materials Engineering
School of Engineering
The University of Tokyo
7-3-1, Hongo, Bunkyo-ku
Tokyo 113-8656
Japan

Junji Watanabe
Department of Materials Engineering
School of Engineering
The University of Tokyo
7-3-1, Hongo, Bunkyo-ku
Tokyo 113-8656
Japan

Ming Zheng
Du Pont Central Research and Development
Experimental Station, E328/B31D
Wilmington, DE 19880
USA

1 Biofunctionalization of Fluorescent Nanoparticles

Michael J. Murcia and Christoph A. Naumann

1.1 Introduction

The current revolution in life sciences is strongly linked to the availability of sophisticated new experimental tools that enable the manipulation of biomolecules and the study of biological processes at the molecular level using state-of-the-art imaging techniques, such as single molecule imaging. Optical microscopy is fundamental to furthering our understanding of the structural, organizational, and dynamic properties of biological systems because a wide variety of complementary, non-invasive optical techniques exemplified by wide-field microscopy techniques, such as brightfield, darkfield, phase contrast, and DIC exist. Among these optical detection techniques, fluorescence microscopy is particularly important because it facilitates highly sensitive and specific imaging experiments. In addition, more sophisticated imaging approaches such as confocal and near-field imaging provide the opportunity for 3D and sub-diffraction limit imaging, respectively.

Optical microscopy is now sensitive enough to track individual molecules if they are conjugated to appropriate imaging probes. Traditionally, such single molecule probes were μm-size colloidal particles and single fluorophores [1]. Colloidal probes such as gold or fluorescently labeled polystyrene beads are typically much larger (0.1–1 μm) than the biomolecule to be studied. However, fluorescent dyes, though smaller, show pronounced photo-instabilities, including blinking (due to fluorescence intensity fluctuations) and photobleaching, thus complicating single molecule tracking experiments and other fluorescence-based long-term studies. From the above description, further progress in the field of optical single molecule imaging obviously depends on the availability of appropriate labels that combine small size and high photostability with the ability to be used in multicolor studies. Fluorescent nanoparticles fulfill these important criteria. To be used in a biological environment, these nanoprobes need to be biofunctionalized appropriately, which remains a significant challenge.

The main focus of this chapter is to provide an overview of recent developments addressing the bioconjugation of fluorescent nanoparticles and their surface modification using biocompatible coatings. Section 1.2 summarizes the different types

Nanotechnologies for the Life Sciences Vol. 1
Biofunctionalization of Nanomaterials. Edited by Challa S. S. R. Kumar

ISBN: 3-527-31381-8

of fluorescent nanoparticles, including dye-doped nanoparticles, quantum dots (QDs), metal nanoparticles, and μm-size hybrids comprising fluorescent nanoprobes. Section 1.3 describes recent developments concerning the conjugation of biomolecules to fluorescent nanoparticles, and compares the different conjugation approaches for nanoparticles consisting of polymeric, semiconductor, or metallic materials. An overview of published design architectures of biocompatible surface coatings as applied to fluorescent nanoparticles is given in Section 1.4. Finally, Section 1.5 lists representative examples of how biofunctionalized nanoprobes can be applied to problems in biosensing, as well as single cell and biological tissue imaging.

1.2
Fluorescent Nanoparticle Probes

Gold nanoparticles that are surface-functionalized with proteins have been used in electron microscopy (EM) applications for quite some time [2]. A prominent example is the specific labeling of tissue by use of antibody-conjugated Au-nanoprobes (10–40 nm diameter) and their imaging by use of transmission electron microscopy (TEM). Such EM studies can achieve the detection of Au-probes with a resolution of less than 10 nm [3]. Though this demonstrates a great sensitivity, EM is limited by its inability to image living biological systems. Optical microscopy may overcome this limitation. For example, colloidal gold of 30–40 nm diameter has been used as an optical imaging label on multiple single molecule tracking experiments at the cellular level [1, and references therein]. Here, colloidal gold is used as a Rayleigh scatterer, for which the scattering $\propto d^6$ (d = diameter), thus making tracking experiments with probe diameters of less than 30 nm extremely challenging or even impossible.

Fluorescent nanoparticles are highly attractive imaging probes because, in contrast to scattering probes, their detection is not limited by the Rayleigh scattering condition. As a consequence, fluorescent nanoprobes > 1 nm can be detected if appropriate imaging setups are used. Importantly, at this size range, such nanoprobes do not exceed the size of individual proteins, thus addressing an important condition for high-quality imaging at the molecular level. In addition, single molecule detection is improved because the weak scattering of the probes lowers the optical background and thus enhances the imaging sensitivity. Figure 1.1 illustrates the size range of these probes in comparison with that of other nanoparticles. The most common types of fluorescent nanoparticles, dye-doped nanospheres and luminescent quantum dots (QDs), are described below in more detail, together with some recently introduced hybrid architectures of fluorescent nanoprobe-containing μm-size particles. Also included is an overview of optically active metal nanoparticles because these probes are highly relevant in single molecule spectroscopy.

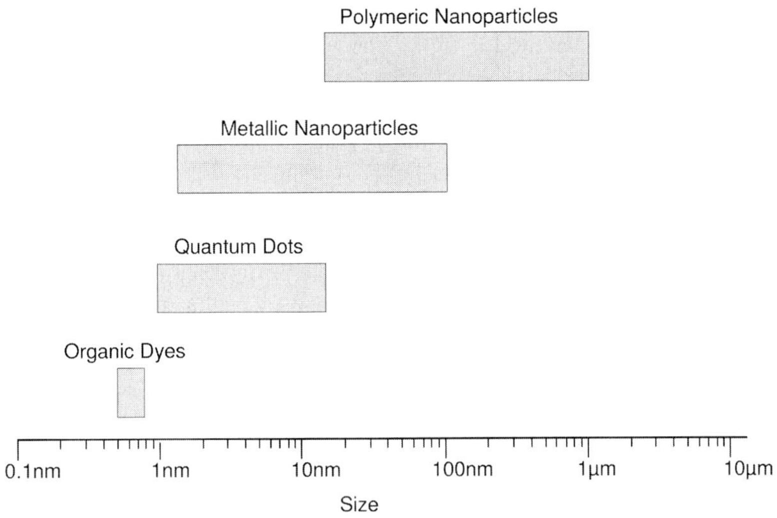

Fig. 1.1. Size ranges of commonly used fluorescent nanoprobes.

1.2.1
Dye-doped Nanoparticles

Dye-doped nanoparticles are polymer or silica-based particles containing organic or inorganic dyes [4, 5]. Dyes can be attached to the nanoparticle surface or can be embedded inside the particles either noncovalently or covalently. For imaging applications, dye-doped nanoparticles containing embedded dyes are particularly attractive because their photostability can be enhanced due to the better protection of the dyes from oxygen. For example, incorporation of pyrene dyes into polystyrene particles using a normal microemulsion approach led to a 40-fold increase in emission intensity with respect to the pure dye at the identical concentration [6]. Brightness of the fluorescence signal from such imaging probes can be controlled by the number of dye molecules per nanoparticle, with the maximum dye density limited only by self-quenching. Therefore, dye-doped nanoparticles can be quite photostable without showing fluorescence intensity fluctuations (blinking).

Typical polymer-based dye-doped nanoparticles are made of hydrophobic polymers. The hydrophobic dye molecules are kept within such nanoparticles through noncovalent hydrophobic interactions, thus preventing the gradual release and photooxidation of the dyes. Dye-doped polymeric nanoparticles have been applied down to a size of ~20 nm [7]. Although they are reasonably photostable, the hydrophobic nature of these probes complicates imaging applications in aqueous environments, which are required for studies on biological systems. Common unwanted phenomena are clustering and non-specific binding. To overcome these problems, the hydrophobic core particles can be surface-functionalized with hydro philic coatings such as polymers like poly(ethylene glycol) (PEG), polysaccharides such as dextran, or proteins such as bovine serum albumin (BSA).

Dye-doped silica nanoparticles are attractive imaging probes because their hydrophilic nature reduces the problems of non-specific binding and clustering. Silica shows several additional properties beneficial for optical imaging applications in biological systems, including chemical inertness, transparency, and the ability to act as stabilizers in protecting the embedded dyes from the outside environment [4]. In addition, the surface hydroxyl groups can be chemically modified, allowing for the straightforward surface modification with amines, carboxyls, or thiols. In addition, pH changes do not lead to swelling and porosity changes, and silica particles are less prone to attack from microbes [8]. However, the incorporation of hydrophobic dyes into the hydrophilic silica matrix is challenging, requiring specific modifications of either the dye molecules or the silica. For example, dyes can be modified with a hydrophilic molecule such as dextran or a hydrophobic silica-precursor can be used during nanoparticle synthesis [9]. Dye-doped silica particles were first synthesized using the Stoeber method [10]. However, this method leads to polydispersity and average particle sizes of >100 nm. More recently, these limitations have been overcome by use of a reverse microemulsion method that can create monodisperse dye-doped silica particles down to a size of 15 nm (Fig. 1.2) [11]. Notably, this elegant approach facilitates the size-tuning via adjustment of the microemulsion composition and does not require elevated temperatures and pressures [11, 12]. Silica also has been used to create hollow silica nanospheres filled with dye molecules [13].

Rare-earth-doped $LaPO_4$ nanoparticles are another interesting class of nanoprobes that show promising properties for diagnostic and imaging applications [14]. These systems combine small size (<10 nm), high chemical stability, very good quantum yield, and high photostability. Furthermore, they are expected to show low cytotoxicity. Recently, such rare-earth-doped $LaPO_4$ nanoparticles were successfully surface-functionalized to allow their subsequent coupling to biomole-

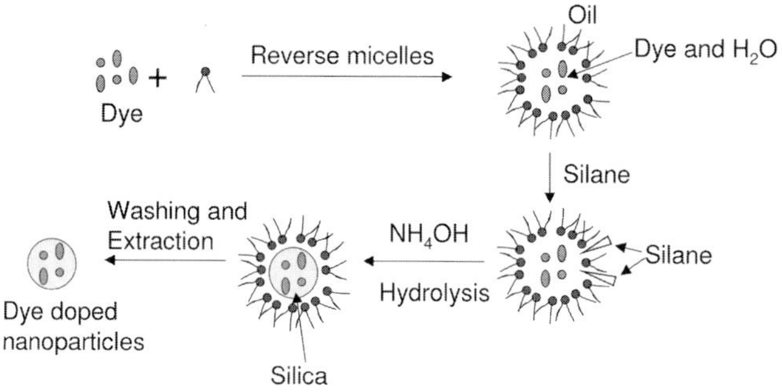

Fig. 1.2. Schematic of the reverse microemulsion method for the synthesis of dye-doped silica nanoparticles (adapted from Bagwe et al., 2004) [11]. In this method, nm-sized water droplets, which are stabilized by surfactant molecules, are formed in a continuous oil phase, thus forming a thermodynamically stable oil–water–surfactant microemulsion.

cules [15]. The nanoparticle surface was first functionalized with aminohexanoic acid and then linked to avidin using EDC coupling.

1.2.2
Quantum Dots (QDs)

Nanocrystals based on semiconductor materials began attracting the interest of physicists three decades ago because of their interesting quantum properties. These properties are the result of size-dependent band gaps, which cause the color emitted by a semiconductor nanocrystal of a specific composition to be a function of its diameter. Physically, quantum properties (in this case a size-dependent fluorescence emission) are expected to occur if electron–hole pairs (excitons) are confined to dimensions that are smaller than the electron–hole distance (exciton diameter) [16–19]. As a result of this condition, the state of free charge carriers within a nanocrystal is quantized and the spacing of the discrete energy states (emission colors) is linked to the size of the nanoparticle. It is this quantum confinement effect that led to the term "quantum dot".

Quantum dots can be based on metallic or semiconductor materials. Most widely used are CdSe and CdTe quantum dots because their quantum confinement region spans the entire optical spectrum. More recently, there has been growing interest in quantum dots with near-infrared emission properties, such as CdTe/CdSe, InAs, or PbS (which are of use in animal imaging studies) [20, and references therein]. In addition, several groups have studied silicon nanocrystals [21–23]. Quantum dots also show other fascinating optical properties, including broad absorption and narrow emission bands, which allows a single laser to excite dots of a wide size-range, with each dot emitting its own specific color. This is in contrast to organic-based fluorophores, which are characterized by narrow Stokes shifts (difference between maximum wavelengths of absorption and emission bands). To protect their surface from photobleaching, quantum dots can be passivated by use of a higher-bandgap semiconductor shell or an organic layer [24]. In fact, successfully passivated, quantum dots show dramatically enhanced photostability, enabling their long-term observation in optical experiments [25]. Furthermore, quantum dots can be brighter than their dye counterparts at an equivalent quantum yield [26] because of their notably higher extinction coefficients [20]. Given the above properties, quantum dots bring fascinating possibilities for single molecule cellular imaging studies because they combine small size, broad absorption, narrow size-tunable emission (covering the entire optical spectrum), and excellent photostability. These features outperform traditional fluorescent dyes in many respects.

The traditional approach to synthesizing quantum dots relies on heating specific organic solvents and injection of semiconductor precursors. In a typical preparation [27], $Cd(CH_3)_2$ and elemental Se are combined with trioctylphosphine oxide (TOPO), which acts as a solvent and stabilizing agent. This mixture is subjected to high temperature (about 350 °C) for 24 hours at which time the mixture is cooled and $Zn(CH_3)_2$ and $S(SiMe_3)_2$ added to form a stabilizing ZnS shell. To create nanocrystals of a narrow size distribution, an additional size-selective precipitation step needs to be included. Because dialkylmetal compounds are very sensitive to oxygen and water and become pyrophoric upon exposure to air, alternative approaches of quantum dot synthesis have been explored. Consequently, CdSe quantum dots can be formed using CdO, selenium, and hexylphosphonic acid or tetradecylphosphonic acid [28]. This synthesis reduces the reaction times to less than 30 min, but still uses temperatures upwards of 300 °C. In another example, our group has synthesized CdSe/ZnS quantum dots by use of sonochemistry [29]. This low-temperature approach not only produces spherical high-quality quantum dots with quantum yields of up to 70% and emission bands of less than 50 nm (FWHM), but also allows for straightforward control of the synthesis parameters. Figure 1.3 shows the photoluminescence spectra of CdSe core quantum dots and

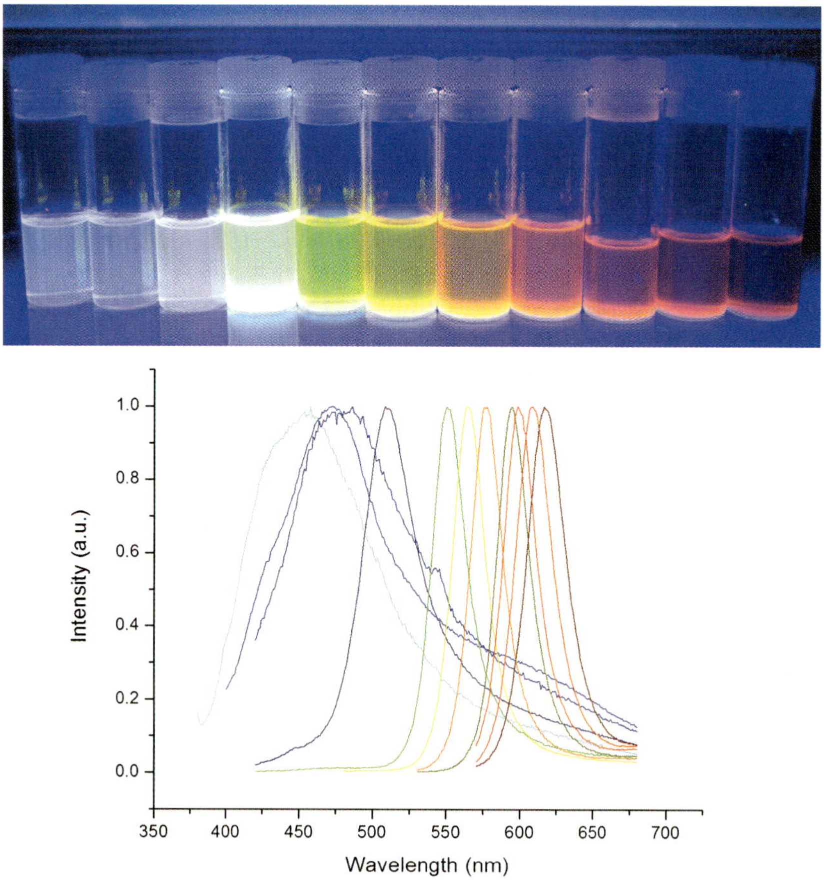

Fig. 1.3. Quantum dots show size-tunable emission properties. The samples represent different sizes of quantum dots, which produce different colors upon UV light. Within the quantum confinement region, an increase in particle sizes produces a redshift in the emission spectrum. Spectra and photograph were obtained from CdSe quantum dots synthesized sonochemically [29].

the colors of these samples upon UV illumination, which are representative of this procedure.

To be of use in biological imaging applications, quantum dots need to be water-soluble. Indeed, synthetic approaches for CdTe [30–32] and CdS [30, 33–38] have utilized aqueous solvent conditions. However, these nanocrystals usually lack the quantum yield and narrow size distribution observed for TOPO-synthesized quantum dots. TOPO-stabilized quantum dots, however, show hydrophobic surface properties. To disperse TOPO-stabilized quantum dots in aqueous solution, several surface modification strategies have been pursued (Fig. 1.4). A common approach is to synthesize quantum dots in TOPO and replace the hydrophobic TOPO layer with bifunctional molecules containing thiol and hydrophilic moieties separated by a molecular spacer (Fig. 1.4: approach I) [39, 40]. The thiol groups bind to the CdSe or ZnS surface, while the hydrophilic moieties radiate from the surface of the corresponding semiconductor. Unfortunately, thiols bind less strongly to ZnS than to Au, which leads to a dynamic equilibrium between bound and unbound thiols. This behavior reduces the long-term water solubility of ZnS-capped quantum dots. To shift the equilibrium towards bound moieties, monothiols have been replaced with molecules containing more than one thiol group (Fig. 1.4: approach II) [41–43]. Another stabilization concept is to enhance binding via surface cross-linking of bound molecules. On the basis of this concept, ZnS-shelled quantum dots have been made water-soluble by adding a silica shell to the nanoparticles by using alkoxysilanes during the polycondensation (Fig. 1.4: approach III) [44–48]. Two types of silanes have been used to stabilize quantum dots in aqueous solution. The first includes silanes whose surface functional groups are positively or negatively charged at neutral pH [48]. The second type includes silanes with poly(ethylene glycol) chains [48, 49]. TOPO-coatings also can be made water-soluble without their replacement by adding amphiphilic molecules such as lipopolymers or amphiphilic diblock copolymers, whose hydrophobic moiety stabilizes the TOPO-coating via hydrophobic forces and whose hydrophilic moiety is exposed to the solvent environment, guaranteeing water-solubility (Fig. 1.4: approach IV). The last approach has the advantage of not exposing the sensitive surface of the quantum dot during a surface exchange step.

1.2.3
Metal Nanoparticles

In contrast to noble metals in bulk, nanoparticular forms of such materials result in interesting photochemical and electronic properties [50]. Three strategies have been pursued to study the photochemical activity of metal nanoparticles: (a) direct excitation of the metal nanoparticles; (b) indirect excitation of the metal nanoparticles via surface-conjugated dye molecules; and (c) photocatalytic processes in semiconductor–metal nanocomposites [50]. After excitation with UV or visible light, metal nanoparticles show several interesting phenomena, including photoluminescence [51–53], nonlinear optical phenomena [54, 55], and surface-enhanced

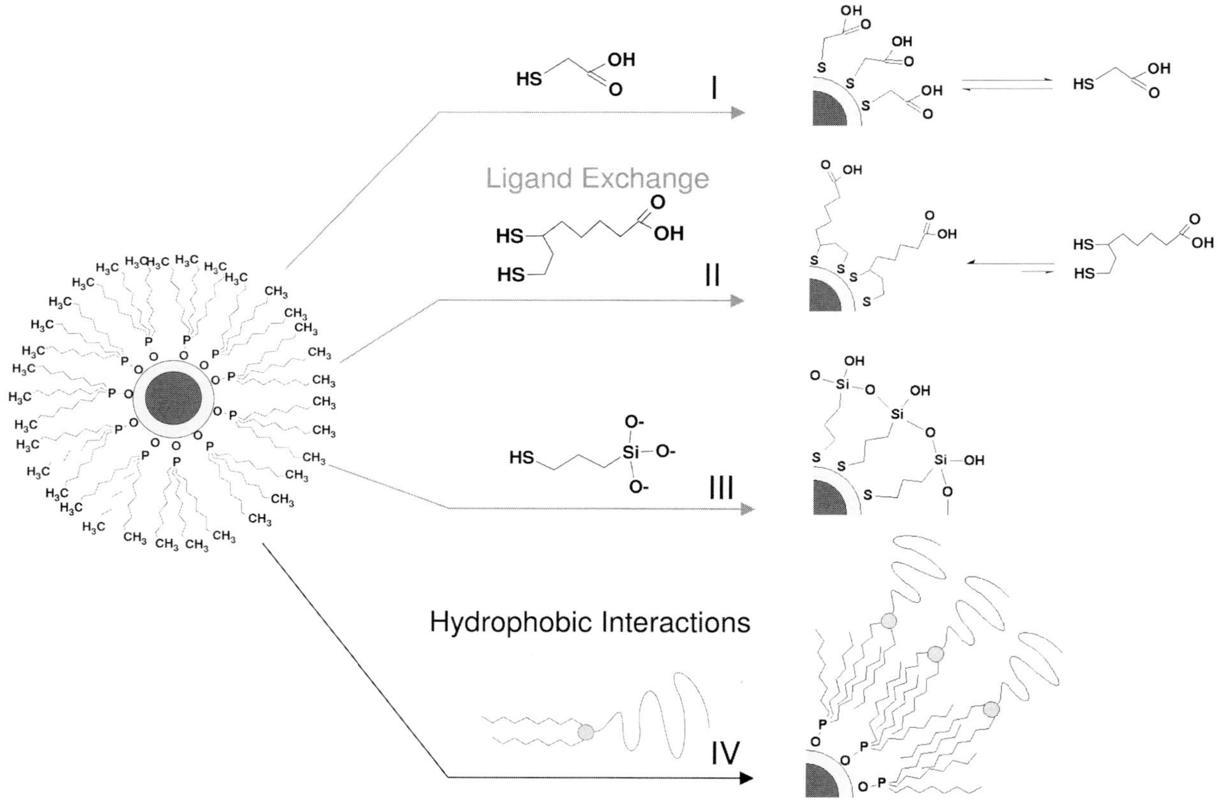

Fig. 1.4. Schematic representation of four common approaches to hydrophilic surface modification of TOPO-stabilized quantum dots. Approach I: TOPO replacement with a heterobifunctional linker consisting of a thiol end group, a spacer, and a hydrophilic end group such as carboxylic acid. II: TOPO replacement with a linker consisting of two thiol groups on one end and a hydrophilic end group on the other end. Approach III: TOPO replacement with a silane forming a stable shell via crosslinking. Approach IV: Stabilization of TOPO layer using amphiphilic molecules such as PEG lipopolymers or amphiphilic diblock copolymers that are held on the surface by hydrophobic interaction with the octyl chains of TOPO.

Raman scattering (SERS) [56–61]. Due to the significant field enhancement, SERS can be used as an extremely sensitive analytical tool, thereby exceeding the sensitivity from luminescence-detecting techniques. For example, biomolecules can be detected with 1000-fold better sensitivity if they are bound to Au nanoparticles [62]. Silver nanoparticles also are useful in this respect. The main experimental challenge in SERS is to keep the surface roughness uniform and reproducible.

There are multiple strategies for synthesizing metal nanoparticles [50]. For example, they can be synthesized using a biphasic reduction approach [63–69]. In this procedure, a noble metal salt such as $HAuCl_4$ is dissolved in water and phase-transfer extracted into an organic solvent followed by reduction with $NaBH_4$. Metal nanoparticles also have been synthesized using reverse micelle procedures where the size and size distribution of nanospheres can be controlled by the micelle composition [12, 70–73]. Gold nanoparticles are particularly attractive for studies in a biological environment because they show no surface oxidation and high biocompatibility without any surface modification. In addition, thiol chemistry can be applied to conjugate molecules to the gold surface.

1.2.4 Hybrid Architectures Involving Fluorescent Nanoprobes

1.2.4.1 Metal–Dye

Another interesting application of metal nanoparticles is their use in combination with conjugated dye molecules (Fig. 1.5). Such hybrid systems are attractive because they can be studied by use of electron microscopy in addition to fluorescence-based techniques such as fluorescence microscopy and spectroscopy. Importantly, if conjugated to biomolecules, metal nanoparticle–dye hybrids can be used as very sensitive biomolecular imaging probes [74, 75]. Interestingly, dye molecules attached to metal nanoparticles can show enhanced emission. For example, Py-CH_2NH_2 molecules bound to gold particles show pronounced emission that is much stronger than that for unbound Py-CH_2NH_2 in THF [50]. The main disadvantage of this approach is that the surface-exposure of the dyes promotes their photooxidation.

1.2.4.2 Dye-doped Silica Shells

To reduce photooxidation, dyes also can be embedded within the nanoparticle. As illustrated in Fig. 1.5(B), dyes can be incorporated into a nanoparticle-capping silica shell. For example, up to 12 alternating fluorescent and nonfluorescent silica shells have been added to silica core particles, where the shells were doped with six dyes of different emission wavelengths. Dyes of multiple colors have been incorporated previously in silica beads throughout the matrix of the particle [76], but not in an ordered fashion [77]. This multi-shell approach helps to reduce unwanted energy transfer. As a multiplexing probe, the system is not as simple to analyze as a quantum dot-based one. Re absorption of the fluorescence emission,

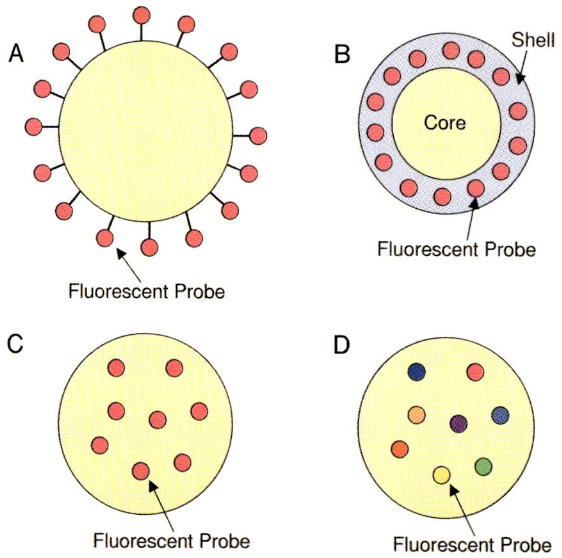

Fig. 1.5. Common hybrid architectures containing fluorescent nanoprobes include (A) dyes bound to a nanoparticle surface; (B) dyes incorporated into the silica shell of a nanoparticle; (C) fluorescent probes such quantum dots or dyes incorporated into the core of microparticles; and (D) a multiplexing approach by embedding probes of different colors.

which is related to the identity of the fluorophore, alters the emission intensity. As a result, it is difficult to determine the possible number of spectral combinations in a designed system, and a flow cytometer must be used to identify the number of individual species in the mixture. This shelling approach has also been reported for single dye systems for enhanced fluorescence [10].

1.2.4.3 **Quantum Dot-containing Microspheres**

An interesting hybrid architecture that has been developed recently is the quantum dot embedded microsphere. Unlike a dye embedded polymeric bead, the quantum dot microbeads utilize the narrow emission of quantum dots combined with their broad absorption characteristics to perform multicolor detection experiments with one excitation wavelength [78–81]. By incorporating up to six different colors of quantum dots and ten intensities of those colors, the quantum dot microbeads can, theoretically, optically "bar code" biomolecules with one million possible spectral signatures. Realistically, the number is likely to be substantially lower due to spectral overlap, fluorescence intensity variations, and signal-to-noise requirements. The multiplexing approach has been tried with organic dyes, but was limited to two colors due to spectral overlapping and the inability to excite more than two or three dyes with the same wavelength [82].

1.3
Bioconjugation of Fluorescent Nanoparticles

1.3.1
General Considerations

1.3.1.1 Overview

To apply fluorescent nanoparticles to biosensing and biomedical imaging applications, it is crucial to develop strategies towards their biofunctionalization. These include the proper linkage of biomolecules to nanoparticles (bioconjugation) and the design of appropriate biocompatible coatings. This section outlines the different aspects of bioconjugation, and Section 1.4 provides a corresponding discussion of biocompatible coatings.

Bioconjugation can be described as any procedure that links a nanoparticle to a biomolecule under mild conditions [83]. As described above, the synthesis of nanoparticles often does not render them capable of attachment to biomolecules, because their surface-chemical properties are not appropriate. Therefore, nanoparticles frequently must undergo surface transformations to create the chemistry needed for coupling to biomolecules under mild (physiological) conditions. There are a few key requirements for successful bioconjugation reactions [4]. Crucially, the conjugation process must avoid compromising the activity of biomolecules. In addition, the bioconjugation ideally should not hinder the signal of the nanoparticle. Another requirement is the ability to control the number of linkage sites on the nanoparticle surface where biomolecules can bind. This requirement can be quite challenging. In addition, the biomolecule–nanoparticle coupling should be stable and, for crystalline particles, the surface should be covered to avoid free valence states. Finally, the thickness of any nanoparticle shell should remain as small as possible relative to the nanoparticle size.

Figure 1.6 illustrates several possible strategies to bioconjugate nanoparticles. Simple adsorption of biomolecules to the nanoparticle surface via noncovalent forces represents the least demanding approach (Fig. 1.6A). However, in this case, the activity of bound biomolecules may be compromised and the amount of bound biomolecules per nanoparticle is difficult to control. In addition, this bioconjugation approach does not target one protein preferentially. Another concept is based on the physisorption (noncovalent coupling) of biomolecules to molecules (e.g., other biomolecules) acting as mediators between biomolecule and nanoparticle surface (Fig. 1.6B). This design may be advantageous over the first one, because it may help biomolecules to bind in a proper orientation. Figure 1.6(C) is based on the chemical coupling between reactive groups of biomolecules (e.g., thiols and primary amines) and crosslinker molecules. These crosslinkers may bind to the nanoparticle surface via physisorption or chemisorption (covalent coupling). However, there are frequently multiple active sites on the target biomolecule to which the probe can bind, thus preventing controlled binding. Furthermore, uncontrolled

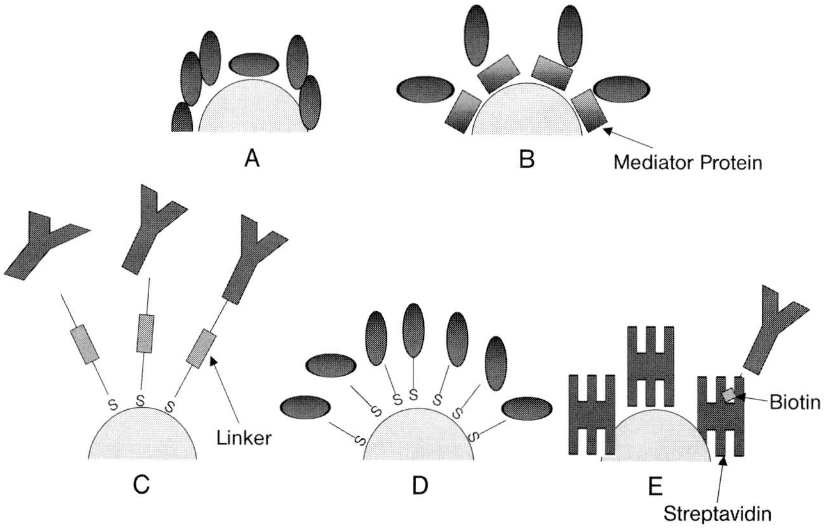

Fig. 1.6. Common strategies for the conjugation of biomolecules to nanoparticles include direct physisorption of biomolecules (A), assisted physisorption using pre-bound molecules (B), chemical linkage of biomolecules to crosslinkers either physisorbed or chemisorbed on the nanoparticle surface (C), direct chemical coupling of biomolecules to nanoparticles (D), and the targeted binding of biotinylated biomolecules to streptavidin-coated nanoparticles via biotin–streptavidin coupling (E).

binding may interfere with the biologically active sites of biomolecules. To overcome this limitation, a ligand (typically an antibody) can be bound to the nanoparticle via the crosslinker. This ligand then facilitates coupling to the biomolecule of interest with high specificity. These crosslinker-based bioconjugation strategies are best executed if appropriate heterobifunctional crosslinkers are used. A large variety of such crosslinker molecules is now commercially available. Alternatively, homobifunctional crosslinkers can be used where one reactive end group is protected. Here, nanoparticle and biomolecule are coupled by binding of the partially protected linker to either nanoparticle or biomolecule and by deprotecting the linker prior to bioconjugation. Unprotected homobifunctional crosslinkers are always problematic because they can induce the clustering of nanoparticles. Figure 1.6(D) shows a facile approach for the chemical coupling of biomolecules to nanoparticles. This approach is particularly useful for attaching oligonucleotides to nanoparticles, e.g., via mercapto groups [84–86]. Still, control over the number of bound biomolecules per nanoparticle remains a challenging endeavor. To achieve such control, a separation step, such as nanoparticle separation using gel electrophoresis, must be added [87]. Another popular approach is to link biotinylated ligands or target biomolecules to streptavidin (or avidin)-functionalized nanoparticles with high specificity (Fig. 1.6E). In this case, the biotin-binding proteins, avidin or streptavidin, act as linker molecules [88, 89].

1.3.1.2 Common Coupling Reactions

The bioconjugation of nanoparticles is critically dependent on the availability of effective covalent coupling procedures. Figure 1.7 lists the most common coupling procedures. The reaction between primary amine and carboxylic acid groups is a very popular coupling procedure (Fig. 1.7A). In a first step, a carboxylic acid reacts with 1-ethyl-3-(3-dimethylaminopropyl)carbodiimide (EDAC) and *N*-hydroxysulfosuccinimide (NHS) to form an acyl amino ester that subsequently reacts with the primary amine to create a stable amide bond. This approach also is attractive because preparation of the ligands is less demanding. A widely used approach is based on the reaction between thiol and maleimide groups (Fig. 1.7B). This affords a stable thioether bond, typically with good yield at physiological pH. Most prominently, this reaction can be used to directly link maleimide-functionalized ligands to thio-groups of proteins. If no thiols are available, they can be created by using heterobifunctional crosslinkers with one thiol endgroup or by reducing disulfide bonds within the target protein. The coupling of two thiols to form a disulfide linkage is another straightforward reaction approach (Fig. 1.7C). Unfortunately, the resulting disulfide bond is relatively labile in biological fluids like serum. Another useful reaction scheme is based on the covalent linkage between aldehyde and hydrazide groups to form a hydrazide bond (Fig. 1.7D). Reactive aldehyde groups can be created by oxidation of carbohydrate groups. Obviously, mild oxidation conditions have to be used for the oxidation reaction on relatively unstable molecules like antibodies. Chemical reaction between two primary amines is another approach for bioconjugation applications (Fig. 1.7E). In this case, coupling can be achieved using homobifunctional crosslinkers such as glutaraldehyde [90, 91].

1.3.2
Bioconjugation of Polymeric Nanoparticles

From a bioconjugation perspective, polymeric nanoparticles are attractive because they can be prepared with various different reactive groups on their surface. The obvious benefit is that a comparably broad spectrum of conjugation chemistry approaches can be used, including covalent and noncovalent ones (Fig. 1.6). These different bioconjugation strategies are reviewed below.

1.3.2.1 Noncovalent Approaches

One of the most widely applied approaches in bioconjugating polymeric nanoparticles is simple physisorption of the biomolecules on the particle surface (Fig. 1.6A) [93–97]. Because biomolecule activity is compromised by uncontrolled adsorption, spacer molecules have been introduced (Fig. 1.6B). For example, nanoparticles first coated with Protein A (isolated from the cell wall of *Staphylococcus aureus*), which attaches specifically to the Fc fragment of the IgG antibody, have proper Fab orientation for antibody binding [97]. Unfortunately, such simple adsorption approaches are only of limited use when applied in serum. This is because serum proteins compete with antibodies for adsorption sites [93–95]. Furthermore, *in vivo* experiments have revealed that such simply designed nanoparticles tend to accumulate

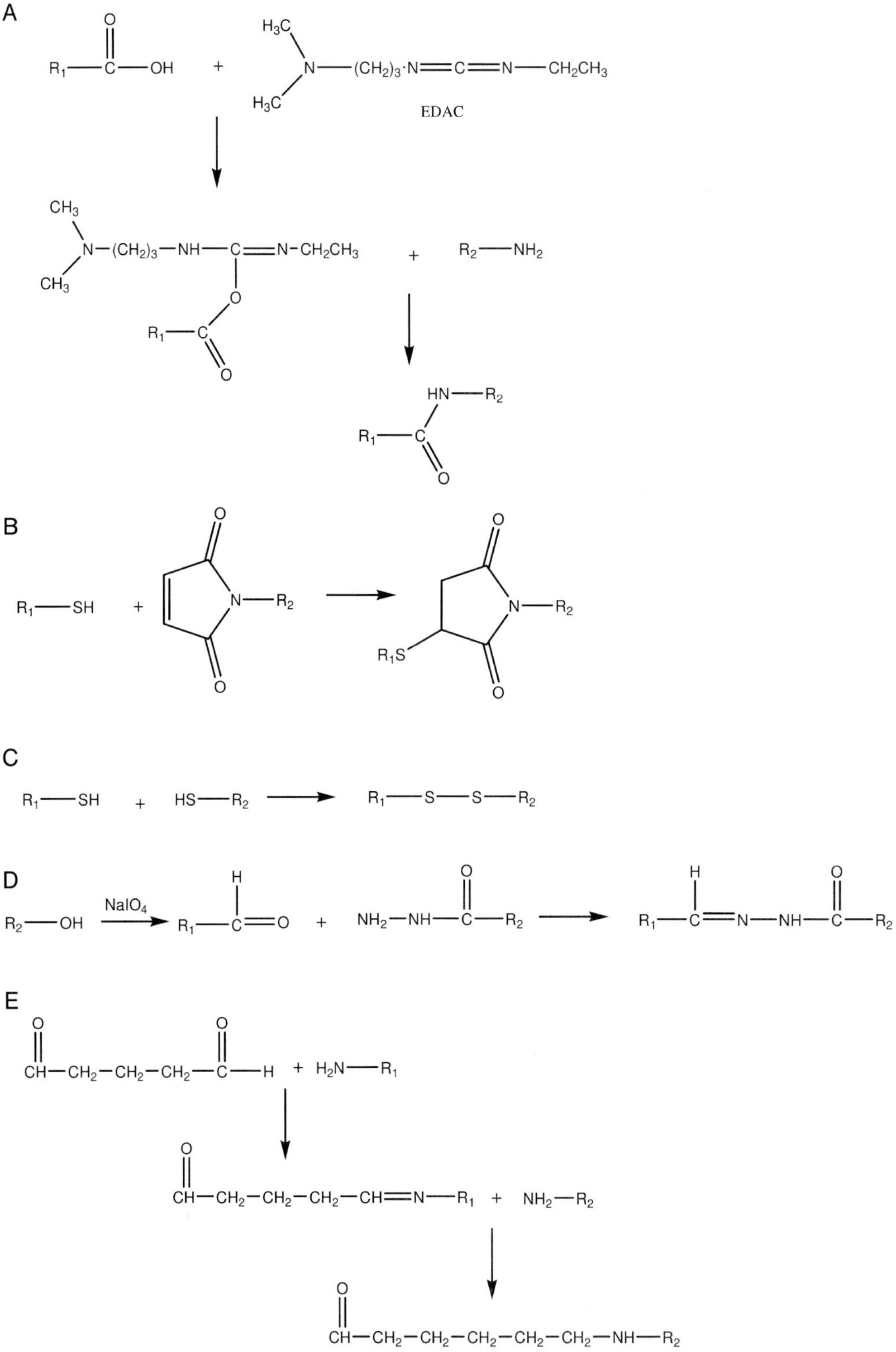
A
EDAC
B
C
D
NaIO4
E

in the liver and spleen. Using a similar design strategy, polystyrene nanoparticles have been functionalized with humanized mAB HuEP5C7.g2 [98]. These delivery systems target cells expressing E and P-selectin.

1.3.2.2 **Covalent Approaches**

Obviously, the activity of ligands bound to nanoparticles strongly depends on the stability of the ligand–nanoparticle linkage and the proper orientation of the ligand. To address these needs, ligands have been bound covalently to polymeric nanoparticles using several different conjugation approaches (Fig. 1.6E) [7, 99–102]. For example, an amide linkage strategy was pursued to bind lactose to the poly(vinylamine)-grafted nanoparticles [99]. Such lactose-functionalized carrier systems are useful because they specifically bind to lectin RCA_{120}. The same amide-based linkage chemistry was used to bind proteins to dye encoded latex particles [7]. In another approach, transferrin was conjugated to PEG coated poly(cyanoacrylate) nanocrystals, with the transferrin bound to PEG via periodate oxidation [100]. A heterobifunctional linker was used to bind antibodies to BSA-containing nanoparticles [101, 102]. In this case, the crosslinker (glutaraldehyde) was bound to BSA to provide free aldehyde groups, which could then be linked to the primary amines of the antibodies. Another interesting strategy is based on formation of ligand-carrying nanoparticles via polymerization of monomers with bound ligands. Such a strategy has been applied to create nanoparticles with biotin groups, which then allowed for specific linkage to avidin [103, 104]. The grafting of carbohydrates to poly(L-lysine) was also reported [105]. This carrier can bind to carbohydrate-binding proteins on the surface of target cells.

1.3.3
Bioconjugation of Quantum Dots

Though quantum dots are very small, their surface area is large enough for linking to multiple biomolecules [106]. There are several ways to bind biomolecules to quantum dots. These involve either direct binding to the quantum dot surface or attachment via a stabilizing layer acting as a crosslinker between the ligand and reactive surface of the nanoparticle. In the first case, ligand binding can be achieved covalently or noncovalently. Direct covalent coupling is accomplished commonly by use of thiol coupling chemistry, although a silane-based coupling is needed if quantum dots carry a stabilizing silica shell. Noncovalent ligand-quantum dot coupling, however, is typically pursed using electrostatic or hydrophobic forces. On the basis of these general concepts, several bioconjugation strategies have been pursued. These are discussed below.

Fig. 1.7. Commonly used chemical reactions in the bioconjugation of fluorescent nanoparticles. Shown are the coupling chemistries between (A) carboxylic acid and primary amine, (B) thiol and maleimide groups, (C) two thiols to form a disulfide bond, (D) hydrazide and aldehyde groups, and (E) two primary amines. (Adapted from Nobs et al., 2004 [92].)

1.3.3.1 Noncovalent Approaches

An electrostatic coupling approach has been applied to link negatively charged CdTe quantum dots and positively charged enzymes [107]. Electrostatic coupling also was pursued in several applications to bind positively charged protein domains (pentahistadine segment) to oppositely charged alkyl-COOH-capped quantum dots [31, 42, 88, 108–112]. An alternative electrostatic-based coupling strategy has been used to bind nanocrystals coated with trimethoxysilylpropyl-urea and acetate groups with high affinity in the cell nucleus [44]. Here the binding of the silanized nanocrystal surface is controlled with an anionic silane reagent. Negatively charged quantum dots have also been electrostatically bound to positively charged Maltose Binding Protein [113]. Quite often, adsorbed proteins show a stabilizing effect on the quantum dot surface, thereby improving the optical properties of the probes. For example, a two-fold increase in fluorescence was observed after adsorption of 10–15 Maltose-Binding Protein Pentahistadine (MBP-5HIS) to the quantum dot surface [114].

1.3.3.2 Covalent Approaches

A relatively straightforward covalent bioconjugation approach is based on the replacement of thiol acids present on the quantum dot surface with thiolated biomolecules. This strategy has been used to attach oligonucleotides, DNA [41, 84] and bovine serum albumin (BSA) [86] to quantum dots. Proteins also have been conjugated to quantum dots by reacting carboxylic acid groups on the nanoparticle surface with amine groups of the proteins [115]. A similar strategy was used to covalently attach IgG and streptavidin to quantum dots. The IgG system was applied as a cancer marker, whereas the streptavidin system was utilized for labeling actin, microtubules and the cell nucleus [116].

In another application, antibodies have been bound to quantum dots via sulfo-NHS crosslinking [117]. In a different approach, reactive biotin was covalently linked to either surface sulfhydryl or amine functionalities, thus allowing for the biotinylation of the quantum dot surface and the subsequent binding to streptavidin [44]. A biotin–streptavidin coupling approach was chosen, for example, to bind quantum dots to fibroblasts [44]. In this case, the nanocrystals were functionalized with biotinamidocaproic acid 3-sulfo-*N*-hydroxysuccinimide ester and then allowed to bind to fibroblasts previously incubated with phalloidin–biotin and streptavidin. A combination of covalent and noncovalent coupling strategies was pursued by conjugating quantum dots stabilized with amphiphilic PEG lipids to DNA. Here, the DNA coupling was achieved by replacing $\frac{1}{2}$ of the PEG-PE phospholipids with amino PEG-PE. Thiol modified DNA was then covalently coupled to the amines on the surface of the quantum dot [118].

1.3.4 Bioconjugation of Metallic Nanoprobes

Most conjugation concepts described for the linkage of ligands to quantum dots can also be applied to metal nanoparticles, such as Au or Ag nanoprobes. Again, surface modification is accomplished using thiol-coupling chemistry. The binding of biomolecules to these nanoparticles can be covalent or noncovalent. With respect to biofunctionalization, gold nanospheres are particularly attractive because gold shows excellent biocompatibility properties, and does not require additional surface chemical modification prior to bioconjugation. In addition, gold nanoparticles can be made with very narrow size distribution. This is advantageous if accurate control of the number of bound biomolecules per nanoparticle is required.

1.3.4.1 Noncovalent Approaches

One option for bioconjugation is the direct attachment of a biomolecule to the metallic nanoparticle surface. Short peptide chains such as tiopronin [119] and the tripeptide glutathione [120] have been conjugated directly to a gold surface. Globular proteins have also been directly conjugated. Miziani et al. conjugated globular proteins directly to the surface of silver sulfide nanoparticles [121]. In another application, gold nanoparticles were coated with BSA via electrostatic interactions under mild conditions [122]. Due to the bioinertness of gold, biomolecules directly bound on the gold surface can retain their activity, as shown, for example, for redox enzymes [123] and cytochrome c [124]. Biotin–streptavidin coupling concepts have also been used. For example, disulfide-modified biotin was conjugated to gold nanoparticles and subsequently reacted with streptavidin [125].

1.3.4.2 Covalent Approaches

Direct coupling of biomolecules to the surface of metal nanoparticles represents a very facile bioconjugation strategy. Among the different metals, this conjugation strategy is best suited for gold because of its excellent bioinertness. For example, thiol-modified DNA has been conjugated directly to gold particles [74, 126–128]. Direct thiol coupling was also pursued to conjugate SH modified PEG to gold-shelled silica nanoparticles [129]. Covalent bioconjugation to the nanoparticle can also be mediated by heterobifunctional crosslinker molecules. One example is the surface modification of iron oxide nanoparticles with a trifluoroethylester-terminal poly(ethylene glycol) (PEG) silane and the subsequent coupling of biomolecules via their terminal amine or carboxyl groups [130].

1.4 Design of Biocompatible Coatings

1.4.1 General Considerations

1.4.1.1 Overview

Though multiple bioconjugation strategies have been worked out, the routine application of fluorescent nanoparticles in biomedical imaging remains challenging. This is largely because not only appropriate conjugation between biomolecules to nanoparticles is required but other important criteria concerning biocompatibility

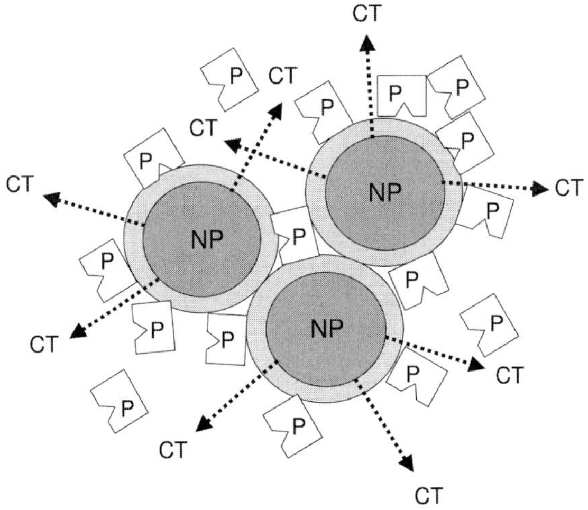

Fig. 1.8. Potential problems compromising the biocompatibility of fluorescent nanoparticles, including nanoparticle (NP) clustering, non-specific adsorption of proteins (P), and release of cytotoxic ions (CT).

have to be fulfilled. These criteria include (a) prevention of nanoparticle aggregation in a biological environment, (b) effective suppression of non-specific adsorption of biomolecules at the nanoparticle surface or their accumulation close to the surface, and (c) low cytotoxicity (Fig. 1.8). To address these criteria, nanoparticles need to be capped with protective coatings that show passivating surface properties. Notably, the first criterion, good colloidal stability, does not guarantee the biocompatibility of nanoparticles as, firstly, ions and proteins may be accumulated on or near the nanoparticle surface, thus varying the complex molecular composition nearby. Secondly, especially with heavy metal-containing quantum dots (e.g., CdSe, CdTe), individual nanoparticles may remain cytotoxic if the coating does not protect the biological environment from released heavy metals ions.

1.4.1.2 **Colloidal Stability**

The dispersion stability of nanoparticles is well-described by the Derjaguin–Landau–Verwey–Overbeek (DLVO) theory, which predicts that such stability is determined by the balance between attractive van der Waals and repulsive electrostatic forces. As a result, nanoparticles are expected to remain stable (show no particle aggregation) if the strength of the repulsive electrostatic force exceeds that of the attractive van der Waals (vdW) force. In other words, nanoparticles show no aggregation if they contain a sufficient density of surface charges. Indeed, particles with charged surface properties do not aggregate in ion-free solutions. At the same time, this balance can clearly be shifted in favor of vdW forces if the charges on the particle surface are screened by counter ions in the solution. This is an important aspect to consider during chemical surface modification, because such

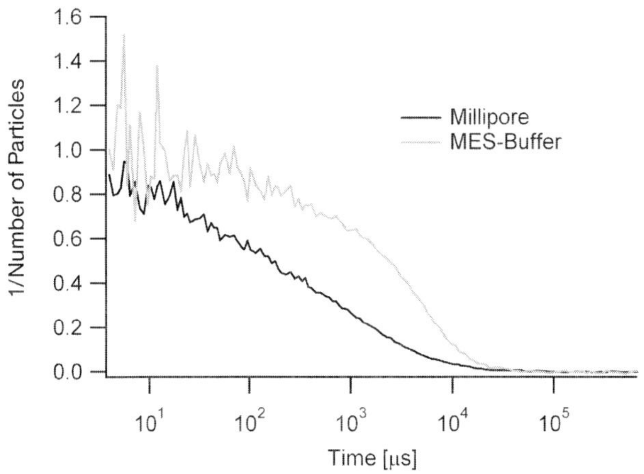

Fig. 1.9. Fluorescence correlation spectroscopy autocorrelation curves of ZnS-capped CdSe quantum dots surface-functionalized with carboxylic acid in Millipore water (dark curve) and 10 mM MES buffer (lighter curve). The notably higher diffusion time obtained for the buffer-based system indicates nanoparticle clustering.

modifications may result in surface charge neutralization, thereby compromising dispersion stability. More importantly, nanoparticles with charged surfaces tend to become unstable (show aggregation) in a biological environment. Figure 1.9 shows the loss of colloidal stability due to charge screening. Here comparative fluorescence correlation spectroscopy (FCS) autocorrelation curves from our laboratory are presented for CdSe/ZnS quantum dots with negatively charged carboxylic acid surface groups in Millipore water and in 10 mM MES buffer. As illustrated, the nanoparticles in MES buffer show notably higher diffusion times, indicating their increasing aggregation. If quantum dots are surface-functionalized with a layer of hydrophilic polymers such as poly(ethylene glycol) (PEG), colloidal stability can be achieved even in the presence of ions in solution. Such particle stabilization via polymer coatings is attributed to the flexibility of polymer chains and their repulsive "entropic spring" effect during particle–particle interaction. Currently, the concept of stabilization of nanoparticles due to the addition of polymeric coatings is widely accepted. Indeed, several experimental results seem to support the concept [131, 132]. Peptides adsorbed to the quantum dot surface can also have a similar stabilizing effect [133]. Conversely, it has been theoretically predicted that homopolymers, if end-grafted to nanoparticles in good solvents, may lead to nanoparticle attraction [134].

1.4.1.3 **Biocompatible Surfaces**

To make fluorescent nanoparticles 'bioinert', their surfaces need to be designed so as to prevent the non-specific adsorption of all relevant molecules in the biological medium. It is challenging to improve the design of surface coatings to a level of sophistication that fulfills this requirement. Fortunately, promising strategies for the creation of bioinert surfaces are known from biomaterials research in the biomedical engineering community. As a result, our understanding about the host response of living tissue with respect to biomaterials has improved significantly and numerous sophisticated biomaterials have been developed [135]. A key aspect for the creation of colloidal solids with sufficient stealth properties in a cellular environment is the understanding of protein adsorption. Like surfactants, proteins have a high tendency to adsorb at interfaces. Interactions between proteins and surfaces are primarily noncovalent and include electrostatic, hydrophobic, and hydrogen-bonding interactions [136]. The different interactions result from the "surface inhomogeneity" of proteins, which typically are characterized by surface patches that may be charged, neutral, hydrophilic, or hydrophobic in character [137]. Consequently, surface properties of biomaterials affect the mechanism, rate, and extent of protein adsorption. Protein adsorption can be suppressed most efficiently on biomaterials whose surfaces are neutral, hydrophilic, and highly dynamic [138]. A paradigm of a protein-resistant surface is a solid substrate surface-functionalized with grafted PEG chains [139]. This is so because PEG is electrically neutral, thus minimizing electrostatic interactions, and highly hydrophilic, thus minimizing hydrophobic interactions. As the PEG chains are highly dynamic in an aqueous environment, the formation of strong hydrogen-bonding between protein and polymer is effectively suppressed. Besides those enthalpic effects, the high dynamics of the PEG chains results in a high entropy, which is also unfavorable for protein adsorption. It has been generally assumed that the surface resistance of PEG functionalized substrates is a result of the steric repulsion grafted PEG chains show for adsorbing proteins [138, 140, 141]. However, this assumption is valid only if the grafted PEG chains are of very high molecular weight and show large enough grafting densities to form polymer brushes [142]. Interestingly, Prime and Whitesides found that protein adsorption is prevented effectively even if the PEG chains have only two ethylene oxide segments, thus indicating that surface coverage is the most important parameter to prevent protein adsorption [143, 144]. In the same context, Single-chain Mean Field Theory (SCMF) calculations and experimental studies showed that protein adsorption on hydrophobic surfaces is prevented because PEG chains bind to the hydrophobic substrate, thereby blocking possible protein binding sites [145]. A later SCMF study by Szleifer and coworkers found that polymers with a low substrate affinity are more effective for kinetic control, whereas those with a higher affinity lead to a lower equilibrium concentration of adsorbed proteins [146]. Obviously, protein adsorption on substrates surface grafted with synthetic polymers is dependent on both the steric hindrance effect of the grafted polymer layer and the affinity of the underlying substrate for proteins and other molecules.

1.4.1.4 **Cytotoxicity**

Several potential processes lead to cytotoxicity. One source of nanoparticle-induced cytotoxicity, rather independent of particle composition, occurs if nanoparticles adsorb to cell surfaces [147, 148] or if they get ingested by cells [149, 150]. The cytotoxicity of CdSe/ZnS quantum dots is suggested to be due mostly to their interaction with cells [151]. Another source of nanoparticle-induced cytotoxicity occurs when the nanoparticle is composed of toxic materials that can be gradually released. A prominent example concerning fluorescent nanoparticles is the gradual release of heavy metal ions such as Cd^{2+} from CdSe or CdSe/ZnS quantum dots [152, 153]. Heavy metal ions are cytotoxic and often show several pathways of cytotoxicity. Indeed, Cd^{2+} may induce hepatotoxicity, immunotoxicity, and nephrotoxicity; apoptosis being a critical part of each toxicity type [154]. Studies concerning Cd-induced hepatotoxicity show, for example, the relevance of direct and indirect cytotoxic pathways [155]. The direct pathway is caused by Cd^{2+} binding to sulfhydryl groups on key mitochondrial molecules, thus damaging the mitochondria. The indirect pathway, though, is assumed to occur via activation of Kupffer cells. However, not all metals show such pronounced cytotoxicity. For example, gold nanoparticles have good biocompatibility properties [156]. From the above information, nanoparticles only show very low cytotoxicity if all potential sources of cytotoxicity are prevented efficiently.

1.4.2
Nanoparticle-stabilizing Coatings

To enhance the biocompatibility of nanoparticles, one popular strategy has been to cap the nanoparticles with polymeric coatings of high biocompatibility. In particular, poly(ethylene glycol) (PEG) has been applied as a coating material because of its excellent biocompatibility properties. Originally studied on flat macroscopic surfaces for biomaterials applications, PEG coatings have been widely applied to sub-micron sized delivery systems and imaging probes [48, 49, 116, 118, 131, 157, 158]. Delivery systems coated with PEG have notably longer circulation times in the blood, thus exceeding traditional non-nanoparticle-based delivery methods for the prolonged delivery of drugs, diagnostics, genes, and vaccines [159–162]. Based on the success of PEG coatings in drug delivery systems, similar coating strategies have been applied to the design of biocompatible coatings of nm-size imaging probes in biological and biomedical imaging. A facile approach for adding a PEG layer to the quantum dot surface is via physisorption of amphiphilic molecules [116, 118]. Here one interesting strategy has been to use PEG-containing lipopolymers, which result in excellent colloidal stability in *Xenopus* embryo cells over several days [118]. In an alternative amphiphilic passivation approach, block copolymers have been utilized to enable colloidal stability of quantum dots [116, 163, 164].

Chemically coupled PEG coatings have even greater stability. Wuelfing et al. reported the surface functionalization of gold nanoparticles using CH_3O-PEG-SH [131]. Covalent PEG coatings were also used to increase the colloidal stability of CdSe [49], CdS, [158] and SiO_2-capped CdS [48] quantum dots. However, in these cases, the PEG coatings lack reactive surface groups, thus preventing the further immobilization of ligands on the PEG layer. To overcome this limitation, nanoparticles need to be surface-functionalized via mixtures of mono-functional PEGs and other linker molecules [48] or via heterobifunctional PEG-linkers. Heterobifunc-

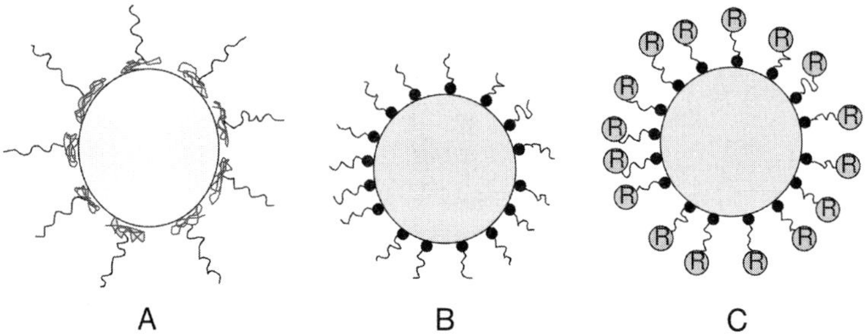

Fig. 1.10. Design of nanoparticles with stabilizing, biocompatible coatings, including (A) adsorption of amphiphilic molecules such as amphiphilic diblock copolymers; (B) chemical coupling of hydrophilic polymeric systems; and (C) linkage of spacer molecules with hydrophilic surface groups.

tional PEG-linkers can be synthesized via monoprotected symmetric PEG linkers, such as monoprotected diamines derived from tetraethylene glycol [165–167]. Another strategy for the synthesis of heterobifunctional PEG linkers is based on the ring-opening polymerization of ethylene oxide using a metal alkoxide initiator [168–171]. For example, α-acetal-PEG-SH has been synthesized using this strategy [172]. Here the facile modification of the acetal group into a reactive aldehyde allowed the immobilization of ligand molecules on the surface of PEGylated gold particles [173]. Meanwhile, various heterobifunctional PEG linkers are also commercially available. Figure 1.10 shows the design of a biocompatible surface coating where a few linkers support the targeted immobilization of ligand molecules. Such a design can be accomplished by using a mixture of homofunctional and heterobifunctional PEGs. An excess of homofunctional PEG molecules, which have no reactive surface groups after surface coating, suppresses the non-specific binding of proteins, whereas the heterobifunctional linkers facilitate the targeted coupling to ligands. Notably, however, a PEG layer does not prevent cytotoxic side reactions due to the leaching of toxic heavy metal ions from quantum dots. In those cases, an additional protective layer preventing the egress of harmful ions is essential [153].

PEG-based coatings are not the only biocompatible polymeric coatings. For example, poly(acrylic acid) has been used to stabilize luminescent silicon nanoparticles [174]. Because this anionic polyelectrolyte has a high density of carboxylic acid moieties, the immobilization of amine-containing molecules is straightforward. A similar concept has been applied to conjugate CdS quantum dots with aminodextran [175]. Dendrimers have also been used as stabilizing coating material [176]. Quantum dots have been embedded into larger polymeric spheres via a facile procedure using block copolymers [163, 177], and CdSe-ZnS quantum dots have been incorporated into glyconanospheres via electrostatic coupling with carboxymethyldextran and polylysine [178]. Several other procedures have afforded gold glyconanospheres [173, 179, 180]. Quantum dots capped with specific peptide coatings have recently been shown to be quite promising biocompatible imaging probes that can be designed for targeted labeling of biomolecules [20, and references therein].

1.4.3
Low Cytotoxicity Coatings

As stated before, successful application of fluorescent nanoparticles in a biological environment requires not only high dispersion stability and the suppression of non-specific biomolecule adsorption, but also should show low cytotoxicity. This topic is particularly important for applications involving quantum dots where toxic heavy metal ions can be released [152]. If properly passivated, quantum dots seem to show no significant cytotoxicity. For example, a study on *Xenopus* embryos did not reveal significant cytotoxicity after injection of 2×10^9 and 5×10^9 CdSe/ZnS quantum dots per cell [118].

Several strategies have been pursued to suppress this oxidation process. One approach is simply to passivate the quantum dot surface with binding ligands [181]. Importantly, such a passivation not only lowers the cytotoxicity of nanoprobes, but also enhances their quantum yields. Quantum dots can be further passivated by adding a protecting semiconductor shell. Such coatings also significantly lower the cytotoxicity of CdSe quantum dots, but do not completely eliminate the problem [152]. Surface silanization is another promising approach to suppressing surface oxidation [44, 46, 182–184]. The stability of the coating is provided by crosslinks within the siloxane shell. Importantly, such shells are quite stable in a biological environment [46]. Furthermore, CdSe/ZnS quantum dots with a protective shell of crosslinked silica significantly reduce the release of Cd^{2+}, thus lowering the cytotoxicity of fluorescent nanoparticles [153]. Interestingly, the addition of a bovine serum albumin (BSA) layer further reduced the cytotoxicity of CdSe/ZnS quantum dots [152]. The BSA, added to the mercaptoacetic acid-functionalized quantum dot surface using EDC coupling, may act as a diffusion barrier for O_2 molecules.

Based on the above discussion, the appropriate biofunctionalization of nanoparticles clearly must address the features of colloidal stability, bioinertness, specificity with respect to target biomolecules, and low cytotoxicity. Figure 1.11 shows a biofunctionalization architecture where these crucial features are considered in its design.

1.5
Applications

Our growing ability to synthesize and surface-functionalize nanoparticles has provided new opportunities in bioanalytical and biological imaging applications. Metallic nanoparticles have been used primarily in bioanalytical projects. Nanoparticle-based imaging applications, however, rely more on dye-doped polymeric nanoparticles and quantum dots due to their excellent fluorescence proper-

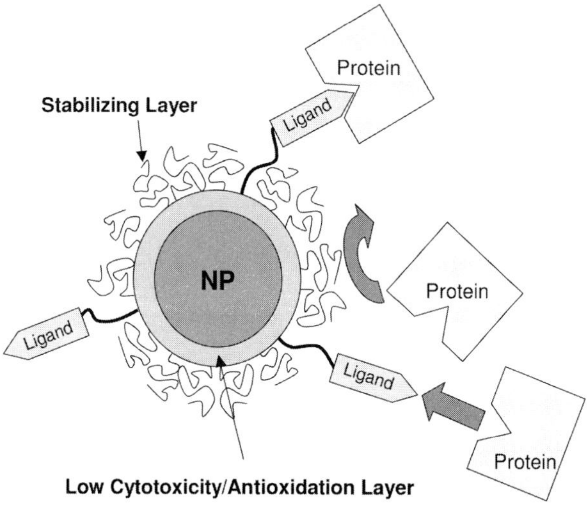

Fig. 1.11. Schematic of an appropriately biofunctionalized quantum dot. The inner coating protects from surface oxidation whereas the outer coating guarantees dispersion stability and biocompatibility. Immobilized ligands mediate the specific binding to biomolecules.

ties and photostability. While dye-doped systems have been used initially in such imaging applications, quantum dots have recently increasingly become the nanoparticle systems of choice. It is fair to say that further progress in bioanalytical and imaging applications is strongly linked to the availability of novel biofunctionalized nanoparticles of improved designs. Though developing rapidly, this highly interdisciplinary field is still in its infancy. The rapidly growing number of publications over the last decade reflect its relevance.

Though this chapter focuses primarily on the relevant *concepts* of biofunctionalization, this section describes recent *applications* using biofunctionalized fluorescent nanoparticles. We do not claim to review all published applications where such particles have been used because this is clearly beyond the scope of the chapter. Instead, the intent is to provide a representative overview of recent nanoparticle-related applications in the fields of diagnostics and live cell and *in vivo* imaging.

1.5.1
Biosensing

Fluorescent nanoparticles are highly promising probes for bioanalytical applications. In particular, their use in the field of biosensors is attractive because fluorescence-based techniques are extremely sensitive and nanoparticle probes show high photostability, thus allowing for long-term observations.

1.5.1.1 Polymeric Sensors

Bioanalytical applications based on polymeric nanoparticles are now well established. In one application, the combination of two silica precursors, tetraethylorthosilicate and phenyltriethoxysilane, was used to synthesize organic dye-doped silica nanoparticles. The nanoparticles were coated with avidin to determine biotinylated bovine serum albumin. In addition, a glutamate sensor was designed by immobilizing glutamate dehydrogenase on the nanoparticle surfaces [185]. In another application, a BODIPY-doped polymeric nanoparticle was designed for the detection of Cu^{2+}. Here the metal-chelating receptor, cyclam, was covalently bound to the surface of the nanoparticle. In the presence of Cu^{2+} the fluorescence emission of the BODIPY is quenched by the overlapping adsorption band of the metal–chelator complex [186]. Fluorescent polymeric nanoparticles have also been used for the intracellular monitoring of key biological components. Using three different nanoparticle fabrication technologies, sensors based on polyacrylamide, cross-linked decyl methacrylate, and silica-based sol–gel have been characterized in aqueous solution and intracellular surroundings. Each matrix can be combined with specific "free dyes", ionophores, or enzymes to produce sensors selective for the biological component of interest. These nano-optodes are termed PEBBLEs (probes encapsulated by biol. localized embedding). Spherical sensors less than 600 nm in diam. (and reducible to below 100 nm) have been made from all three matrices. Acrylamide-based sensors have been used to monitor intracellular pH and calcium (with proven selectivity over Mg^{2+}). Decyl methacrylate has been successfully applied to intracellular potassium monitoring with probes 1000× more selective for potassium than sodium. Such a sol–gel-based approach has also proven useful for monitoring intracellular oxygen at physiologically interesting concentrations. PEBBLEs, with a wide range of both simple and complex sensing schemes, provide a unique tool for minimally invasive intracellular monitoring, with many significant advantages over free dyes as well as over fiber-optic sensors [187–189].

1.5.1.2 Quantum Dot Sensors

The great potential of quantum dots for sensing applications has been demonstrated in several instances. In one application, quantum dots have been utilized as maltose sensors [114]. Here quantum dots were surface-functionalized with a maltose-binding protein (MBP) containing β-cyclodextrin-QSY-9 attached to the binding site to quench the quantum dot emission. The senor concept is that maltose displaces the β-cyclodextrin-QSY-9, thus inducing quantum dot emission. Another reported quantum dot-based maltose sensor using MBP acts as a double FRET sensor [114]. Here the quantum dot emission excites Cy3 that is adsorbed on the surface of the MBP. The Cy3 emission then excites the β-cyclodextrin–Cy3.5 whose emission is observed. Once maltose is introduced to the sensor, the Cy3 emission is no longer quenched by the Cy3.5, because the β-cyclodextrin–Cy3.5 has been displaced by maltose [114].

Quantum dots also show great promise in immunoassays. For example, an immunoassay has been performed by binding an antibody covalently to a glass chip, followed by binding of the antigen. The antigen was then detected with the addition of antibody labeled quantum dots, which bound selectively to the captured antigen [190]. In another application, Tran et al. prepared quantum dot conjugates with the immunoglobin G (IgG) binding domain of streptococcal protein G (PG) appended with a basic leucine zipper attachment domain (PG-zb). They also demonstrated that the quantum dot/PG conjugates retain their ability to bind IgG antibodies, and that a specific antibody coupled to quantum dots via the PG functional domain efficiently binds its antigen. Preliminary results indicated that electrostatically self-assembled quantum dot/PG-zb/IgG bioconjugates can be used in fluoro-immunoassays [191]. Quantum dot–antibody conjugates were again successfully used in fluoro-immunoassays to detect both a protein toxin (staphylococcal enterotoxin B) and a small molecule (2,4,6-trinitrotoluene) [108]. Goldman et al. described a conjugation strategy employing an engineered molecular adaptor protein, attached to the quantum dots via electrostatic/hydrophobic self-assembly, to link quantum dots with antibodies. Quantum dots can also be used as sensors for sugars; a quantum dot FRET application using adsorbed MBP has been mentioned [114].

Powerful sensor concepts can also be designed using the multiplexing capability of quantum dots. This results from the broad excitation and narrow, size-dependent emission bands of quantum dots. This concept has been used, for example, to embed quantum dots of six different colors and ten intensities per color in nanoparticles composed of styrene, divinylbenzene, and acrylic acid. This combination can, theoretically, code one million nucleic acids or protein sequences [80]. In another application, a high-throughput assay has been developed for the parallel detection of antibodies using quantum dot microbeads. In this case, a custom designed microfluidic chip with multiple micro-wells was utilized for capturing of microbeads, antib... n into each micro-well, QD injection, and fluo-
... ads could be identified with a standard flow
... [193].

... n used to recognize and detect specific DNA
... Detection is based on fluorescently tagged,
... d to the surface of the gold nanoparticle.
... arch toward the gold surface, quenching the
... priate target sequence, the oligonucleotide
... moving it away from the gold nanoparticle
... e [194]. Another interesting approach to
... idization is based on Au nanoparticle-
... PR). Interestingly, even without further op-
... que begins to approach that of traditional
... bridization and oligonucleotide detection
... used in the detection of glucose and glu-
... oparticles requires H_2O_2 and converts it
... glucose oxidase and glucose, O_2 is converted into

H_2O_2, allowing the Au nanoparticles to grow, thus giving a shift in absorbance over time [195]. Finally, Ag has also been employed for surface plasmon-based nanosensors concerning the detection of Alzheimer's disease. Autopsied brain samples of humans with Alzheimer's disease show elevated levels of amyloid-derived diffusible ligands (ADDLs), which suggest that a definitive chemical diagnosis of Alzheimer's could be achieved with a sensitive method to detect ADDL or anti-ADDL antibodies. The λ_{max} of silver nanoparticles conjugated with anti-ADDL was monitored before and after the incubation with ADDL. The resulting $\Delta\lambda_{max}$ indicated that it is possible to monitor the interaction between ADDL and anti-ADDL using Ag nanoparticles. While undergoing a promising initial trial, the practicality of the system as a sensor is limited because its specificity becomes low at nM concentrations of anti-ADDLs [196].

1.5.2 Fluorescent Nanoparticles as Labels in Biological Imaging

1.5.2.1 Dye-doped Nanoparticles

Though very small, fluorescent dyes are only of limited applicability in biological imaging because of their poor photostability and limited brightness. To improve the photostability, initially, dye-doped nanoparticles have been used as photostable imaging probes. For example, 20 nm dye-doped latex nanoparticles have been linked to DNA-binding proteins (restriction enzyme EcoR1) to probe specific sequences on stretched DNA [7]. In addition, ruthenium bipyridyl-doped silica nanoparticles can be used to stain and image leukemia cells [4]. More recently, Ru(bpy)-doped silica nanoparticles have been applied successfully in several fluorescent imaging applications, including immunocytochemistry, immunohistochemistry, and DNA and protein microarrays [197]. Here the nanoparticles were surface-functionalized with avidin, thus allowing straightforward coupling to biotinylated antibodies. In one case, avidin-capped, dye-doped silica nanoparticles were conjugated with biotinylated mouse anti-hIgM to stain human peripheral blood mononuclear cells. In another case, these photostable nanoprobes were coupled to biotinylated goat anti-ChAT antibodies to label choline acetyltransferase to image mouse brain tissue. Interestingly, these dye-doped silica nanoparticles are not outperformed by quantum dots with respect to photostability.

1.5.2.2 Quantum Dots

Among the different types of fluorescent nanoparticles, quantum dots seem to show the greatest promise as labels in biological imaging applications. Since their introduction as labels in cellular imaging in 1998 [44, 115], multiple reports have shown the strengths of these nanoprobes for tagging and imaging applications in biological systems. This strength is based on the impressive photostability of quantum dots and on their broad excitation and narrow size-dependent emission properties. Most importantly, the high photostability guarantees the observation of biomolecules over longer time periods. Dubertret et al. have reported a very elegant example of such a long-term observation of biological processes [118]. Here, quantum dots with biocompatible coatings were injected into *Xenopus* embryos and their movement into different cells during tadpole development was monitored over several days.

Quantum dot multi-color imaging in cells is another fascinating imaging approach. For example, quantum dots biofunctionalized with streptavidin and IgG have been used to label the breast cancer marker Her2 on fixed and live cancer cells, to tag actin and microtubules, and to stain nuclear antigens inside the nucleus [116]. Quantum dots have also been shown to be useful in studying ATP driven biological processes. The *in vitro* sliding of quantum dot labeled actin filaments was observed over periods of 10–12 s [198]. The chaperonin proteins GroEL (from *Escherichia coli*) and T.th ('T.th cpn', from *Thermus thermophilus* HB8) typically encapsulate denatured proteins within a cavity and release them in the presence of ATP. This encapsulation and release technique was used to give quantum dots high thermal and chemical stability in various aqueous mediums, while also allowing the controlled release of quantum dots [199].

Quantum dot labels are particularly advantageous over traditional organic dyes in single-molecule tracking applications because dye-based tracking experiments are limited by very short observation times [200, 201]. Quantum dot-based single molecule tracking in biological systems represents a fascinating emerging research area. The first results indicate great promise. Dahan et al. have successfully tracked individual quantum dot-tagged glycine receptors in the neuronal membrane of live cells and analyzed the diffusion properties [202]. Furthermore, this technique allowed them to observe the entry of individual glycine receptors into the synapse, which was confirmed by electron microscopy experiments. The ability to detect quantum dots not only optically but also by electron microscopy is clearly a very powerful feature. Another recent single-molecule application was related to the monitoring of quantum dot-labeled epidermal growth factor. In this case, a new transport process was discovered [203].

Fluorescent nanoparticles have also been applied in animal imaging experiments; again, quantum dots seem to show great promise. Proper biocompatible surface coating is essential for long-term stability of the probes in a biological environment [204]. In another application, quantum dots have been targeted *in vivo* via peptides immobilized on the quantum dot surface [205]. Here, several types of peptides were used to label different regions of the mice tissue. Thus, quantum dots with lung-targeting peptides were shown to accumulate in the lungs of mice whereas other peptides targeted quantum dots to blood or lymphatic vessels in tumors. Targeted quantum dot transport in live animals was recently reported in mice [164]. In this case, PEG-coated nanoprobes were used that carried conjugated antibodies directed against prostate-specific membrane antigens. A clear boost in animal imaging should be expected from the recent development of quantum dots with emission bands in the near-infrared (NIR) because this wavelength range offers an optical window for tissue imaging. Indeed, NIR quantum dots have been applied successfully to conduct imaging experiments on rat and porcine tissue [206, 207]. In one case, rat coronary vasculature was studied. In the other case, porcine sentinel lymph nodes were imaged. Interestingly, when injected interdermally on the thigh of a 35 kg pig, doctors could visualize the nearby sentinel lymph nodes within 3–4 min and use the infrared signal as a guide during surgery. Despite the relatively low power NIR excitation used (5 mW cm^{-2}) the sentinel lymph nodes were observed as deep as 1 cm below the skin surface.

References

1 SAXTON, M. J., JACOBSON, K., Single particle tracking: Applications to membrane dynamics. *Annu. Rev. Biophys. Biomol. Struct.* **1997**, *26*, 373–399.

2 KREUTER, J., in *Microcapsules and Nanoparticles in Medicine and Pharmacy* (Ed.: N. DOMBROW), CRC, Boca Raton, FL, **1992**.

3 NIEMEYER, C. M., Nanoparticles, proteins, nucleic acids: Biotechnology meets Materials Science. *Angew. Chem. Int. Ed.* **2001**, *40*, 4128–4158.

4 BAGWE, R. P., ZHAO, X., TAN, W., Bioconjugated luminescent nanoparticles for biological applications. *J. Dispers. Sci. Technol.* **2003**, *3&4*, 453–464.

5 SANTRA, S., WANG, K., TAPEC, R., TAN, W. H., Development of novel dye doped silica nanoparticles for biomarker applications. *J. Biomed. Opt.* **2001**, 6, 160–166.

6 GAO, H., ZHAO, Y., FU, S., LI, B., LI, M., Preparation of novel polymeric fluorescent nanoparticles. *Colloid Polym. Sci.* **2002**, *280*, 653–660.

7 TAYLOR, J. R., FANG, M. M., NIE, S., Probing specific sequences on single DNA molecules with bioconjugated fluorescent nanoparticles. *Anal. Chem.* **2000**, *72*, 1979–1986.

8 JAIN, T. K., ROY, I., DE, T. K., MAITRA, A. N., Nanometer silica particles encapsulating active compounds: a novel ceramic drug carrier. *J. Am. Chem. Soc.* **1998**, *120*, 11092–11095.

9 ZHAO, X. J., TAPEC-DYTIOCO, R., WANG, K. M., TAN, W. H., Collection of trace amounts of DNA/mRNA molecules using genomagnetic nanocapturers. *Anal. Chem.* **2003**, *75*, 3476–3483.

10 VAN BLAADEREN, A., VRJI, A., Synthesis and characterization of colloidal dispersions of fluorescent, monodisperse silica spheres. *Langmuir* **1992**, *8*, 2921–2931.

11 BAGWE, R. P., YANG, C., HILLARD, L. R., TAN, W., Optimization of dye-doped silica nanoparticles prepared using a reverse microemulsion method. *Langmuir* **2004**, *20*, 8336–8342.

12 BAGWE, R. P., KHILAR, K. C., Effects of intermicellar exchange rate on the formation of silver nanoparticles in reverse microemulsions of AOT. *Langmuir* **2000**, *16*, 906–910.

13 MAKAROVA, A. V., OSTAFIN, A. E., MIYOSHI, H., NORRIS, J. R., MEISEL, D., Adsorption and encapsulation of fluorescent probes in nanoparticles. *J. Phys. Chem. B* **1999**, *103*, 9080–9084.

14 MEYSSAMY, H., RIWOTZKI, R., KORNOWSKI, A., NAUSED, S., HAASE, M., Wet-chemical synthesis of doped colloidal nanomaterials: Particles and fibers of $LaPO_4$:Eu, $LaPO_4$:Ce, and $LaPO_4$:Ce,Tb. *Adv. Mater.* **1999**, *11*, 840–844.

15 MEISER, F., CORTEZ, C., CARUSO, F., Biofunctionalization of fluorescent rare-earth-doped lanthanum phosphate colloidal nanoparticles. *Angew. Chem. Int. Ed.* **2004**, *43*, 5954–5957.

16 BRUS, L. E., A simple model for the ionization potential, electron affinity, and aqueous redox potentials of small semiconductor crystallites. *J. Chem. Phys.* **1983**, *79*, 5566–5571.

17 BRUS, L. E., Electron-electron and electron-hole interactions in small semiconductor crystallites: the size dependence of the lowest excited

electronic state. *J. Chem. Phys.* **1983**, *80*, 4403–4409.

18 Chestnoy, N., Harris, T. D., Hull, R., Brus, L. E., Luminescence and photophysics of cadmium sulfide semiconductor clusters: the nature of the emitting electronic state. *J. Phys. Chem.* **1986**, *90*, 2555–2560.

19 Bawendi, M. G., Steigerwald, M. W., Brus, L. E., The quantum mechanics of larger semiconductor clusters ("quantum dots"). *Annu. Rev. Phys. Chem.* **1990**, *41*, 477–496.

20 Michalet, X., Pinaud, F. F., Bentolila, L. A., Tsay, J. M., Doose, S., Li, J. J., Sundaresan, G., Wu, A. M., Gambhir, S. S., Weiss, S., Quantum dots for live cells, in vivo imaging, and diagnostics. *Science* **2005**, *307*, 538–544.

21 Wilson, W. L., Szajowski, P. F., Brus, L. E., Quantum confinement in size-selected surface-oxidised silicon nanocrystals. *Science* **1993**, *262*, 1242–1244.

22 Bley, R. A., Kauzlarich, S. M., A Low-temperature solution phase route for the synthesis of silicon nano-clusters. *J. Am. Chem. Soc.* **1996**, *118*, 12461–12462.

23 Holmes, J. D., Ziegler, K. J., Doty, R. C., Pell, L. E., Johnston, K. P., Korgel, B. A., Highly luminescent silicon nanocrystals with discrete optical transitions. *J. Am. Chem. Soc.* **2001**, *123*, 3743–3748.

24 Hines, M. A., Guyot-Sionnest, P., Synthesis and characterization of strongly luminescing ZnS-capped CdSe nanocrystals. *J. Phys. Chem.* **1996**, *100*, 468–471.

25 Stsiapura, V., Sukhanova, A., Artemyev, M., Pluot, M., Cohen, J. H. M., Baranov, A. V., Oleinikov, V., Nabiev, I., Functionalized nanocrystal-tagged fluorescent polymer beads: synthesis, physicochemical characterization, and immunolabeling application. *Anal. Biochem.* **2004**, *334*, 257–265.

26 Reiss, P., Bleuse, J., Pron, A., Highly luminescent CdSe/ZnSe core/shell nanocrystals of low size dispersion. *Nano Lett.* **2002**, *2*, 781–784.

27 Peng, X., Wickham, J., Alivisatos, A. P., Epitaxial growth of highly luminescent CdSe/CdS core/shell nanocrystals with photostability and electronic accessibility. *J. Am. Chem. Soc.* **1998**, *120*, 5343–5344.

28 Peng, Z. A., Peng, X., Kinetics of II–VI and III–V colloidal semiconductor nanocrystal growth: "Focusing" of size distributions. *J. Am. Chem. Soc.* **2001**, *123*, 183–184.

29 Murcia, M. J., Shaw, D. L., Woodruff, H., Naumann, C. A., Young, B. A., Long, E. C., Facile sonochemical synthesis of highly-luminescent ZnS-shelled CdSe quantum dots. Submitted to *Chem. Mater.*

30 Rogach, A. L., Katsikas, L., Kornowski, A., Su, D., Eychmueller, A., Weller, H., Bunsenges, B., Synthesis, morphology, and optical properties of thiol-stabilized CdTe nanoclusters in aqueous solution. *Berich. Bunsen Gesell.* **1997**, *101*(11), 1668–1670.

31 Mamedova, N. N., Kotov, N. A., Rogach, A. L., Studer, J., Albumin-CdTe nanoparticle bioconjugates: Preparation, structure, and interunit energy transfer with antenna effect. *Nano Lett.* **2001**, *1*, 281–286.

32 Lakowicz, J. R., Gryczynski, I., Gryczynski, Z., Murphy, C. J., Luminescence spectral properties of CdS nanoparticles. *J. Phys. Chem. B* **1999**, *103*, 7613–7620.

33 Torimoto, T., Yamashita, M., Kuwabata, S., Sakata, T., Mori, H., Yoneyama, H., Fabrication of CdS nanoparticle chains along DNA double strands. *J. Phys. Chem. B* **1999**, *103*, 8799–8803.

34 Lakowicz, J. R., Gryczynski, I., Gryczynski, Z., Nowaczyk, K., Murphy, C. J., Luminescence spectral properties of CdS nanoparticles. *Anal. Biochem.* **2000**, *280*, 128–136.

35 Bigham, S. R., Coffer, J. L., Thermochemical passivation of DNA-stabilized Q-cadmium sulfide nanoparticles. *J. Cluster Sci.* **2000**, *11*, 359–372.

36 Li, X., Coffer, J. L., Effect of pressure

on the photoluminescence of polynucleotide-stabilized cadmium sulfide nanocrystals. *Chem. Mater.* **1999**, *11*, 2326–2330.

37 Willner, I., Patolsky, F., Wasserman, J., Photoelectrochemistry with controlled DNA-cross-linked CdS nanoparticle arrays. *Angew. Chem. Int. Ed.* **2001**, *40*, 1861–1864.

38 Chen, H. M., Huang, X. F., Xu, L., Xu, J., Chen, K. J., Feng, D., Self-assembly and photoluminescence of CdS-mercaptoacetic clusters with internal structures. *Superlatt., Microstruct.* **2000**, *27*, 1–5.

39 Peng, X., Schlamp, M. C., Kadavanich, A. V., Alivisatos, A. P., Epitaxial growth of highly luminescent CdSe/CdS core/shell nanocrystals with photostability and electronic accessibility. *J. Am. Chem. Soc.* **1997**, *119*, 7019–7029.

40 Passow, T., Leonardi, K., Hommel, D., Optical and structural properties of CdSe/Zn(S)Se quantum dot stacks. *Phys. Stat. Sol. B* **2001**, *224*, 143–146.

41 Pathak, S., Choi, S. K., Arnheim, N., Thompson, M. E., Hydroxylated quantum dots as luminescent probes for in situ hybridization. *J. Am. Chem. Soc.* **2001**, *123*(17), 4103–4104.

42 Mattoussi, H., Mauro, J. M., Goldman, E. R., Anderson, G. P., Sundar, V. C., Mikulec, F. V., Bawendi, M. G., Bioconjugation of highly luminescent colloidal CdSe-ZnS quantum dots with an engineered two-domain recombinant protein. *J. Am. Chem. Soc.* **2000**, *122*, 12142–12150.

43 Mattoussi, H., Mauro, J. M., Goldman, E. R., Green, T. M., Anderson, G. P., Sundar, V. C., Bawendi, M. G., Bioconjugation of highly luminescent colloidal CdSe-ZnS quantum dots with an engineered two-domain recombinant protein. *Phys. Stat. Sol. B* **2001**, *224*(1), 277–283.

44 Brunchez, M. J., Moronne, M., Gin, P., Weiss, S., Alivisatos, A. P., Semiconductor nanocrystals as fluorescent labels. *Science* **1998**, *281*, 2013–2016.

45 Liz-Marzán, L. M., Giersig, M., Mulvaney, P., Synthesis of nanosized gold-silica core-shell particles. *Langmuir* **1996**, *12*, 4329–4335.

46 Gerion, D., Pinaud, F., Williams, S. C., Parak, W. J., Zanchet, D., Weiss, S., Alivisatos, A. P., Synthesis and properties of biocompatible water-soluble silica-coated CdSe/ZnS semiconductor quantum dots. *J. Phys. Chem. B* **2001**, *105*, 8861–8871.

47 Schroedter, A., Weller, H., Ligand design and bioconjugation of colloidal gold nanoparticles. *Angew. Chem. Int. Ed.* **2002**, *41*, 3218–3221.

48 Parak, W. J., Gerion, D., Zanchet, D., Woerz, A. S., Pellegrino, T., Micheel, C., Williams, S. C., Seitz, M., Bruehl, R. E., Bryant, Z., Bustamante, C., Bertozzi, C. R., Alivisatos, A. P., Conjugation of DNA to silanized colloidal semiconductor nanocrystalline quantum dots. *Chem. Mater.* **2002**, *14*, 2113–2119.

49 Skaff, H., Emrick, T., The use of 4-substituted pyridines to afford amphiphilic, pegylated cadmium selenide. *Chem. Commun.* **2003**, 52–53.

50 Kamat, P. V., Photophysical, photochemical and photocatalytic aspects of metal nanoparticles. *J. Phys. Chem. B* **2002**, *106*, 7729–7744.

51 Wilcoxon, J. P., Martin, J. E., Parsapour, F., Wiedenman, B., Kelley, D. F., Photoluminescence from nanosize gold clusters. *J. Chem. Phys.* **1998**, *108*(21), 9137–9143.

52 Moffitt, M., Vali, H., Eisenberg, A., Spherical assemblies of semiconductor nanoparticles in water-soluble block copolymer aggregates. *Chem. Mater.* **1998**, *10*, 1021–1028.

53 Huang, T., Murray, R. W., Visible Luminescence of water-soluble monolayer-protected gold clusters. *J. Phys. Chem. B* **2001**, *105*, 12498–12502.

54 Sato, T., Ichikawa, T., Ito, T., Yonezawa, Y., Kadono, K., Sakaguchi, T., Miya, M., Nonlinear optical properties of silver sols prepared by photoreduction method. *Chem. Phys. Lett.* **1995**, *242*, 310–314.

55 François, L., Mostafavi, M., Belloni, J., Delouis, J. F., Delaire, J., Feneyrou, P., Optical limitation induced by gold clusters: 1. Size effect. *J. Phys. Chem. B* **2000**, *104*, 6133–6137.

56 Keating, C. D., Kovaleski, K. K., Natan, M. J., Heightened electromagnetic fields between metal nanoparticles: Surface enhanced raman scattering from metal-cytochrome c-metal sandwiches. *J. Phys. Chem. B* **1998**, *102*, 9414–9425.

57 Hulteen, J. C., Treichel, D. A., Smith, M. T., Duval, M. L., Jensen, T. R., Van, R. P., Nanosphere lithography: Size-tunable silver nanoparticle and surface cluster arrays. *J. Phys. Chem. B* **1999**, *103*, 3854–3863.

58 Michaels, A. M., Jiang, J., Brus, L., Ag nanocrystal junctions as the site for surface-enhanced Raman scattering of single rhodamine 6G molecules. *J. Phys. Chem. B* **2000**, *104*, 11965–11971.

59 Oldenburg, S. J., Westcott, S. L., Averitt, R. D., Halas, N. J., Surface enhanced Raman scattering in the near infrared using metal nanoshell substrates. *J. Chem. Phys.* **1999**, *111*, 4729–4735.

60 Lee, P. C., Meisel, D., Adsorption and surface-enhanced Raman of dyes on silver and gold sols. *J. Phys. Chem.* **1982**, *86*(17), 3391–3395.

61 Freeman, R. G., Hommer, M. B., Grabar, K. C., Jackson, M. A., Natan, M. J., Ag-clad Au nanoparticles: Novel aggregation, optical, and surface-enhanced Raman scattering Properties. *J. Phys. Chem.* **1996**, *100*, 718–724.

62 He, L., Musick, M. D., Nicewarner, S. R., Salias, F. G., Benkovic, S. J., Natan, N. J., Keating, C. D., Colloidal Au-enhanced surface plasmon resonance for ultrasensitive detection of DNA hybridization. *J. Am. Chem. Soc.* **2000**, *122*, 9071–9077.

63 Brust, M., Walker, M., Bethell, D., Schiffrin, D. J., Whymann, R. J., Synthesis of thiol-derivatised gold nanoparticles in a two-phase liquid–liquid system. *J. Chem. Soc., Chem. Commun.* **1994**, *7*, 801–802.

64 Brust, M., Fink, J., Bethell, D., Schiffrin, D. J., Kiely, C. J., Synthesis and reactions of functionalised gold nanoparticles. *J. Chem. Soc., Chem. Commun.* **1995**, *16*, 1655–1656.

65 Kolb, U., Quasier, S. A., Winter, M., Reetz, M. T., Investigation of tetra-alkylammonium bromide stabilized palladium/platinum bimetallic clusters using extended X-ray absorption fine structure. *Chem. Mater.* **1996**, *8*, 1889–1894.

66 Fink, J., Kiely, C., Bethell, D., Schiffrin, D. J., Self-organization of nanosized gold particles. *Chem. Mater.* **1998**, *10*, 922–926.

67 Perez, M., Pradeau, J. P., Albouy, P. A., Perez-Omil, J., Synthesis and characterization of functionalized platinum nanoparticles. *Chem. Mater.* **1999**, *11*, 3460–3463.

68 Subramanian, V., Wolf, E., Kamat, P. V., Semiconductor-metal composite nanostructures. To what extent do metal nanoparticles improve the photocatalytic activity of TiO_2 films. *J. Phys. Chem. B* **2001**, *105*, 11439–11446.

69 Niidome, Y., Hori, A., Sato, T., Yamada, S., Enormous size growth of thiol-passivated gold nanoparticles induced by near-IR laser light. *Chem. Lett.* **2000**, 310–311.

70 Bagwe, R. P., Mishra, B. K., Khilar, K. C., Effect of chain length of oxyethylene group on particle size and absorption spectra of silver nanoparticles prepared in non-ionic water-in-oil microemulsions. *J. Disp. Sci. Technol.* **1999**, *20*(6), 1569–1579.

71 Bagwe, R. P., Khilar, K. C., Effects of intermicellar exchange rate on the formation of silver nanoparticles in reverse microemulsions of AOT. *Langmuir* **1997**, *13*(24), 6432–6438.

72 Shah, D. O., Bagwe, R. P., Parmar, B. S., The effects of interfacial viscosity on the kinetics of formation of silver nanparticles using water-in-oil microemulsions as nanoreactors. *Mater. Res. Soc. Symp. Proc.* **2002**, *704*, W10.1.1–W10.1.8.

73 SCHLUPEN, J., HAEGEL, F. H., KUHLMANN, J., GEISLER, H., SCHWUGER, M. J., Synthesis of nano-sized gold-silica core-shell particles. *Colloid Surf. A* **1999**, *156*, 335–347.

74 ELGHANIAN, R., STORHOFF, J. J., MUCIC, R. C., LETSINGER, R. L., MIRKIN, C. A., Selective colorimetric detection of polynucleotides based on the distance-dependent optical properties of gold nanoparticles. *Science* **1997**, *277*, 1078–1080.

75 HAINFELD, J. F., FURUYA, F. R., A 1.4 nm gold cluster covalently attached to antibodies improves immunolabeling. *J. Histochem. Cytochem.* **1992**, *40*, 177–184.

76 MATTHEWS, D. C., GRONDAHL, L., BATTERSBY, B. J., TRAU, M., Multi-fluorescent silica colloids for encoding large combinatorial libraries. *Aust. J. Chem.* **2001**, *54*(9 & 10), 649–656.

77 LAWRIE, G. A., BATTERSBY, B. J., TRAU, M., Synthesis of optically complex core-shell colloidal suspensions: Pathways to multiplexed biological screening. *Adv. Funct. Mater.* **2003**, *13*(11), 887–896.

78 GOLDMAN, E. R., CLAPP, A. R., ANDERSON, G. P., UYEDA, H. T., MAURO, J. M., MEDNITZ, I. L., MATOUSSI, H., Multiplexed toxin analysis using four colors of quantum dot fluororeagents. *Anal. Chem.* **2004**, *76*, 684–688.

79 ROSENTHAL, S. J., Bar-coding biomolecules with fluorescent nanocrystals., *Nat. Biotechnol.* **2001**, *19*(7), 621–622.

80 HAN, M., GAO, X., SU, J. Z., NIE, S., Quantum-dot-tagged microbeads for multiplexed optical coding of biomolecules. *Nat. Biotechnol.* **2001**, *19*(7), 631–635.

81 XU, H., SHA, M. Y., WONG, E. Y., UPHO, J., XU, Y., TREADWAY, J. A., TRUONG, A., O'BRIEN, E., ASQUITH, S., STUBBINS, M., SPURR, N. K., LAI, E. H., MAHONEY, W., Multiplexed SNP genotyping using the Qbead system: a quantum dot-encoded microsphere-based assay. *Nucleic Acids Res.* **2003**, *31*, e43/1–e43/10.

82 FULTON, R. J., MCDADE, R. L., SMITH, P. L., KIENKER, L. J., KETTMAN JR., L. R., Advanced multiplexed analysis with the FlowMetrix^{TM} system. *Clin. Chem.* **1997**, *43*, 1749–1756.

83 VERONESE, F. M., MORPURGO, M., Bioconjugation in pharmaceutical chemistry. *Farmaco* **1999**; *54*(8), 497–516.

84 MITCHELL, G. P., MIRKIN, C. A., LETSINGER, R. L., Programmed assembly of DNA functionalized quantum dots. *J. Am. Chem. Soc.* **1999**, *121*(35), 8122–8123.

85 ZHANG, C. Y., MA, H., NIE, S. M., DING, Y., JIN, L., CHEN, D. Y., Quantum dot-labeled trichosanthin. *Analyst* **2000**, *125*, 1029–1031.

86 WILLARD, D. M., CARILLO, L. L., JUNG, J., ORDEN, A. V., CdSe-ZnS quantum dots as resonance energy transfer donors in a model protein-protein binding assay. *Nano Lett.* **2001**, *1*(9), 469–474.

87 PARAK, W. J., GERION, D., PELLEGRINO, T., ZANCHET, D., MICHEEL, C., WILLIAMS, S. C., BOUDREAU, R., LE GROS, M. A., LARABELL, C. A., ALIVISATOS, A. P., Biological applications of colloidal nanocrystals. *Nanotechnology* **2003**, *14*, R15–R27.

88 GOLDMAN, E. R., BALIGHAIAN, E. D., MATTOUSSI, H., KUNO, M. K., MAURO, J. M., TRAN, P. T., ANDERSON, G. P., Avidin: A natural bridge for quantum dot-antibody conjugates. *J. Am. Chem. Soc.* **2002**, *124*, 6378–6382.

89 BAEUMLE, M., STAMOU, D., SEGURA, J. M., HOVIUS, R., VOGEL, H., Vitro sliding of actin filaments labelled with single quantum dots. *Langmuir* **2004**, *314*(2), 529–534.

90 TORCHILIN, V. P., KHAW, B. A., SMIRNOV, V. N., HABER, E., Preservation of antimyosin antibody activity after covalent coupling to liposomes. *Biochem. Biophys. Res. Commun.* **1979**, *85*, 1114–1119.

91 MAGNANI, P., PAGANELLI, G., MODORATI, G., ZITO, F., SONGINI, C., SUDATI, F., KOCH, P., MAECKE, H. R., BRANCATO, R., SICCARDI, A. G., FAZIO, F., Quantitative comparison of direct antibody labeling and tumor

pretargeting in uveal melanoma. *J. Nucleic Med.* **1996**, *37*, 967–971.

92 Nobs, L., Buchegger, F., Gurny, R., Allémann, E., Current methods for attaching targeting ligands to liposomes and nanoparticles. *J. Pharm. Sci.* **2004**, *93*, 1980–1992.

93 Illum, L., Jones, P. D. E., Kreuter, J., Baldwin, R. W., Davis, S. S., Adsorption of monoclonal antibodies to polyhexylcyanoacrylate nanoparticles and subsequent immunospecific binding to tumour cells in vitro. *Int. J. Pharm.* **1983**, *17*, 65–76.

94 Illum, L., Jones, P. D., Baldwin, R. W., Davis, S. S., Tissue distribution of poly(hexyl 2-cyanoacrylate) nanoparticles coated with monoclonal antibodies in mice bearing human tumor xenografts. *J. Pharmacol. Exp. Ther.* **1984**, *230*, 733–736.

95 Kubiak, C., Manil, L., Couvreur, P., Sorptive properties of antibodies onto cyanoacrylic nanoparticles. *Int. J. Pharm.* **1988**, *41*, 181–187.

96 Manil, L., Roblot-Treupel, L., Couvreur, P., Isobutyl cyanoacrylate nanoparticles as a solid phase for an efficient immunoradiometric assay. *Biomaterials* **1986**, *7*, 212–216.

97 Couvreur, P., Aubry, J., Breimer, D. D., Speises, P., Monoclonal antibodies for the targeting of drugs: Application to nanoparticles. *Top. Pharmaceut. Sci.* **1983**, 305–316.

98 Blackwell, J. E., Dagia, N. M., Dickerson, J. B., Berg, E. L., Goetz, D. J., Ligand coated nanosphere adhesion to E- and P-selectin under static and flow conditions. *Ann. Biomed. Eng.* **2001**, *29*, 523–533.

99 Serizawa, T., Uchida, T., Akashi, M., Synthesis of polystyrene nanospheres having lactose-conjugated hydrophilic polymers on their surfaces and carbohydrate recognition by proteins. *Biomater. Sci. Polym. Ed.* **1999**, *10*, 391–401.

100 Li, Y., Ogris, M., Wagner, E., Pelisek, J., Rüffer, M., Nanoparticles bearing polyethylenglycol-coupled transferrin as gene carriers: preparation and in vitro evaluation. *Int. J. Pharm.* **2003**, *259*, 93–101.

101 Akasaka, Y., Ueda, H., Takayama, K., Machida, Y., Nagai, T., Preparation and evaluation of bovine serum albumin nanospheres coated with monoclonal antibodies. *Drug Des. Disc.* **1988**, *3*, 85–97.

102 Rolland, A., Bourel, D., Genetet, B., Le Verge, R., Monoclonal antibodies covalently coupled to polymethacrylic nanoparticles: in vitro specific targeting to human T lymphocytes. *Int. J. Pharm.* **1987**, *39*, 173–180.

103 Gautier, S. N., Grudzielski, N., Goffinet, G., de Hassonville, S. H., Delattre, L., Jérôme, R., Preparation of poly(D,L-lactide) nanoparticles assisted by amphiphilic poly(methyl methacrylate-co-methacrylic acid) copolymers. *J. Biomater. Sci. Polym.* **2001**, *12*, 429–450.

104 Gref, R., Couvreur, P., Barratt, G., Mysiakine, E., Surface-engineered nanoparticles for multiple ligand coupling. *Biomaterials* **2003**, *24*, 4529–4537.

105 Maruyama, A., Ishihara, T., Kim, J. S., Kim, S. W., Akaike, T., Nanoparticle DNA carrier with poly(L-lysine) grafted polysaccharide copolymer and poly(D,L-lactic acid). *Bioconjug. Chem.* **1997**, *8*, 735–742.

106 Chan, W. C. W., Maxwell, D. J., Gao, X., Bailey, R. E., Han, M., Nie, S., Luminescent quantum dots for multiplexed biological detection and imaging. *Curr. Opin. Biotechnol.* **2002**, *13*(1), 40–46.

107 Lin, Z., Cui, S., Zhang, H., Chen, Q., Yang, B., Su, X., Zhang, J., Jin, Q., Studies on quantum dots synthesized in aqueous solution for biological labeling via electrostatic interaction. *Anal. Biochem.* **2003**, *319*(2), 239–243.

108 Goldman, E. R., et al., Conjugation of luminescent quantum dots with antibodies using an engineered adaptor protein to provide new reagents for fluoroimmunoassays. *Anal. Chem.* **2002**, *274*, 841–847.

109 Mattoussi, H., et al. in *Optical Biosensors: Present and Future* (Ed.: F. S. Ligler, C. A. Rowe Taitt), Elsevier, The Netherlands, **2002**.

110 Kagan, C. R., Murray, C. B., Bawendi, M. G., Long-range resonance transfer of electronic excitations in close-packed CdSe quantum-dot solids. *Phys. Rev. B* **1996**, *54*, 8633–8643.
111 Wang, L. Y., Kan, X. W., Zhang, M. C., Zhu, C. Q., Wang, L., Fluorescence for the determination of protein with functionalized nano-ZnS. *Analyst* **2002**, *127*, 1531–1534.
112 Hanaki, K., Momo, A., Oku, T., Komoto, A., Maenosono, S., Yamaguchi, Y., Yamamoto, K., Semiconductor quantum dot/albumin complex is a long-life and highly photostable endosome marker. *Biochem. Biophys. Res. Commun.* **2003**, *302*, 496–501.
113 Tran, P. T., Goldman, E. R., Anderson, G. P., Mauro, J. M., Mattoussi, H., Use of luminescent CdSe-ZnS nanocrystal bioconjugates in quantum dot-based nanosensors. *Phys. Stat. Sol. B* **2002**, *229*(1), 427–432.
114 Medintz, I. L., Clapp, A. R., Mattoussi, H., Goldman, E. R., Fisher, B., Mauro, J. M., Self-assembled nanoscale biosensors based on quantum dot FRET donors. *Nat. Mater.* **2003**, *2*(9), 630–638.
115 Chan, W. C. W., Nie, S., Quantum dot bioconjugates for ultrasensitive nonisotopic detection. *Science* **1998**, *281*(5385), 2016–2018.
116 Wu, X., Liu, J., Liu, H., Haley, K. N., Treadway, J. A., Larson, J. P., Ge, N., Peale, F., Bruchez, M. P., Immunofluorescent labeling of cancer marker Her2 and other cellular targets with semiconductor quantum dots. *Nat. Biotechnol.* **2003**, *21*, 41–46.
117 Wang, S. P., Mamedova, N., Kotov, N. A., Chen, W., Studer, J., Antigen/antibody immunocomplex from CdTe nanoparticle bioconjugates. *Nano Lett.* **2002**, *2*, 817–822.
118 Dubertret, B., Skourides, P., Norris, D. J., Noireaux, V., Brivanlou, A. H., In vivo imaging of quantum dots encapsuled in phospholipid micelles. *Science* **2002**, *298*, 1759–1762.
119 Templeton, A. C., Chen, S., Gross, S. M., Murray, R. W., Water-soluble, isolable gold clusters protected by tiopronin and coenzyme A monolayers. *Langmuir* **1999**, *15*, 66–76.
120 Schaaff, T. G., Knight, G., Shafigullin, M. N., Borkman, R. F., Whetten, R. L., Isolation and selected properties of a 10.4 kDa gold: Glutathione cluster compound. *J. Phys. Chem. B* **1998**, *102*, 10643–10646.
121 Miziani, M. J., Sun, Y. P., Protein-conjugated nanoparticles from rapid expansion of supercritical fluid solution into aqueous solution. *J. Am. Chem. Soc.* **2003**, *125*, 8015–8018.
122 Burt, J. L., Gutierrez-Wing, C., Miki-Yoshida, M., Jose-Yacaman, M., Noble-metal nanoparticles directly conjugated to globular proteins. *Langmuir* **2004**, *20*(26), 11778–11783.
123 Crumbliss, A. L., Perine, S. C., Stonehuerner, J., Tubergen, K. R., Zhao, Junguo, Henkens, R. W., O'Daly, J. P., Colloidal gold as an enzyme immobilization matrix for electrochemical biosensors. *Biotechnol. Bioeng.* **1992**, *40*, 483–490.
124 Brown, K. R., Fox, A. P., Natan, M. J., Morphology-dependent electrochemistry of cytochrome c at Au colloid-modified SnO_2 electrodes. *J. Am. Chem. Soc.* **1996**, *118*, 1154–1157.
125 Sastry, M., Lala, N., Patil, V., Chavan, S. P., Chittiboyina, A. G., Optical absorption study of the biotin-avidin interaction on colloidal silver and gold particles. *Langmuir* **1998**, *14*(15), 4138–4142.
126 Alivisatos, A. P., Johnsson, K. P., Peng, X., Wilson, T. E., Loweth, C. J., Bruchez Jr., M. P., Schultz, P. G., Organization of 'nanocrystal molecules' using DNA. *Nature* **1996**, *382*, 609–611.
127 Mucic, R. C., Storhoff, J. J., Mirkin, C. A., Letsinger, R. L., DNA-directed synthesis of binary nanoparticle network materials. *J. Am. Chem. Soc.* **1998**, *120*, 12674–12675.
128 Zanchet, D., Micheel, C. M., Paral, W. J., Gerion, D., Alivisatos, A. P.,

Electrophoretic isolation of discrete Au nanocrystal/DNA conjugates. *Nano Lett.* **2001**, *1*, 32–35.
129 Hirsch, L. R., Stafford, R. J., Bankson, J. A., Sershen, S. R., Rivera, B., Price, R. E., Hazle, J. D., Halas, N. J., West, J. L., Nanoshell-mediated near-infrared thermal therapy of tumors under magnetic resonance guidance. *Proc. Natl. Acad. Sci. U.S.A.* **2003**, *100*(23), 13549–13554.
130 Kohler, N., Fryxell, G. E., Zhang, M., A bifunctional poly(ethylene glycol) silane immobilized on metallic oxide-based nanoparticles for conjugation with cell targeting agents. *J. Am. Chem. Soc.* **2004**, *126*(23), 7206–7211.
131 Wuelfing, W. P., Gross, S. M., Miles, D. T., Murray, R. W., Nanometer gold clusters protected by surface-bound monolayers of thiolated poly(ethylene glycol) polymer electrolyte. *J. Am. Chem. Soc.* **1998**, *120*, 12696–12697.
132 Quaroni, L., Chumanov, G., Preparation of polymer-coated functionalized silver nanoparticles. *J. Am. Chem. Soc.* **1999**, *121*, 10642–10643.
133 Pinaud, F., King, D., Moore, H. P., Weiss, S., Bioactivation and cell targeting of semiconductor CdSe/ZnS nanoscrystals with phytochelation-related peptides. *J. Am. Chem. Soc.* **2004**, *126*(19), 6115–6123.
134 Roan, J. R., Attraction between nano-particles by end-grafted homopolymers in good solvent. *Phys. Rev. Lett.* **2001**, *86*, 1027–1030.
135 Okano, T., *Biorelated Polymers and Gels*, Academic Press, Boston, **1998**.
136 Horbett, T. A., Brash, T. J. L., *Proteins at Interfaces II.*, ACS Symposium Series 602, Washington, DC, **1995**.
137 Andrade, J. D., Hlady, V., Wei, A. P., Adsorption of complex proteins at interfaces. *Pure Appl. Chem.* **1992**, *64*, 1777–1781.
138 Jeon, S. I., Lee, J. H., Andrade, J. D., de Gennes, P. G., Protein-surface interactions in the presence of polyethylene oxide. I. Simplified theory. *J. Colloid Interface Sci.* **1991**, *142*, 149–158.
139 Harris, J. M., *Poly(ethylene glycol) Chemistry, Biotechnical and Biomedical Applications*, Plenum Press, New York, **1992**.
140 Ikada, Y., Blood-compatible polymers. *Adv. Polym. Sci.* **1984**, *57*, 104–140.
141 Amiji, M., Park, K., Surface modification of polymeric biomaterials with poly(ethylene oxide), albumin, and heparin for reduced thrombogenicity. *J. Biomater. Sci. Polym. Ed.* **1993**, *4*, 217–234.
142 Szleifer, I., Polymers and proteins: interactions at interfaces. *Curr. Opin. Solid State Mater. Sci.* **1997**, *2*, 337–344.
143 Prime, K. L., Whitesides, G. M., Self-assembled organic monolayers: model systems for studying adsorption of proteins at surfaces. *Science* **1991**, *252*, 1164–1167.
144 Ostuni, E., Chapman, R. G., Holmlin, R. E., Takayama, S., Whitesides, G. M., A survey of structure-property relationships of surfaces that resist the adsorption of protein. *Langmuir* **2001**, *17*, 5605–5620.
145 McPearson, T., Kidane, A., Szleifer, I., Park, K., Prevention of protein adsorption by tethered poly(ethylene oxide) layers: experiments and single-chain mean-field analysis. *Langmuir* **1998**, *14*, 176–186.
146 Satulovsky, J., Carigano, M. A., Szleifer, I., Kinetic and thermodynamic control of protein adsorption. *Proc. Natl. Acad. Sci. U.S.A.* **2000**, *10*, 9037–9041.
147 Ghitescu, L., Fixman, A., Surface charge distribution on the endothelial cell of liver sinusoids. *J. Cell Biol.* **1984**, *99*, 639–647.
148 Jordan, A., Scholz, R., Wust, P., Schirra, H., Schiestel, T., Schmidt, H., Felix, R., Visualization and registration of three-dimensional E-field distributions in annual-phased-array applicators. *J. Magn. Magn. Mater.* **1999**, *194*, 185–196.
149 Wilhelm, C., Billotey, C., Roger, J.,

Bittoun, J., Pons, J. N., Bacri, J. C., Gazeau, F., Intracellular uptake of anionic superparamagnetic nanoparticles as a function of their surface coating. *Biomaterials* **2003**, *24*, 1001–1011.

150 Kloepfer, J. A., Mielke, R. E., Wong, M. S., Nealson, K. H., Stucky, G., Nedeau, J. L., Quantum dots as strain- and metabolism-specific microbiological labels. *Appl. Environ. Microbiol.* **2003**, *69*, 4205–4213.

151 Hoshino, A., Fujioka, K., Oku, T., Suga, M., Sasaki, Y. F., Ohta, T., Yasuhara, M., Suzuki, K., Yamamoto, K., Physicochemical properties and cellular toxicity of nanocrystal quantum dots depend on their surface modification. *Nano Lett.* **2004**, *4*, 2163–2169.

152 Derfus, A. M., Chan, W. C. W., Bhatia, S. N., Probing the cytotoxicity of semiconductor quantum dots. *Nano Lett.* **2004**, *4*, 11–18.

153 Kirchner, C., Liedl, T., Kudera, S., Pellegrino, T., Javier, A. M., Gaub, H. E., Stoelzle, S., Fertig, N., Parak, W. J., Cytotoxicity of colloidal CdSe and CdSe/ZnS nanoparticles. *Nano Lett.* **2005**, *5*(2), 331–338.

154 Kondoh, M., Araragi, S., Sato, K., Higashimoto, M., Takiguchi, M., Sato, M., Cadmium induces apoptosis partly via caspapase-9 activation in HL-60 cells. *Toxicology* **2002**, *170*, 111–117.

155 Rikans, L. E., Yamano, T., Mechanisms of cadmium-induced acute hepatotoxicity. *J. Biochem. Mol. Toxicol.* **2000**, *14*, 110–117.

156 Hayat, M., *Colloidal Gold: Principles, Methods and Applications*, Academic, San Diego, **1989**.

157 Otsuka, H., Nagasaki, Y., Kataoka, K., PEGylated nanoparticles for biological and pharmaceutical applications. *Adv. Drug Deliv.* **2003**, *55*, 403–419.

158 Qi, L., Colfen, H., Antonietti, M., Synthesis and characterization of CdS nanoparticles stabilized by double-hydrophilic block copolymers. *Nano Lett.* **2001**, *1*, 61–65.

159 Mumper, R. J., Ledebur, H. C., Dendritic cell delivery of plasmid DNA: applications for genetic vaccines. *Mol. Biotechnol.* **2001**, *19*, 79–95.

160 MacLaughlin, F. C., Mumper, R. J., Wang, J., Tagliaferri, J. M., Roland, A. P., Nanotemplate engineering of cell specific nanoparticles. *J. Controlled Rel.* **1998**, *4*(56), 259–272.

161 Kreuter, J., Nanoparticles as adjuvants for vaccines. *Pharm. Biotechnol.* **1995**, *6*, 463–472.

162 Douglas, S. J., Davis, S. S., Illum, L., Nanoparticles in drug delivery. *Crit. Rev. Ther. Drug Carrier Syst.* **1987**, *3*, 233–261.

163 Wang, C. W., Moffitt, M. G., Surface-tunable photoluminescence from block copolymer-stabilized cadmium sulfide quantum dots. *Langmuir* **2004**, *20*(26), 11784–96.

164 Gao, X., Cui, Y., Levenson, R. M., Chung, L. W. K., Nie, S., In vivo cancer targeting and imaging with semiconductor quantum dots. *Nat. Biotechnol.* **2004**, *22*(8), 969–976.

165 Bertozzi, C. R., Bednarski, M. D., The synthesis of heterobifunctional linkers for the conjugation of ligands to molecular probes. *J. Org. Chem.* **1991**, *56*, 4326–4329.

166 Cook, R. M., Adams, J. H., Hudson, D., The preparation and synthetic application of heterobifunctional biocompatible spacer arms. *Tetrahedron Lett.* **1994**, *35*, 6777–6780.

167 Schwabacher, A. W., Lane, J. W., Schiesher, M. W., Leigh, K. M., Johnson, C. W., Desymmetrization reactions: Efficient preparation of unsymmetrically substituted linker molecules. *J. Org. Chem.* **1998**, *63*, 1727–1729.

168 Nagasaki, Y., Kutsuna, T., Iijima, M., Kato, M., Kataoka, K., Formyl-ended heterobifunctional poly(ethylene oxide): synthesis of poly(ethylene oxide) with a formyl group at one end and a hydroxyl group at the other. *Bioconj. Chem.* **1995**, *6*, 231–233.

169 Nagasaki, Y., Iijima, M., Kato, M., Kataoka, K., Primary amino-terminal heterobifunctional poly(ethylene

oxide). Facile synthesis of poly(ethylene oxide) with a primary amino group at one end and a hydroxylgroup at the other. *Bioconj. Chem.* **1995**, 6, 702–704.

170 NAGASAKI, Y., OGAWA, R., YAMAMOTO, S., KATO, M., KATAOKA, K., Synthesis of heterotelechelic poly(ethylene glycol) macromonomers. Preparation of poly(ethylene glycol) possessing a methacryloyl group at one end a formyl group at the other end. *Macromolecules* **1997**, *30*, 6489–6493.

171 NAKAMURA, T., NAGASAKI, Y., KATAOKA, K., Synthesis of heterobifunctional poly(ethylene glycol) with a reducing monosaccharide residue at one end. *Bioconj. Chem.* **1998**, *9*, 300–303.

172 AKIYAMA, Y., OTSUKA, H., NAGASAKI, Y., KATAOKA, K., Selective synthesis of heterobifunctional poly(ethylene glycol) derivatives containing both mercapto and acetal terminals. *Bioconj. Chem.* **2000**, *11*, 947–950.

173 OTSUKA, H., AKIYAMA, Y., NAGASAKI, Y., KATAOKA, K., Quantitative and reversible lectin-induced association of gold nanoparticles modified with α-lactosyl-ω-mercapto-poly(ethylene glycol). *J. Am. Chem. Soc.* **2001**, *123*, 8226–8230.

174 LI, Z. F., RUCKENSTEIN, E., Water-soluble poly(acrylic acid) grafted silicon nanoparticles and their use as fluorescent biological staining labels. *Nano Lett.* **2004**, *4*, 1463–1467.

175 SONDI, I., SIIMAN, O., KOESTER, S., MATIJEVIC, E., Preparation of aminodextran-CdS nanoparticle complexes and biologically active antibody-aminodextran-CdS nanoparticle conjugates. *Langmuir* **2000**, *16*, 3107–3118.

176 WANG, Y. A., LI, J. J., CHEN, H. Y., PENG, X. G., Stabilization of inorganic nanocrystals by organic dendrons. *J. Am. Chem. Soc.* **2002**, *124*, 2293–2298.

177 MOFFITT, M., VALI, H., EISENBERG, A., Spherical assemblies of semiconductor nanoparticles in water-soluble block copolymer aggregates. *Chem. Mater.* **1998**, *10*, 1021–1028.

178 CHEN, Y., JI, T., ROSENZWEIG, Z., Synthesis of glyconanospheres containing luminescent CdSe-ZnS quantum dots. *Nano Lett.* **2003**, *3*, 581–584.

179 DE LA FUENTE, J. M., BARRIENTOS, A. G., ROJAS, T. C., ROJO, J., CANADA, J., FERNÁNDEZ, A., PENADÉS, S., Gold glyconanoparticles as water-soluble polyvalent models to study carbohydrate interactions. *Angew. Chem. Int. Ed.* **2001**, *40*, 2258–2261.

180 ROJAS, T. C., DE LA FUENTE, J. M., BARRIENTOS, A. G., PENADÉS, S., Gold glyconanoparticles as binding blocks for nanomaterials design. *Adv. Mater.* **2002**, *14*, 585–588.

181 ALDANA, J., WANG, Y. A., PENG, X. G., Photochemical instability of CdSe nanocrystals coated by hydrophilic thiols. *J. Am. Chem. Soc.* **2001**, *123*, 8844–8850.

182 CORREA-DUARTE, M. A., GIERSIG, M., LIZ-MARZÁN, L. M., Stabilization of CdS semiconductor nanoparticles against photodegradation by a silica coating procedure. *Chem. Phys. Lett.* **1998**, *286*, 497–501.

183 MULVANEY, P., LIZ-MARZÁN, L. M., GIERSIG, M., UNG, T., Silica encapsulation of quantum dots and metal clusters. *J. Mater. Chem.* **2000**, *10*, 1259–1270.

184 ROGACH, A. L., NAGESHA, D., OSTRANDER, J. W., GIERSIG, M., KOTOV, N. A., "Raisin bun"-type composite spheres of silica and semiconductor nanocrystals. *Chem. Mater.* **2000**, *12*, 2676–2685.

185 TAPEC, R., ZHAO, X. J., TAN, W., Development of organic dye-doped silica nanoparticles for bioanalysis and biosensors. *J. Nanosci. Nanotech.* **2002**, *2*(3–4), 405–409.

186 MEALLET-RENAULT, R., PANSU, R., AMIGONI-GERBIER, S., LARPENT, C., Metal-chelating nanoparticles as selective fluorescent sensor for Cu2+. *Chem. Commun.* **2004**, (20), 2344–2345.

187 BRASUEL, M., KOPELMAN, R., AYLOTT, J. W., CLARK, H., XU, H., HOYER, M., MILLER, T. J., TJALKENS, R., PHILBERT, M. A., Production, characteristics and applications of fluorescent PEBBLE

nanosensors: potassium, oxygen, calcium and pH imaging inside live cells. *Sensors Mater.* **2002**, *14*(6), 309–338.

188 Park, E. J., Brasuel, M., Behrend, C., Philbert, M. A., Kopelman, R., Ratiometric optical PEBBLE nanosensors for real-time magnesium ion concentrations inside viable cells. *Anal. Chem.* **2003**, *75*(15), 3784–3791.

189 Buck, S. M., Xu, H., Brasuel, M., Philbert, M. A., Kopelman, R., Nanoscale probes encapsulated by biologically localized embedding (PEBBLEs) for ion sensing and imaging in live cells. *Talanta* **2004**, *63*(1), 41–59.

190 Sun, B., Xie, W., Yi, G., Chen, D., Zhou, Y., Cheng, J., Microminiaturized immunoassays using quantum dots as fluorescent label by laser confocal scanning fluorescence detection. *J. Immunol. Methods* **2001**, *249*(1–2), 85–89.

191 Tran, P. T., Goldman, E. R., Mattoussi, H., Anderson, G. P., Mauro, J. M., Bioconjugates of luminescent CdSe-ZnS quantum dots with an engineered two-domain protein G for use in fluoroimmunoassays. *Int. Soc. Opt. Eng.* **2001**, *4258*, 1–7.

192 Yun, K. S., Lee, D., Kim, M. S., Kim, H. S., Lee, G. M., Yoon, E., High-throughput bio-molecule detection using microbead-based assay with quantum dot fluorescence in a microfluidic chip, in *Micro Total Analysis Systems 2004*, Vol. 2, (Ed.: Royal Society of Chemistry), Cambridge, UK, **2004**, pp. 222–224.

193 Gao, X., Nie, S., Quantum dot-encoded mesoporous beads with high brightness and uniformity: Rapid readout using flow cytometry. *Anal. Chem.* **2004**, *76*(8), 2406–2410.

194 Maxwell, D. J., Taylor, J. R., Nie, S., Self-assembled nanoparticle probes for recognition and detection of biomolecules. *J. Am. Chem. Soc.* **2002**, *124*(32), 9606–9612.

195 Zayats, M., Baron, R., Popov, I., Willner, I., Biocatalytic growth of Au nanoparticles: From mechanistic aspects to biosensors design. *Nano Lett.* **2005**, *5*(1), 21–25.

196 Haes, A. J., Hall, W. P., Chang, L., Klein, W. L., Van Duyne, R. P., A localized surface plasmon resonance biosensor: First steps toward an assay for Alzheimer's disease. *Nano Lett.* **2004**, *4*(6), 1029–1034.

197 Lian, W., Litherland, S. A., Badrane, H., Tan, W., Wu, D., Baker, H. V., Gulig, P. A., Lim, D. V., Jin, S., Ultrasensitive detection of biomolecules with fluorescent dye-doped nanoparticles. *Anal. Biochem.* **2004**, *334*, 135–144.

198 Mansson, A., Sundberg, M., Balaz, M., Bunk, R., Nicholls, I. A., Omling, P., Tagerud, S., Montelius, L., In vitro sliding of actin filaments labeled with single quantum dots. *Biochem. Biophys. Res. Commun.* **2004**, *314*(2), 529–534.

199 Daisuke, I., Kazushi, K., Yasuhiro, I., Noriyuki, I., Mina, O., Masafumi, Y., Takuzo, A., Chaperonin-mediated stabilization and ATP-triggered release of semiconductor nanoparticles. *Nature* **2003**, *423*, 628–632.

200 Schmidt, T., Schuetz, G. J., Baumgartner, W., Gruber, H. J., Schindler, H., Characterization of photophysics and mobility of single molecules in a fluid lipid membrane. *J. Phys. Chem.* **1995**, *99*, 17662–17668.

201 Deverall, M. A., Gindl, E., Sinner, E. K., Ruehe, J., Saxton, M. J., Naumann, C. A., Membrane lateral mobility obstructed by polymer-tethered lipids studied at the single molecule level. *Biophys. J.* **2005**, *88*, 1875–1886.

202 Dahan, M., Lévi, S., Luccardini, C., Rostaing, P., Riveau, B., Triller, A., Diffusion dynamics of glycine receptors revealed by single-quantum dot tracking. *Science* **2003**, *302*, 442–445.

203 Lidke, D. S., Nagy, P., Heintzmann, R., Arndt-Jovin, D. J., Post, J. N., Greeco, H. E., Jares-Erijman, E. A., Jovin, T. M., Quantum dot ligands provide new insights into erbB/HER receptor-mediated signal transduction. *Nat. Biotechnol.* **2004**, *22*, 198–203.

204 Ballou, B., Lagerholm, B. C., Ernst,

L. A., Brunchez, M. P., Waggoner, A. S., Noninvasive imaging of quantum dots in mice. *Bioconj. Chem.* **2004**, *15*, 79–86.

205 Åkerman, M. E., Chan, W. C. W., Laakonen, P., Bhatia, S. N., Ruoslahti, E., Nanocrystal targeting in vivo. *Proc. Natl. Acad. Sci. U.S.A.* **2002**, *99*, 12617–12621.

206 Kershaw, S. V., Harrison, M., Rogach, A. L., Kornowski, A., Development of IR-emitting colloidal II–VI quantum-dot materials. *IEEE J. Sel. Top. Quantum Electron.* **2000**, *6*, 534–543.

207 Kim, S., Lim, Y. T., Soltesz, E. G., De Grand, A. M., Lee, J., Nakayama, A., Parker, J. A., Mihaljevic, T., Laurence, R. G., Dor, D. M., Cohn, L. H., Bawendi, M. G., Frangioni, J. V., Near-infrared fluorescent type II quantum dots for sentinel lymph node mapping. *Nat. Biotechnol.* **2004**, *22*, 93–97.

2
Biofunctionalization of Carbon Nanotubes

Elena Bekyarova, Robert C. Haddon, and Vladimir Parpura

2.1
Introduction

The decade long history of carbon nanotubes (CNTs) has been largely devoted to investigation of their growth mechanism and physical and chemical properties. This has led to sustained progress in the synthesis of materials of higher purity, to chemically functionalized CNTs with specifically tailored properties, and to the development of technologies for the processing and assembly of CNTs into functional structures and devices. Recent research on the chemical interactions between biological molecules and CNTs has led to the assembly of functional hybrid (CNT-biomolecule) structures for nanoelectronics, scaffolds for cell and tissue growth, and high-performance biosensors. While much remains to be accomplished, this fascinating nanomaterial clearly offers great potential for the development of revolutionary hybrid structures and devices, and work in this field has propelled CNTs to a point that their entry into the realm of nanobiotechnology and nanomedicine is now a reality [1].

In this chapter, we overview the currently available methods for biofunctionalization of CNTs and some of their applications in biology and nanotechnology. We briefly discuss the structure, properties, and most common methods for synthesis of CNTs, focusing on current progress in patterned growth and purification of CNTs. We summarize the achievements in chemical modification of CNTs that are related to the solubilization of CNTs in water, since the dispersion and stabilization of CNTs in aqueous media is a key step in developing biological applications. We present various schemes for noncovalent and covalent modifications of CNTs with biological molecules. Additionally, we review the applicability of the modified CNTs in the assembly of electronic devices, for biosensing, and as scaffolds or substrates for neuronal growth.

Nanotechnologies for the Life Sciences Vol. 1
Biofunctionalization of Nanomaterials. Edited by Challa S. S. R. Kumar

ISBN: 3-527-31381-8

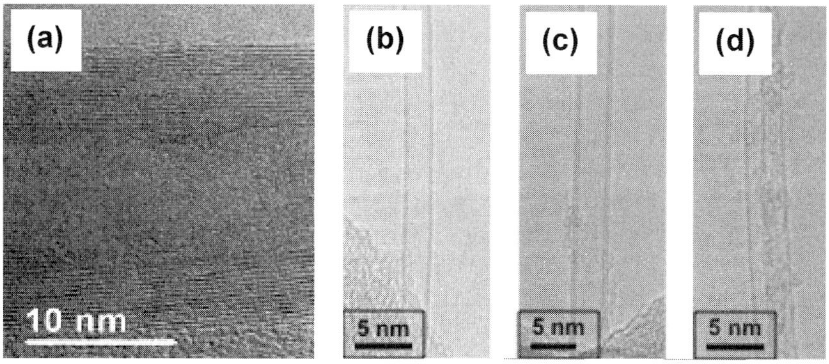

Fig. 2.1. Transmission electron microscopy images of (a) multi-walled carbon nanotubes, (b) single-walled carbon nanotubes, (c) double-walled carbon nanotubes, and (d) a bundle of single-walled carbon nanotubes. (TEM micrographs in (b)–(d) [112] are reproduced by permission of the American Chemical Society Publications.)

2.2
Carbon Nanotubes – Types, Structures and Properties

CNTs can be classified according to the number of concentric graphene cylinders that constitute their structure (Fig. 2.1). Multi-walled CNTs (MWNTs) consist of several concentric graphene cylinders with their ends individually capped with hemispheres of fullerene molecules. Typically, their outer diameter ranges from 2 to 100 nm, while their inner diameter is about 1–3 nm. The MWNTs are from 1 to several hundred μm long. Double-walled CNTs (DWNTs) are composed of two concentric graphene cylinders, and represent an intermediate structure between MWNTs and single-walled CNTs (SWNTs), the later consisting of a single graphene cylinder. Although the smallest SWNTs reported have a diameter of 0.4 nm [2, 3], which corresponds to a hemispherical fragment of the C_{20} dodecahedron, SWNTs are usually produced with a random distribution of diameters (0.7–2 nm) and exist in hexagonally close-packed bundles held together by van der Walls forces.

Based on their hexagonal lattice structure, SWNTs are classified as armchair, zigzag and chiral (Fig. 2.2). The wrapping angle of the graphene sheet determines the electronic properties of SWNTs [4–6]. All armchair nanotubes are conductive (metallic), while the zigzag and chiral nanotubes can be either metallic or semiconducting. Most currently available synthetic methods produce SWNTs with a random distribution of metallic and semiconducting nanotubes in a ratio of 1:2. Because CNTs are either metallic or semiconducting, they provide the necessary building blocks for molecular electronics. In addition, they are ballistic conductors with high effective mobility and can sustain very high current densities. A rope of SWNTs has a room temperature conductivity in the range 10 000–30 000 S cm^{-1} [7]. These properties provide a unique opportunity to develop miniature advanced

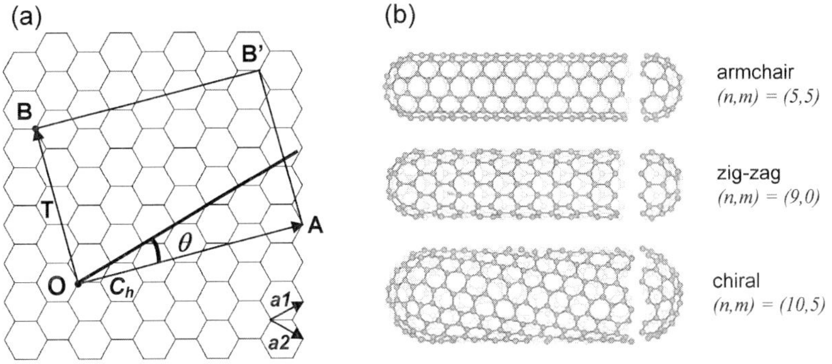

Fig. 2.2. (a) Two-dimensional graphene sheet. A carbon nanotube is formed by rolling up the graphene sheet and superimposing the two ends OA of the chiral vector (C_h). The chiral vector is defined as $C_h = na_1 + ma_2$, where a_1 and a_2 are unit vectors in the two-dimensional hexagonal lattice, and n and m are integers. The pair of integers (n, m) and the chiral angle (θ – the angle between C_h and a_1) define the nanotube type: armchair ($n = m$, $\theta = 30°$), zigzag (n or $m = 0$, $\theta = 0°$) and chiral (θ between 0 and 30°). The diagram is constructed for a (5, 2) carbon nanotube. T is the basic translation vector for the tubule and the unit cell of this tubule is defined by OABB′. (b) Schematic models for the three types of SWNTs. (Courtesy of Riichiro Saito, Tohoku University, Japan.)

sensors [8] for rapid, label-free electronic detection of different biological materials (Section 2.5.2). With a Young's modulus of ~1 TPa [9, 10], CNTs also have exceptional mechanical strength – a useful feature for tissue scaffolds and engineering.

2.3 Synthesis of Carbon Nanotubes

The most widely used techniques for synthesis of CNTs are electric arc discharge, laser ablation, chemical vapor deposition (CVD) and high-pressure carbon monoxide disproportionation (HiPco) [11]. The first two methods involve the vaporization of carbon in an inert atmosphere, whereas CVD and HiPco are based on catalytic decomposition of hydrocarbons. The synthesis of CNTs has advanced to the point that patterns of aligned MWNTs or SWNTs can be engineered. Such patterned growth is of interest in tissue engineering [12]. CNT-based scaffolds have some advantages over bio-degradable synthetic polymers currently used in tissue engineering as they posses the structural integrity and high mechanical stability to support developing tissue and to withstand *in vivo* forces [12].

SWNTs can be aligned by applying an electric field during CVD growth of the nanotubes [13–15], and vertically aligned arrays of MWNTs (Fig. 2.3) are routinely produced in standard CVD experiments [16–19]. Network architectures have been produced by the reassembly of dense CNT arrays using the capillary forces induced

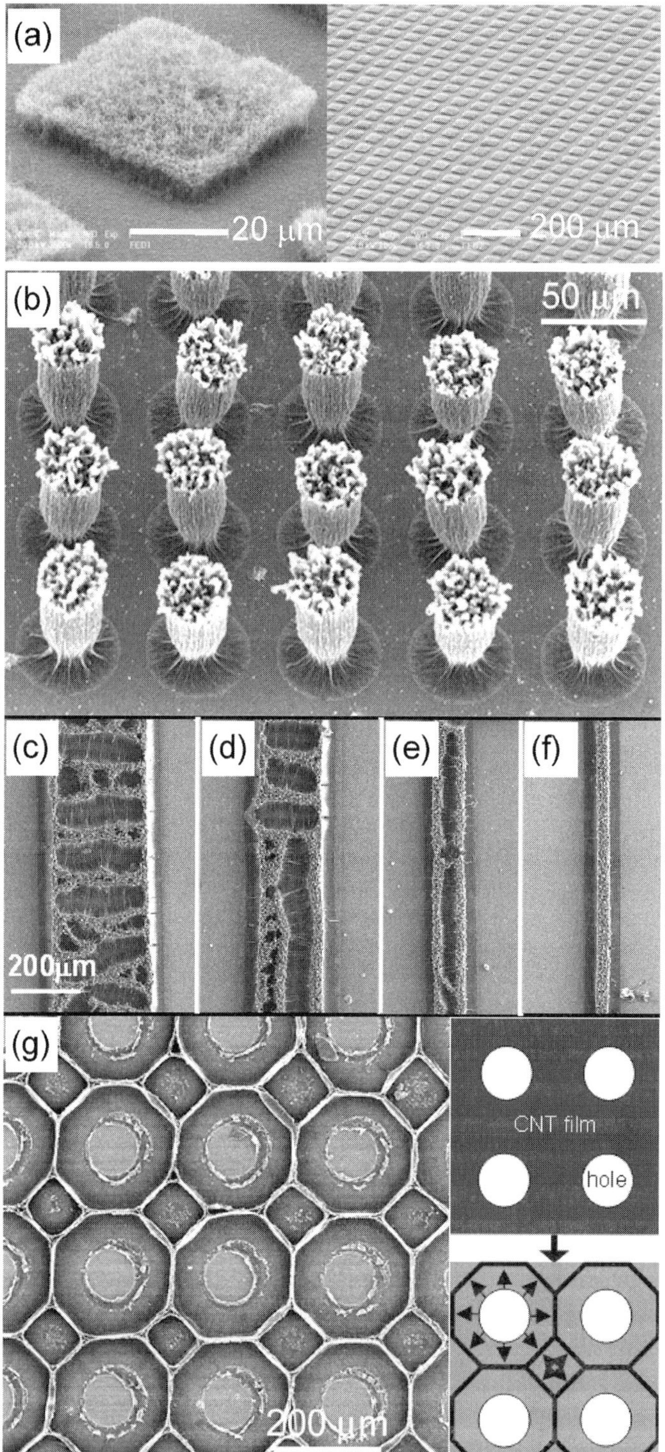
(a)
20 µm
200 µm
(b)
50 µm
(c)
(d)
(e)
(f)
200µm
(g)
200 µm
CNT film
hole

by the evaporation of liquids from the CNT films or mats (Fig. 2.3) [12, 19]. In this process, the nanotubes collapse to cellular structures due to the induced surface tension; the resulting periodic architectures might find applications as scaffolds for tissue engineering. Indeed, similar structures composed of MWNTs (Fig. 2.4) have been used to support the cellular adhesion and growth of mouse fibroblasts [12].

While patterned films and mats that are attractive for cell growth, biosensors, and bioelectronics all require relatively small amounts of material, applications may be envisaged in which bulk quantities of CNTs are necessary. Although bulk production is a necessary step, the purity of the CNT material is an essential prerequisite for further progress. MWNTs of high purity can be readily synthesized. However, SWNTs typically contain a substantial fraction of carbonaceous impurities together with the metal that is used as a catalyst in the synthesis. Quality control in SWNT manufacturing is a major issue, and the absence of widely accepted and established methods for quality assessment has raised questions regarding the purity of commercially available CNT materials [20]. Certainly, high purity material is required if SWNTs are to play an important role in biotechnology. Although quality control is virtually nonexistent in the CNT industry, analytical tools for reliable evaluation of the quality of SWNT materials exist, and efforts to establish standards in the field may help to reform current CNT industrial practices. Solution phase near-infrared (NIR) spectroscopy [21–24], Raman spectroscopy [25, 26], thermogravimetric analysis [25, 27], and combinations of these analytical methods [28] have been used to evaluate SWNT purity. At this point, NIR spectroscopy has been established as the simplest, fastest, most efficient and unambiguous technique for the quantitative assessment of the carbonaceous purity of SWNTs [29], while thermogravimetric analysis can reliably estimate the metal content based on the residue remaining after pyrolysis of the carbon content of the sample.

The quality of CNTs can be improved by progress in the synthesis or purification techniques, and significant achievements in both areas have been reported. Recently, very high purity, metal-free SWNTs (carbonaceous purity of 99.98%) have been synthesized [30]. The purification processes are based on a combination of several steps, which usually include gas or vapor-phase oxidation, wet chemical oxidation, centrifugation, filtration or chromatography (see Refs. [31–35] and references therein).

Fig. 2.3. (a) Patterned MWNTs grown by CVD. (b)–(g) Patterned carbon nanotube films. (b) Wine glass-like structures obtained by the evaporation of liquids from cylindrical MWNT arrays. (c)–(f) Cellular structures of aligned MWNTs formed after immersion of the nanotube sample in acetone and drying under ambient conditions. (g) Carbon nanotube structure of a patterned MWNT array. The consolidation of the rims during the drying of the patterned CNT array affords a structure with mainly square and octagonal cells. The inset represents schematics of this process. Arrows indicate the direction of the CNT collapse due to surface tension [19]. (Reproduced by permission of the National Academy of Sciences U.S.A.)

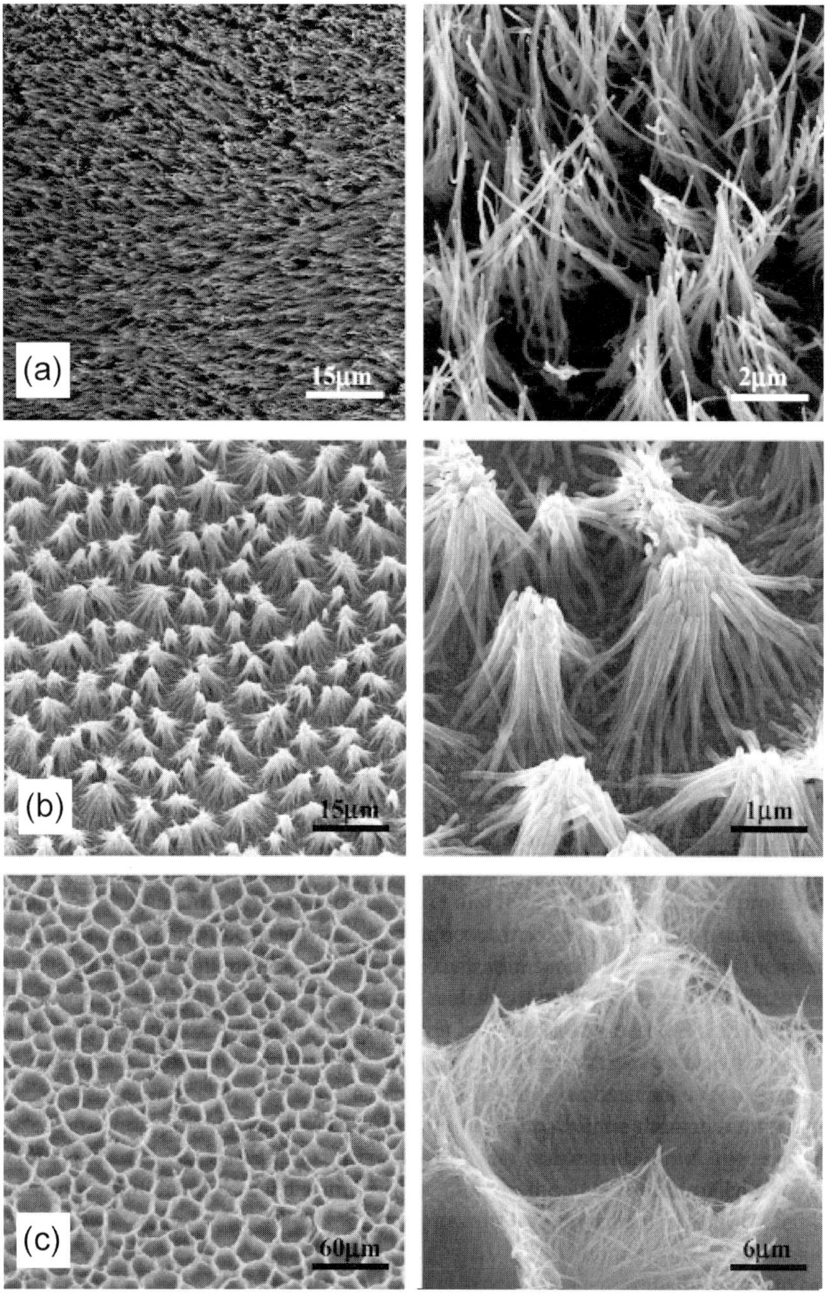

Fig. 2.4. SEM micrographs of MWNT structures used as scaffold for fibroblast growth. Left-hand column, low magnifications; right-hand column, high magnifications. (a) Perpendicularly aligned CNTs. (b) Pyramid-like structures. (c) Network of crosslinked CNT walls forming cavities [12]. (Reproduced by permission of the American Chemical Society.)

2.4
Approaches to Aqueous Solubilization of Carbon Nanotubes

2.4.1
Chemical Modifications

As-prepared SWNTs self-assemble in hexagonally packed bundles, in which the nanotubes are held together by van der Walls forces. The strength of these attractive forces makes the exfoliation of individual CNTs from the bundle and their stabilization in solution difficult. An additional complication arises from the chemical inertness of the CNTs due to the absence of functional groups in their graphitic structure, making their dissolution in a solvent a complex issue. Consequently, chemical functionalization has been used as a valuable route to the solubilization and exfoliation of individual CNTs from the bundles.

One of the most widely used chemical approaches to introduce functionalities onto CNTs involves treatment with strong oxidizing agents such as nitric and sulfuric acids. These strong acids preferentially disrupt the aromatic ring structure at the caps of CNTs and lead to the introduction of carboxylic acid groups at the open ends [21, 31, 34, 36, 37]; this functionality can undergo further reactions to produce a large family of tailored materials. Numerous amidation and esterification reactions of oxidized SWNTs have been reported [36, 38]. Typically, carboxylic acid functionalized SWNTs (SWNT-COOH) are treated with thionyl chloride ($SOCl_2$) to form the acyl chloride intermediate (SWNT-COCl) [31], which is then reacted with an amino derivative. This approach has been used to covalently attach octadecylamine to the open ends of the SWNTs, affording SWNT-CONH$(CH_2)_{17}CH_3$, a form of the carbon nanotubes that proved to be soluble in various organic solvents (Fig. 2.5) [21]. This approach has proved to be applicable to various functionalities. However, the solubilization of CNTs in aqueous solutions – a prerequisite for use in many biological applications – is a more challenging task because of the hydrophobic nature of CNTs. Although stable aqueous solutions of SWNTs have been obtained by ultrasonication in a mixture of sulfuric acid and hydrogen peroxide [39], the more common methods of dispersing CNTs in aqueous solutions involve: (a) coating CNTs with surfactants, (b) functionalization of CNTs with water-soluble polymers, and (c) interaction of CNTs with biological molecules. These methods are detailed below.

2.4.2
Use of Water-compatible Surfactants

Surfactant-induced dispersion of CNTs depends on the presence of hydrophilic and hydrophobic regions in the surfactant molecule. Adsorption of the surfactant on the side walls of the nanotubes occurs through the hydrophobic tail of the surfactant molecule, which can adopt a wide range of orientations with respect to the tube, leaving the hydrophilic moiety oriented towards the aqueous phase. This can induce stable dispersions of surfactant-coated SWNTs in water. SWNTs were

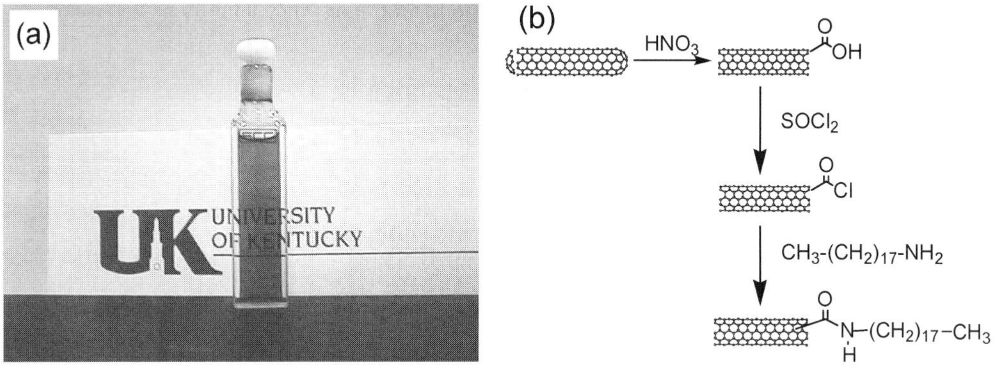

Fig. 2.5. (a) A solution of SWNTs chemically functionalized with octadecylamine [21] by the general functionalization scheme illustrated in (b).

successfully dispersed in water with various surfactants [40–42]. This surfactant detached tubes from the bundles during vigorous sonication and stabilized individual SWNTs in solution [41]. Since the individual nanotube encased in a close-packed SDS micelle had a lower specific gravity than SDS-coated bundles, centrifugation led to their separation. This made it possible to use spectroscopy to study individual SWNTs, which displayed a bright photoluminescence in the NIR [41]. Since then, surfactant-assisted dispersion of nanotubes has been widely used by several research groups for fundamental studies of the electronic properties of individual SWNTs, as these properties give rise to distinctive features in the optical spectra [43–47].

Various anionic, nonionic, and cationic surfactants have been studied for their ability to disperse SWNTs in water [46]. Typically, a solution of a specific surfactant concentration is mixed with the nanotubes using high shear homogenization, followed by ultrasonication, and ultracentrifugation.

Among ionic surfactants, sodium dodecylbenzene sulfonate (SDBS) and SDS are the most efficient dispersing agents. For nonionic systems, surfactants with higher molecular weight suspend higher amounts of SWNT material [46].

2.4.3
Functionalization with Water-soluble Polymers

The covalent attachment of water-soluble polymers is an efficient approach to the dispersion of CNTs in water. By applying the functionalization scheme of Fig. 2.5, poly-*m*-aminobenzene sulfonic acid (PABS) [48, 49] and polyethylene glycol (PEG) [49] have been covalently linked to SWNTs to form water-soluble nanotube-graft copolymers (Fig. 2.6) [48, 49]. Several other types of functionalized SWNTs bearing water-soluble moieties have been synthesized (Scheme 2.1), including the attachment of water-soluble linear polymers, such as monoamine-terminated polyethylene oxide (PEO) [50], diamine terminated polyethylene glycol (PEG_{1500N}) [51],

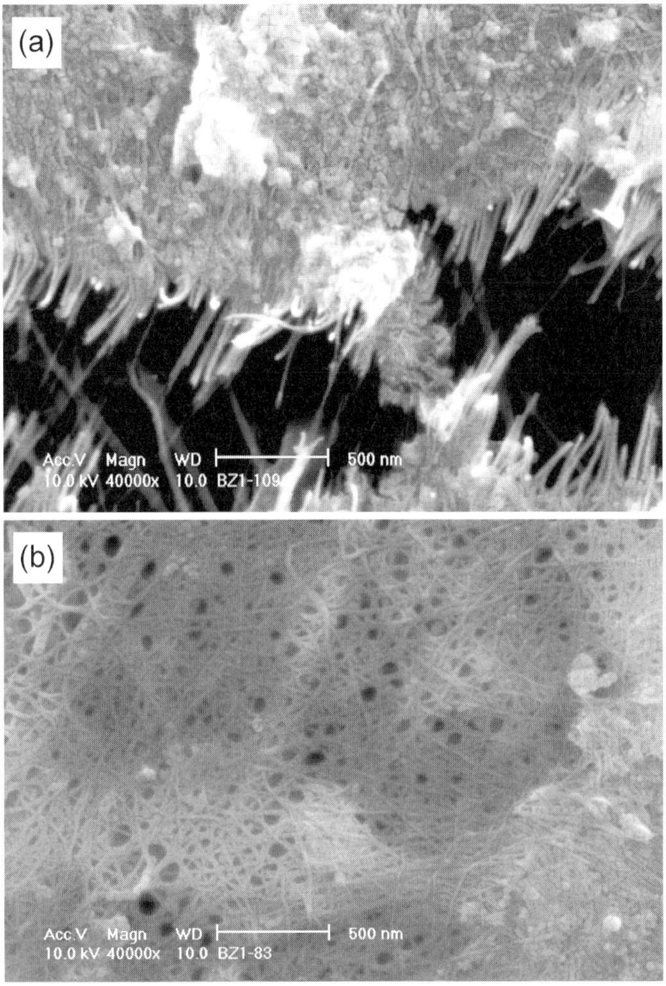

Fig. 2.6. SEM images of (a) SWNT-PABS and (b) SWNT-PEG [49].

poly(propionylethylenimine-*co*-ethylenimine) (PPEI-EI) [51], poly(vinyl alcohol) (PVA) [51], and glucosamine (GA) [52] to CNTs. Since these functionalized nanotubes have high solubility in water (8–89 mg mL^{-1}) [51], this is clearly an efficient route for the aqueous dissolution of carbon nanotubes.

2.4.4 Interaction and Functionalization with Biological Molecules

Interactions of CNTs with biological molecules, such as lipids, DNA and proteins, efficiently disperse the CNTs in water. Noncovalent modification is the preferred method if the electronic characteristics of the nanotubes need to be preserved. Co-

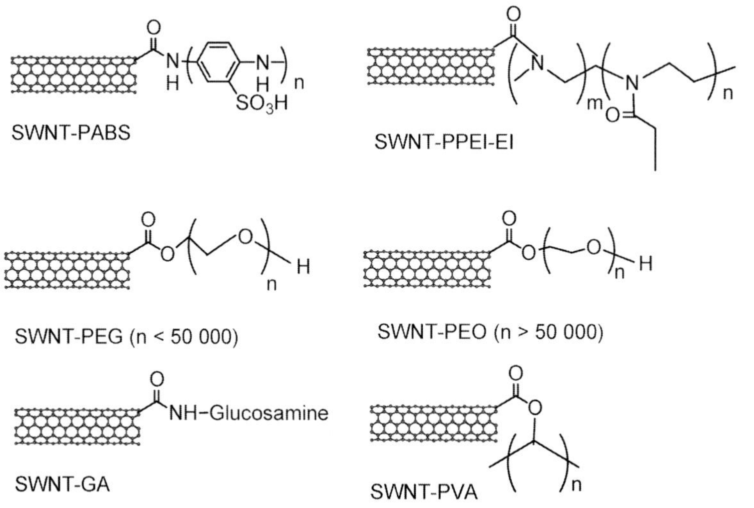

Scheme 2.1. Structures of SWNTs functionalized with polymers: PABS – poly(*m*-aminobenzene sulfonic acid), PEG – poly(ethylene glycol), GA – glucosamine, PPEI-EI – poly(propionylethylenimine-*co*-ethylenimine), PEO – poly(ethylene oxide) and PVA – poly(vinyl alcohol).

valent chemistry, which takes place via modifications of the CNT side walls, disturbs the extended π-network, leading to a localization of electrons at the defect sites that are generated at the point of attachment. However, covalent chemistry at the ends of the SWNTs retains the SWNT electronic properties and provides a robust linkage to the biological molecule, although with some variability in the endogenous properties and functions of these molecules.

2.4.4.1 **Noncovalent Biofunctionalization**

Various lipids and proteins, including enzymes, peptides and nucleic acids, adsorb strongly to CNTs [53–59]. These interactions between CNTs and biological molecules provide a more efficient means to solubilize the nanotubes in water than the use of surfactants and polymers. In a similar manner to surfactants, amphiphilic biological molecules, which possess hydrophobic and hydrophilic moieties, solubilize CNTs in aqueous media. For example, MWNTs form stable dispersions in water upon interaction with specific lipid derivatives composed of a lipidic chain of 12 and 18 carbon atoms and a polar head group [56]. Single-chain lipidic reagents self-organize on the nanotube walls, forming supramolecular assemblies. Similar highly ordered heterogeneous structures have been found upon adsorption of other biological molecules. For example, HupR, a DNA binding protein from the nitrogen-regulatory protein subfamily, and streptavidin interacted strongly with MWNT to form highly ordered helical structures, but the exact solubility in water was not reported [53]. However, an efficient protocol for dispersion of CNTs in water using a specifically designed amphiphilic α-helical peptide, which functioned by wrapping individual CNTs, has been reported and this led to a stable dispersion of CNTs at a concentration of 0.7 mg mL^{-1} [60].

Single-stranded DNA (ssDNA) interacts strongly with CNTs to form stable CNT-DNA hybrids, which efficiently disperse CNTs in aqueous solution [57, 61]. A concentration of CNTs of 0.2–0.4 mg mL^{-1} was readily achieved upon dispersion with DNA, and it was possible to further concentrate the CNTs solution to 4 mg mL^{-1} [61]. It has been suggested that this highly efficient mechanism for dispersion of individual SWNTs in solution involves π-stacking interactions between the nanotube walls and the DNA bases, resulting in helical wrapping of the nanotubes. In addition, the hydrophilic interactions between the sugar-phosphate groups in the backbone of DNA and surrounding water molecules render the hybrid structure soluble in water. The phosphate groups on the SWNT-DNA hybrid provide a negative charge density on the surface of the CNT, enabling the debundling and dispersion of individual SWNTs [57, 61, 62]. The wrapping of the nanotubes with ssDNA was found to be sequence dependent, and the interaction between certain DNA sequences and individual SWNTs allowed ion-exchange chromatography separation based on the electronic characteristics of SWNTs. The separation procedure takes advantage of the different electrostatic charges on the hybrid macromolecules, which are composed of metallic and semiconducting SWNTs [57, 61]. Since the separation of metallic and semiconducting SWNTs is the most important obstacle to the application of carbon nanotubes in nanoelectronics, this DNA-assisted separation demonstrates the power of hybrid CNT-biological molecules for solving problems in nanotechnology.

A combination of surfactants and polymers has also been used for noncovalent attachment of proteins to CNTs, in which the successive adsorption of surfactants (Triton X-100 or Triton X-405) and biotin-functionalized polymer (PEG) provides an interface for binding with streptavidin [63].

Biomolecules can be attached to noncovalently functionalized CNTs. In this approach 1-pyrenebutanoic acid succinimidyl ester (1-PBA) is irreversibly adsorbed on the hydrophobic graphene surface of the CNTs via π-stacking interactions [64]. The protein is then covalently attached to the succinimidyl functionality of 1-PBA through a nucleophilic substitution reaction by an amine group of the protein (Fig. 2.7). This approach for immobilization of proteins onto CNTs has been utilized in development of biosensors based on glucose oxidase-functionalized SWNTs (Section 2.5.2) [55].

An important question that arises is whether the immobilized biological molecules retain their biological activity. Studies regarding this issue are limited. In one study on the structure and functions of proteins adsorbed on SWNTs, it was shown that the proteins undergo conformational changes upon interaction with the carbon walls [59]. The authors used enzymes as highly sensitive probes of the protein functions and found that, depending on the nature of the protein, SWNTs can differentially affect the biological activity of the adsorbed proteins; soybean peroxidase retained 30% of its native activity, while α-chymotrypsin retained only 1% of its native activity, and was denatured when attached to SWNTs [59].

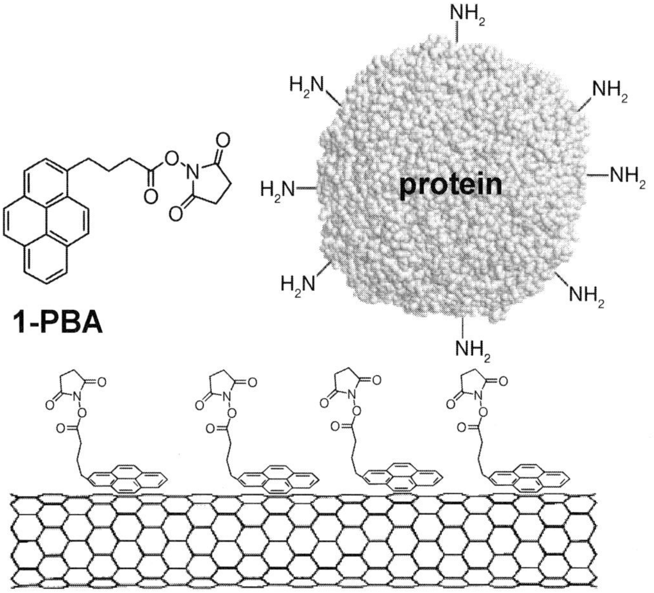

Fig. 2.7. 1-Pyrenebutanoic acid succinimidyl ester (1-PBA), adsorbed on the side-wall of a SWNT via π-stacking, has been used to immobilize protein due to interactions with the protein's amino groups. (Modified from Ref. [64].)

2.4.4.2 **Covalent Biofunctionalization**

Carbodiimide chemistry can be readily applied to covalently link CNTs to various biological molecules. Carbodiimide activates the carboxylic acid groups, which are easily introduced into the CNTs by the oxidative treatments discussed earlier, and it facilitates their reaction with the amino groups present in the biological molecules. Carbodiimide coupling agents commonly utilized for these reactions are the water-soluble derivatives 1-ethyl-3-(3-dimethylaminopropyl)-t-carbodiimide (EDC) (Scheme 2.2, paths a, b) and *N,N′*-dicyclohexylcarbodiimide (DCC) (Scheme 2.2, path c), which are often used with dimethylformamide (DMF) as a solvent. *N*-Hydroxysuccinimine (NHS), which reacts with the carboxylic groups to form an active intermediate ester, is often used to assist amide bond formation in the presence of EDC (Scheme 2.2, path b). These general reactions have been utilized to functionalize CNTs with proteins [65] and amine-terminated DNA [66, 67].

Alternatively, CNTs can be chemically modified by introducing amine moieties [68], which can be further reacted with the biological molecules (Scheme 2.3). In the first step, the carboxylic acid groups of the SWNTs, introduced by oxidation with nitric acid, are reacted with thionyl chloride to form an acyl chloride intermediate, which is then crosslinked with ethylenediamine to produce amine-terminated SWNTs (SWNT-NH_2). These SWNT-NH_2 have been used for covalent attachment of DNA [68]. This was achieved by introducing maleimide groups to SWNT-NH_2

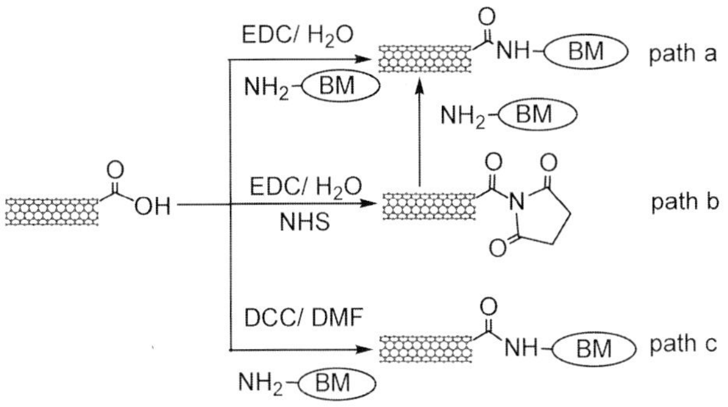

BM - biomolecule (protein, NH_2-terminated DNA)
EDC - 1-ethyl-3-(3-dimethylaminopropyl)-carbodiimide
NHS - N-hydroxysuccinimide
DCC - dicyclohexyl-carbodiimide
DMF - dimethylformamide

Scheme 2.2. Schematic illustration of carbodiimide procedures for covalent functionalization of SWNTs with biological molecules. (Modified from Ref. [1].)

by crosslinking with succinimidyl 4-(*N*-maleimidomethyl)cyclohexane-1-carboxylate (SMCC) and further reacted with thiol-terminated DNA [68]. The resulting DNA-CNT hybridized selectively with complementary DNA sequences, while showing little interaction with non-complementary DNA sequences, indicating that the procedure preserves DNA specificity.

In addition to the chemistry that occurs at the oxidized open ends of CNTs, the side walls undergo 1,3-cycloaddition reactions (Scheme 2.4) [69, 70], and both SWNTs and MWNTs have been covalently linked to N-protected amino acids by this technique, which can be used to prepare water-soluble CNTs [70]. In such functionalization schemes the amino acid is condensed with paraformaldehyde in

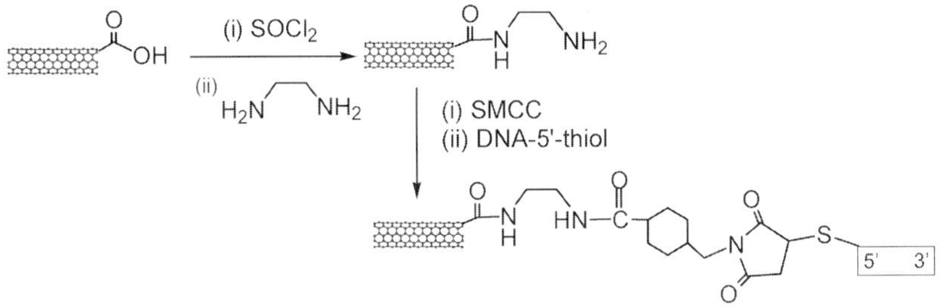

SMCC - Succinimidyl 4-(*N*-maleimidomethyl) cyclohexane-1-carboxylate

Scheme 2.3. Schematic of the maleimide procedure for covalent functionalization of SWNTs with biological molecules.

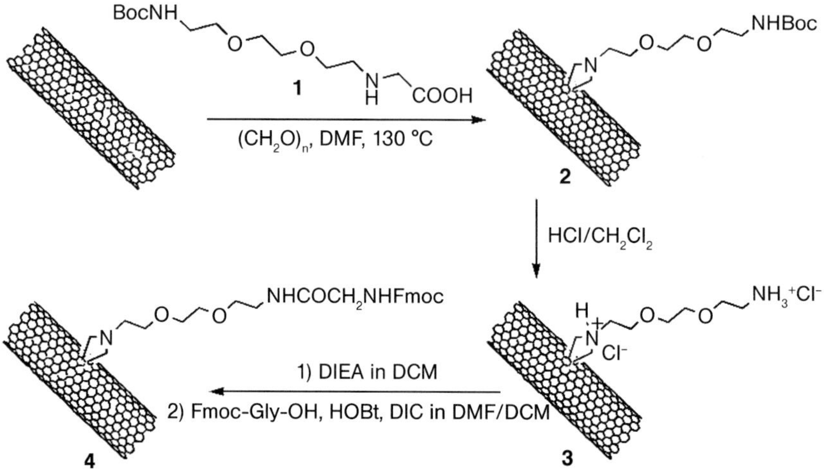

Scheme 2.4. Covalent functionalization of carbon nanotubes with amino acids. Boc – butoxycarbonyl protecting group, DMF – dimethylformamide, DCM –dichloromethane, DIEA – diisopropylethylamine, DIC – diisopropylcarbodiimide, HOBt – *N*-hydroxybenzotriazole, Fmoc – 9-fluorenylmethoxycarbonyl, Gly – glycolic acid [70]. (Reproduced by permission of the Royal Society of Chemistry.)

the presence of CNTs dispersed in DMF (Scheme 2.4; 1); the protecting group, N-tetrabutoxycarbonyl (Boc), in the derivative (Scheme 2.4; 2) is cleaved by reaction with HCl. The resulting amino acid functionalized CNTs (Scheme 2.4; 3) have a remarkable solubility in water (20 mg mL^{-1}). Additionally, amino acid functionalized CNTs can be reacted easily with N-terminal protected amino acid (Fmoc-Gly-OH) via a coupling reaction activated with *N*-hydroxybenzotriazole (HOBt) and diisopropylcarbodiimide (DIC) (Scheme 2.4; 4).

2.5 Applications of Biofunctionalized Carbon Nanotubes

2.5.1 Assembly of Electronic Devices

Biofunctionalization of CNTs can potentially facilitate the use of these materials in functional structures and for the bottom-up design of nanodevices if it is possible to make use of the powerful self-assembly properties of natural substances. Because CNTs are promising building blocks for molecular electronics, the nanofabrication of electronic devices utilizing CNTs based on the self-assembly principles of biology has been attempted. For example, the bottom-up fabrication of field-effect transistors (FETs) based on individual SWNTs has been attempted by using DNA-mediated self-assembly and homologous genetic recombination [71]. A long

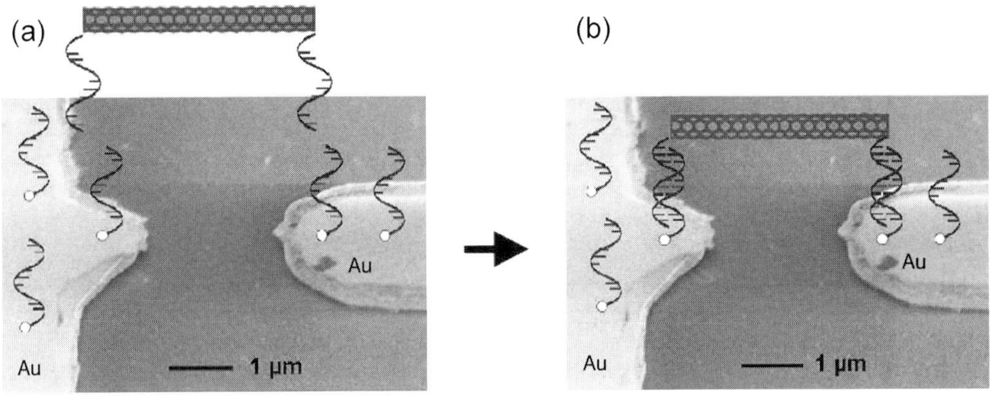

Fig. 2.8. DNA-templated deposition of SWNT between gold electrodes. (a) DNA-bearing gold electrodes immersed in a solution of oligonucleotide-functionalized SWNT. (b) Bridging the two electrodes with a SWNT by hybridization between the complementary strands [72]. (Reproduced by permission of Elsevier.)

DNA molecule was used as a scaffold onto which streptavidin-functionalized SWNTs were assembled, utilizing primary antibodies against RecA, a protein from *Escherichia coli*, and biotinylated secondary antibodies. This allowed a controlled localization of a semiconducting SWNT at a desired address on the DNA scaffold molecule. Electrical contact to the nanotubes may be obtained by metallization of the scaffold DNA molecule. Because the nanotubes are usually a mixture of metallic and semiconducting constituents, the fabrication of devices with reproducible characteristics represents a challenge, although the emerging methods for separating CNTs based on their electronic properties will assist this endeavor [57, 61]. However, the approach involves a complex multi-step process, and thus would lead to a low production yield of devices.

A suggested alternative approach for fabrication of an FET, with a reduced number of reaction steps, could enable the production of devices in high yield. This approach utilized the hybridization between short complementary DNA sequences located on metal contacts and SWNTs (Fig. 2.8) [72]. The thiol-terminated oligonucleotides were deposited on gold contacts, and the devices were immersed in a solution of SWNTs functionalized with complementary oligonucleotides. This allowed the hybridization of the complementary oligonucleotides, with one strand on the electrodes and the other attached to the SWNTs; the success of this operation led to the placement of individual SWNTs or small bundles between the electrodes, with efficient electrical contacts to the SWNTs at both electrodes in about 12% of the devices [72]. Those devices that exhibited efficient electrical contacts had stable electrical characteristics over hundreds of measurements. Indeed, this technique was also implemented to assemble SWNT-FET devices [73]. Although both approaches described above are far from a general technology, they highlight the potential use of biofunctionalized CNTs and self-assembly approach for bottom-up construction of CNT-based electronics.

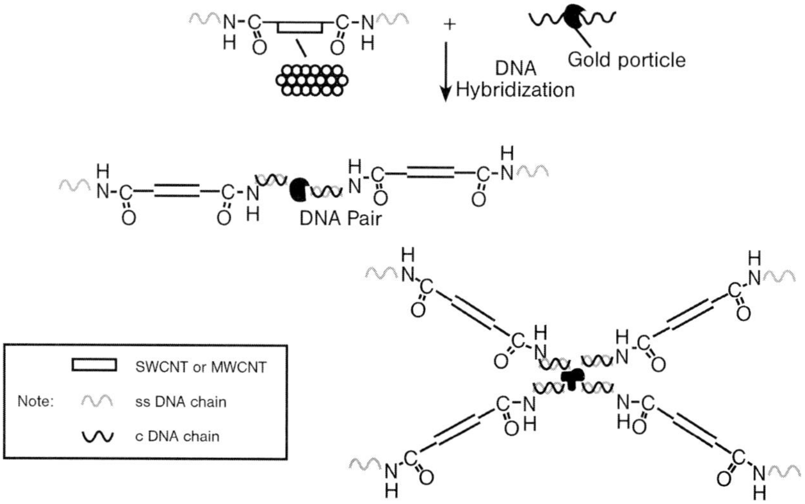

Scheme 2.5. Schematic of procedures for DNA directed self-assembling of multiple carbon nanotubes and gold nanoparticles [75]. (Reproduced by permission of the American Chemical Society Publications.)

Controlled assembly of multifunctional SWNT structures is of interest for development of devices for biosensing. The functionalization of CNTs with biological molecules facilitates the formation of such functional structures and it also increases their versatility. Nanoparticle–CNT structures have been prepared using a DNA-directed self-assembly [74, 75]. In one approach DNA-graft gold nanoparticles have been attached to SWNTs grafted with complementary DNA chains, using the carboxylic group of the SWNT-COOH and amine-terminated DNA [75]. This approach has been used to assemble CNTs into various multicomponent structures, containing interconnected MWNTs and SWNTs, (Scheme 2.5) [75], and multifunctional structures could be obtained by varying the base sequence and the number of complementary DNA chains grafted to the gold nanoparticle.

Besides the assembly of functionalized CNTs (above), it is possible to functionalize pre-formed films of CNTs and prepare CNT film-based devices. Such preparations are readily achieved by spraying [8] or filtration [76, 77]. Additionally, the versatile chemistry at the open ends of the CNTs forming the film [36, 37] affords the opportunity to interconnect the nanotubes and to form patterned multi-layered SWNT films [78, 79]. Thus, carboxylic acid terminated CNTs have been interconnected using 4,4′-oxydianiline as a linker molecule [78]. The functionalized CNTs can be stacked on aminated glass substrates, which allows a diverse patterning of the CNT films and the introduction of various functional groups for further conjugation with biological molecules [78]. For example, DNA oligonucleotides have been attached, using carbodiimide chemistry (Scheme 2.2), to pre-patterned CNT multilayer films to give interfaces that exhibit a high sensitivity in subsequent hybridization (Scheme 2.6) [78]. Although their performance is inferior to individual

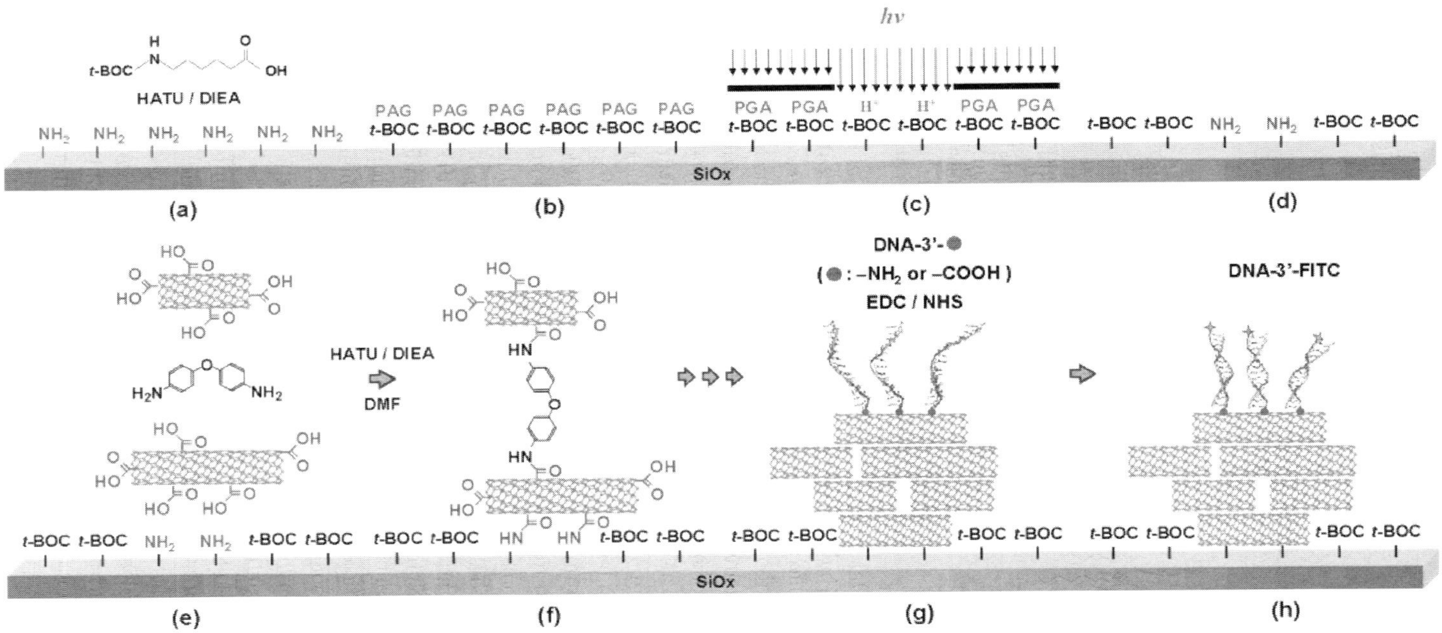

Scheme 2.6. Patterned SWNT multilayer films with selectively immobilized DNA molecules: (a) protection of the surface with *t*-Boc, (b) deposition of a layer of a photoacid generator (PAG). (c) exposure to UV light using a photomask for patterning, (d) development process, (e) selective immobilization of the nanotubes onto the aminated regions of the substrate, (f) covalent functionalization of the SWNT layers using a 4,4′-oxydianiline as a linker molecule and *O*-(7-azabenzotriazol-1-yl)-*N*,*N*,*N*′,*N*′-tetramethyl uranium hexafluorophosphate (HATU) as a condensation agent, (g) covalent immobilization of oligonucleotides onto the patterned SWNT multilayers, and (h) hybridization of the fluorescently (FITC)-labeled complementary oligonucleotide [78]. DIEA – diisopropylethylamine, DMF – dimethylformamide, t-Boc – *t*-butoxycarbonyl, EDC – 1-ethyl-3-(3-dimethylaminopropyl)-*t*-carbodiimide, NHS – *N*-hydroxysuccinimine. (Reproduced with permission from the American Chemical Society Publications.)

CNT devices, film-based devices made of CNTs provide convenient manufacture and have led to a powerful sensor platform [8]. Since this approach can lead to patterning at a specific location on a substrate, it could advance the development of sensors requiring site specificity.

SWNTs functionalized with poly-L-lysine (PLL) have been reported to assemble in functional structures, which have been used as a platform for electrodes with enhanced biosensing properties [80]. Assembly was achieved by reacting carboxylic acid bearing SWNTs with some of the amino groups of PLL (Scheme 2.7). The unreacted amino groups were available for subsequent attachment of the SWNT-PLL graft copolymer to the carboxylic acid bearing gold electrodes and also for conjugation to horseradish peroxidase. Attachment of this enzyme led to the construction of electrodes for amplified sensing of hydrogen peroxide [80]. Indeed, various enzymes could be attached using this method to the PLL-functionalized CNTs for the development of sensor devices. Because PLL is a permissive substrate for cellular adhesion and growth, this methodology could be exploited for development of composite substrates that would serve a dual role; they would support cellular growth and also serve as sensors.

2.5.2 Biosensing

Among the potential usage of CNTs in biology and medicine, the development of advanced biosensor devices has emerged as the most promising short-term application. CNTs offer a unique combination of quasi-1D structure and excellent electronic properties, which can dramatically improve the miniaturization prospects for electronic biosensor devices. Additionally, CNTs offer new opportunities for rapid, sensitive and label-free detection of biological agents, with the selectivity of detection provided by biofunctionalization of the CNTs. Furthermore, the nanotubes can clearly serve both as the transducer and as the platform where the biorecognition event occurs. Taken together, these prospects make CNTs one of the most promising materials for advanced biosensors.

Several groups have already demonstrated the use of SWNTs in biosensors [55, 81–92]. Research on CNT-based biosensors is currently focused on exploiting two major fundamental approaches: the development of CNT electrodes for the electrochemical detection of biological agents and fabrication of transistor devices for electronic detection of binding events.

Electronic detection of biological species is very attractive because it offers a fast and direct, label-free detection, while sampling data in real time. Additionally, it does not require preparation steps and multiple reagents, making the use of these sensors quite simple. Electronic detection is possible because a semiconducting SWNT exhibits a significant conductance change in response to interaction with gas molecules, which can change the electron density on the nanotube [93, 94]. Similar electronic changes in the behavior of SWNTs have been found upon interaction with small biological molecules and proteins [55, 89, 95, 96]. The *in situ* electronic detection of proteins using CNTs has proved to be very sensitive. Adsorp-

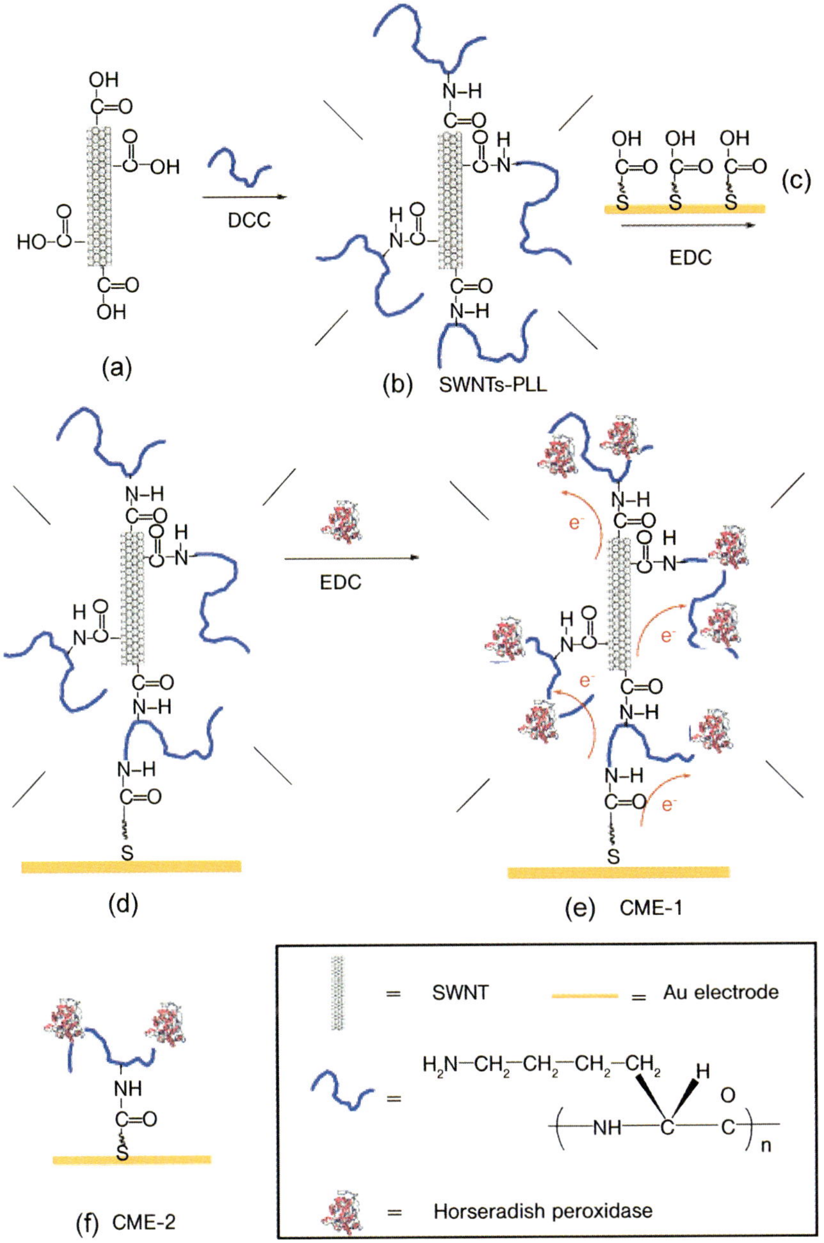

Scheme 2.7. Illustration of the assembling of SWNTs, poly-L-lysine (PLL), and horseradish peroxidase and the fabrication of chemically modified electrodes (CME) [80]. DCC – *N*,*N*′-dicyclohexylcarbodiimide, EDC – 1-ethyl-3-(3-dimethylaminopropyl)-*t*-carbodiimide. (Reproduced with permission from the American Chemical Society Publications.)

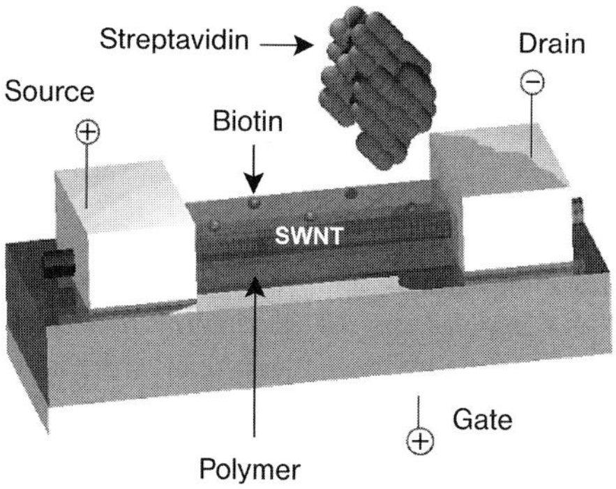

Fig. 2.9. Schematic of a nanotube field-effect transistor (FET). The nanotube (SWNT) is functionalized with biotin using a polymeric functional layer, which coats the nanotubes. (Modified from Ref. [89]; by permission of the American Chemical Society Publications.)

tion of cytochrome *c*, a redox catalyst in the respiratory chain of mitochondria, on an individual SWNT in a transistor configuration induced a sufficient decrease in the conductance of the device to allow the detection of a few tens of molecules [96].

An FET composed of an individual pristine SWNT (Fig. 2.9) has been shown to change its resistance upon exposure to proteins [89]. For example, adsorption of streptavidin on the SWNT shifted the transconductance towards negative gate voltages with little change in the current. Taking into account that the nanotubes before the adsorption exhibited p-type electronic behavior, presumably due to doping from environmental oxygen [94], these changes indicate an electron transfer from the streptavidin molecule to the nanotube. This hybrid, streptavidin-SWNT has been shown to be sensitive to the presence of biotin, which specifically binds to streptavidin, resulting in a decrease of the current. Because the interaction between streptavidin and SWNTs is non-specific it is necessary to impart selectivity to the device and to prevent non-specific interactions; this can be accomplished by coating the SWNTs with hydrophilic polymers, PEG and polyethyleneimine (PEI), containing biotin. The polymer coated/biotin functionalized SWNTs devices are very sensitive in the detection of streptavidin – down to as few as 10 protein molecules [89].

Although the mechanism of chemical sensing exhibited by SWNTs has not been unambiguously identified, as discussed above it seems probable that the resistance change in the devices originates from doping of the CNTs as a result of charge-transfer processes that are associated with interactions between the SWNTs and the analyte [8]. In some cases the conductance change originates from electronic effects occurring at the metal–nanotube contacts during adsorption [97].

In addition to direct sensing with SWNTs, biologically functionalized SWNTs also show promise as sensors. For example, glucose oxidase (GO) has been covalently attached to a semiconducting SWNT and used as the conducting channel in an FET [55]; the attached GO retained its enzymatic activity and imparted sensitivity to the nanotubes towards glucose. Importantly, the increase in conductance measured with such devices in the presence of glucose was rapid, which has implications for real time studies of enzymatic activity at molecular level. The GO-coated SWNT devices were very sensitive to pH, whereas the conductance of pristine SWNT was pH independent in the range 4–5.5; after modification of the nanotube with GO, a strong increase in conductance with decreasing pH was observed [55]. On changing the pH from 4 to 5.5, the effective gate voltage changed by 20 mV, which corresponded to a 30 μS change in the conductance of the nanotube. These measurements show that it is possible to detect the doping induced by the binding of about 50 protein molecules to a ~600 nm long semiconducting SWNT.

Several research groups have explored the electrochemical detection of biological molecules with electrodes consisting of CNTs in their pristine or modified forms; details of the achievements in electrochemical biosensing using CNTs have been outlined in a recent review [98]. Since their introduction into electrochemistry, CNT electrodes have demonstrated an enhanced sensitivity compared with conventional carbon electrodes. For example, detection of transmitter dopamine exhibited characteristic cyclic voltammograms at conventional electrodes such as glassy carbon and pyrolytic carbon fibers, as well as at CNT electrodes [81]. However, the conventional electrodes suffered from poor reversibility, while CNT electrodes exhibited excellent reversibility and were also very sensitive in the analysis of goat brain tissue. This illustrates the potential to use CNT electrodes for *in vivo* and *in vitro* neurotransmitter investigations involving dopamine, and possibly with other oxidizable transmitters. Similarly, the ultrasensitivity of CNT electrodes in electrochemical detection of proteins and DNA has been reported [91]. Covalent coupling of the alkaline phosphatase (ALP) enzyme to CNTs has led to the highest sensitivity (detection limit 1 pg L^{-1}) reported thus far for electrical detection of DNA. This CNT-ALP-linked assay can be modified for antigen detection by using specific antibody–antigen recognition, which could provide a fast, simple solution for molecular diagnosis in pathologies where molecular markers exist, such as DNA or protein.

Ultrasensitive DNA detection has been also achieved with a nanoelectrode array composed of aligned MWNTs embedded in silicon dioxide. The nanoelectrodes have been fabricated by a bottom-up approach, which resulted in precisely positioned and well-aligned MWNTs embedded in the silicon dioxide matrix. This configuration provided structural integrity to the electrodes and allowed the sensitivity of the array to be tailored by controlling the nanotube density [83]. The sensitivity was increased dramatically upon lowering the nanotube density in the array, allowing for the detection of less than a few attomoles of oligonucleotide.

A similar approach has been used to develop a MWNT-based nanoelectrode array for selective detection of glucose [85]. Nanotubes in the array were embedded in an epoxy matrix. The exposed nanotube tips were functionalized with glucose oxidase using carbodiimide chemistry. The devices showed a linear response to glucose up to a concentration of about 30 mM with the detection limit down to 0.08 mM, achieving a much wider range than necessary for sampling glucose in human blood and urine.

Alternative approaches for the development of glucose biosensors involve conducting polymer coated CNT arrays [86, 87]. In this approach GO was incorporated into a layer of conducting polymer, such as polypyrrole [87] or polyaniline [86], which coated aligned nanotubes. The amperometric response from these aligned nanotube–polymer nanowires was much higher than that of conventional electrodes using conducting polymers.

An additional advantage of CNT-based biosensors is the possibility of the favorable improvement of screen-printed graphite sensors by their modification with CNTs [92]. MWNTs have been used for modification of working graphite ink electrodes; the nanotubes were deposited on the graphite surface by evaporation of a solution of MWNTs in DMF, and the electrodes were further modified by adsorption of organophosphorus hydrolase, which allowed detection of the pesticide paraoxon with greater sensitivity than for previous detection methods [92].

Atomic force microscopy (AFM) is a CNTs biosensing application that also impacts structural biology; due to their high aspect ratio, strength and chemical versatility, CNTs can be used to improve upon standard AFM tips in several ways. The most obvious is to enhance the image resolution as the tip size is significantly reduced when SWNTs are utilized. Standard commercial silicon-based tips have radial curvatures of about 5–10 nm, while SWNT AFM tips with a diameter in the range of 1–3 nm have already been fabricated [99, 100]. The improved resolution of the CNT tips has been demonstrated clearly in an AFM study of isolated proteins at room temperature in which a MWNT tip reproducibly resolved the distinct Y-shape of an isolated immunoglobulin G (IgG) [101], while previous images obtained with conventional tips yielded only a heart-shaped structure. Similarly, SWNT tips were used for high-resolution imaging of isolated DNA molecules [102]. This method has been implemented for determination of haplotypes on UGT1A7 [101], a gene suggested to be a cancer risk factor. Using SWNTs as a tip gives a resolution of approximately 10 bases, which enables direct reading of DNA sequences, and the utilization of SWNT tips in haplotyping clearly could be applied to the understanding and diagnosis of genetic diseases.

AFM probes with functionalized SWNTs as tips have been proposed as the ideal high-resolution probe for mapping chemical domains by using chemical force microscopy [103]. SWNT tips are extremely sensitive to surface polarity, pH and many other chemical characteristics of the sample, as demonstrated by tapping mode AFM studies using a tip of CNTs with terminal carboxylic groups [104], where it was possible to chemically map the patterned substrate containing areas of methyl and carboxylic groups (Fig. 2.10). The ability of AFM tips to detect biological molecules has also been demonstrated, and biotin-modified SWNT AFM tips have been used to study biotin interaction with streptavidin immobilized on a mica surface [104]. This method offers the opportunity to detect the spatio-temporal location of a specific molecule; in this approach the temporal resolution would be limited by the scanning speed and biosensor properties, while the spatial resolution would be limited by the diameter of the nanotube. For example, nanotubes capable of sensing glucose [105, 106] or neurotransmitters could be used to scan for the uptake and release of these compounds from specific cells under various stimuli.

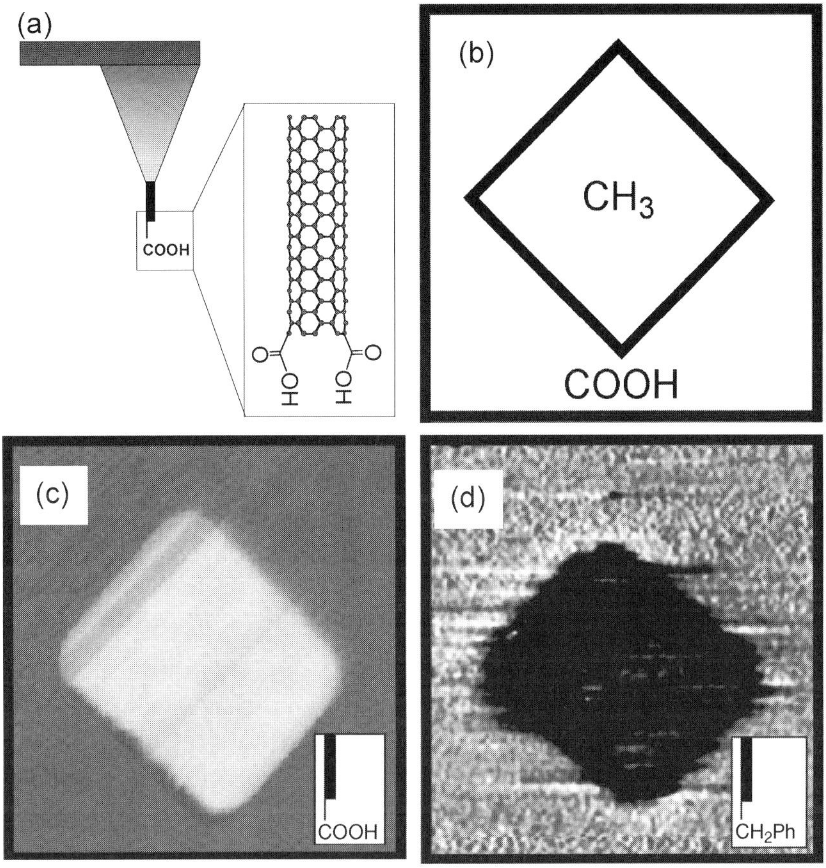

Fig. 2.10. (a) Schematic of a SWNT tip with attached carboxylic acid groups. (b)–(d) Chemical mapping with functionalized SWNT tip. (b) Schematic of a patterned substrate consisting of a self-assembled monolayer (SAM) region terminated with methyl groups and surrounded by carboxylic acid-terminated SAM. (c) Tapping mode phase image of the patterned SAM in (b) imaged with a carboxylic acid-terminated SWNT tip, and (d) phase image of a similar substrate imaged with a C_6H_5-terminated SWNT tip. (Courtesy of Charles M. Lieber, Harvard University, USA.)

2.5.3
Substrates for Neuronal Growth

The first use of CNTs in contact with living cells made use of carbon nanotubes as a substrate for neuronal growth [107]. In this work, cultured hippocampal neurons were grown on MWNTs deposited on PEI-coated coverslips. Scanning electron microscopy was used to visualize the morphological parameters of neuronal growth. The neuronal bodies adhered to the surface of the MWNTs, showing outgrowth of neurites that elaborated into many small branches. The neurons remained alive on the MWNTs for at least 11 days.

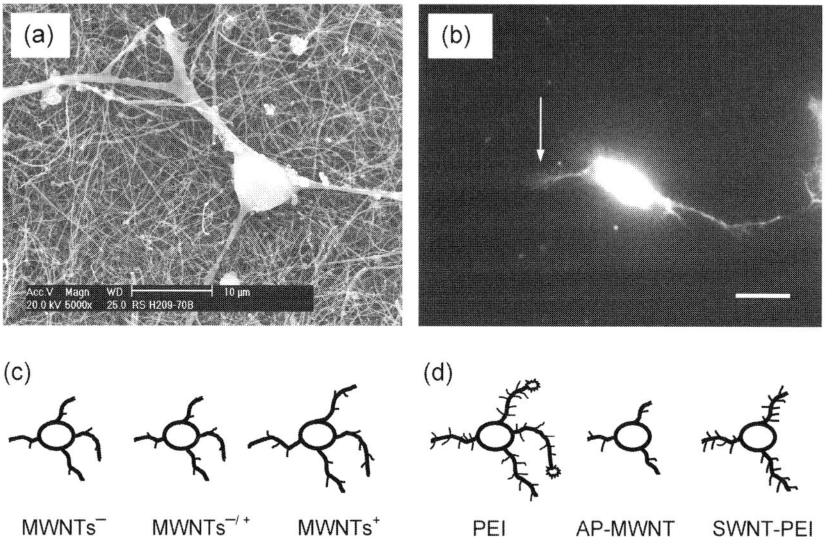

Fig. 2.11. (A) SEM image of a neuron grown on as-prepared MWNTs (AP-MWNTs). (b) Fluorescence image showing a live neuron on AP-MWNTs, which accumulated the vital stain, calcein. Arrow indicates a growth cone. Scale bar, 20 μm. (c) Drawing summarizing the effects of MWNT charges and (d) the effects of graft copolymer SWNT-PEI on growth cones, neurite outgrowth and branching. PEI, polyethyleneimine. (Modified from Refs. [108, 109].)

More recently, this work was extended by characterizing the morphological features of live neurons labeled with the fluorescent dye calcein, and visualized with a fluorescence microscope (Fig. 2.11) [108]. Neuronal growth was systematically controlled by modified MWNTs, prepared by covalently conjugating CNTs with functionalities designed to carry negative, neutral or positive charges at physiological extracellular pH. By using these CNTs as the scaffold for neuronal growth, it was found that the neurons grown on positively charged MWNTs showed more numerous growth cones, longer neurite outgrowth and more successful neurite branching than neurons grown on negatively charged CNTs (Fig. 2.11). Thus, by varying the electrostatic charge on the MWNTs it was possible to manipulate the growth pattern of the neurons. Similarly, neuronal growth was also modulated by using a SWNT-PEI graft copolymer as a scaffold or substrate for cultured neurons [109]. SWNT-PEI promoted neurite outgrowth and branching; neurons grown on SWNT-PEI showed more extensive neurite branching than neurons grown on as-prepared (AP-) MWNT, but having quantitatively similar neurite branching to those of neurons grown on PEI. The number of their growth cones was comparable to those on neurons grown on AP-MWNTs; the neurite lengths were intermediate and fell between those of neurons grown on AP-MWNTs and PEI (Fig. 2.11). Where PEI was combined with SWNTs, the positive charge on the PEI was reduced, perhaps by $\sim$20%, in proportion to the SWNT loading in the copolymer. The surface charge reduction could be the basis for the effect of the copolymer on neuronal growth characteristics. Besides giving new information on the sensitivity of neuron growth parameters to substrate quality and charge, the data gathered may provide the basis for the development of materials where the ratio of SWNT/PEI in the copolymer could control neurite outgrowth and branching.

Taken together these studies demonstrate that CNTs can be used as a scaffold or substrate for neuronal growth and that modifications of CNTs, including graft copolymers with PEI, can be employed to modulate the arborization of neuronal processes and their outgrowth. This suggests that it may become possible to employ suitably functionalized CNTs as neural prostheses in neurite regeneration.

2.6 Concluding Remarks

It is apparent from the body of work detailed in this chapter that there is already an impressive array of currently available methods for biofunctionalization of CNTs and of CNT applications in biology and nanotechnology. As a result of their unique properties and the sophistication of the chemistries available for their modification, CNTs have immense potential in biotechnology and biomedicine that are only now starting to be realized – although their toxicity remains a concern [110, 111]. Presently, CNTs are mainly under investigation in research laboratories, but if there is widespread commercialization of CNTs, the exposure of the general populace to this material must not occur without adequate testing. At this point there is no indication that CNTs will be any more hazardous than other forms of carbon, and their enormous potential in nanomedicine mandates the continued investigation of this unique nanomaterial from the biological standpoint.

Acknowledgments

We thank Erik Malarkey for his comments on an earlier version of this manuscript. The authors' work is supported by the National Institute of Mental Health (MH 069791) and by DOD/DARPA/DMEA under Award No. DMEA90-02-2-0216. V.P. is an Institute for Complex Adaptive Matter Senior Fellow.

References

1 Bekyarova, E., Ni, Y., Malarkey, E.B., Montana, V., McWilliams, J.L., Haddon, R.C., Parpura, V., Applications of carbon nanotubes in biotechnology and biomedicine. *J. Biomed. Nanotechnol.* **2005**, *1*, 3–17.

2 Qin, L.-C., Zhao, X., Hirahara, K., Miyamoto, Y., Ando, Y., Iijima, S., The smallest carbon nanotube. *Nature* **2000**, *408*, 50.

3 Wang, N., Tang, Z.K., Li, G.D., Chen, J.S., Single-walled 4 Å carbon

nanotube arrays. *Nature* **2000**, *408*, 50–51.

4 Mintmire, J.W., Dunlap, B.I., White, C.T., Are fullerene tubules metallic? *Phys. Rev. Lett.* **1992**, *68*, 631–634.

5 Hamada, N., Sawada, S.I., Oshiyama, A., New one-dimensional conductors: graphitic microtubules. *Phys. Rev. Lett.* **1992**, *68*, 1579–1581.

6 Saito, R., Fujita, M., Dresselhaus, G., Dresselhaus, M.S., Electronic structure of chiral graphene tubules. *Appl. Phys. Lett.* **1992**, *60*, 2204–2206.

7 Fischer, J.E., Dai, H., Thess, A., Lee, R., Hanjani, N.M., Dehaas, D.L., Smalley, R.E., Metallic resistivity in crystalline ropes of single-wall carbon nanotubes. *Phys. Rev. B* **1997**, *55*, R4921–R4924.

8 Bekyarova, E., Davis, M., Burch, T., Itkis, M.E., Zhao, B., Sunshine, S., Haddon, R.C., Chemically functionalized single-walled carbon nanotubes for ammonia sensors. *J. Phys. Chem. B* **2004**, *108*, 19717–19720.

9 Salvetat, J.P., Briggs, G.A.D., Bonard, J.M., Basca, R.R., Kulik, A.J., Stockli, T., Burnham, N.A., Forro, L., Elastic and shear moduli of single-walled carbon nanotube ropes. *Phys. Rev. Lett.* **1999**, *82*, 944–947.

10 Yu, M.F., Files, B.S., Arepalli, S., Ruoff, R.S., Tensile loading of ropes of single wall carbon nanotubes and their mechanical properties. *Phys. Rev. Lett.* **2000**, *84*, 5552–5555.

11 Journet, C., Bernier, P., Production of carbon nanotubes. *Appl. Phys. A* **1998**, *67*, 1–9.

12 Correa-Duarte, M.A., Wagner, N., Rojas-Chapana, J., Morsczeck, C., Thie, M., Giersig, M., Fabrication and biocompatibility of carbon nanotube-based 3D networks as scaffolds for cell seeding and growth. *Nano Lett.* **2004**, *4*, 2233–2236.

13 Zhang, Y., Chang, A., Cao, J., Wang, Q., Kim, W., Li, Y., Morris, N., Yenilmez, E., Kong, J., Dai, H., Electric-field-directed growth of aligned single-walled carbon nanotubes. *Appl. Phys. Lett.* **2001**, *79*, 3155–3157.

14 Joselevich, E., Lieber, C.M., Vectorial growth of metallic and semiconducting single-wall carbon nanotubes. *Nano Lett.* **2002**, *2*, 1137–1141.

15 Yu, Z., Li, S., Burke, P.J., Synthesis of aligned arrays of millimeter long, straight single-walled carbon nanotubes. *Chem. Mater.* **2004**, *16*, 3414–3416.

16 Dai, H., Carbon nanotubes: synthesis, integration, and properties. *Acc. Chem. Res.* **2002**, *35*, 1035–1044.

17 Rao, A.M., Jacques, D., Haddon, R.C., Zhu, W., Bower, C., Jin, S., In situ-grown carbon nanotube arrays with excellent field emission characteristics. *Appl. Phys. Lett.* **2000**, *76*, 3813–3815.

18 Geohegan, D.B., Schittenhelm, H., Fan, X., Pennycook, S.J., Puretzky, A.A., Guillorn, M.A., Blom, D.A., Joy, D.C., Condensed phase growth of single-wall carbon nanotubes from laser annealed nanoparticulates. *Appl. Phys. Lett.* **2001**, *78*, 3307–3309.

19 Chakrapani, N., Wei, B., Carrillo, A., Ajayan, P.M., Kane, R.S., Capillary-driven assembly of two-dimensional cellular carbon nanotube foams. *Proc. Nat. Acad. Sci. U.S.A.* **2004**, *101*, 4009–4012.

20 Giles, J., Growing nanotech trade hit by questions over quality. *Nature* **2004**, *432*, 791.

21 Chen, J., Hamon, M.A., Hu, H., Chen, Y., Rao, A.M., Eklund, P.C., Haddon, R.C., Solution properties of single-walled carbon nanotubes. *Science* **1998**, *282*, 95–98.

22 Itkis, M.E., Niyogi, S., Meng, M., Hamon, M., Hu, H., Haddon, R.C., Spectroscopic study of the Fermi level electronic structure of single walled carbon nanotubes. *Nano Lett.* **2002**, *2*, 155–159.

23 Itkis, M.E., Perea, D., Niyogi, S., Rickard, S., Hamon, M., Hu, H., Zhao, B., Haddon, R.C., Purity evaluation of as-prepared single-walled carbon nanotube soot by use of solution phase near-IR spectroscopy. *Nano Lett.* **2003**, *3*, 309–314.

24 Nishide, D., Kataura, H., Suzuki, S., Tsukagoshi, K., Aoyagi, Y., Achiba,

Y., High-yield production of single-wall carbon nanotubes in nitrogen gas. *Chem. Phys. Lett.* **2003**, *372*, 45–50.

25 Dillon, A.C., Gennett, T., Parilla, P.A., Alleman, J.L., Jones, K.M., Heben, M.J., Evaluating the purity of single-wall nanotube materials. *Mater. Res. Soc. Symp. Proc.* **2001**, *633*, A5.2.1–A5.2.6.

26 Dresselhaus, M.S., Dresselhaus, G., Jorio, A., Souza Filsho, A.G., Pimenta, M.A., Saito, R., Single nanotube Raman spectroscopy. *Acc. Chem. Res.* **2002**, *35*, 1070–1078.

27 Zhang, M., Yudasaka, M., Koshio, A., Iijima, S., Thermogravimetric analysis of single-wall carbon nanotubes ultrasonicated in monochlorobenzene. *Chem. Phys. Lett.* **2002**, *364*, 420–426.

28 Arepalli, S., Nikolaev, P., Gorelik, O.P., Nadjiev, V.G., Holmes, W., Files, B., Yowell, L., Protocol for the characterization of single-wall carbon nanotube material quality. *Carbon* **2004**, *42*, 1783–1791.

29 Itkis, M.E., Perea, D., Jung, R., Niyogi, S., Haddon, R.C., Comparison of analytical techniques for purity evaluation of single-walled carbon nanotubes. *J. Am. Chem. Soc.* **2005**, *127*, 3439–3448.

30 Hata, K., Fubata, D.N., Mizuno, K., Namai, T., Yumura, M., Iijima, S., Water-assisted highly efficient synthesis of impurity-free single-walled carbon nanotubes. *Science* **2004**, *306*, 1362–1364.

31 Liu, J., Rinzler, A.G., Dai, H., Hafner, J.H., Bradley, R.K., Boul, P.J., Lu, A., Iverson, T., Shelimov, K., Huffman, C.B., Rodriguez-Macias, F., Shon, Y.-S., Lee, T.R., Colbert, D.T., Smalley, R.E., Fullerene pipes. *Science* **1998**, *280*, 1253–1256.

32 Chiang, I.W., Brinson, B.E., Smalley, R.E., Margrave, J.L., Hauge, R.H., Purification and characterization of single-wall carbon nanotubes. *J. Phys. Chem. B* **2001**, *105*, 1157–1161.

33 Niyogi, S., Hu, H., Hamon, M.A., Bhowmik, P., Zhao, B., Rozenzhak, S.M., Chen, J., Itkis, M.E., Meier, M.S., Haddon, R.C., Chromatographic purification of soluble single-walled carbon nanotubes (s-SWNTs). *J. Am. Chem. Soc.* **2001**, *123*, 733–734.

34 Hu, H., Zhao, B., Itkis, M.E., Haddon, R.C., Nitric acid purification of single-walled carbon nanotubes. *J. Phys. Chem. B* **2003**, *107*, 13838–13842.

35 Haddon, R.C., Sippel, J., Rinzler, A.G., Papadimitrakopoulos, F., Purification and separation of carbon nanotubes. *MRS Bull.* **2004**, *29*, 252–259.

36 Niyogi, S., Hamon, M.A., Hu, H., Zhao, B., Bhowmik, P., Sen, R., Itkis, M.E., Haddon, R.C., Chemistry of single-walled carbon nanotubes. *Acc. Chem. Res.* **2002**, *35*, 1105–1113.

37 Zhao, B., Hu, H., Bekyarova, E., Itkis, M.E., Niyogi, S., Haddon, R.C., Carbon nanotubes: Chemistry. *Encycloped. Nanosci. Nanotechnol.* **2004**, 493–506.

38 Sun, Y.P., Fu, K., Lin, Y., Huang, W., Functionalized carbon nanotubes: properties and applications. *Acc. Chem. Res.* **2002**, *35*, 1096–1104.

39 Zhao, W., Song, C., Pehrsson, P.E., Water-soluble and optically pH-sensitive single-walled carbon nanotubes from surface modification. *J. Am. Chem. Soc.* **2002**, *124*, 12418–12419.

40 Rinzler, A.G., Liu, J., Dai, H., Nikolaev, P., Huffman, C.B., Rodriguez-Macias, F.J., Boul, P.J., Lu, A.H., Heymann, D., Colbert, D.T., Lee, R.S., Fischer, J.E., Rao, A.M., Eklund, P.C., Smalley, R.E., Large-scale purification of single-wall carbon nanotubes: process, product and characterization. *Appl. Phys. A* **1998**, *67*, 29–37.

41 O'Connell, M.J., Bachilo, S.M., Huffman, C.B., Moore, V.C., Strano, M.S., Haroz, E.H., Rialon, K.L., Boul, P.J., Noon, W.H., Kittrell, C., Ma, J., Hauge, R.H., Weisman, B.R., Smalley, R.E., Band gap fluorescence from individual single-walled carbon nanotubes. *Science* **2002**, *297*, 593–596.

42 O'Connell, M.J., Boul, P., Ericson, L.M., Huffman, C., Wang, Y., Haroz, E., Kuper, C., Tour, J., Ausman, K.D., Smalley, R.E., Reversible water-solubilization of single-walled carbon nanotubes by polymer wrapping. *Chem. Phys. Lett.* **2001**, *342*, 265–271.

43 Dyke, C.A., Tour, J.M., Unbundled and highly functionalized carbon nanotubes from aqueous reactions. *Nano Lett.* **2003**, *3*, 1215–1218.

44 Heller, D.A., Barone, P.W., Swanson, J.P., Mayrhofer, R.M., Strano, M.S., Using Raman spectroscopy to elucidate the aggregation state of single-walled carbon nanotubes. *J. Phys. Chem. B* **2004**, *108*, 6905–6909.

45 Zhang, X., Lu, Z., Wen, M., Liang, H., Zhang, J., Liu, Z., Single-walled carbon nanotube-based coaxial nanowires: synthesis, characterization, and electrical properties. *J. Phys. Chem. B* **2005**, *109*, 1101–1107.

46 Moore, V.C., Strano, M.S., Haroz, E.H., Hauge, R.H., Smalley, R.E., Schmidt, J., Talmon, Y., Individually suspended single-walled carbon nanotubes in various surfactants. *Nano Lett.* **2003**, *3*, 1379–1382.

47 Riggs, J.E., Walker, D.B., Carroll, D.L., Sun, Y.-P., Optical limiting properties of suspended and solubilized carbon nanotubes. *J. Phys. Chem. B* **2000**, *104*, 7071–7076.

48 Zhao, B., Hu, H., Haddon, R.C., Synthesis and properties of a water soluble single-walled carbon nanotube-poly (m-aminobenzene sulphonic acid) graft copolymer. *Adv. Funct. Mater.* **2004**, *14*, 71–76.

49 Zhao, B., Hu, H., Yu, A., Perea, D., Haddon, R.C., Synthesis and characterization of water soluble single-walled carbon nanotube graft copolymers. *J. Am. Chem. Soc.* **2005**, *127*, 8197–8203.

50 Sano, M., Kamino, A., Okamura, J., Shinkai, S., Self-organization of PEO-graft-single-walled carbon nanotubes in solutions and Langmuir-Blodgett films. *Langmuir* **2001**, *17*, 5125–5128.

51 Fernando, K.A.S., Lin, Y., Sun, Y.P., High aqueous solubility of functionalized single-walled carbon nanotubes. *Langmuir* **2004**, *20*, 4777–4778.

52 Pompeo, F., Resasco, D.E., Water solubilization of single-walled carbon nanotubes by functionalization with glucosamine. *Nano Lett.* **2002**, *2*, 369–373.

53 Balavoine, F., Schultz, P., Richard, C., Mallouh, V., Ebbesen, T.W., Mioskowski, C., Helical crystallization of proteins on carbon nanotubes: A first step towards the development of new biosensors. *Angew. Chem. Int. Ed.* **1999**, *38*, 1912–1915.

54 Erlanger, B.F., Chen, B.X., Zhu, M., Brus, L., Binding of an anti-fullerene IgG monoclonal antibody to single wall carbon nanotubes. *Nano Lett.* **2001**, *1*, 465–467.

55 Besteman, K., Lee, J.-O., Wiertz, F.G., Heering, H.A., Dekker, C., Enzyme-coated carbon nanotubes as single-molecule biosensors. *Nano Lett.* **2003**, *3*, 727–730.

56 Richard, C., Balavoine, F., Schultz, P., Ebbesen, T.W., Mioskowski, C., Supramolecular self-assembly of lipid derivatives on carbon nanotubes. *Science* **2003**, *300*, 775–778.

57 Zheng, M., Jagota, A., Strano, M.S., Santos, A.P., Barone, P., Chou, S.G., Diner, B.A., Dresselhaus, M.S., Mclean, R.S., Onoa, G.B., Samsonidze, G.G., Semke, E.D., Usrey, M.L., Walls, D.J., Structure-based carbon nanotube sorting by sequence-dependent DNA assembly. *Science* **2003**, *302*, 1545–1548.

58 Zorbas, V., Ortiz-Acevedo, A., Dalton, A.B., Yoshida, M.M., Dieckmann, G.R., Draper, R.K., Baughman, R.H., Jose-Yacaman, M., Musselman, I.H., Preparation and characterization of individual peptide-wrapped single-walled carbon nanotubes. *J. Am. Chem. Soc.* **2004**, *126*, 7222–7227.

59 Karajanagi, S.S., Vertegel, A.A., Kane, R.S., Dordick, J.S., Structure and function of enzymes adsorbed onto single-walled carbon nanotubes. *Langmuir* **2004**, *20*, 11594–11599.

60 Dieckmann, G.R., Dalton, A.B.,

Johnson, P.A., Razal, J., Chen, J., Giordano, G.M., Munoz, E., Musselman, I.H., Baughman, R.H., Draper, R.K., Controlled assembly of carbon nanotubes by designed amphiphilic peptide helices. *J. Am. Chem. Soc.* **2003**, *125*, 1770–1777.

61 Zheng, M., Jagota, A., Semke, E.D., Diner, B.A., McLean, R.S., Lustig, S.R., Richardson, R.E., Tassi, N.G., DNA-assisted dispersion and separation of carbon nanotubes. *Nature Mater.* **2003**, *2*, 338–342.

62 Strano, M.S., Zheng, M., Jagota, A., Onoa, G.B., Heller, D.A., Barone, P.W., Usrey, M.L., Understanding the nature of the DNA-assisted separation of single-walled carbon nanotubes using fluorescence and Raman spectroscopy. *Nano Lett.* **2004**, *4*, 543–550.

63 Shim, M., Kam, N.W.S., Chen, R.J., Li, Y., Dai, H., Functionalization of carbon nanotubes for biocompatibility and biomolecular recognition. *Nano Lett.* **2002**, *2*, 285–288.

64 Chen, R.J., Zhang, Y., Wang, D., Dai, H., Noncovalent sidewall functionalization of single-walled carbon nanotubes for protein immobilization. *J. Am. Chem. Soc.* **2001**, *123*, 3838–3839.

65 Huang, W., Taylor, S., Fu, K., Lin, Y., Zhang, D., Hanks, T.W., Rao, A.M., Sun, Y.-P., Attaching proteins to carbon nanotubes via diimide-activated amidation. *Nano Lett.* **2002**, *2*, 311–314.

66 Dwyer, C., Guthold, M., Falvo, M., Washburn, S., Superfine, R., Erie, D., DNA-functionalized single-walled carbon nanotubes. *Nanotechnology* **2002**, *13*, 601–604.

67 Williams, K.A., Veenhuizen, P.T.M., de la Torre, B.G., Eritja, R., Dekker, C., Nanotechnology: Carbon nanotubes with DNA recognition. *Nature* **2002**, *420*, 761.

68 Baker, S.E., Cai, W., Lasseter, T.L., Weidkamp, K.P., Hamers, R.J., Covalently bonded adducts of deoxyribonucleic acid (DNA) oligonucleotides with single-wall carbon nanotubes: synthesis and hybridization. *Nano Lett.* **2002**, *2*, 1413–1417.

69 Georgakilas, V., Kordatos, K., Prato, M., Guldi, D.M., Holzinger, M., Hirsch, A., Organic functionalization of carbon nanotubes. *J. Am. Chem. Soc.* **2002**, *124*, 760–761.

70 Georgakilas, V., Tagmatarchis, N., Pantarotto, D., Bianco, A., Briand, J.P., Prato, M., Amino acid functionalization of water soluble carbon nanotubes. *Chem. Commun.* **2002**, 3050–3051.

71 Keren, K., Berman, R.S., Buchstab, E., Sivan, U., Braun, E., DNA-templated carbon nanotube field-effect transistor. *Science* **2003**, *302*, 1380–1382.

72 Hazani, M., Hennrich, F., Kappes, M., Naaman, R., Peled, D., Sidorov, V., Shvarts, D., DNA-mediated self-assembly of carbon nanotube-based electronic devices. *Chem. Phys. Lett.* **2004**, *391*, 389–392.

73 Hazani, M., Shvarts, D., Peled, D., Sidorov, V., Naaman, R., Self-assembled carbon-nanotube-based field-effect transistors. *J. Appl. Phys.* **2004**, *85*, 5025–5027.

74 Moghaddam, M.J., Taylor, S., Gao, M., Huang, S., Dai, L., McCall, M.J., Highly efficient binding of DNA on the sidewalls and tips of carbon nanotubes using photochemistry. *Nano Lett.* **2004**, *4*, 89–93.

75 Li, S., He, P., Dong, J., Guo, Z., Dai, H., DNA-directed self-assembling of carbon nanotubes. *J. Am. Chem. Soc.* **2005**, *127*, 14–15.

76 Hu, L., Hecht, D.S., Gruner, G., Percolation in transparent and conducting carbon nanotube networks. *Nano Lett.* **2004**, *4*, 2513–2517.

77 Wu, Z., Chen, Z., Du, X., Logan, J.M., Sippel, J., Nikolou, M., Kamaras, K., Reynolds, J.R., Tanner, D.B., Hebard, A.F., Rinzler, A.G., Transparent, conductive carbon nanotube films. *Science* **2004**, *305*, 1273–1276.

78 Jung, D.-H., Kim, B.H., Ko, Y.K., Jung, M.S., Jung, S., Lee, S.Y., Jung, H.-T., Covalent attachment and

hybridization of DNA oligonucleotides on patterned single-walled carbon nanotube films. *Langmuir* **2004**, *20*, 8886–8891.

79 Jung, D.H., Jung, M.S., Ko, Y.K., Seo, S.J., Jung, H.-T., Carbon nanotube conducting arrays by consecutive amidation reactions. *Chem. Commun.* **2004**, 526–527.

80 Zhang, Y., Li, J., Shen, Y., Wang, M., Li, J., Poly-L-lysine functionalization of single-walled carbon nanotubes. *J. Phys. Chem. B* **2004**, *108*, 15343–15346.

81 Britto, P.J., Santhaman, S.K.V., Ajayan, P.M., Carbon nanotube electrode for oxidation of dopamine. *Bioelectrochem. Bioenerg.* **1996**, *41*, 121–125.

82 Guiseppi-Elie, A., Lei, C., Baughman, R.H., Direct electron transfer of glucose oxidase on carbon nanotubes. *Nanotechnology* **2002**, *13*, 559–564.

83 Li, J., Ng, H.T., Cassell, A., Fan, W., Chen, H., Ye, Q., Koehne, J., Han, J., Meyyappan, M., Carbon nanotube nanoelectrode array for ultrasensitive DNA detection. *Nano Lett.* **2003**, *3*, 597–602.

84 Gooding, J.J., Wibowo, R., Liu, J., Yang, W., Losic, D., Orbons, S., Mearns, F.J., Shapter, J.G., Hibbert, D.B., Protein electrochemistry using aligned carbon nanotube arrays. *J. Am. Chem. Soc.* **2003**, *125*, 9006–9007.

85 Lin, Y., Lu, F., Tu, Y., Ren, Z., Glucose biosensors based on carbon nanotube nanoelectrode ensembles. *Nano Lett.* **2004**, *4*, 191–195.

86 Soundarrajan, P., Patil, A., Dai, L., Surface modification of aligned carbon nanotube array for electrochemical sensing applications. *J. Vac. Sci. Technol. A* **2003**, *21*, 1198–1201.

87 Gao, M., Dai, L., Wallace, G.G., Biosensors based on aligned carbon nanotubes coated with inherently conducting polymers. *Electroanalysis* **2003**, *15*, 1089–1094.

88 Wang, J., Musameh, M., Carbon nanotube/Teflon composite electrochemical sensors and biosensors. *Anal. Chem.* **2003**, *75*, 2075–2079.

89 Star, A., Gabriel, J.-C.P., Bradley, K., Gruner, G., Electronic detection of specific protein binding using nanotube FET devices. *Nano Lett.* **2003**, *3*, 459–463.

90 Luong, J.H., Hrapovic, S., Wang, D., Bensebaa, F., Simard, B., Solubilization of multiwall carbon nanotubes by 3-aminopropyltriethoxysilane towards the fabrication of electrochemical biosensors with promoted electron transfer. *Electroanalysis* **2004**, *16*, 132–139.

91 Wang, J., Liu, G., Jan, M.R., Ultrasensitive electrical biosensing of proteins and DNA: Carbon-nanotube derived amplification of the recognition and transduction events. *J. Am. Chem. Soc.* **2004**, *126*, 3010–3011.

92 Trojanowicz, M., Mulchandani, A., Mascini, M., Carbon nanotubes-modified screen-printed electrodes for chemical sensors and biosensors. *Anal. Lett.* **2004**, *37*, 3185–3204.

93 Kong, J., Franklin, N.R., Zhou, C.W., Chapline, M.G., Peng, S., Cho, K.J., Dai, H.J., Nanotube molecular wires as chemical sensors. *Science* **2000**, *287*, 622–625.

94 Collins, P.G., Bradley, K., Ishigami, M., Zettl, A., Extreme oxygen sensitivity of electronic properties of carbon nanotubes. *Science* **2000**, *287*, 1801–1804.

95 Bradley, K., Briman, M., Star, A., Gruner, G., Charge transfer from adsorbed proteins. *Nano Lett.* **2003**, *4*, 253–256.

96 Boussaad, S., Tao, N.J., Zhang, R., Hopson, T., Nagahara, L.A., In situ detection of cytochrome c adsorption with single walled carbon nanotube device. *Chem. Commun.* **2003**, 1502–1503.

97 Chen, R.J., Choi, H.C., Bangsaruntip, S., Yenilmez, E., Tang, X., Wang, Q., Chang, Y.-L., Dai, H., An investigation of the mechanism of electronic sensing of protein adsorption on carbon nanotube devices. *J. Am. Chem. Soc.* **2004**, *126*, 1563–1568.

98 Zhao, O., Gan, Z., Zhuang, Q., Electrochemical sensors based on

carbon nanotubes. *Electroanalysis* **2002**, *14*, 1609–1613.
99 Hafner, J.H., Cheung, C.L., Lieber, C.M., Direct growth of single-walled carbon nanotube scanning probe microscopy tips. *J. Am. Chem. Soc.* **1999**, 9750–9751.
100 Hafner, J.H., Cheung, C.-L., Oosterkamp, T.H., Lieber, C.M., High-yield assembly of individual single-walled carbon nanotube tips for scanning probe microscopies. *J. Phys. Chem. B* **2000**, *105*, 743–746.
101 Wooley, A.T., Cheung, C.L., Hafner, J.H., Lieber, C.M., Structural biology with carbon nanotube AFM probes. *Chem. Biol.* **2000**, *7*, R193–R204.
102 Chen, L., Cheung, C.L., Ashby, P.D., Lieber, C.M., Single-walled carbon nanotube AFM probes: Optical imaging resolution of nanoclusters and biomolecules in ambient and fluid environments. *Nano Lett.* **2004**, *4*, 1725–1731.
103 Wong, S.S., Woolley, A.T., Joselevich, E., Cheung, C.L., Lieber, C.M., Covalently-functionalized single-walled carbon nanotube probe tips for chemical force microscopy. *J. Am. Chem. Soc.* **1998**, *120*, 8557–8558.
104 Wong, S.S., Joselevich, E., Wooley, A.T., Cheung, C.L., Lieber, C.M., Covalently functionalized nanotubes as nanometre-sized probes in chemistry and biology. *Nature* **1998**, *394*, 52–55.
105 Wang, S.G., Zhang, Q., Wang, R., Yoon, S.F., A novel multi-walled carbon nanotube based biosensor for glucose detection. *Biochem. Biophys. Res. Commun.* **2003**, *311*, 572–576.
106 Tang, H., Chen, J., Yao, S., Nie, L., Deng, G., Kuang, Y., Amperometric glucose biosensor based on adsorption of glucose oxidase at platinum nanoparticle-modified carbon nanotube electrode. *Anal. Biochem.* **2004**, *331*, 89–97.
107 Mattson, M.P., Haddon, R.C., Rao, A.M., Molecular functionalization of carbon nanotubes and use as substrates for neuronal growth. *J. Mol. Neurosci.* **2000**, *14*, 175–182.
108 Hu, H., Ni, Y., Montana, V., Haddon, R.C., Parpura, V., Chemically functionalized carbon nanotubes as substrates for neuronal growth. *Nano Lett.* **2004**, *4*, 507–511.
109 Hu, H., Ni, Y., Mandal, S.K., Montana, V., Zhao, B., Haddon, R.C., Parpura, V., Polyethyleneimine functionalized single-walled carbon nanotubes as substrates for neuronal growth. *J. Phys. Chem. B* **2005**, *109*, 4285–4289.
110 Service, R.F., Nanotechnology. Sorting technique may boost nanotube research. *Science* **2003**, *300*, 2018.
111 Service, R.F., Nanotoxicology. Nanotechnology grows up. *Science* **2004**, *304*, 1732–1734.
112 Chikkannanavar, S.B., Luzzi, D.E., Paulson, S., Johnson, A.T., Jr., Synthesis of peapods using substrate-grown SWNTs and DWNTs: An enabling step toward peapod devices. *Nano Lett.* **2005**, *5*, 151–155.

3
Biofunctionalization of Magnetic Nanoparticles

Yong Gao

3.1
Introduction

Advances in information storage technologies since the 1950s have led to tremendous progress in the preparation of magnetic particles of nanometer dimensions with defined properties [1, 2]. Since then, magnetic nanoparticles have found applications in biomedicine [3]. Magnetic particles with a grain size down to the nanometer scales have been used for *in vitro* cell/protein bio-separation, and chem-/bio-syntheses of pharmaceutical drug molecules. They have also been employed for *in vivo* magnetic drug targeting, magnetic resonance imaging (MRI) and magnetic hyperthermia tumor therapy [4–12]. More recently, due to rapid advances in nanotechnology, novel synthetic routes for fabricating magnetic nanoparticles with the ability to rigorously control the microstructures of magnetic nanoparticles, for example, coating, crystallinity and size uniformity, have been reported [13–38]. The development of these new types of magnetic nanomaterials has led to renewed research efforts on the functionalization of magnetic nanoparticles for their expanded biomedical applications.

In vitro and *in vivo* applications of magnetic nanoparticles in biomedicine are due to numerous beneficial factors associated with the unique nanometer-scale magnetic and physiological properties of magnetic nanospheres. Below a critical size, magnetic nanoparticles become single-domain and exhibit phenomena that differ from those of micrometer-sized counterparts, such as superparamagnetism, quantum tunneling of the magnetization, and unusually large coercivities, [1, 39–41]. Superparamagnetic iron oxide nanoparticles have been used as MRI contrast agents because of their very large magnetic moments – typically three orders of magnitude greater than those of other paramagnetic materials [4–6]. In addition to endowing them with unique magnetic properties, the small dimensions of magnetic nanoparticles, which range from several nanometers to hundreds of nanometers, typically smaller than those of proteins, cells and viruses, allow magnetic nanoparticles to have "close" contacts with a biological entity of interest. Thereby, magnetic nanoparticles can be utilized as a support for immobilization of bioactive molecules for bio-separation and bio-labeling applications since these nano-

Nanotechnologies for the Life Sciences Vol. 1
Biofunctionalization of Nanomaterials. Edited by Challa S. S. R. Kumar

ISBN: 3-527-31381-8

particular supports present minimal steric hindrance to the surface-loaded proteins and cells. Magnetic nanoparticles also have advantages over their micrometer counterparts in *in vivo* bioapplications due to their small sizes. For example, *in vivo* applications of magnetic particles usually prefer a particle dimension below 20 nm for high tissue penetration [42]. The small sizes can also help magnetic nanoparticles evade hepatic clearance from the bloodstream by the mononuclear phagocyte system (MPS). This will increase the plasma half-life of nanoparticles and, thus, increase the probability of attaining the desired target inside the body with magnetic nanoclusters [43].

A core/shell structure is usually required in many biomedical applications of magnetic nanoparticles. Such nanoclusters have an inorganic core, e.g., iron oxide, surrounded by an outer layer of shell wall that consists of long-chain organic ligands or inorganic/organic polymers. For many biomedical applications, the inorganic cores need to be superparamagnetic. For instance, the Food and Drug Administration (FDA) approved iron oxide MRI contrast agents have a superparamagnetic nano-core coated with dextran polymers. Superparamagnetism is also preferred for bio-separation and bio-labeling applications of magnetic nanoparticles. This is because (1) superparamagnetic cores will respond to an external magnetic field, but retain no magnetic properties once the field is removed [7]. The lack of magnetic remanence will allow magnetic materials to be repeatedly dispersed and concentrated in solution without forming magnetized clusters; and (2) superparamagnetic materials have large magnetic moments, permitting the use of low-field magnets for efficiently concentrating nanoparticles. Recently, progress has been made on the synthesis of monodisperse and structurally well defined iron oxide and other types of magnetic nanoparticles [13–33]. These new materials can be employed for constructing the interior cores of the core/shell magnetic nanoparticles – potentially endowing them with improved magnetic properties. Hyeon has recently reviewed developments in the chemical synthesis of magnetic nanoparticles [44].

The shell wall of core/shell magnetic nanoparticles is of particular importance to the bioapplications, stability and magnetic properties of nanoparticular complexes. Due to anisotropic dipolar attraction, nanoparticles tend to aggregate into large clusters that cause the loss of specific properties associated with single-domain nanostructures. Consequently, long-chain organic ligands or a layer of polymers are usually introduced to coat the inorganic cores to prevent core aggregations. In addition to improving the stability of nanoparticles, the shells also determine the solubility of nanocomplexes in aqueous buffer media and provide a platform for the functionalization of nanoclusters. Bio-active molecules, e.g., antibodies and proteins, can be immobilized onto the surface of shell walls and interact with a biological entity in surrounding solutions. However, as the size of nanoparticles decreases, the influence of surface interactions upon the magnetic properties of magnetic nanoparticles becomes more significant due to the increased volume fraction of surface atoms. The symmetry is reduced for the chemical surroundings of magnetic metal cations at the surface due to the incomplete coordination sphere. As a consequence, the magnetic properties of the nanoparticle surfaces usually differ from those in the body of the nanoparticle, and surface effects could become increasingly important to the overall magnetic properties of magnetic nanoparticle as its size decreases [45–50].

The present chapter focuses on recent developments in the synthesis and biofunctionalization of core/shell magnetic nanoparticles as well as their applications in biological and medical sciences. Although widely used in bio-separation applications, micrometer-sized magnetic particles are outside the scope of this review. This chapter is divided into three sections: functionalization of magnetic nanoparticles for (a) *in vitro* protein/cell separation (Section 3.2); (b) *in vitro* biochemical/chemical synthesis of therapeutic drugs and their intermediates (Section 3.3); and (c) *in vivo* bio-imaging, drug targeting and tumor hyperthermia treatments (Section 3.4), which includes some recent work on molecular imaging and gene therapy using functionalized magnetic nanoparticles. Although most reported molecular imaging and gene therapy experiments were carried out under *in vitro* environments, the ultimate goal in these two areas is to develop novel techniques using magnetic nanoclusters for *in situ* cellular visualization and gene therapy in living animals. Therefore, functionalization of magnetic nanoparticles for cellular imaging and gene therapy is listed under the *in vivo* applications of magnetic nanoparticles.

3.2
Functionalization of Magnetic Nanoparticles for *In Vitro* Protein/Cell Separation

The synthesis of core/shell magnetic nanoclusters and the attachment of bio-active ligands to the surface of the outer shells are key to bioapplications of magnetic nanoparticles. Several strategies have been developed recently for coating magnetic cores. The most common method is to use long-chain organic ligands to wrap up the inorganic cores. Hydrophobic interactions between ligands from neighboring nanoparticles will prevent adjacent inorganic cores agglomerating into a larger cluster. However, biological applications usually require magnetic nanoparticles to have good solubility in aqueous media. Hydrophobic long-chain alkanes will lower the solubility of magnetic nanoparticles in aqueous buffers. To solve this problem, our group has investigated the employment of charged bipyridinium carboxylic acids for coating iron oxide cores to make these nanoparticles water-soluble (Fig. 3.1) [51]. The positive charges on the surface of nanoparticles not only stabilize nanoparticles, by repelling neighboring clusters from forming aggregation, but also improve the solubility of nanoparticles in aqueous media. This is particularly important with biotin-functionalized maghemite nanoparticles since biotin is practically insoluble in distilled water. Both biotin and bipyridinium ligands were anchored to the surface of inorganic cores, having an average dimension of about 13 nm due to interactions between carboxyl groups and iron oxide. Such biotin-functionalized maghemite nanocomposites have been utilized for affinity isolation of fluorescein-labeled protein avidin.

A similar strategy using a bidentate enediol dopamine as a stable anchor of mag-

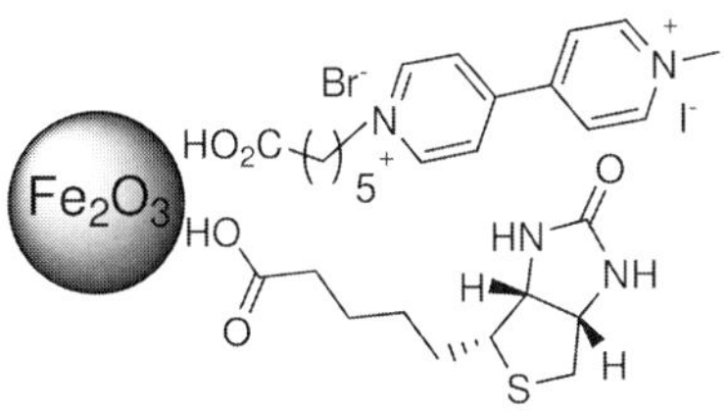

Fig. 3.1. Structure of maghemite nanoparticles coated with biotin and bipyridinium carboxylic acids. (Adapted from Fan et al. [51].)

netite nanoparticles for protein separation has been reported by Xu (Fig. 3.2A) [52]. Two types of superparamagnetic nanoparticles were synthesized and tested as supports for immobilization of nitrilotriacetic acid: one has a cobalt core with a Fe_2O_3 shell, and the other has a $SmCo_{5.2}$ core surrounded by an Fe_2O_3 shell. Dopamine was anchored to magnetic nanoparticles via interactions between its bidentate enediol functional group and surface iron oxide. Nitrilotriacetic acid was linked to dopamine through a long tether. Upon chelation to Ni^{2+}, dopamine-functionalized magnetic nanoparticles separated histidine-tagged proteins from a cell lysate with high efficiency and capacity. Histidine-tagged proteins were segregated from the solution due to interactions between a histidine tag and Ni^{2+} complexed with nitrilotriacetic acid. The separation process was readily achieved by applying an external small magnet. A similar bidentate enediol functional group, *C*-undecylcalix[4]resorcinaren, has also been reported for coating cobalt magnetic nanoparticles that self-assemble into bracelet-like rings [53].

Interactions between a sulfur group and FePt have been utilized to immobilize nitrilotriacetic acid for the separation of histidine-tagged proteins from a cell lysate

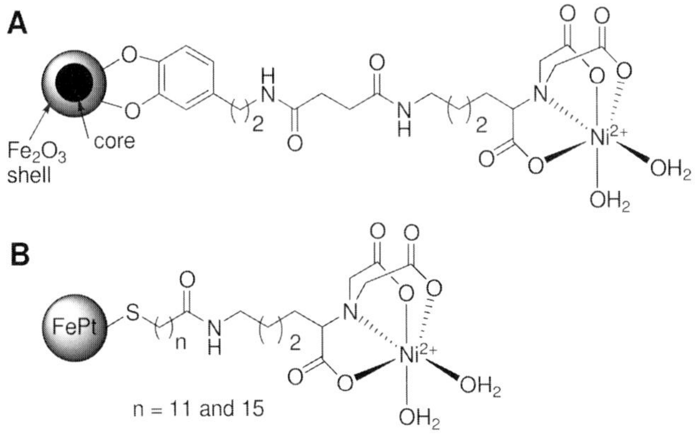

Fig. 3.2. Structures of magnetic nanocomposites using dopamine (A) and sulfur (B) to anchor nitrilotriacetic acid for separating histidine-tagged proteins. (Adapted from Xu [52, 54].)

(Fig. 3.2B) [54]. Many other functional groups, such as –OH, –SH and $–NH_2$, have also been tested for their interactions with metals and metal oxides as capping agents of magnetic metal and metal oxide cores. For instance, the amino groups of vancomycin have been employed for immobilizing the antibiotic to the surface of FePt nanoparticles [55]. Such complexes could capture and detect vancomycin-resistant enterococci and other Gram-positive bacteria at concentrations of 10^1 cfu mL^{-1} within an hour. Additional examples of using amino groups for the functionalization of magnetic nanoparticles have also been reported [56, 57]. A similar nanocomposite of IgG and magnetite has also been employed by Chen's group as an effective affinity probe to concentrate target bacteria selectively [58]. IgG was immobilized onto the surface of a magnetite core via an ester bond. Other than antibodies, DNA/RNA-functionalized magnetic nanoparticles have also been used for the isolation and extraction of DNA/RNA targets [59]. The surfaces of these nanoparticles were usually coated with molecular beacon DNA probes for specific recognition of DNA/RNA targets in solution.

The –OH, –SH and $–NH_2$ functional groups are usually introduced through a surface exchange reaction with pre-synthesized magnetic nanoparticles coated with a different functional group [31, 60, 61], or by co-precipitation of an aqueous solution of metal ion salts such as Fe^{2+}/Fe^{3+} in the presence of these organic capping groups [42]. For example, iron oxide nanoparticles coated with α-cyclodextrin (CD) were obtained by a surface exchange reaction from iron oxide nanoparticles protected by oleate [62]. α-CD was added to the surface of nanoparticles by vigorously stirring, at room temperature, mixtures of hexane suspensions of iron oxide nanoparticles coated with oleate and an equal volume of α-CD aqueous solution. Oleate-stabilized nanoparticles were transferred from organic into aqueous phase by surface modification using α-CD. CD molecules have –OH groups that can bind to the surface of iron oxide cores.

An interesting way of capping magnetic iron oxide cores is to use phospholipids to form nanometer-sized magnetoliposomes. An example [63] of such phospholipid-coated magnetite nanoparticles, employing 1,2-myristoyl-*sn*-glycero-3-phosphoglycerol, sodium salt and 1,2-dimyristoyl-*sn*-glycerol-3-phosphocholine, had an iron oxide core dimension of 8 nm and a phospholipids/surfactant shell of 4 nm. These particles were effective ion exchange media for the recovery and separation of proteins from protein mixtures. These nanocomposites demonstrated high adsorptive capacities of proteins and exhibited none of the diffusion resistances offered by conventional porous ion exchange media.

Due to strong interactions with metal oxide, organosilane groups have also been explored for anchoring bioactive molecules onto the surface of iron oxide nanocores. Zhang has reported a novel approach using bifunctional trifluoroethylester polyethylene glycol (PEG) silane for the functionalization of iron oxide nanoparticles (Fig. 3.3) [64]. Folate acid, a widely used targeting agent for cancer therapies [65], was attached to the outer terminus of the PEG chain to demonstrate the effectiveness of bio-active ligand immobilization by this strategy. Silylation of magnetite is key to the functionalization of magnetic nanoparticles in this route. Introduction of PEG molecules as a linker will potentially benefit *in vivo* applications of these

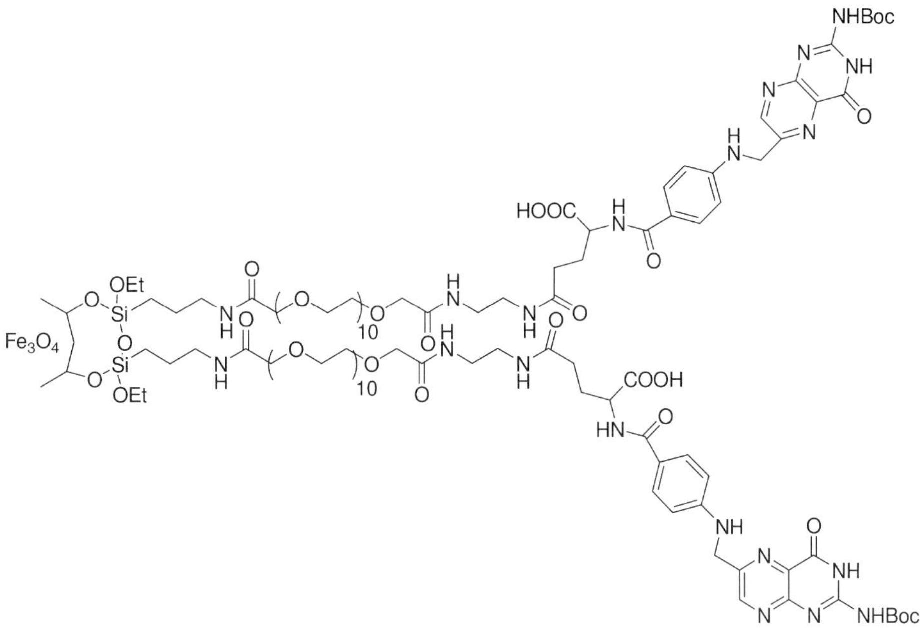

Fig. 3.3. Structure of magnetite nanoparticles coated with PEG and folic acid. (Adapted from Kohler et al. [64].)

nanoparticles since PEG molecules are nonimmunogenic, nonantigenic and protein resistant and can increase particulate circulation time in the blood. Willner has used the silylation of magnetic metal oxide surfaces for the immobilization of redox functions to magnetite particles. Such complexes were used in constructing a magneto-switchable bioelectrocatalysis sensor [66].

Sol–gel approaches have been examined for coating magnetic metal oxide cores to form a core/shell structure having an inorganic metal oxide core wrapped with a layer of silica [67–76]. Two different strategies have been investigated to generate silica coatings on the surface of iron oxide particles. The first method relies on the well-known Stöber process [77], in which silica is formed *in situ* through the hydrolysis and condensation of a sol–gel precursor. For example, Xia has reported the use of tetraethyl orthosilicate (TEOS) for coating mixed-crystalline iron oxide nanoparticles (water-soluble ferrofluid) [74]. Because the iron oxide surface has a strong affinity towards silica, no primer was required to promote the deposition and adhesion of silica, allowing magnetic nanoparticles directly coated with amorphous silica to be formed via the hydrolysis of TEOS. A second sol–gel approach is based on a microemulsion strategy, in which micelles or inverse micelles are used to confine and control the coating of silica on core nanoparticles. The microemulsion approach can control the thickness of the silica shell wall coating so that the stability and solubility of the formed magnetic nanoparticles in aqueous media can, presumably, be tuned for different bio-applications. An example is discussed in Section 3.3 (Fig. 3.7 below) [75]. Core/shell magnetite/silica nanoparticles were synthesized by a microemulsion approach and functionalized with protein β-lactamase to promote hydrolysis.

Natural polymers and their derivatives have been widely utilized for coating magnetic metal and metal oxide nanocore surfaces. In particular, natural biopolymers such as dextrans, proteins/peptides and PEG are usually the materials of choice for the synthesis of core/shell magnetic nanoparticles designated for *in vivo* applications. This is because such natural polymers are inexpensive and are known to be nonimmunogenic and nonantigenic in the body. Natural polymers are usually anchored onto the surfaces of magnetic metal oxide cores through carboxylate groups on their side chains. Section 3.4 includes detailed discussions and examples of using these natural polymer-functionalized magnetic nanoparticles for *in vivo* applications.

Tremendous research efforts have focused on the employment of synthetic polymers for coating the surfaces of magnetic inorganic cores to generate core/shell magnetic nanoparticles. For example, layer-by-layer deposition of charged polymers onto the surfaces of magnetic inorganic cores in sequence has been reported [78]. Although progress has been made, the layer-by-layer assembly strategy has yet to become the method of choice for coating very small, sub-20 nm magnetic nanoparticle cores because of the curvature of nanoparticle surfaces and the mechanical strength of the polymeric chains. Unfortunately, magnetic nanoparticles with an overall dimension below 20 nm are usually preferred for some *in vivo* applications due to their high tissue penetration capability and long blood circulation time [42, 43]. Here we focus on two alternative strategies that can potentially be utilized and expanded for synthesizing magnetic nanoparticles of various sizes and shapes.

The first approach is to utilize surface-initiated polymerization to grow polymer chains on the surface of inorganic cores. Free radical initiators are first immobilized onto the surfaces of metal and metal oxide cores followed by polymer growth outwards to give rise to a radius structure. Among many polymerization routes, living free radical polymerization, especially atom transfer radical polymerization (ATRP), has become the method of choice for the surface-initiated polymerization synthesis of core/shell magnetic nanoparticles (Fig. 3.4) [79]. ATRP is a versatile technique that offers several advantages over other polymerization routes, including control over molecular weight and molecular weight distribution for the synthesis of well-defined and complex macromolecular architectures of magnetic nanoparticles [80]. For example, by manipulating reaction time and the concentration of polymerizable ligands in solution one can control the shell wall polymer molecular weight and, thus, the thickness of the polymeric shell wall of core/shell magnetic nanoparticles. ATRP also allows the polymers to be end-functionalized or block copolymerized upon the addition of other monomers. Not only does this feature offer tailorability of the polymer coating with various compositions and functionalities, but also provides the platform for functionalization of the polymeric shell wall with bio-active functional groups. As a consequence, extensive research has been carried out by many groups using ATRP for the synthesis of core/shell polymer magnetic nanoparticles [79, 81, 82]. Our group has examined

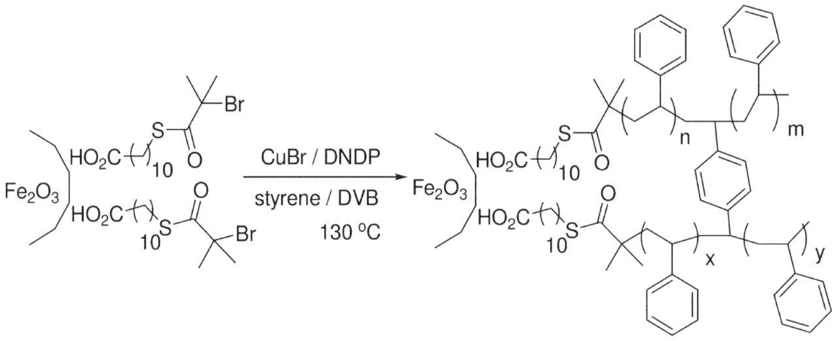

Fig. 3.4. Surface-initiated ATRP synthesis of polymeric core/shell nanoparticles using divinylbenzene (DVB) as a crosslinking agent. (Reproduced by permission of the American Chemical Society.)

recently an ATRP method for the preparation of core/shell maghemite/polystyrene nanocrystals (Fig. 3.4) [79]. Our inorganic cores have an average size of about 11 nm while the thickness of the crosslinked polystyrene shells were maintained to only about 4.7 nm (Fig. 3.5). However, further work is needed to adapt ATRP techniques for the synthesis of hydrophilic and water-soluble magnetic nanoparticles for biomedical applications. A recent paper from Armes [83] on the synthesis of hydrophilic polymer-grafted ultrafine inorganic oxide particles suggested that such water-soluble polymeric magnetic nanoparticles can potentially be achieved through a different ATRP method.

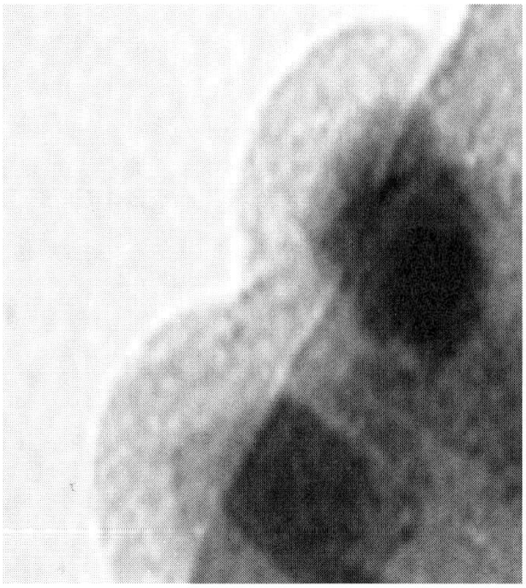

Fig. 3.5. TEM micrograph of 10% DVB-crosslinked Fe_2O_3/polystyrene core/shell nanoparticles on a lacey carbon film coated copper grid (300 mesh) consisting of woven-mesh-like holes. The polystyrene shells are visible at the edge of a hole. Dark spots on the carbon film are Fe_2O_3 cores. (Reproduced by permission of the American Chemical Society.)

A second, extensively researched, approach to synthesizing polymeric core/shell magnetic nanoparticles is to use pre-formed synthetic polymers as a matrix to confine and control the formation of magnetic cores. For example, core/shell magnetic nanoparticles have been produced by chemical co-precipitation of iron salts in an aqueous solution of the poly(ethylene oxide) (PEO)/poly(propylene oxide) (PPO)–poly(acrylic acid) (PAA) graft copolymers [84]. After magnetite nucleation begins, carboxylic acid groups on the PAA backbone bind to the particle surface, limiting the magnetic core growth. The bifunctional polymer shell is formed from the hydrophilic PEO and hydrophobic PPO side chains in the graft copolymer. These nanoparticles are stable and soluble in organic solutions. Similar magnetite nanoparticles coated with long poly(vinyl-*N*-alkylpyridinium) chains have also been synthesized by this strategy [85]. Alkylated polyethylenamines made these materials highly bactericidal toward both Gram-positive and Gram-negative pathogenic bacteria. Other types of polymers such as poly(vinylpyrrolidone) [86, 87], polylactide [88], poly(isopropylacrylamide) [89], polyacrylate [90], poly(methacrylate) [91], poly(vinyl alcohol) [92] and polysiloxane block copolymers [93] have also been reported as matrices for the synthesis of core/shell magnetic nanoparticles.

3.3
Functionalization of Magnetic Nanoparticles for Biochemical/Chemical Synthesis of Therapeutic Drugs and Their Intermediates

Catalysts are widely used in pharmaceutical and chemical industries in producing therapeutical drug molecules and their intermediates. Catalysts such as biocatalysts (enzymes) and metal catalysts (homogeneous and heterogeneous catalysts) can promote organic and biological reactions that are otherwise too slow for industrial standards. Recycling and reuse of industrial catalysts is particularly important for cutting industrial operation costs and minimizing environmental pollutions, especially when expensive and toxic heavy metals are used [94].

Recently, efforts have been directed towards the use of magnetic nanoparticles as supports for immobilization of biocatalysts [75, 95, 96]. Core/shell magnetic nanoparticles are usually covalently attached with biocatalyst enzymes on their shell surfaces. Due to the small sizes of particles, nanoparticle-immobilized proteins are usually soluble in aqueous buffers, which differs from other supports such as polystyrene beads, in which proteins are usually suspended in solution. The magnetic, usually superparamagnetic cores will allow these biofunctionalized particles to be magnetically concentrated with the assistance of an external magnetic field. This could allow immobilized enzymes to be used repeatedly or continuously in various reactors. Enzymes can be easily separated from soluble reaction products and unreacted substrates, thus simplifying work-up and preventing protein contamination of the final products. This will also simplify the control of microbial contamination in immobilized proteins.

Candida rugosa lipase (E.C.3.1.1.3) has been immobilized on maghemite nanoparticles with an average size of about 20 ± 10 nm (Fig. 3.6) [95]. A carboxylate

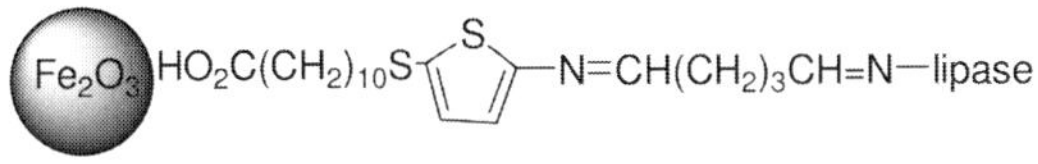

Fig. 3.6. Representative structure of magnetic nanoparticles immobilized with *Candida rugosa* lipase. (Adapted from Dayal [95].)

group was used to anchor a 2-thiophene thiolate linker and the enzyme was chemically bonded to the nanoparticle surface through a C=N bond using glutaraldehyde. The amount of immobilized enzyme was determined by standard BCA protein assays of the original lipase solution, the supernatants and washing solutions after immobilization, respectively. The presence of protein on the surface of nanoparticles was also confirmed by AFM measurements of a small amount of the enzyme-functionalized magnetic nanoparticles on a thin layer of glue deposited on a steel disk. Enzymatic activity of the immobilized lipase was determined by following the ester cleavage of *p*-nitrophenol butyrate aqueous solution with UV spectroscopy. The enzymatic activity for *Candida rugosa* lipase immobilized on maghemite nanoparticles was lower than that of the free enzymes, but the loss in activity on nanoparticles was significantly lower than that reported for enzyme immobilized on micrometer-sized polymeric beads using physisorption. The most significant advantage of the nanoparticle-immobilized enzyme is its long-term stability. The hybrid enzyme–nanoparticle composites showed only a ~2% decrease in activity over 14 days due to desorption or denaturation. This long-term stability illustrates the advantages of attaching enzymes chemically to the nanoparticles.

A similar investigation was also reported recently using magnetic nanoparticles for immobilization of β-lactamase I (Fig. 3.7) [75]. Here, a layer of silica coating was placed on the surface of an iron oxide core. TEM images determined the average size inorganic core to be about 9.1 nm, with a silica shell of about 3.5 nm. β-Lactamase I was immobilized onto the surface through glutaraldehyde and C=N bonds. An assay evaluation, using a UV spectrometer, of active β-lactamase I on nanoparticle composites was carried out at room temperature using phenoxymethylpenicillin as the substrate in a buffer. The nanoparticle-immobilized enzyme showed an activity of about 53.76% of that of the free enzyme in solution. However, a kinetic study has shown that the K_M of the immobilized enzyme matches well that of the parent free enzyme. This suggests that nanoparticle-immobilized enzymes do not suffer from the mass-transfer problems frequently encountered with insoluble supports used for immobilizing enzymes.

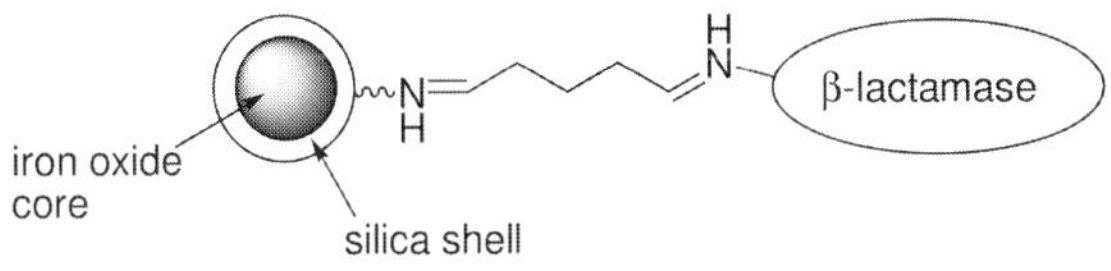

Fig. 3.7. Immobilization of enzyme β-lactamase I to core/shell iron oxide/silica nanoparticles. (Adapted from Gao [75].)

Other than biocatalysts, metal catalysts, especially homogeneous metal catalysts, have also been immobilized onto the surfaces of core/shell magnetic nanoparticles. Due to their small sizes, the solubility of magnetic nanoparticles in organic media can be tuned by controlling the structure of organic and polymer coatings of nanoparticles. Such soluble supports could be magnetically concentrated and isolated from reaction media by applying an external magnetic field. Magnetic nanoparticles are an ideal soluble support, providing a unique solution to the problem of recycling homogeneous catalysts in pharmaceutical and chemical industries. The reader is referred to two recent papers in this emerging field [97, 98].

3.4 Functionalization of Magnetic Nanoparticles for *In Vivo* Bio-imaging, Drug Targeting and Tumor Hyperthermia Treatments

Magnetic nanoparticles have been explored extensively as contrast agents for *in vivo* magnetic resonance imaging (MRI), magnetic guides for drug targeting and mediators for magnetic hyperthermia treatments of a large variety of diseases. With proper coatings, superparamagnetic nanoparticles can interact with an external magnetic field and deliver radiotherapeutic and chemotherapeutic agents to a target area – minimizing the cytotoxicity of tumor therapeutic agents to healthy body compartments. This is important in the treatment and diagnosis of certain types of cancers due to, for example, their lack of specific tumor markers and the presence of the blood–brain barrier (BBB). A further medical use of magnetic nanoparticles is to utilize superparamagnetic nanoclusters as MRI contrast agents for cancer diagnosis and detection. A third major *in vivo* application of magnetic nanoparticles is magnetic hyperthermia therapy. Magnetic nanoparticles can be made to resonantly respond to a time-varying magnetic field, with advantageous results related to the transfer of energy from the exciting field to the nanoparticles. This is utilized to make magnetic nanoparticles heat up, which leads to their use as hyperthermia mediators, delivering toxic amounts of thermal energy to targeted tumor cells.

Typical magnetic nanoparticles used in *in vivo* studies consist of a magnetic core surrounded by a biocompatible polymeric coating. Iron oxide particles such as magnetite or its oxidized form maghemite are by far the most commonly employed for *in vivo* applications. Highly magnetic materials such as cobalt and nickel are toxic and susceptible to oxidation and hence are often overlooked for *in vivo* biomedical applications. Iron oxide nanoparticles are physiologically well tolerated. For example, dextran-magnetite has no measurable toxicity index LD_{50} [99–101]. This is partially because the body is designed to process excess iron. In the human body iron is stored primarily in the core of the iron storage protein ferritin. Iron contained in endosomes and lysosomes is metabolized into elemental iron and oxygen by hydrolytic enzymes, where the iron joins normal body stores [101]. Iron homeostasis is well controlled by adsorption, excretion and storage. As a consequence, iron from iron nanoparticles in the body can be processed and iron oxide can be tolerated by the body. However, notably, iron has a rather limited bioavailability, and in some situations it can also be toxic to cells [102].

In vivo applications require that these magnetic nanoparticles have a long-circulating time in the body in order to reach the target sites [43] before being eliminated from the blood circulation through clearance by the mononuclear phagocyte system (MPS) [103]. The MPS, also known as the reticuloendothelial system, is defined as the cell family consisting of bone marrow progenitors, blood monocytes and tissue macrophages such as Kupffer cells in the liver. These macrophages are widely distributed and strategically placed in many tissues of the body to recognize and clear senescent cells, invading microorganisms and particles [104]. The first step of the clearance mechanism is the opsonization process. Opsonins, circulating plasma proteins, adsorb themselves spontaneously onto the surface of an invading entity. Particles of different surface characteristics, size and morphology attract different arrays of opsonins, which can interact with the specialized plasma membrane receptors on monocytes and macrophages [105]. Then, endocytosis/phagocytosis of the particles by the circulating monocytes or the fixed macrophages leads to the elimination of particles from circulation.

Previous studies of liposomes and polymeric nanoparticle systems have shown that, among many surface factors, the size, surface charge density and hydrophilicity/hydrophobicity have a profound effect on opsonization [43]. Therefore, significant efforts have been directed at exploring various biocompatible coating materials to increase plasma half-life as long as possible in order to increase the probability of reaching the desired targets in the body [106]. Neutral and hydrophilic natural and synthetic polymers have become the materials of choice. For example, dextrans have been frequently used for coating iron oxide nanocrystals [43]. Other biological macromolecules such as heparin and polysaccharides that complement regular proteins have also been investigated [107, 108]. Among synthetic polymers, poloxamers, poloxamines and their block-copolymers increase their circulation time [109, 110], and can potentially be utilized for coating iron oxide nanoparticle cores for this purpose. An alternative approach is to covalently anchor PEG macromolecules onto the nanoparticle surfaces. PEG is an effective polymer for suppressing the protein adsorption-opsonization process [65]. Immobilization of PEG to drug carrier surface is well known in liposome drug delivery where PEG macromolecules are conjugated to the surfaces of liposomes to improve their circulation lifetime, bioavailability and decrease their immunogenicity [111]. Recent successes using this PEG strategy in a quantum dots biodistribution study [112] has offered the possibility of extending this method to other nanomaterials, including iron oxide nanoparticles.

3.4.1
MR Imaging

Superparamagnetic nanoparticles represent a class of MRI contrast agents that are usually referred to as T_2 (transversal relaxation time) or T_2^* contrast agents [113] as opposed to T_1 (longitudinal relaxation time) agents such as paramagnetic gadolinium chelates [114]. MRI is based on the NMR (nuclear magnetic resonance) signal of protons from water in tissues and organs through the combined effects of a strong static magnetic field (B_0) and a transverse radiofrequency field (rf field) [115]. After rf excitation, hydrogen nuclei attempt to return to their ground states through two independent relaxation processes: (1) longitudinal relaxation, which is also called T_1-recovery or "spin–lattice" relaxation; hydrogen atoms release the previously absorbed energy to the surrounding tissue (lattice) in their attempt to re-align with B_0. (2) Transverse relaxation, also called T_2 decay or "spin–spin" relaxation, which is due to the exchange of energy between spinning hydrogens in tissues. MR images of biological tissues are constructed from relaxation data collected by a computer applying a two-dimensional Fourier transformation to give the amplitudes of NMR signals [116–118]. While, in many clinical situations, the intrinsic differences in relaxivity ($1/T$) between tissues are small, exogenous contrast agents can be utilized to improve greatly the diagnostic value of MRI for a better delineation of tissues [100]. Gadolinium complexes are the most commonly used T_1 contrast agents while superparamagnetic iron oxide nanoparticles are FDA-approved T_2 agents.

Depending on their size, colloidal iron oxide nanoparticles of magnetite (Fe_3O_4) to maghemite (γ-Fe_2O_3) are often called SPIO (superparamagnetic iron oxide) with a particle size typically larger than 50 nm, and USPIO (ultra-small superparamagnetic nanoparticles), with a dimension < 50 nm [6, 119]. Hydrophilic polymers such as heparin [107], dextran [120], chitosan [121], starch [122], DNA [123], and cyclodextrian [124] have been employed for coating the iron oxide cores. These water-soluble macromolecules are employed to stabilize nanoclusters by preventing aggregation of their inorganic cores and reduce opsonization process. However, the structure of surface coating materials greatly influences the magnetic properties of magnetic nanoparticles [45–50]. Adoption of different polymers for coating iron oxide cores could significantly alter MR relaxation properties of the overall nanoparticle contrast agents [124].

Due to their size, SPIOs usually can be cleared out of the blood circulation and accumulated in MPS organs very quickly, especially in liver and spleen [113, 125]. For example, about 80% of the injected SPIO doses were found in liver and 5–10% in the spleen with a plasma half-life of less than 10 min [4]. As a consequence, SPIOs can decrease the liver and spleen signals within several minutes after i.v. administration, and this type of agent is usually used for liver and spleen imaging [126–129]. USPIOs, however, are smaller than SPIOs. They usually have longer plasma life, higher than 2 hours, and therefore remain in the blood long enough to act as blood-pool agents for MR angiography [113]. Also because of their small sizes, USPIOs can leak into the interstitium, where they can be accumulated in the lymph nodes and thereby used for imaging lymphatic systems [130–135].

Progress has been made on the functionalization of core/shell magnetic nanoparticles for tissue/organ-specific *in vivo* imaging. Antibodies such as human polyclonal IgG and L6 antibodies have been physically adsorbed or covalently attached to iron oxide nanoparticles [136–138]. Investigations in rodents revealed that antibodies led to a high concentration of magnetic nanoparticles at specific sites. Recently, Moore has reported using a peptide [139] for the functionalization of iron oxide nanoparticles for tissue-specific *in vivo* imaging. The synthetic peptide EPPT1(YCAREPPTRTFAYWG) – a short fragment of the CDR3 V_h region of a monoclonal antibody ASM2 – was covalently linked to the surface of aminated crosslinked superparamagnetic iron oxide nanocomplexes (CLIO-NH_2). CLIO-NH_2 consists of a core of superparamagnetic iron oxide and a crosslinked coating of dextran with amino groups [140, 141]. EPPT1 peptide has significant affinity towards under-glycosylated mucin-1 antigen (uMUC-1), which is overexpressed on many cancer cell lines. A Cy5.5 dye was also immobilized onto the surface of CLIO-NH_2 as a near-infrared fluorescence optical probe. *In vivo* MRI and near-infrared-imaging experiments on tumor-bearing mice showed specific accumulation of the probe in uMUC-1-positive tumors and no signal in control tumors. The high specific concentration of magnetic nanoparticles at the target sites was due to the presence of EPPT1 peptide on the surface of dextran–iron oxide nanoparticles. Similar experiments using folate-labeled magnetic nanoparticles for *in vivo* imaging of tumors with overexpressed folate receptors have also been reported recently [142].

Cellular imaging has long attracted a great deal of research interest [143]. Studies using unfunctionalized iron oxide nanoparticles for labeling various types of cell lines such as leukocytes, lymphocytes and monocytes for MR imaging of cells have been reported [124, 144–146]. If a cell can be sufficiently loaded with magnetic materials, then MRI can be adopted for use in cell tracking with a resolution of 20–25 μm or higher, approaching the size of single cells [6]. However, cellular uptake of dextran-coated iron oxide nanoparticles was low. Improvements are still needed to increase the cellular uptake of magnetic nanoparticles. Recently, progress has been made towards this goal for high-efficiency internal labeling of large numbers of cells. Iron oxide nanoparticles with a HIV-1 tat peptide fragment attached at the outer surface of their dextran coating (CLIO-NH_2) increase the cellular uptake of nanoparticles over 100-fold into lymphocytes when compared to untagged particles [147, 148]. HIV-1 tat peptide carries a transmembrane and a nuclear localization signal within its sequence and is, therefore, capable of translocating exogenous nanoparticles into cells [149]. Folic acid has also been immobilized onto iron oxide nanoparticles for targeting the folate receptor-bearing cells [150, 151]. Folate-mediation internalized folate-labeled nanoparticles and increased the cellular uptake of iron oxide nanoparticles that were used as contrast agents for cellular imaging. Iron oxide nanoparticles functionalized with the C_2 domain of synaptotagmin I [152] and dendrimers [153] have also been synthesized and utilized for MRI studies of cells. A further goal in this area is to exploit the use of MRI techniques to image transgene expression. Research in this area has focused on depicting the activity of endocytotic receptors for cellular uptake of functionalized iron oxide nanoparticles [154, 155]. A growing number of cell biologists, molecular biologists and experts in MRI are working together to develop techniques for the *in situ* visualization of gene expression in living animals [143].

3.4.2
Targeted Drug Delivery

Magnetic drug targeting has attracted a great deal of attention. This approach is an alternative to antibody-directed drug targeting, offering additional advantages for the treatment and diagnosis of certain types of cancers due to, for example, their lack of specific tumor markers and presence of the BBB [156]. *In vivo* experiments of magnetic drug targeting have usually been performed in rodents [157], but investigations using swine [158] and rabbits [159] have also been reported. Generally, iron oxide cores are coated with silica, and polymers such as PVA and dextran. The first clinical trials in humans with a magnetic drug targeting were reported by Lübbe et al. [160, 161]. They used a ferrofluid (size about 100 nm) coated with starch polymers and anionic phosphate groups for loading the drug epirubicin. The shell phosphate group forms strong anionic interactions with the positively charged amino sugars of epirubicin. During infusion and for 45 min afterwards, a magnetic field was applied about less than 0.5 cm from the tumor site. It took about only 30 min in half of the patients before the ferrofluids could be successfully directed to the tumors. Similar investigations using liposomes containing magnetic nanoparticles and drugs have also been reported [162]. Magnetic drug targeting has been employed to deliver cytotoxic drugs to brain tumors, which are difficult to treat due to the BBB. Pulfer and Gallo demonstrated that particles as large as 1–2 μm could be concentrated at the site of intracerebral rat glioma-2 tumors [156].

Despite early success, magnetic drug targeting still needs to be improved to make it more effective. Limitations [161] include (1) difficulties in scaling up from small rodent models to humans or large animals due to the requirement of much stronger external magnetic fields; (2) the possibility of embolization of the blood vessels in the target region due to accumulation of the magnetic carriers; and (3) difficulties in controlling the release of drug molecules from carriers and the molecular uptake of these therapeutic agents by tumor cells.

Some of the aforementioned limitations can be overcome if magnetic nanoparticle carriers are utilized for delivering radiotherapeutic agents for tumor radiotherapy. In contrast to chemotherapeutical drugs, radioisotopes can be delivered close to the tumor sites and exert their cytotoxicity over a defined, radioisotope-dependent distance – the chelated metals do not need to be released from the carriers so that they can bind to or enter the cells to be cytotoxic. The effectiveness of this technique has been confirmed by several investigations using yttrium-90 [163] and rhenium-188 [164] in both animal and cell culture studies.

Arbab et al. have recently demonstrated the possibility of using iron oxide nanoparticles for delivering mesenchymal stem cells (MSCs) to a targeted area in an animal model by applying an external magnet [165]. MSCs were labeled with iron oxide nanoparticles and the resulting magnetic cell complexes were intravenously injected into two groups of rats with or without a magnet placed over the livers. Experiments showed that the external magnets influenced the movement of labeled MSCs as higher iron concentration and increased labeled cell numbers were detected in rat livers with external magnets. These results demonstrated that cells could be retained in the region of interest inside the body using magnetic forces, and magnetic drug targeting can be utilized for *in vivo* delivery of stem cells or genetically altered cells to the target sites.

A further area of interest in the use of targeted magnetic nanoparticles is in the field of gene therapy. One of the impediments to successful gene therapy is the inefficient delivery of genes because of low transfection efficiencies. This can be addressed by using a viral vector carrying the therapeutic gene loaded on magnetic carrier surface. An external magnetic field was applied to allow the viral vector a longer of period of time in contact with the tissues, thereby increasing the efficiency of gene transfection and expression [166–168]. Research in this area has recently attracted a great deal of interest – a review article is listed here [169] for interested readers.

3.4.3
Magnetic Hyperthermia

Magnetic hyperthermia is a promising form of cancer therapy aside from the well-known methods of surgery, chemotherapy and radiotherapy [170, 171]. Magnetic nanoparticles are used as mediators for magnetic hyperthermia. In broad terms, magnetic hyperthermia involves dispersing magnetic particles through the targeted tissue, and then applying an AC magnetic field of sufficient strength and frequency to cause the particle to heat. This heat conducts into the immediately surrounding diseased tissue. Hyperthermia treatment of cancers is based on observations that some cancer cells are more sensitive to temperatures in excess of 41 °C than their normal healthy counterparts. Two kinds of heat treatment are currently distinguished: mild hyperthermia is performed between 41 and 46 °C to stimulate the immune response for non-specific immunotherapy of cancers, and thermo-ablation between 46 and 56 °C for thermal destruction of tumors by direct cell necrosis, coagulation or carbonization [170, 171].

Generally, two types of magnetic nanoparticles have been used for magnetic hyperthermia, via two different mechanisms: (a) heating of ferromagnetic nanoparticles when exposed to a time varying magnetic field, which is essentially due to hysteresis losses and Brownian relaxation losses of the particles; and (b) Brown and Néel heating mechanisms that contribute to the heating of superparamagnetic nanoparticles. The heating power of the particles is quantified as the specific absorption rate (SAR) and describes the energy amount converted into heat per time and mass. Superparamagnetic nanoparticles usually give higher SAR than ferromagnetic nanoparticles because the hysteresis loop of ferromagnetic nanoparticles can rarely be fully used because of physiological and technical restrictions on the external field amplitude [4]. Consequently, dispersions of superparamagnetic nanoparticles appear to be the most promising since they are used as ferrofluids. This technique is termed magnetic fluid hyperthermia (MFH) [170]. However, ferromagnetic nanoparticles remain potentially useful due to their Curie temperature – providing one of the more powerful methods for controlling the maximal temperature *in vivo*.

Maghemite nanoparticles encapsulated in polymer matrix beads have been tested successfully for the treatment of macroscopic liver tumors [172, 173], which were introduced through the arterial embolization method, taking advantage of the fact that liver tumors take their blood supply from the hepatic arterial system. Such beads appear to be safe and well-tolerated as there was no significant hepatic clearance 28 days after injection [174]. Under inductive applicator conditions of 53 kHz and 30 kA^{-1}, an intratumoral temperature of 48 °C was reached after 5 min. Smaller magnetic nanoparticles have also been investigated for magnetic hyperthermia. Magnetite nanoparticles from ferrofluids coated with dextran can be taken up by carcinoma cells. However, cellular uptake of these dextran-iron oxide nanoparticles was low. To solve this problem, magnetic nanoparticles were coated with aminosilane groups; *in vitro* cellular uptake of such nanoparticles in globlastoma cells was found to be 1000× higher than for their dextran-magnetite counterparts [175]. To further improve mediator uptake by cancer cells for better intracellular hyperthermia treatment efficacy, monoclonal IgG antibody was immobilized onto the surface of PEG-coated magnetite nanoparticles [176]. These particles exhibited an improved *in vitro* specificity for cancer cells and, thus, higher cellular uptake by tumor cells than non-functionalized PEG-magnetite nanoparticles. Similar investigations using various antibodies and their fragments for labeling magnetoliposomes have also been tested for improving the cellular uptake of magnetic liposomes during hyperthermia experiments [177–179]. *In vivo* experiments were performed by injecting these magnetic liposomes into the tumor-harboring mice. Most of the mediators accumulated in the tumor tissue while the rest were distributed in liver and spleen. After these mice were exposed to an AC magnetic field, the temperature of the tumor tissue increased and the growth of tumor usually ceased over a period of time [177–179]. However, few studies have been reported on the administration of mediators through i.v. injections. Functionalization of magnetic nanoparticles for *in vivo* hyperthermia is still in its early stages. Collaboration between materials scientists and hyperthermia experts is needed to further develop this promising therapy.

3.5 Conclusions

This chapter has summarized recent advances in the synthesis of functional biomolecule–magnetic nanoparticle hybrid systems. The uses of such biofunctionalized nanoparticles for *in vitro* protein/cell isolation and immobilization of biocatalysts for drug synthesis as well as *in vivo* applications such as drug targeting, MR imaging and hyperthermia therapies have been discussed. Nanometer-sized magnetic particles have many advantages over their micrometer counterparts in biomedical applications due to the unique physical, chemical and physiological properties associated with their small dimensions. A combination of the unusual properties of nanomaterials and biomaterials provides a unique opportunity for physicists, chemists, biologists, material scientists and experts from many other fields to mold this new area of nanobiotechnology. Based on recent advances in the field, exciting new science and novel systems can be anticipated from such an interdisciplinary effort.

Acknowledgments

Financial support from the SIU Materials Technology Center, American Cancer Society and the NSF through a career award to Y.G. is acknowledged.

References

1 Cornell, R. M., Schwertmann, U. *The Iron Oxides: Structure, Properties, Reactions, Occurrence and Uses*, VCH, New York, 1996.

2 Schmid, G. *Nanoparticles: From Theory to Applications*, Wiley-VCH, Weinheim, 2004.

3 Häfeli, U., Schütt, W., Teller, J., Zborowski, M. *Scientific and Clinical Applications of Magnetic Carriers*, Plenum, New York, 1996.

4 Mornet, S., Vasseur, S., Grasset, F., Duguet, E., Magnetic nanoparticle design for medical diagnosis and therapy. *J. Mater. Chem.* **2004**, *14*, 2161–2175.

5 Pankhurst, Q. A., Connolly, J., Jones, S. K., Dobson, J., Applications of magnetic nanoparticles in biomedicine. *J. Phys. D: Appl. Phys.* **2003**, *36*, R167–R181.

6 Berry, C. C., Curtis, A. S. G., Functionalisation of magnetic nanoparticles for applications in biomedicine. *J. Phys. D: Appl. Phys.* **2003**, *36*, R198–R206.

7 Bauer, L. A., Birenbaum, N. S., Meyer, G. J., Biological applications of high aspect ratio nanoparticles. *J. Mater. Chem.* **2004**, *14*, 517–526.

8 Katz, E., Willner, I., Integrated nanoparticle-biomolecule hybrid systems: synthesis, properties and applications. *Angew. Chem. Int. Ed.* **2004**, *43*, 6042–6108.

9 Tartaj, P., Morales, M. D. P., Veintemillas-Verdaguer, S., González-Cappreño, T., Serna, C. J., The preparation of magnetic nanoparticles for applications in biomedicine. *J. Phys. D: Appl. Phys.* **2003**, *36*, R182–R197.

10 Niemeyer, C. M., Nanoparticles, proteins, and nucleic acids: biotechnology meets materials science. *Angew. Chem. Int. Ed.* **2001**, *40*, 4128–4158.

11 Landfester, K., Pamírez, L. P., Encapsulated magnetic particles for biomedical applications. *J. Phys.: Condens. Matter.* **2003**, *15*, S1345–S1361.

12 Matsunaga, T., Okamura, Y., Tanaka, T., Biotechnological applications of nano-scale engineered bacterial magnetic particles. *J. Mater. Chem.* **2004**, *14*, 2099–2115.

13 Puntes, A. F., Krishnan, K. M., Alivisatos, A. P., Colloidal nanocrystal shape and size control: the case of cobalt. *Science* **2001**, *291*, 2115–2117.

14 Sun, S., Murray, C. B., Weller, D., Folks, L., Moser, A., Monodisperse FePt nanoparticles and ferromagnetic FePt nanocrystal superlattices. *Science* **2000**, *287*, 1989–1992.

15 Park, J., An, K., Hwang, Y., Park, J.-G., Noh, H.-J., Kim, J.-Y., Park, J.-H., Hwang, N.-M., Hyeon, T., Ultra-large-scale synthesis of mono-

disperse nanocrystals. *Nat. Mater.* **2004**, *3*, 891–895.
16 Redl, F. X., Cho, K.-S., Murray, C. B., O'Brien, S., Three-dimensional binary superlattices of magnetic nanocrystals and semiconductor quantum dots. *Nature*, **2003**, *423*, 968–971.
17 Song, Q., Zhang, Z. J., Shape control and associated magnetic properties of spinel cobalt ferrite nanocrystals. *J. Am. Chem. Soc.* **2004**, *126*, 6164–6168.
18 Ngo, A. T., Pileni, M. P., Nanoparticles of cobalt ferrite: influence of the applied field on the organization of the nanocrystals on a substrate and on their magnetic properties. *Adv. Mater.* **2000**, *12*, 276–279.
19 Shafi, K. V. P., Ulman, A., Yan, X., Yang, N.-L., Estournes, C., White, H., Rafailovich, M., Sonochemical synthesis of functionalized amorphous iron oxide nanoparticles. *Langmuir*, **2001**, *17*, 5093–5097.
20 Jana, N. R., Chen, Y., Peng, X., Size- and shape-controlled magnetic (Cr, Mn, Fe, Co, Ni) oxide nanocrystals via a simple and general approach. *Chem. Mater.* **2004**, *16*, 3931–3935.
21 Li, Z., Chen, H., Bao, H., Gao, M., One-pot reaction to synthesize water-soluble magnetic nanocrystals. *Chem. Mater.* **2004**, *16*, 1391–1393.
22 Sun, S., Zeng, H., Robinson, D. B., Raoux, S., Rice, P. M., Wang, S. X., Li, G., Monodisperse MFe_2O_4 (M = Fe, Co, Mn) nanoparticles. *J. Am. Chem. Soc.* **2004**, *126*, 273–279.
23 Tartaj, P., Serna, C. J., Synthesis of monodisperse superparamagnetic Fe/Silica nanospherical composites. *J. Am. Chem. Soc.* **2004**, *125*, 15754–15755.
24 Teng, X., Yang, H., Synthesis of face-centered tetragonal FePt nanoparticles and granular films from $Pt@Fe_2O_3$ core-shell nanoparticles. *J. Am. Chem. Soc.* **2003**, *125*, 14559–14563.
25 Ji, T., Jian, W.-B., Fang, J., The first synthesis of $Pb_{1-x}Mn_xSe$ nanocrystals. *J. Am. Chem. Soc.* **2003**, *125*, 8448–8449.
26 Shevchenko, E. V., Talapin, D. V., Schnablegger, H., Kornowski, A., Festin, Ö., Svedlindh, P., Haase, M., Weller, H., Study of nucleation and growth in the organometallic synthesis of magnetic alloy nanocrystals: the role of nucleation rate in size control of $CoPt_3$ nanocrystals. *J. Am. Chem. Soc.* **2003**, *125*, 9090–9101.
27 Li, Q., Li, H., Pol, V. G., Bruckental, I., Koltypin, Y., Calderon-Moreno, J., Nowik, I., Gedanken, A., Sonochemical synthesis, structural and magnetic properties of air-stable Fe/Co alloy nanoparticles. *New. J. Chem.* **2003**, *27*, 1194–1199.
28 Carnes, C. L., Klabunde, K. J., Unique chemical reactivities of nanocrystalline metal oxides toward hydrogen sulfide. *Chem. Mater.* **2002**, *14*, 1806–1811.
29 Fried T., Shemer, G., Markovich, G., Ordered two-dimensional arrays of ferrite nanoparticles. *Adv. Mater.* **2001**, *13*, 1158–1161.
30 Bourlinos, A. B., Simopoulos, A., Petridis, D., Synthesis of capped ultrafine γ-Fe_2O_3 particles from iron(III) hydroxide caprylate: a novel starting material for readily attainable organosols. *Chem. Mater.* **2002**, *14*, 899–903.
31 Lu, J., Fan, J., Xu, R., Roy, S., Ali, N., Gao, Y., Synthesis of alkyl sulfonate/alcohol-protected γ-Fe_2O_3 nanocrystals with narrow size distributions. *J. Colloid Interface Sci.* **2003**, *258*, 427–431.
32 Lyon, J. L., Fleming, D. A., Stone, M. B., Schiffer, P., Williams, M. E., Synthesis of Fe oxide core/Au shell nanoparticles by iterative hydroxylamine seeding. *Nano Lett.* **2004**, *4*, 719–723.
33 Vaucher, S., Fielden, J., Li, M., Dujardin, E., Mann, S., Molecule-based magnetic nanoparticles: synthesis of cobalt hexacyanoferrate, cobalt pentacyanonitrosylferrate, and chromium hexacyanochromate coordination polymers in water-in-oil microemulsions. *Nano Lett.* **2002**, *2*, 225–229.

34 Mooney, K. E., Nelson, J. A., Wagner, M. J., Superparamagnetic cobalt ferrite nanocrystals synthesized by alkalide reduction. *Chem. Mater.* **2004**, *16*, 3155–3161.

35 Gu, H., Zheng, R., Zhang, X., Xu, B., Facile one-pot synthesis of bifunctional heterodimers of nanoparticles: a conjugate of quantum dot and magnetic nanoparticles. *J. Am. Chem. Soc.* **2004**, *126*, 5664–5665.

36 Kang, Y. S., Risbud, S., Rabolt, J. F., Stroeve, P., Synthesis and characterization of nanometer-sized Fe_3O_4 and γ-Fe_2O_3 particles. *Chem. Mater.* **1996**, *8*, 2209–2211.

37 Elkins, K. E., Vedantam, T. S., Liu, J. P., Zeng, H., Sun, S., Ding, Y., Wang, Z. L., Ultrafine FePt nanoparticles prepared by the chemical reduction method. *Nano Lett.* **2003**, *3*, 1647–1649.

38 Hou, Y., Kondoh, H., Kogure, T., Ohta, T., Preparation and characterization of monodisperse FePd nanoparticles. *Chem. Mater.* **2004**, *16*, 5149–5152.

39 Majetich, S. A., Jin, Y., Magnetization directions of individual nanoparticles. *Science* **1999**, *284*, 470–473.

40 Gambardella, P., Rusponi, S., Veronese, M., Dhesi, S. S., Grazioli, C., Dallmeyer, A., Cabria, I., Zeller, R., Dederichs, P. H., Kern, K., Carbone, C., Brune, H., Giant magnetic anisotropy of single cobalt atoms and nanoparticles. *Science* **2003**, *300*, 1130–1133.

41 Dormann, J. L., Fiorani, D. *Magnetic Properties of Fine Particles*, North-Holland, New York, 1991.

42 Portet, D., Denizot, B., Rump, E., Lejeune, J.-J., Jallet, P., Nonpolymeric coatings of iron oxide colloids for biological use as magnetic resonance imaging contrast agents. *J. Colloid Interface Sci.* **2001**, *238*, 37–42.

43 Moghimi, S. M., Hunter, A. C., Murray, J. C., Long-circulating and target-specific nanoparticles: theory to practice. *Pharmacol. Rev.* **2001**, *2*, 283–318.

44 Hyeon, T., Chemical synthesis of magnetic nanoparticles. *Chem. Commun.* **2003**, 927–934.

45 Vestal, C. R., Zhang, J., Effects of surface coordination chemistry on the magnetic properties of $MnFe_2O_4$ spinel ferrite nanoparticles. *J. Am. Chem. Soc.* **2003**, *125*, 9828–9833.

46 Mikhaylova, M., Kim, D. K., Bobrysheva, N., Osmolowsky, M., Semenov, V., Tsakalakos, T., Muhammed, M., Superparamagnetism of magnetic nanoparticles: dependence on surface modification. *Langmuir* **2004**, *20*, 2472–2477.

47 Gradmann, U., Surface magnetism. *J. Magn. Magn. Mater.* **1991**, *100*, 481–496.

48 Tronc, E., Ezzir, A., Cherkaoui, R., Chaneac, C., Nogues, M., Kachkachi, H., Fiorani, D., Testa, A. M., Greneche, J. M., Jolivet, J. P., Surface-related properties of γ-Fe_2O_3 nanoparticles. *J. Magn. Magn. Mater.* **2000**, *221*, 63–79.

49 Gazeau, F., Bacri, J. C., Gendron, F., Perzynski, R., Raikher, Y. L., Stepanov, V. I., Dubois, E., Magnetic resonance of ferrite nanoparticles: evidence of surface effects. *J. Magn. Magn. Mater.* **1998**, *186*, 175–187.

50 Kodama, R. H., Berkowitz, A. E., McNiff, E. J., Jr., Foner, S., Surface spin disorder in ferrite nanoparticles. *J. Appl. Phys.* **1997**, *81*, 5552–5557.

51 Fan, J., Lu, J., Xu, R., Jiang, R., Gao, Y., Use of water-dispersible Fe_2O_3 nanoparticles with narrow size distributions in isolating avidin. *J. Colloid Interface Sci.* **2003**, *266*, 215–218.

52 Xu, C., Xu, K., Gu, H., Zheng, R., Liu, H., Zhang, X., Guo, Z., Xu, B., Dopamine as a robust anchor to immobilize functional molecules on the iron oxide shell of magnetic nanoparticles. *J. Am. Chem. Soc.* **2004**, *126*, 9938–9939.

53 Tripp, S. L., Pusztay, S. V., Ribbe, A. E., Wei, A., Self-assembly of cobalt nanoparticle rings. *J. Am. Chem. Soc.* **2002**, *124*, 7914–7915.

54 Xu, C., Xu, K., Gu, H., Zhong, X., Guo, Z., Zheng, R., Zhang, X., Xu, B., Nitrilotriacetic acid-modified

magnetic nanoparticles as a general agent to bind histidine-tagged proteins. *J. Am. Chem. Soc.* **2004**, *126*, 3392–3393.

55 Gu, H., Ho, P.-L., Tsang, K. W. T., Wang, L., Xu, B., Using biofunctional magnetic nanoparticles to capture vancomycin-resistant enterococci and other gram-positive bacteria at ultralow concentration. *J. Am. Chem. Soc.* **2003**, *125*, 15702–15703.

56 Kumar, C. S. S. R., Leuschner, C., Doomes, E. E., Henry, L., Juban, M., Hormes, J., Efficacy of lytic peptide-bound magnetite nanoparticles in destroying breast cancer cells. *J. Nanosci. Nanotech.* **2004**, *4*, 245–249.

57 Chen, D. W., Liao, M. H., Preparation and characterization of YADH-bound magnetic nanoparticles. *J. Mol. Catal. B: Enzym* **2002**, *16*, 283–291.

58 Ho, K.-C., Tsai, P.-J., Lin, Y.-S., Chen, Y.-C., Using biofunctionalized nanoparticles to probe pathogenic bacteria. *Anal. Chem.* **2004**, *76*, 7162–7168.

59 Zhao, X., Tapec-Dytioco, R., Wang, K., Tan, W., Collection of trace amounts of DNA/mRNA molecules using genomagnetic nanocapturers. *Anal. Chem.* **2003**, *75*, 3476–3483.

60 Boal, A. K., Das, K., Gray, M., Rotello, V. M., Monolayer exchange chemistry of γ-Fe_2O_3 nanoparticles. *Chem. Mater.* **2002**, *14*, 2628–2636.

61 Bourlinos, A. B., Bakandritsos, A., Georgakilas, V., Petridis, D., Surface modification of ultrafine magnetic iron oxide particles. *Chem. Mater.* **2002**, *14*, 3226–3228.

62 Wang, Y., Wong, J. F., Teng, X., Lin, X. Z., Yang, H., "Pulling" nanoparticles into water: phase transfer of oleic acid stabilized monodisperse nanoparticles into aqueous solutions of α-cyclodextrin. *Nano Lett.* **2003**, *3*, 1555–1559.

63 Bucak, S., Jones, D. A., Laibinis, P. E., Hatton, T. A., Protein separation using colloidal magnetic nanoparticles. *Biotechnol. Prog.* **2003**, *19*, 477–484.

64 Kohler, N., Fryxell, G. E., Zhang, M., A bifunctional poly(ethylene glycol) silane immobilized on metallic oxide-based nanoparticles for conjugation with cell targeting agents. *J. Am. Chem. Soc.* **2004**, *126*, 7206–7211.

65 Reddy, J. A., Low, P. S., Folate-mediated targeting of therapeutic and imaging agents to cancers. *Crit. Rev. Ther. Drug Carrier Syst.*, **1998**, *15*, 587–627.

66 Hirsch, R., Katz, E., Willner, I., Magneto-switchable bioelectrocatalysis. *J. Am. Chem. Soc.* **2000**, *122*, 12053–12054.

67 Ennas, G., Musinu, A., Piccaluga, G., Zedda, D., Gatteschi, D., Sangregorio, C., Stanger, J. L., Concas, G., Spano, G., Characterization of iron oxide nanoparticles in an Fe_2O_3-SiO_2 composite prepared by a sol-gel method. *Chem. Mater.* **1998**, *10*, 495–502.

68 Grasset, F., Labhsetwar, N., Li, D., Park, D. C., Saito, N., Haneda, H., Cador, O., Roisnel, T., Mornet, S., Duguet, E., Portier, J., Etourneau, J., Synthesis and magnetic characterization of zinc ferrite nanoparticles with different environments: powder, colloidal solution, and zinc ferrite-silica core-shell nanoparticles. *Langmuir* **2002**, *18*, 8209–8216.

69 Vestal, C. R., Zhang, Z. J., Synthesis and magnetic characterization of Mn and Co spinel ferrite-silica nanoparticles with tunable magnetic core. *Nano Lett.* **2003**, *3*, 1739–1743.

70 Lu, H., Yi, G., Zhao, S., Chen, D., Guo, L.-H., Cheng, J., Synthesis and characterization of multi-functional magnetic, up-conversion fluorescence and bio-affinity properties. *J. Mater. Chem.* **2004**, *14*, 1336–1341.

71 del Monte, F., Morales, M. P., Levy, D., Fernandez, A., Ocaña, M., Roig, A., Molins, E., O'Grady, K., Serna, C. J., Formation of γ-Fe_2O_3 isolated nanoparticles in a silica matrix. *Langmuir* **1997**, *13*, 3627–3634.

72 Hutlova, A., Niznansky, D., Rehspringer, J.-L., Estournès, C., Kurmoo, M., High coercive field for nanoparticles of $CoFe_2O_4$ in

amorphous silica sol-gel. *Adv. Mater.* **2003**, *15*, 1622–1625.

73 Kobayashi, Y., Horie, M., Konno, M., Rodríguez-González, B., Liz-Martzán, L. M., Preparation and properties of silica-coated cobalt nanoparticles. *J. Phys. Chem. B.* **2003**, *107*, 7420–7425.

74 Lu, Y., Yin, Y., Mayers, B. T., Xia, Y., Modifying the surface properties of superparamagnetic iorn oxide nanoparticles through a sol-gel approach. *Nano Lett.* **2002**, *2*, 183–186.

75 Gao, X., Yu, K. M. K., Tam, K. Y., Tsang, S. C., Colloidal stable silica encapsulated nano-magnetic composite as a novel bio-catalyst carrier. *Chem. Commun.* **2003**, 2998–2999.

76 Aliev, F. G., Correa-Duarte, M. A., Mamedov, A., Ostrander, J. W., Giersig, M., Liz-Marzán, L. M., Kotov, N. A., Layer-by-layer assembly of core/shell magnetite nanoparticles: effect of silica coating on interparticle interactions and magnetic properties. *Adv. Mater.* **1999**, *11*, 1006–1010.

77 Stöber, W., Fink, A., Bohn, E., Controlled growth of monodisperse silica spheres in the micron size range. *J. Colloid Interface Sci.* **1968**, *26*, 62–69.

78 Caruso, F. in *Colloids and Colloid Assemblies*, Caruso, F. (Ed.), Wiley-VCH: Weinheim, 2004, pp. 246–283.

79 Li, G., Fan, J., Jiang, R., Gao, Y., Cross-linking the linear polymeric chains in the ATRP synthesis of iron oxide/polystyrene core/shell nanoparticles. *Chem. Mater.* **2004**, *16*, 1835–1837.

80 Matyjaszewski, K., Xia, J., Atom transfer radical polymerization. *Chem. Rev.* **2001**, *101*, 2921–2990.

81 Vestal, C. R., Zhang, Z. J., Atom transfer radical polymerization synthesis and magnetic characterization of $MnFe_2O_4$/polystyrene core/shell nanoparticles. *J. Am. Chem. Soc.* **2002**, *124*, 14312–14313.

82 Wang, Y., Teng, X., Wang, J.-S., Yang, H., Solvent-free atom transfer radical polymerization in the synthesis of Fe_2O_3@polystyrene core-shell nanoparticles. *Nano Lett.* **2003**, *3*, 789–793.

83 Chen, X. Y., Armes, S. P., Greaves, S. J., Watts, J. F., Synthesis of hydrophilic polymer-grafted ultrafine inorganic oxide particles in protic media at ambient temperature via atom transfer radical polymerization: use of an electrostatically adsorbed polyelectrolytic macroinitiator. *Langmuir* **2004**, *20*, 587–595.

84 Moeser, G. D., Green, W. H., Laibinis, P. E., Linse, P., Hatton, T. A., Structure of polymer-stabilized magnetic fluids: small-angle neutron scattering and mean-field lattice modeling. *Langmuir* **2004**, *20*, 5223–5234.

85 Jin, J., Qiu, S., Lewis, K., Klibanov, A. M., Bactericidal properties of flat surfaces and nanoparticles derivatized with alkylated polyethylenimines. *Biotechnol. Prog.* **2002**, *18*, 1082–1086.

86 Sun, Y.-P., Rollins, H. W., Guduru, R., Preparation of nickel, cobalt, and iron nanoparticles through the rapid expansion of supercritical fluid solutions (RESS) and chemical reduction. *Chem. Mater.* **1999**, *11*, 7–9.

87 Sun, S., Anders, S., Hamann, H. F., Thiele, J.-U., Baglin, J. E. E., Thomson, T., Fullerton, E. E., Murray, C. B., Terris, B. D., Polymer mediated self-assembly of magnetic nanoparticles. *J. Am. Chem. Soc.* **2002**, *12*, 2884–2885.

88 Gómez-Lopera, S. A., Plaza, R. C., Delgado, A. V., Synthesis and characterization of spherical magnetite/biodegradable polymer composite particles. *J. Colloid Interface Sci.* **2001**, *240*, 40–47.

89 Deng, Y., Yang, W., Wang, C., Fu, S., A novel approach for preparation of thermoresponsive polymer magnetic microspheres with core-shell structure. *Adv. Mater.* **2003**, *15*, 1729–1732.

90 Liao, M.-H., Chen, D.-H., Preparation and characterization of a novel magnetic nano-adsorbent. *J. Mater. Chem.* **2002**, *12*, 3654–3659.

91 Yu, S., Chow, G. M., Carboxyl group ($-CO_2H$) functionalized ferromagnetic

iron oxide nanoparticles for potential bio-applications. *J. Mater. Chem.* **2004**, *14*, 2781–2786.

92 Tong, X.-D., Xue, B., Sun, Y., A novel magnetic affinity support for protein adsorption and purification. *Biotechnol. Prog.* **2001**, *17*, 134–139.

93 Rutnakornpituk, M., Thompson, M. S., Harris, L. A., Farmer, K. E., Esker, A. R., Riffle, J. S., Connolly, J., St. Pierre, T. G., Formation of cobalt nanoparticle dispersions in the presence of polysiloxane block copolymers. *Polymer* **2002**, *43*, 2337–2348.

94 Cole-Hamilton, D. J., Homogeneous catalysis-new approaches to catalyst separation, recovery, and recycling. *Science* **2003**, *299*, 1702–1706.

95 Dayal, A., Loos, K., Noto, M., Chang, S. W., Spagnoli, C., Shafi, K. V. P. M., Ulman, A., Cowman, M., Gross, R. A., Activity of *Candida rugosa* lipase immobilized on γ-Fe_2O_3 magnetic nanoparticles. *J. Am. Chem. Soc.* **2003**, *125*, 1684–1685.

96 Koneracka, M., Kopcansky, P., Timko, M., Ramchand, C. N., de Sequeira, A., Trevan, M., Direct binding procedure of proteins and enzymes to fine magnetic particles. *J. Mol. Catal. B: Enzym.* **2002**, *18*, 13–18.

97 Yoon, T.-J., Lee, W., Oh, Y.-S., Lee, J.-K., Magnetic nanoparticles as a catalyst vehicle for simple and easy recycling. *New. J. Chem.* **2003**, *27*, 227–229.

98 Stevens, P. D., Fan, J., Gardimalla, H. M. R., Yen, M., Gao, Y., Superparamagnetic nanoparticle-supported catalysis of Suzuki cross-coupling reactions, *Org. Lett.* **2005**, *11*, 2085–2088.

99 Babincova, M., Sourivong, P., Leszczynska, D., Babinec, P., Blood-specific whole-body electromagnetic hyperthermia. *Med. Hypoth.* **2000**, *55*, 459–460.

100 Muller, R. N., Roch, A., Colet, J.-M., Ouakssim, A., Gillis, P. in *The Chemistry of Contrast Agents in Medical Magnetic Resonance Imaging*, Merbach, A. E., Tóth, E. (Eds.), Wiley: Chichester, 2001, pp. 417–435.

101 Pantopoulos, K., Iron metabolism and the IRE/IRP regulatory system: an update. *Ann. N. Y. Acad. Sci.* **2004**, *1012*, 1–13.

102 Dobson, J., Nanoscale biogenic iron oxides and neurodegenerative disease. *FEBS Lett.* **2001**, *496*, 1–5.

103 Hume, D. A., Ross, I. L., Himes, S. R., Sasmono, R. T., Wells, C. A., Ravasi, T., The mononuclear phagocyte system revisited. *J. Leukocyte Biol.* **2002**, *72*, 621–627.

104 Davis, S. S., Biomedical applications of nanotechnology – implications for drug targeting and gene therapy. *Trends Biotechnol.* **1997**, *15*, 217–224.

105 Moghimi, S. M., Patel, H. M., Serum-mediated recognition of liposomes by phagocytic cells of the reticuloendothelial system. The concept of tissue specificity. *Adv. Drug Delivery Rev.* **1998**, *32*, 45–60.

106 Gaur, U., Sahoo, S. K., De, T. K., Ghosh, P. C., Maitra, A., Ghosh, P. K., Biodistribution of fluoresceinated dextran using novel nanoparticles evading reticuloendothelial system. *Int. J. Pharm.* **2000**, *202*, 1–10.

107 Arbab, A. S., Yocum, G. T., Kalish, H., Jordan, E. K., Anderson, S. A., Khakoo, A. Y., Read, E. J., Frank, J. A., Efficient magnetic cell labeling with protamine sulfate complexed to ferumoxides for cellular MRI. *Blood* **2004**, *104*, 1217–1223.

108 Berry, C. C., Charles, S., Wells, S., Dalby, M. J., Curtis, A. S. G., The influence of transferrin stabilised magnetic nanoparticles on human dermal fibroblasts in culture. *Int. J. Pharm.* **2004**, *269*, 211–225.

109 Moghimi, S. M., Hunter, A. C., Poloxamers and poloxamines in nanoparticle engineering and experimental medicine. *Trends Biotechnol.* **2000**, *18*, 412–420.

110 Moghimi, S. M., Prolonging the circulation time and modifying the body distribution of intravenously injected polystyrene nanospheres by prior intravenous administration of poloxamine-908. A 'hepatic-blockade' event or manipulation of nanosphere surface in vivo? *Biochim. Biophys. Acta* **1997**, *1336*, 1–6.

111 Molineux, G., PEGylation: engineering improved pharmaceuticals for enhanced therapy. *Cancer Treatment Rev.* **2002**, *28*, 13–16.

112 Gao, X., Cui, Y., Levenson, R. M., Chung, L. W. K., Nie, S., *In vivo* targeting and imaging with semiconductor quantum dots. *Nat. Biotechnol.* **2004**, *22*, 969–976.

113 Bonnemain, B., Superparamagnetic agents in magnetic resonance imaging. Physicochemical characteristics and clinical applications. A review. *J. Drug Targeting* **1998**, *6*, 167–174.

114 Lauffer, R. B., Paramagnetic metal complexes as water proton relaxation agents for NMR imaging: theory and design. *Chem. Rev.* **1987**, *87*, 901–927.

115 Brown, M. A., Semelka, R. C. *MRI: Basic Principles and Applications*, Wiley, New York, 2003.

116 Bulte, J. W. M., Brooks, R. A., Moskowitz, B. M., Bryant, L. H., Jr., Frank, J. A., Relaxometry and magnetometry of the MR contrast agent MION-46L. *Magn. Reson. Med.* **1999**, *42*, 379–384.

117 Gillis, P., Koenig, S. H., Transverse relaxation of solvent protons induced by magnetized spheres: application to ferritin, erythrocytes, and magnetite. *Magn. Reson. Med.* **1987**, *5*, 323–345.

118 Muller, R. N., Gillis, P., Moiny, F., Roch, A., Transverse relaxivity of particulate MRI contrast media: from theories to experiments. *Magn. Reson. Med.*, **1991**, *22*, 178–182.

119 Brigger, I., Dubernet, C., Couvreur, P., Nanoparticles in cancer therapy and diagnosis. *Adv. Drug Delivery Rev.* **2002**, *54*, 631–651.

120 Molday, R. S., MacKenzie, D., Immunospecific ferromagnetic iron-dextran reagents for the labeling and magnetic separation of cells. *J. Immunol. Methods* **1982**, *52*, 353–367.

121 Grüttner, C., Teller, J., Schütt, W., Westphal, F., Schümichen, C., Paulke, B.-R. in *Scientific and Clinical Applications of Magnetic Carriers*, Häfeli, U., Schütt, W., Teller, J., Zborowski, M. (Eds.), Plenum: New York, 1996, pp. 53–67.

122 Kim, D. K., Mikhaylova, M., Wang, F. H., Kehr, J., Bjelke, B., Zhang, Y., Tsakalakos, T., Muhammed, M., Starch-coated superparamagnetic nanoparticles as MR contrast agents. *Chem. Mater.* **2003**, *15*, 4343–4351.

123 Byrne, S. J., Corr, S. A., Gun'ko, Y. K., Kelly, J. M., Brougham, D. F., Ghosh, S., Magnetic nanoparticle assemblies on denatured DNA show unusual magnetic relaxivity and potential applications for MRI. *Chem. Commun.* **2004**, 2560–2561.

124 Kalish, H., Arbab, A. S., Miller, B. R., Lewis, B. K., Zywicke, H. A., Bulte, J. W. M., Bryan, L. H., Jr., Frank, J. A., Combination of transfection agents and magnetic resonance contrast agents for cellular imaging: relationship between relaxivities, electrostatic forces, and chemical composition. *Magn. Reson. Med.* **2003**, *50*, 275–282.

125 Van Beers, B. E., Pringot, J., Gallez, B., Iron oxides as contrast agents for MRI of the liver. *J. Radiol.* **1995**, *76*, 991–995.

126 Kubaska, S., Sahani, D. V., Saini, S., Hahn, P. F., Halpern, E., Dual contrast enhanced magnetic resonance imaging of the liver with superparamagnetic iron oxide followed by gadolinium for lesion detection and characterization. *Clin. Radiology* **2001**, *56*, 410–415.

127 Halavaara, J., Tervahartiala, P., Isoniemi, H., Hockerstedt, K., Efficacy of sequential use of superparamagnetic iron oxide and gadolinium in liver MR imaging. *Acta Radiol.* **2002**, *43*, 180–185.

128 Reimer, P., Balzer, T., Ferucarbotran (Resovist): a new clinically approved RES-specific contrast agent for contrast-enhanced MRI of the liver: properties, clinical development, and applications. *Eur. Radiol.* **2003**, *13*, 1266–1276.

129 Fahlvik, A. K., Holtz, E., Klaveness, J., Relaxation efficacy of paramagnetic and superparamagnetic microspheres in liver and spleen. *Magn. Res. Imaging* **1990**, *8*, 363–369.

130 Gellissen, J., Axmann, C., Prescher,

A., Bohndorf, K., Lodemann, K.-P., Extra- and intracellular accumulation of ultrasmall superparamagnetic iron oxides (USPIO) in experimentally induced abscesses of the peripheral soft tissues and their effects on magnetic resonance imaging. *Magn. Reson. Imaging* **1999**, *17*, 557–567.

131 Muhler, A., Zhang, X., Wang, H., Lawaczeck, R., Weinmann, H. J., Investigation of mechanisms influencing the accumulation of ultrasmall superparamagnetic iron oxide particles in lymph nodes. *Invest. Radiol.* **1995**, *30*, 98–103.

132 Moore, A., Marecos, E., Bogdanov, A., Jr., Weissleder, R., Tumoral distribution of long-circulating dextran-coated iron oxide nanoparticles in a rodent model. *Radiology* **2000**, *214*, 568–574.

133 Guimaraes, R., Clement, O., Bittoun, J., Carnot, F., Frija, G., MR lymphography with superparamagnetic iron nanoparticles in rats: pathologic basis for contrast enhancement. *Am. J. Roentgenol.* **1994**, *162*, 201–207.

134 Bellin, M. F., Lebleu, L., Meric, J. B., Evaluation of retroperitoneal and pelvic lymph node metastases with MRI and MR lymphangiography. *Abdom. Imaging* **2003**, *28*, 155–163.

135 Réty, F., Clément, O., Siauve, N., Cuénod, C.-A., Carnot, F., Sich, M., Buisine, A., Frija, G., MR lymphography using iron oxide nanoparticles in rats: pharmacokinetics in the lymphatic system after intravenous injection. *J. Magn. Reson. Imaging* **2000**, *12*, 734–739.

136 Cerdan, S., Lotscher, H. R., Kunnecke, B., Seelig, J., Monoclonal antibody-coated magnetite particles as contrast agents in magnetic resonance imaging of tumors. *Magn. Reson. Med.* **1989**, *12*, 151–163.

137 Weissleder, R., Lee, A. S., Fischman, A. J., Reimer, P., Shen, T., Wilkinson, R., Callahan, R. J., Brady, T. J., Polyclonal human immunoglobulin G labeled with polymeric iron oxide: antibody MR imaging. *Radiology* **1991**, *181*, 245–249.

138 Remsen, L. G., McCormick, C. I., Roman-Goldstein, S., Nilaver, G., Weissleder, R., Bogdanov, A., Hellstrom, I., Kroll, R. A., Neuwelt, E. A., MR of carcinoma-specific monoclonal antibody conjugated to monocrystalline iron oxide nanoparticles: the potential for noninvasive diagnosis. *Am. J. Neuroradiol.* **1996**, *17*, 411–418.

139 Moore, A., Medarova, Z., Potthast, A., Dai, G., In vivo targeting of underglycosylated MUC-1 tumor antigen using a multimodal imaging probe. *Cancer Res.* **2004**, *64*, 1821–1827.

140 Palmacci, S., Josephson, L., Synthesis of polysaccharide covered superparamagnetic oxide colloids. *U.S. Pat.* 5,262,176, 1993.

141 Josephson, L., Tung, C.-H., Moore, A., Weissleder, R., High-efficiency intracellular magnetic labeling with novel superparamagnetic-Tat peptide conjugates. *Bioconjugate Chem.* **1999**, *10*, 186–191.

142 Choi, H., Choi, S. R., Zhou, R., Kung, H. F., Chen, I.-W., Iron oxide nanoparticles as magnetic resonance contrast agent for tumor imaging via folate receptor-targeted delivery. *Acad. Radiol.* **2004**, *11*, 996–1004.

143 Lok, C., Picture perfect. *Nature* **2001**, *412*, 372–374.

144 Sipe, J. C., Filippi, M., Martino, G., Furlan, R., Rocca, M. A., Rovaris, M., Bergami, A., Zyroff, J., Scotti, G., Comi, G., Method for intracellular magnetic labeling of human mononuclear cells using approved iron contrast agents. *Magn. Reson. Imaging* **1999**, *17*, 1521–1523.

145 Moore, A., Marecos, E., Bogdanov, A., Jr., Weissleder, R., Tumoral distribution of long-circulating dextran-coated iron oxide nanoparticles in a rodent model. *Radiology* **2000**, *214*, 568–574.

146 Schulze, E., Ferrucci, J. T., Jr., Poss, K., Lapointe, L., Bogdanova, A., Weissleder, R., Cellular uptake and trafficking of a prototypical

magnetic iron oxide label in vitro. *Invest. Radiol.* **1995**, *30*, 604–610.

147 Zhao, M., Kircher, M. F., Josephson, L., Weissleder, R., Differential conjugation of Tat peptide to superparamagnetic nanoparticles and its effects on cellular uptake. *Bioconjugate Chem.* **2002**, *13*, 840–844.

148 Koch, A. M., Reynolds, F., Kircher, M. F., Merkle, H. P., Weissleder, R., Josephson, L., Uptake and metabolism of a dual fluorochrome Tat-nanoparticle in HeLa cells. *Bioconjugate Chem.* **2003**, *14*, 1115–1121.

149 Frankel, A. D., Pabo, C. O., Cellular uptake of the tat protein from human immunodeficiency virus. *Cell* **1988**, *55*, 1189–1193.

150 Zhang, Y., Kohler, N., Zhang, M., Surface modification of superparamagnetic magnetite nanoparticles and their intracellular uptake. *Biomaterials* **2002**, *23*, 1553–1561.

151 Stella, B., Arpicco, S., Peracchia, M. T., Desmaële, D., Hoebeke, J., Renoir, M., D'Angelo, J., Cattel, L., Couvreur, P., Design of folic-aid nanoparticles for drug targeting. *J. Pharm. Sci.* **2000**, *11*, 1452–1464.

152 Zhao, M., Beauregard, D. A., Loizou, L., Davletov, B., Brindle, K. M., Non-invasive detection of apoptosis using magnetic resonance imaging and a targeted contrast agent. *Nat. Med.* **2001**, *7*, 1241–1244.

153 Bulte, J. W., Douglas, T., Witwer, B., Zhang, S. C., Strable, E., Lewis, B. K., Zywicke, H., Miller, B., van Gelderen, P., Moskowitz, B. M., Duncan, I. D., Frank, J. A., Magnetodendrimers allow endosomal magnetic labeling and in vivo tracking of stem cells. *Nat. Biotechnol.* **2001**, *19*, 1141–1147.

154 Hogemann, D., Josephson, L., Weissleder, R., Basilion, J. P., Improvement of MRI probes to allow efficient detection of gene expression. *Bioconj. Chem.* **2000**, *11*, 941–946.

155 Moore, A., Josephson, L., Bhorade, R. M., Basilion, J. P., Weissleder, R., Human transferrin receptor gene as a marker gene for MR imaging. *Radiology* **2001**, *221*, 244–250.

156 Pulfer, S. K., Gallo, J. M. in *Scientific and Clinical Applications of Magnetic Carriers*, Häfeli, U., Schütt, W., Teller, J., Zborowski, M. (Eds.), Plenum: New York, 1996, pp. 445–455.

157 Widder, K. J., Morris, R. M., Poore, G. A., Howard, D. P., Senyei, A. E., Selective targeting of magnetic albumin microspheres containing low-dose doxorubicin: total remission in Yoshida sarcoma-bearing rats. *Eur. J. Cancer Clin. Oncol.* **1983**, *19*, 135–139.

158 Goodwin, S. C., Bittner, C. A., Peterson, C. L., Wong, G., Single-dose toxicity study of hepatic intra-arterial infusion of doxorubicin coupled to a novel magnetically targeted drug carrier. *Toxicol. Sci.* **2001**, *60*, 177–183.

159 Alexiou, C., Arnold, W., Klein, R. J., Parak, F. G., Hulin, P., Bergemann, C., Erhardt, W., Wagenpfeil, S., Lubbe, A. S., Locoregional cancer treatment with magnetic drug targeting. *Cancer Res.* **2000**, *60*, 6641–6648.

160 Lübbe, A. S., Alexiou, C., Bergemann, C., Clinical applications of magnetic drug targeting. *J. Surg. Res.* **2001**, *95*, 200–206.

161 Lübbe, A. S., Bergemann, C. in *Scientific and Clinical Applications of Magnetic Carriers*, Häfeli, U., Schütt, W., Teller, J., Zborowski, M. (Eds.), Plenum: New York, 1996, pp. 457–480.

162 Müller-Schulte, D., Füssl, F., Lueken, H., De Cuyper, M. in Ref. [161], pp. 517–526.

163 Häfeli, U., Pauer, G. J., Roberts, W. K., Humm, J. L., Macklis, R. M. in Ref. [161], pp. 501–516.

164 Häfeli, U., Pauer, G., Failing, S., Tapolsky, G., Radiolabeling of magnetic particles with rhenium-188 for cancer therapy. *J. Magn. Magn. Mater.* **2001**, *225*, 73–78.

165 Arbab, A. S., Jordan, E. K., Wilson, L. B., Yocum, G. T., Lewis, B. K., Frank, J. A., *In vivo* trafficking and targeted delivery of magnetically

labeled stem cells. *Human Gene Therapy* **2004**, *15*, 351–360.

166 Bergemann, C., Muller-Schulte, D., Oster, J., Brassard, L., Lübbe, A. S., Magnetic ion-exchange nano- and microparticles for medical, biochemical and molecular biological applications. *J. Magn. Magn. Mater.* **1999**, *194*, 45–52.

167 Hughes, C., Galea-Lauri, J., Farzaneh, F., Darling, D., Streptavidin paramagnetic particles provide a choice of three affinity-based capture and magnetic concentration strategies for retroviral vectors. *Mol. Therapy* **2001**, *3*, 623–630.

168 Scherer, F., Anton, M., Schillinger, U., Henke, J., Bergemann, C., Kruger, A., Gansbacher, B., Plank, C., Magnetofection: enhancing and targeting gene delivery by magnetic force in vitro and in vivo. *Gene Therapy* **2002**, *9*, 102–109.

169 Plank, C., Schillinger, U., Scherer, F., Bergemann, C., Remy, J.-S., Kroetz, F., Anton, M., Lausier, J., Rosenecker, J., The magnetofection method: Using magnetic force to enhance gene delivery. *Biol. Chem.* **2003**, *384*, 737–747.

170 Jordan, A., Scholz, R., Wust, P., Fähling, H., Felix, R., Magnetic fluid hyperthermia (MFH): cancer treatment with AC magnetic field induced excitation of biocompatible superparamagnetic nanoparticles. *J. Magn. Magn. Mater.* **1999**, *210*, 413–419.

171 Moroz, P., Jones, S. K., Gray, B. N., Magnetically mediated hyperthermia: current status and future directions. *Int. J. Hyperthermia* **2002**, *18*, 267–284.

172 Moroz, P., Jones, S. K., Gray, B. N., Arterial embolization hyperthermia in porcine renal tissue. *J. Surg. Res.*, **2002**, *105*, 209–214.

173 Moroz, P., Jones, S. K., Gray, B. N., Tumor response to arterial embolization hyperthermia and direct injection hyperthermia in a rabbit liver tumor model. *J. Surg. Oncol.* **2002**, *80*, 149–156.

174 Moroz, P., Jones, S. K., Metcalf, C., Gray, B. N., Hepatic clearance of arterially infused ferromagnetic particles. *Int. J. Hyperthermia* **2003**, *19*, 23–34.

175 Jordan, A., Scholz, R., Wust, P., Schirra, H., Schiestel, T., Schmidt, H., Felix, R., Endocytosis of dextran and silica-coated magnetite nanoparticles and the effect of intracellular hyperthermia on human mammary carcinoma cells in vitro. *J. Magn. Magn. Mater.* **1999**, *194*, 185–196.

176 Suzuki, M., Shinkai, M., Kamihira, M., Kobayashi, T., Preparation and characteristics of magnetite-labeled antibody with the use of poly(ethylene glycol) derivatives. *Biotechnol. Appl. Biochem.* **1995**, *21*, 335–345.

177 Ito, A., Kuga, Y., Honda, H., Kikkawa, H., Horiuchi, A., Watanabe, Y., Kobayashi, T., Magnetite nanoparticle-loaded anti-HER2 immunoliposomes for combination of antibody therapy with hyperthermia. *Cancer Lett.* **2004**, *212*, 167–175.

178 Le, B., Shinkai, M., Kitade, T., Honda, H., Yoshida, J., Wakabayashi, T., Kobayashi, T., Preparation of tumor-specific magnetoliposomes and their application for hyperthermia. *J. Chem. Eng. Jpn.* **2001**, *34*, 66–72.

179 Shinkai, M., Le, B., Honda, H., Yoshikawa, K., Shimizu, K., Saga, S., Wakabayashi, T., Yoshida, J., Kobayashi, T., Targeting hyperthermia for renal cell carcinoma using human MN antigen-specific magnetoliposomes. *Jpn. J. Cancer Res.* **2001**, *92*, 1138–1145.

4
Biofunctionalization of Gold Nanoparticles

Ming Zheng and Xueying Huang

4.1
Introduction

Gold (Au) as a precious material was first extracted in the 5th millennium BC [1]. The "soluble" gold, which we now call colloid gold, was developed around the 5th or 4th century BC [1]. Even though several scientists studied the formation and synthesis of colloid Au, such as using phosphorous in CS_2 to reduce chloroaurate ($AuCl_4^-$) [2], colloid Au did not gain wide attention or became a subject of broad interest in the scientific community until very recently, especially in the last decade. The interest in such tiny Au particles partially arises from the commercial and industrial needs for new, advanced materials. These particles are nanometer size materials with unique optic, electronic, and magnetic properties. Macrobiological molecules, also in the nanometer size range, possess functionalities that enable recognition and self-assembly. The integration of nanoparticles and biological molecules is very attractive and has gained tremendous attention from academics and industry, because such a combination could create new materials for electronics and optics, and lead to new applications in genomics, proteomics, and biomedical and bioanalytical areas [3–8]. To be integrated with biological molecules or be used in biological systems, Au nanoparticles (NPs) have to be soluble in aqueous solution. This chapter, therefore, is mainly focused on the synthesis of water-soluble Au NPs, their surface functionality and modification, and biological applications. Section 4.2 reviews two general synthetic routes for obtaining monolayer-protected Au nanoparticles. Examples of programmable assembly of these particles using biomolecules, i.e. DNA and proteins, are covered in Section 4.3. The problem of nonspecific binding between nanoparticles and biomolecules is discussed in Section 4.5. Finally, Section 4.6 reviews biological and biomedical applications of Au nanoparticles.

4.2
General Synthetic Routes

Generally, Au nanoparticles are synthesized by reduction of aurate salts, usually chloroaurate ($AuCl_4^-$) with reducing agents, such as sodium borohydride ($NaBH_4$),

Nanotechnologies for the Life Sciences Vol. 1
Biofunctionalization of Nanomaterials. Edited by Challa S. S. R. Kumar

ISBN: 3-527-31381-8

thiocyanate, phosphorus, citrate, ascorbic acid, and even ethyl alcohol [9]. The synthesized Au NPs have particle sizes ranging from sub-nanometer, e.g. 0.8 to 80 nm with their color changing from yellow-orange to red-purple to blue-green. The size of Au NPs determines their unique optical and electronic properties. Au NPs synthesized by the reduction of aurate salts are composed of an internal core of pure Au that is surrounded by a surface layer of adsorbed $AuCl^{2-}$ ions [9]. These negatively charged surfaces prevent Au NPs aggregating. However, these Au NPs are very sensitive to their environmental factors such as pH, temperature, electrolytes, and solvent. For these Au NPs to be utilized, a key issue is their surface chemistry and functionalization that determine their stability, functionality and applications. To solve this issue, various ligand-protected Au NPs have been synthesized recently, mainly by direct synthesis and ligand exchange reaction.

4.2.1
Direct Synthesis of Ligand-protected Au NPs

In the past three decades, two major classes of ligand-protected Au NPs have been developed. The first is phosphine-protected Au NPs, which were originally reported by McPartlin et al. in 1969 [10] and then modified by Cariati et al. in 1971 [11]. Synthesis was achieved through reduction by $NaBH_4$ of either an aurate salt, such as $HAuCl_4$ in the presence of triarylphosphine in a two-phase system of toluene and water, or Au(L)X (here L is triarylphosphine and X is an anion, such as I^-, SCN^-, or CN^-) in an organic solvent such as ethanol. As Au–P bonding is very weak the phosphine ligand could be easily replaced by other ligands. Apart from being used as the starting materials for other functionalized Au NPs, phosphine ligand-protected Au NPs have very limited use. The second class is thiol- or amine-ended ligand-protected Au NPs, first developed by Brust et al. in 1994 [12]. In their initial report, Brust et al. synthesized toluene-stable dodecanethiol-protected Au NP by using $NaBH_4$ to reduce $HAuCl_4$ in a two-phase system with tetraoctylammonium bromide as the phase-transfer, [Fig. 4.1(route a)]. Subsequently, they developed a one-phase synthesis by using methanol as the reaction solvent [13] [Fig. 4.1(route b)]. These Au NPs are mainly organic-soluble. Since

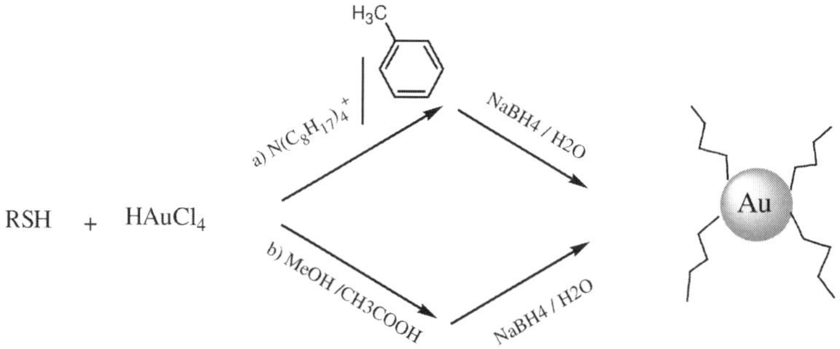

Fig. 4.1. Au NPs synthesized through a two-phase route (a) and a one-phase route (b).

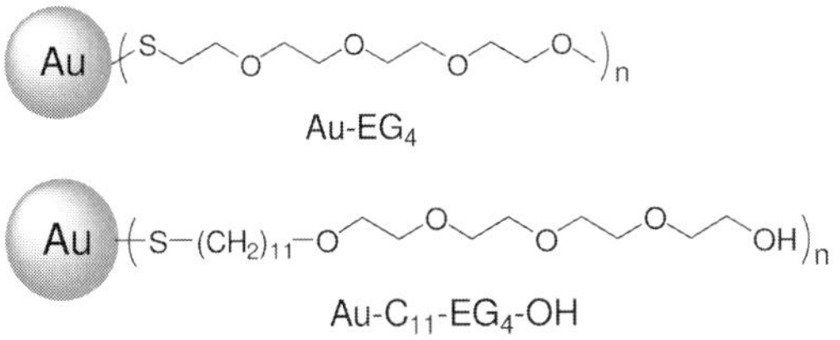

Fig. 4.2. Schematic structures of tetra(ethylene glycol) and thioalkylated oligo(ethylene glycol) protected Au NPs.

1998, this synthetic strategy has been extended, initially by Schaaff et al. [14] and Murray et al. [15] and then by many other researchers, to the synthesis of various water-soluble Au NPs. Compared with phosphine ligand-protected Au NPs, thio-protected Au NPs have a much more stable Au–S bond, giving the nanoparticles higher stability and wider utility.

A few authors have proposed a mechanism for the formation of the thiol monolayer on protected Au NP [12, 16, 17]. As shown in Eqs. (1) and (2), the electron-rich thiol group (HS–) in R–SH reacts with $AuCl_4^-$ to form a polymer intermediate. The polymer is then reduced by BH_4^- to form the nanoparticle.

$$AuCl_4^- + HSR \rightarrow (-Au^{I}SR-)_n \text{ (polymer)} \tag{1}$$

$$(-Au^{I}SR-)_n + BH_4^- \rightarrow Au_p(SR)_q \tag{2}$$

Although the synthetic methods developed by Brust et al. and Murray et al. provide guidelines for preparing ligand-protected Au NPs, the details for NP formation, such as solvent selection, control of nucleation and aggregation, are still not well understood. There is still an element of art in the synthesis of a new ligand-protected Au NP. Among various reaction conditions to be optimized, solvent selection for the synthesis is especially important. This is demonstrated by the synthesis of tetra(ethylene glycol) protected Au NP (Au–EG_4) (Fig. 4.2). Foos et al. first reported the synthesis of short ethylene oxide chain protected gold nanoparticles by ligand exchange reaction [18]. The procedure involved synthesis of hexanethiol (C6) protected gold nanoparticles followed by two steps of replacing C6 with ethylene glycol thiol molecules. Direct synthesis of ethylene glycol protected nanoparticle was, unsuccessfully, also attempted by Foos et al. using published methods. Bartz et al. synthesized Au–EG_4 NP directly in aqueous phase with a very low molar ratio of reducing agent ($NaBH_4$) and tetrachloroauric acid, resulting in partial reduction [19]. With increasing amount of $NaBH_4$, the reaction increased aggregation. The yield was very low. We also synthesized Au–EG_n ($n = 2$–4) using methanol as the solvent. The reagents $HAuCl_4$ and EG_4–SH, for example, were dissolved in a mixture of methanol and acetic acid; a freshly prepared $NaBH_4$ solution in methanol was then added with rapid stirring. Au–EG_4 nanoparticles formed as soon as the $NaBH_4$ methanol solution was added. After purifying and drying, the nanoparticle is readily redissolved in water to form a clear red/purple solution. However, the yield is very low (>10%). No precipitation was observed in the reaction mixture, meaning that the reduction reaction of $HAuCl_4$ was not complete. The mechanism of partial reduction in methanol was not investigated. After many trials, we established a direct synthesis of ethylene glycol [$HS-(CH_2CH_2O)_n-CH_3$, $n = 2-4$] protected gold nanoparticles in a mixed solvent of methanol and water by utilizing the $NaBH_4$ reduction method, with much improved yield [20, 21]. The key for this synthesis is the control of water content in the reaction mixture. A water content of 9–18% (v/v) is the optimum for the formation of stable, water-soluble nanoparticles. Instead of Au–EG_4, Brust et al. successfully synthesized a thioalkylated oligo(ethylene glycol) ligand-protected Au NP by using a mixed solvent of 2-propanol and methanol (Fig. 4.2) [22].

Even though the solvent effect on the synthesis of water-soluble nanoparticles was not systematically investigated in our original work, the polarity and solubility of the ligand are relevant to solvent selection for the synthesis. The solubility of Au NPs is determined by the capping ligand. Capping ligands for preparing water-soluble Au NPs can be classified into three categories: cationic, anionic, and neutral based on the charge on the molecules. In view of synthetic conditions for preparing Au NPs, we divide the capping ligands into different categories: strongly ionic, weakly ionic, and neutral. Here we briefly review solvent selection in each category of Au NP synthesis. Such a review should be beneficial as a reference for synthesizing new ligand-protected Au NPs.

4.2.1.1 Strongly Ionic Ligand-protected Au NPs

For strongly ionic ligands, including strong cationic and strong anionic, water as the single solvent is sufficient for synthesizing water-soluble nanoparticles. Examples include the synthesis of gold nanoparticles capped with coenzyme A [23], *N,N*-trimethyl(undecylmercapto)ammonium [24], 5-mercapto-2-benzimidazole sulfonic acid sodium salt [25], and the zwitterionic ligand cysteine [26].

4.2.1.2 Weakly Ionic Ligand-protected Au NPs

For weakly ionic ligands, a mixture of water and a water-miscible organic solvent, such as methanol, is usually used for the synthesis. Examples include the synthesis of gold nanoparticles protected with tiopronin [14], glutathione (GSH) [15], and mercaptosuccinic acid [27, 28]. In the synthesis of tiopronin-protected gold nanoparticles, using water as the only solvent leads to a water-insoluble product [14]. For the synthesis of GSH protected gold nanoparticle, a 2:3 water–methanol medium is used to prevent uncontrolled reduction reaction [15]. Presumably, the ratio of water to organic solvent in the mixed solvent system is related to the structure and polarity of the ligand. When a weak anionic ligand is highly polar and water soluble, water as the sole solvent could be sufficient for the synthesis of NPs. Examples include synthesis of Au NPs protected with meso-2,3-dimercaptosuccinic acid [29], and L-cysteine [30].

4.2.1.3 Au NPs Protected with Neutral Ligands

A mixed solvent of water and a water-miscible organic, such as methanol or ethanol, is usually a good start to synthesize neutral ligand protected Au NPs. Neutral ligands for coating nanoparticles include ethylene glycol small molecules, as described above, and poly(ethylene glycol) (PEG) molecules. With increasing units of ethylene glycol from 2 to 4 to 70 [31], or aldehyde derivatized PEG ($M_n = 3090$) [32], the solvent used in the synthesis of nanoparticles changes from a mixture of water and methanol to simply water. Sugar molecules and oligosaccharides are another important type of water-soluble ligand. Glyco-Au NPs have been synthesized in a mixed solvent of water and methanol [33–37]. Apparently, the solubility of the ligand molecules plays a major role in choosing the right solvent for the synthesis. Although the mechanistic reasons for this correlation are not clear, this summary should nevertheless provide a useful guidance for the synthesis of new types of water-soluble Au NPs.

4.2.2
Ligand Exchange Reaction

Au–X (X = P, S, or N) is quite labile. This unique character can be utilized to synthesize versatile surface functionality. One of the earliest examples, demonstrated by Schmid et al., replaced the triarylphosphine ligand on Au NP with a sulfonated triarylphosphine ligand [38]. Murray et al. pioneered the thiol ligand exchange reaction [39], a general route for the preparation of ligand-protected Au NPs. Since then, ligand exchange or S_N2 reactions have been widely used for preparing nanoparticles protected with either a homogeneous monolayer or a heterogeneous monolayer (also called mixed monolayer). Mixed monolayer protected Au NPs are especially important because they are used most in applications in electrochemistry [40, 41], conductivity [42, 43], fluorescence [44, 45], biological bindings [46, 47], and coatings [48]. Synthetically, the ligand replacement reaction has both advantages and disadvantages compared with direct synthesis. Versatility is its biggest advantage. By using ligand replacement reaction, various different mixed monolayer protected Au NPs can be synthesized that do not heavily depend on the nature of the ligands and the reaction conditions. However, the ligand replacement reaction certainly has several disadvantages. First, unlike direct synthesis, it is a multi-step process. Secondly, for the preparation of mixed monolayer protected Au NPs, it is difficult to control the number of ligands on a nanoparticle. The composition of the mixed monolayer is essential and directly responsible for the surface properties and interactions with the target molecules.

4.3
Preparative-scale Synthesis and Solution-phase Characterization of DNA-directed Nanoparticle Assemblies

In the previous section, we reviewed synthetic strategies for preparing ligand-protected Au NPs. These materials serve as building blocks for the assembly of higher order nanoparticle structures that could be used for applications as well as for fundamental studies. One assembly strategy involves using DNA molecules.

DNA has the unique self-assembly capability, i.e. hybridization. In addition, DNA is very hydrophilic and negatively charged. Unless the nanoparticles are positively charged, there is not much nonspecific binding between DNA and nanoparticles. Those two unique features have allowed many successful routes for the controlled assembly of nanoparticles using DNA functionalized Au NPs. These include nanoparticle assemblies through either specific hybridization of a single strand DNA attached on the nanoparticle [49, 50] or by electrostatic interaction of positively charged nanoparticles with DNA molecules [51, 52]. In addition, Niemeyer et al. have prepared nanoscale networks and aggregates using biotinylated DNA and streptavidin [53, 54]. DNA functionalized nanoparticles have been used successfully for DNA detection and as biosensors [55, 56].

Bio-based assembly of nano-scale materials into higher order structures is an active area of research. Previous studies by Alivisatos et al. [50, 57] and Mirkin et al. [49, 58] have demonstrated the power of using DNA hybridization to assemble nanoparticles into higher order structures. Work from Alivisatos et al. in particular has demonstrated the possibility of using DNA-directed assembly to make small-scale finite nanoparticle complexes that resemble artificial molecules. These structures may serve as model systems for studying nano-scale phenomena, and have potential applications in nanoelectronic circuits, optoelectronics and biosensors. One critical issue that needs to be addressed is the scale of the synthesis of these nanoparticle-based artificial molecules. Also lacking is the direct solution characterization of such assemblies, so that structure–function relationships can be established for these artificial molecules. We describe here our methods for solving the scaling-up problem, and the solution characterization of some simple nanoparticle assemblies we have made.

For this study, we first developed ligand-protected Au NPs with high stability and relatively uniform-size distributions. Following known synthetic routes, we have made glutathione and tiopronin [*N*-(2-mercaptopropionyl)glycine] monolayer-protected Au NPs [14, 59]. However, these particles, as synthesized, still have a size distribution that is too broad for our subsequent assembly studies. We have, thus, developed a non-solvent precipitation method as a very efficient way to fractionate particles of different sizes to obtain highly monodispersed nanoparticles [60]. By adding increasing amounts of either methanol or ethanol, particles of larger to smaller sizes are precipitated out of solution. After centrifugation, particles of a particular size can be selected for further assembly. A typical example for fractionation of Au-Tp NPs is given here. Au-Tp NPs (0.3 g) were dissolved in 50 mL of a 100 mM sodium chloride solution. The first fraction of the nanoparticles was precipitated out by adding methanol to the nanoparticle solution to a final content of 10% by volume. Nanoparticles were collected by centrifugation at 4000 rpm for 1 min in a Sorvall® RT7 PLUS centrifuge (Kendro Laboratory Products, Newtown, CT). More methanol was then added to the supernatant to a final content of 20% by volume and the precipitated nanoparticles were collected as described above, as the second fraction, which was used for the following experiments.

To label nanoparticles with single-stranded DNA (ssDNA), we chose the ligand

Tab. 4.1. Stoichiometry for attaching ssDNA to Au NPs by using ligand replacement reaction (volume unit = μL).

	Rxn 1	*Rxn 2*	*Rxn 3*	*Rxn 4*	*Rxn 5*	*Rxn 6*
Au-Tp (60 μM)	3	3	3	3	3	3
SsDNA (40 μM)	0	1	2	4	8	1.6 (400 μM)
NaCl (1 M)	1.5	1.5	1.5	1.5	1.5	1.5
H_2O	10.5	9.5	8.5	6.5	2.5	8.9
Total (μL)	15	15	15	15	15	15

replacement reaction described in Section 4.2. A typical example is as follows. Single-stranded DNA (ssDNA) oligo nucleotides were purchased from Integrated DNA Technologies, Inc. (Coralville, IA), with 5′ C6 SH modification. Materials were used as-received without further treatment. For this example, a ssDNA with sequence AAA AAA GCG TGG GCG TGG GCG TGG GCG TGG GCG was used. The gold particles had a concentration of 60 μM in H_2O. To determine the optimal ratio of Au-Tp vs. ssDNA for labeling reaction, a titration experiment was set up by mixing appropriate amounts of Au-Tp, ssDNA, NaCl, and H_2O (Table 4.1). Each reaction was carried out in a 1.5 mL volume test tube. The reaction mixture was incubated at 60 °C for 15 min and allowed to slowly cool to room temperature over 30 min. Products were analyzed by gel electrophoresis using a 4% agarose/Tris-Borate-EDTA (TBE) gel (BioWhittaker, Rockland, ME). The gel was immersed in 1X TBE running buffer (89 mM Tris, 89 mM boric acid, 2 mM EDTA, pH 8.3), and electrophoresis was carried out at a constant voltage of 90 V for 80 min in an Horizon 58 gel box (Life Technologies, Rockville, MD). The gel image (Fig. 4.3A) was recorded using a HP ScanJet 6300C scanner (Agilent Technologies, Wilmington, DE). Lanes 1–6 correspond to reactions 1–6, respectively, in Table 4.1.

This experiment showed that Au particles with different numbers of ssDNAs labels can be clearly resolved by a 4% agarose gel (Fig. 4.3A). As the ratio of ssDNA vs. Au-Tp increases, more ssDNAs can be found on a particle. Thus, the stoichiometry of ssDNA and Au-Tp can be used to control the average number of ssDNAs on the surface of Au particles.

Due to the narrow size distribution of our nanoparticles, we were able to use liquid chromatography to obtain Au particles with an exact number of ssDNAs attached. After the labeling reaction, we separated reaction mixture with a size exclusion gel filtration column. A typical example of the separation of Au NPs with different numbers of single-stranded DNAs is given here. Here, the labeling reaction was performed as follows: 400 μM ssDNA (986-ZF) (8 μL) and 1 M NaCl (12 μL) were added to 100 μL of Au-Tp (60 μM). The reaction mixture was incubated at 60 °C for 15 min and allowed to slowly cool to room temperature over 30 min. This mixture was then injected into a Superdex 200 gel filtration column (Amersham Biosciences, Piscataway, NJ) mounted on a BioCAD/SPRINT HPLC system (PerSeptive Biosystems, Framingham, MA), and eluted with 0.05 NaCl/0.15 M $NaHPO_4$ buffer (pH 7) at 0.5 mL min^{-1}. The elution profile is shown in

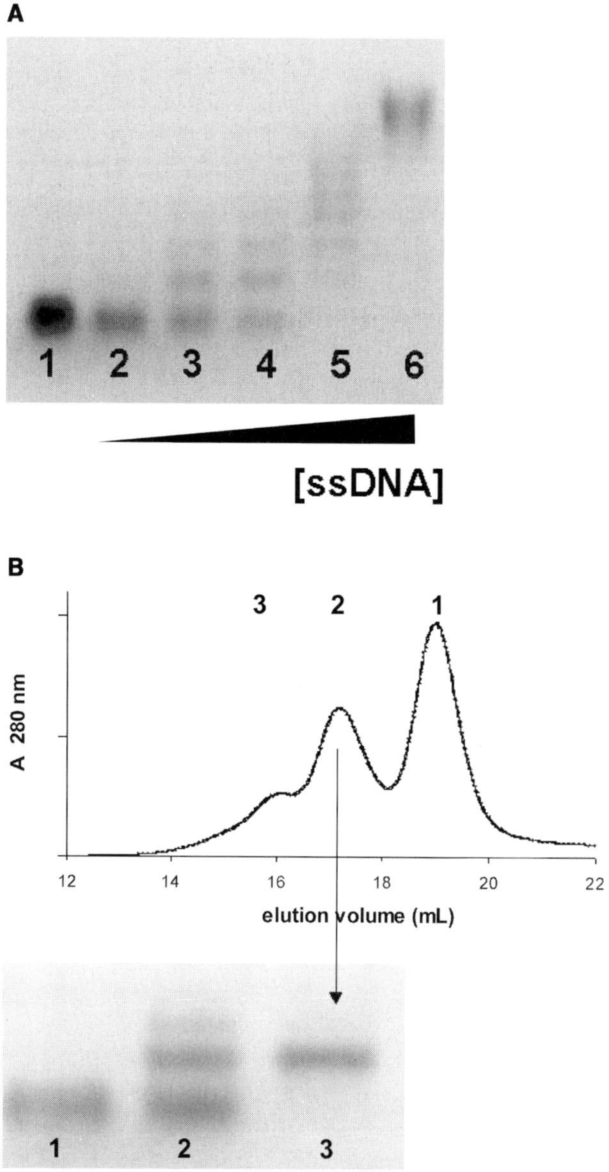

Fig. 4.3. (A) Gel electrophoresis (4% agarose gel) of gold nanoparticles reacted with increasing amounts of ssDNA molecules (Table 4.1). (B) Gel filtration separation and subsequent gel electrophoresis of gold nanoparticles labeled with different numbers of ssDNA molecules. A Superdex 200 gel filtration column (Amersham Biosciences, Piscataway, NJ) mounted on a BioCAD/SPRINT HPLC system (PerSeptive Biosystems, Framingham, MA) was used. Elution was performed with 0.05 M NaCl/0.15 M $NaHPO_4$ buffer (pH 7) at 0.5 mL min^{-1}. Peaks 1–3 correspond to nanoparticles labeled with 0, 1 and 2 ssDNA, respectively. The gel image compares Au-Tp (lane1), Au-Tp/ssDNA reaction mix (lane 2), and the column fraction corresponding to peak 2 (lane 3).

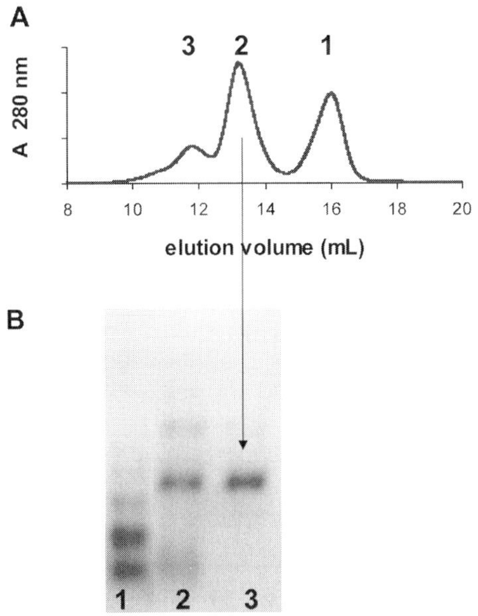

Fig. 4.4. (A) Gel filtration separation of a hybridization reaction of ssDNA-labeled gold particles, with conditions similar to those described in Fig. 4.3. (B) Gel electrophoresis of the separated fractions from (A).

Fig. 4.3(B). Peaks 1–3 correspond to nanoparticles labeled with 0–2 ssDNA, respectively. The gel image at the bottom of Fig. 4.3(B) compares Au-Tp (lane1), Au-Tp/ssDNA reaction mix (lane 2), and the column fraction corresponding to peak 2 (lane 3). The gel mobility of the peak 2 fraction is consistent with the material being a one-particle/one-ssDNA species. By following the above procedure, we have labeled Au particles with two different ssDNA sequences that are complementary. The hybridization reaction was then carried out by mixing these two types of particles. The hybridization mixture was separated again by size exclusion gel filtration. A typical elution profile is shown in Fig. 4.4(A). In addition to the major product eluted in peak 2, side-products represented by peaks 1 and 3 are noticeable. These arise from impurities in the starting materials, which contain a small fraction of particles with 0, 2 and more ssDNA attached. Figure 4.4(B) shows a gel image, comparing the Au-Tp/ssDNA reaction mix (lane 1), the hybridization reaction mix (lane 2), and the column fraction corresponding to peak 2 in Fig. 4.4(A) (lane 3). The gel mobility of the peak 2 fraction is consistent with it being a dimer species. This material was analyzed by transmission electron microscopy (TEM) [Fig. 4.5(A)]. Quantitatively, over 90% of the purified species is dimeric Au NPs. Figure 4.5(B) provides an enlarged view of some dimer structures.

The synthetic procedure we have developed could be used to construct more complex structures. As a demonstration, we have synthesized a triatomic structure

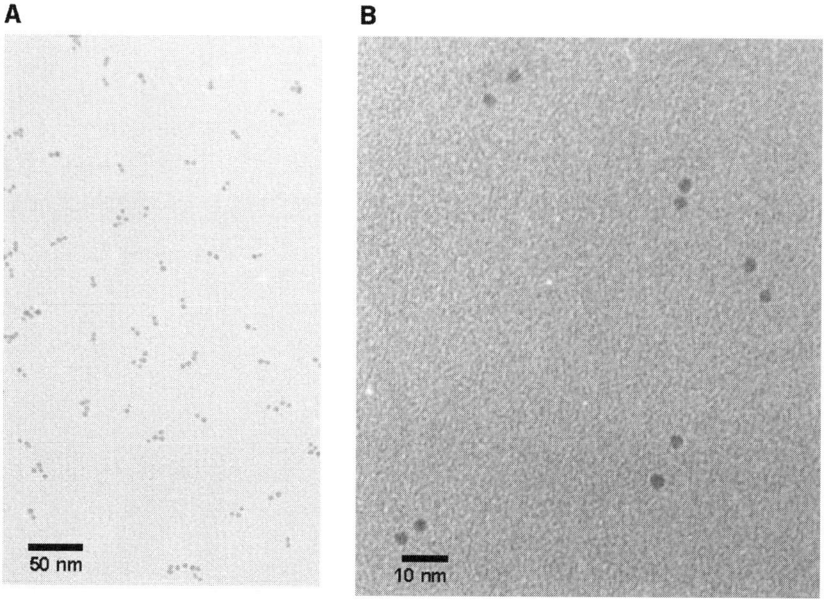

Fig. 4.5. TEM images of gold nanoparticle dimer structures prepared according to Fig. 4.4.

involving hybridization of three ssDNAs, each of which contain two segments that are complementary to part of the other two sequences (Fig. 4.6). Using the ligand exchange reaction and size exclusion separation techniques described above, we first obtained Au particles labeled with each of the three ssDNAs (lane 2 in Fig. 4.6). Hybridization between two types of Au particles labeled with two different ssDNA yielded a two-particle assembly (lane 3 of Fig. 4.6). The complete trimer structure (lane 4) was obtained by mixing the purified two-particle assembly with third-type ssDNA labeled Au particles. TEM images of the purified final hybridization mixture confirmed formation of the designed product.

Large-scale preparation has allowed us to measure directly solution structures of nanoparticle assemblies by small angle X-ray scattering (SAXS). Previous studies of nanoparticle assemblies have relied on TEM, which has the advantage of requiring small samples. However, TEM is performed under vacuum conditions and the projection nature of the TEM image prevents a direct measure of the geometric parameters of particle assembles. Large-scale synthesis allows us for the first time to use solution methods to measure directly the geometry of nanoparticle assemblies we have made. SAXS spectroscopy proved to be ideal for our Au nanoparticle complexes, because of the large electron density on Au particles. We have measured two dimer structures of different bond lengths (Fig. 4.7). Dimer A was constructed with a 24 base pair long dsDNA with a C6 spacer on each side. Dimer B was similarly constructed with a 33 base pair long DNA. The measured Au–Au separation is 11.5 and 13.7 nm for dimers A and B, respectively. In both cases, the monomer diameter, as measured by the position of the first peak, is 3.6 nm. Assuming

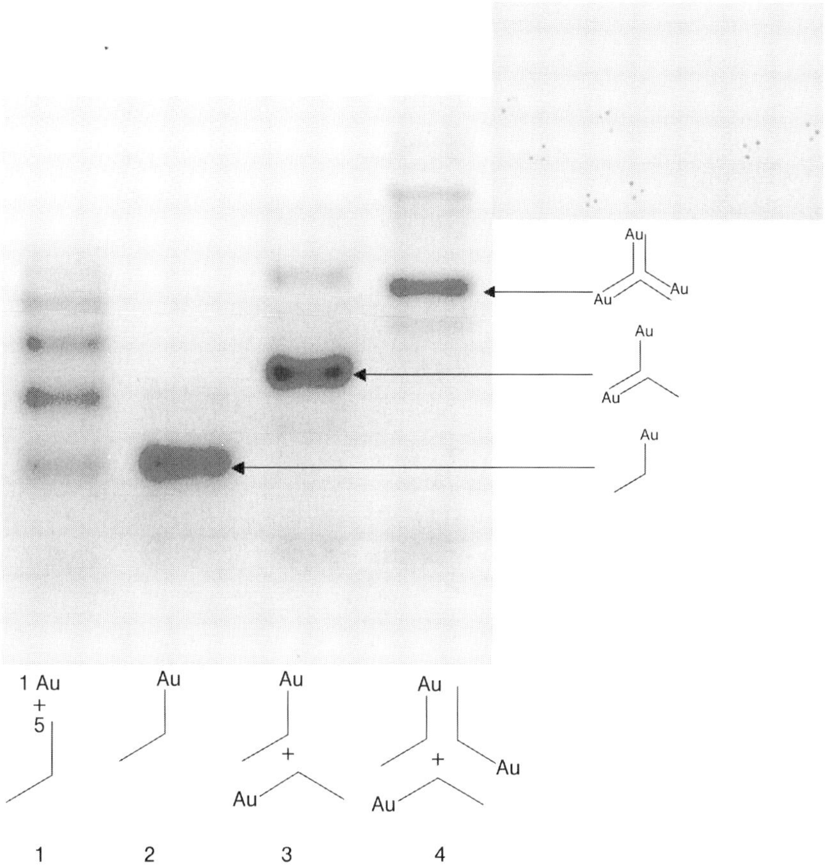

Fig. 4.6. Gel electrophoresis and TEM image of gold particle trimer structures prepared by the DNA hybridization process. Lane 1 is from a DNA labeling reaction mixture. Lanes 2–4 are monomeric, dimeric and trimeric Au particle complexes, respectively.

the C6 spacer is 1 nm long and the diameter of Au particles is 3.6 nm, then from the measured length of either dimer one obtains 0.246 nm bp^{-1} (dimer A) or 0.245 nm bp^{-1} (dimer B). However, C6 might be flexible, and the estimated 1 nm might be a source of error. Thus, the base-separation parameter was also calculated by the length difference between the two dimers: the length difference of 2.2 nm between two dimers can be attributed to the 9 base pair difference. This gives 0.244 nm bp^{-1}, which is consistent with the previous estimation. Table 4.2 lists the derived structure parameters. To our surprise, the particle–particle separations in these dimer structures are consistent with the A- instead of the B-form DNA structure (the latter is expected under normal physiological conditions).

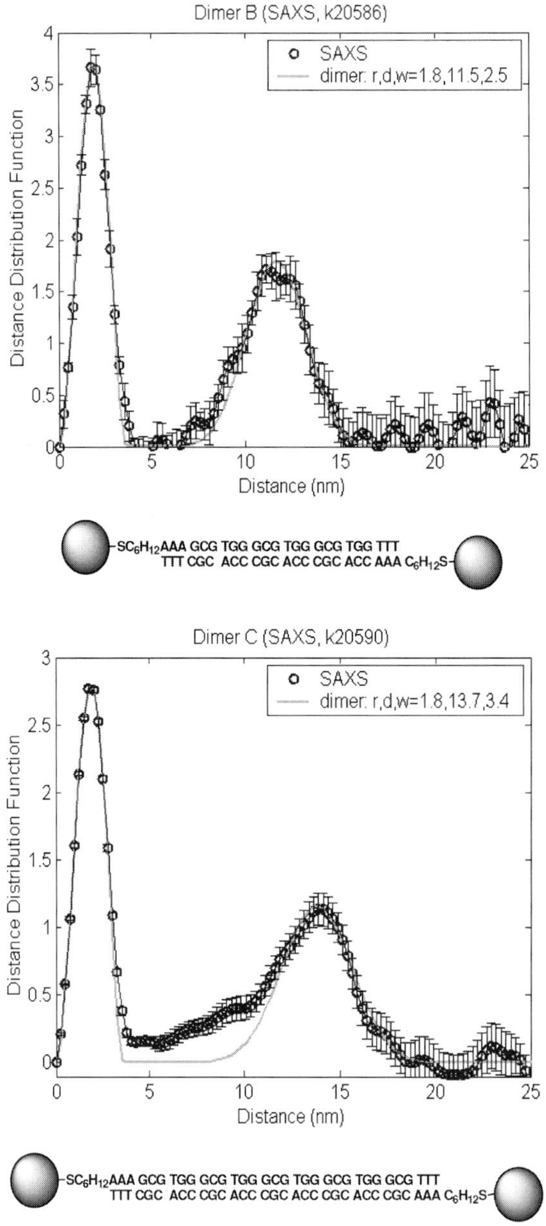

Fig. 4.7. SAXS measurements of two gold particle dimer structures linked with different lengths of DNA. In the two data plots, open circles are the experimental data, and the solid lines are simulations using the parameters shown.

Tab. 4.2. Geometrical parameters of two Au particle dimers obtained by SAXS measurement.

Dimer	*Number of base pairs*	*Expected Au–Au separation (assuming A-form DNA, 0.25 nm per bp) (nm)*	*Expected Au–Au separation (assuming B-form DNA, 0.34 nm per bp) (nm)*	*Measured Au–Au separation (nm)*
A	24	11.6	13.8	11.5
B	33	13.9	16.8	13.7

In summary, we have established a simple yet effective way to make large quantities of nanoparticle-based diatomic and triatomic artificial molecules. Monodispersed Au-Tp NPs are obtained through direct synthesis, followed by fractionation using an alcohol precipitation procedure. Au-Tp particles with one DNA oligonucleotide molecule per particle are obtained in large quantity by size exclusion chromatography. From these particles, simple diatomic and triatomic artificial molecules are self-assembled through DNA hybridization reactions. Relatively large quantities of pure diatomic and triatomic structure are obtained after fractionation and purification by size exclusion chromatography, allowing for the first time characterization of these structures in solution. SAXS data revealed that double-stranded DNA bridging two gold nanoparticles adopts, unexpectedly, the A-type conformation, illustrating the dramatic effect of environmental conditions on DNA structures.

4.4
Bifunctional Proteins for Programmable Assembly of Nanoparticles

DNA hybridization is only one of many possible ways to assemble nanoparticles. We have explored the possibility of using DNA as a template to define spatial locations for the assembly of nanoparticles. As one such way of using DNA, we sought to create a protein that has bifunctionality: it would bind with high affinity and specificity to DNA as well as nanoparticles. Our approach is to create a fusion protein composed of a DNA binding domain and a nanoparticle binding domain (Fig. 4.8).

There are many proteins that recognize a specific sequence of DNA. Transcription factors involved in gene regulation possess such a property. We decided to use the class of DNA binding proteins called Zn fingers, owing to their high binding affinity and specificity, and because many such proteins are available. Comparison of the human genome sequence with a few other sequenced mammalian species showed that the Zn finger domain is the most frequently observed protein domain in mammalian cells [61, 62]. One can even evolve Zn finger proteins to bind DNA sequences of one's choice. A well-characterized Zn-finger protein Zif268 [63, 64] was chosen here for demonstration. For the nanoparticle binding domain, we chose well-characterized ligand binding protein domains to bind to

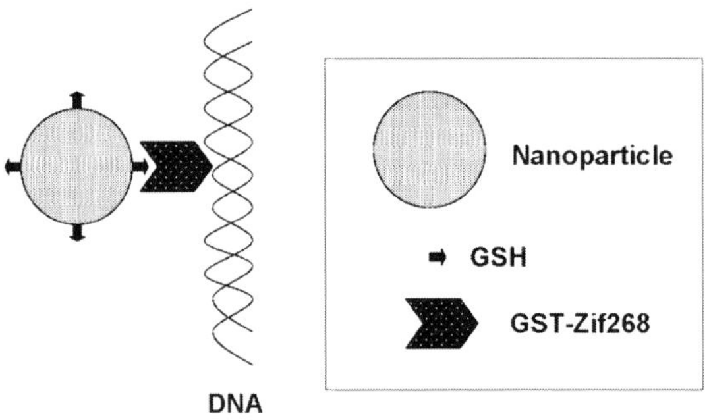

Fig. 4.8. Design of bifunctional proteins to assemble nanoparticles onto DNA.

nanoparticles that are surface coated with the cognate ligands. The GST (glutathione S-transferase)-GSH (glutathione) pair was chosen for demonstration (Fig. 4.8). We constructed the bifunctional protein following conventional molecular biology protocol, overexpressed it in *E. coli* cells, and purified the protein using GST affinity purification.

We performed a set of protein functional assays to demonstrate that, indeed, the designed protein has bifunctional binding capabilities. The Zif268 DNA binding site was defined by sequence 5′-GCGTGGGCG-3′. When the purified protein was incubated with a DNA construct that contains multiple Zif268 binding sites, we observed a clear band shift in a gel electrophoresis assay, indicating that the purified GST-Zif268 fusion protein binds to the target DNA sequence. Similarly, we showed that the protein binds to GSH-modified Au NPs (Fig. 4.9).

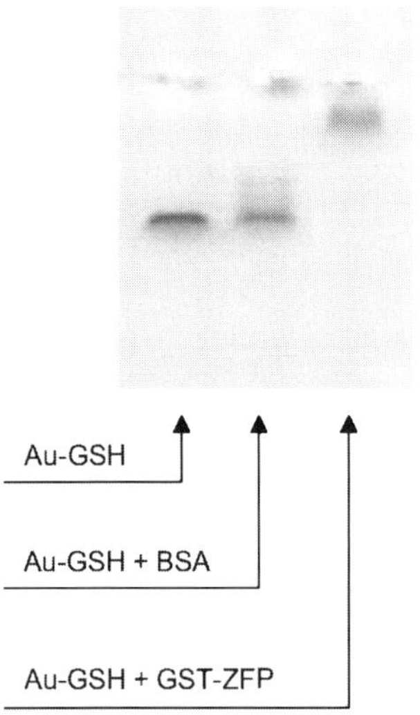

Fig. 4.9. Gel electrophoresis analysis of protein binding to Au-GSH particles.

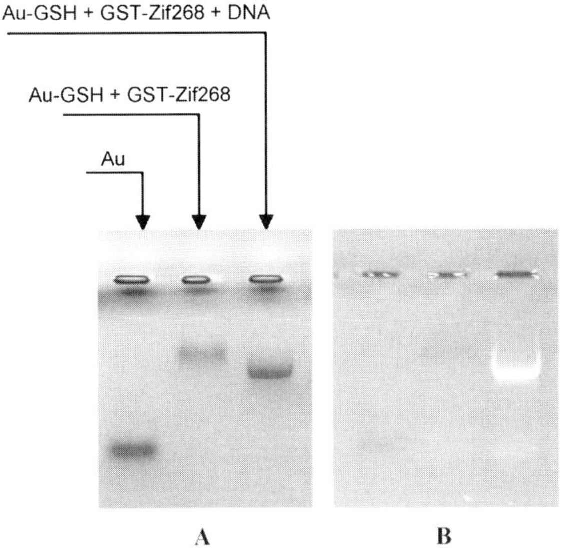

Fig. 4.10. Gel electrophoresis analysis of GST-Zif268 and DNA binding to Au-GSH particles. (A) Is a direct gel image, whereas (B) is the gel image under UV illumination.

Evidence for the bifunctional binding activity was provided by an experiment shown in Fig. 4.10(A) and 10(B). This is a gel shift assay on the purified GST-Zif268 protein binding to both Au-GSH nanoparticles and DNA. Figure 4.10(A) is a direct gel image, whereas Fig. 4.10(B) is the gel image under UV illumination, indicating where the DNA band is located. As can be seen in Fig. 4.10, addition of a piece of DNA that contains protein recognition sequence caused the protein–particle complex to migrate at a different speed, and DNA co-migrated with Au particles. These results indicate that the bifunctional protein can indeed direct particles onto DNA. However, we also noticed a problem in this system that limits the efficiency of assembly by the bifunctional protein: the positively charged Zif268 has a tendency to nonspecifically bind to the negatively charged Au-GSH nanoparticles. Effectively, the Au-GSH particles compete with the DNA for the Zif268 binding site, and reduce the efficiency of the intended assembly. Such a problem triggered us to look into the general issue of nonspecific binding, which will be discussed in detail in the next section.

4.5
Strategies for Eliminating Nonspecific Interactions and Enabling Specific Binding with Biomolecules

It is very attractive to integrate nanoparticles with biological molecules such as DNA, and proteins to create new materials for potential new applications in electronics, optics, genomics, proteomics, and biomedical and bioanalytical areas. However, for proteins, nonspecific binding could be a serious issue. Proteins are much more complicated than DNA. They can be either hydrophobic or hydrophilic, with either positive or negative charge, making it extremely challenging to avoid nonspecific binding with nanoparticles. To fully utilize the potential of protein–nanoparticle hybrids, we synthesized ethylene glycol monolayer protected gold nanoparticles that are very stable in aqueous media and have complete resistance to nonspecific bindings with proteins, DNA and RNA [20]. However, these biologically inert nanoparticles do not provide functionality. To allow specific interactions or bindings with biological entities, a specific binding functionality has to be introduced onto the nanoparticles. For this purpose, we designed nanoparticles protected with a mixed monolayer of an ethylene glycol molecule and a ligand. The ethylene glycol short chains with well-defined lengths function as a shielding component to minimize nonspecific interaction between nanoparticles and biological molecules, whereas the ligand acts as a capture agent to engage biological molecules specifically. To demonstrate this method, we prepared a Au NP protected with a mixed monolayer of tri(ethylene glycol) and glutathione [Au–$(S{-}EG_3)_nGSH$] by adding a reducing agent ($NaBH_4$) to a mixture of $HAuCl_4$, $EG_3{-}SH$, GSH, methanol and acetic acid in a one-step direct synthesis (Fig. 4.11). We discovered

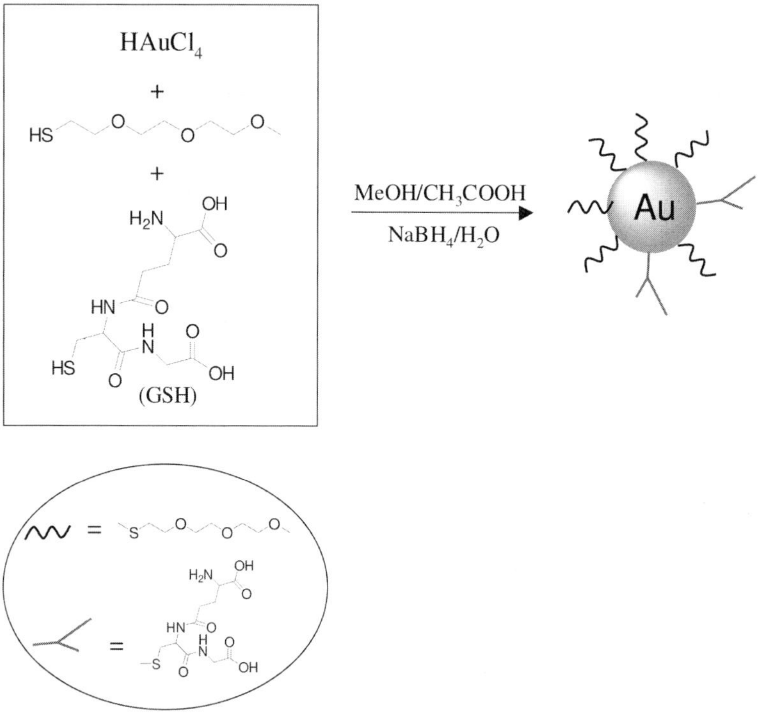

Fig. 4.11. Reaction scheme for making $(EG_3{-}S{-})$/GSH mixed monolayer protected nanoparticles.

that in a one-step direct synthesis the water content in the reaction mixture was critical for synthesizing Au NPs in high yield. The optimum water concentration is 9–18%. This method also applies to the synthesis of other Au NPs protected with a mixed monolayer in which ethylene glycol is the major component. The synthesis utilized the optimum condition such that water for dissolving $NaBH_4$ was added into the mixture of reagents to a final concentration of 12.5% (v/v). Under this condition, the reaction went well and no precipitation was seen. The yield was about 40%. The purified nanoparticles were very stable in pure water as well as concentrated electrolyte solutions, such as 1.0 M aqueous NaCl. These nanoparticles did not degrade after one-year storage in water.

In such a mixed monolayer protected Au NP system, GSH as a ligand molecule enables specific binding to a target. However, GSH might also contribute to the nonspecific binding. Thus, quantitative control of the ligand number or percentage is crucial to achieve specific interaction. The feeding ratio of EG_3–SH and GSH is easily controlled in the direct synthesis approach, but the essential information is the relative amount of EG_3–S– and GSH on the nanoparticle surface, which is directly responsible for the surface properties and interactions with the target molecules. To control the relative amount of the shielding component (EG_3–S–) and the capture component (SGH), we envisage two approaches. The first is to study the relative reactivities of EG_3–SH and GSH by synthesizing a series of Au NPs with controlled feeding molar ratios of the shielding and capture components, followed analysis of the surface composition. The measured surface composition can be plotted against the feeding ratio to determine the relative reactivity of the shielding and capture components, which could be used to control the surface composition. For example, we have used ^1H NMR spectroscopy as an analytical tool for measuring the surface composition of EG_3–S–/tiopronin on Au NPs and determined that the EG_3–SH is three times more reactive than tiopronin [59]. However, in many cases of mixed monolayer protected Au NPs, it is not easy to determine an accurate surface composition. In addition, NMR analysis is very tedious and needs sophisticated equipment.

For most applications, accurate understanding of the surface composition might not be necessary. The correlation of the feeding ratio of EG_3–SH and the ligand with the nanoparticle binding performance should be sufficient information to design the synthesis of nanoparticle with only specific interactions. Based on this consideration, we developed the second approach by using gel electrophoresis analysis to identify a critical feeding ratio for the nanoparticle to avoid nonspecific interactions and in the meantime to provide maximum binding to a specific target. We used $Au(–S–EG_3)_n GSH$ as an example. With a constant ratio of $HAuCl_4$ and capping agents (EG_3–SH and GSH) at 2.0, a series of nanoparticles were synthesized with the feeding ratio of $[EG_3–SH]/[GSH]$ at 1, 4, 14, and 19, respectively. $Au(–S–EG_3)_{4fr}GSH$ represents the nanoparticle synthesized when the feeding ratio of $[EG_3–SH]/[GSH] = 4$. The charge density of $Au(–S–EG_3)_{nfr}GSH$ nanoparticles representing the surface density of GSH was characterized qualitatively with their migration speed in the gel electrophoresis [Fig. 4.12(a)]. Lane 1 is $Au(–S–EG_3)_{1fr}GSH$ nanoparticles with an EG_3–SH/GSH feeding ratio of 1:1.

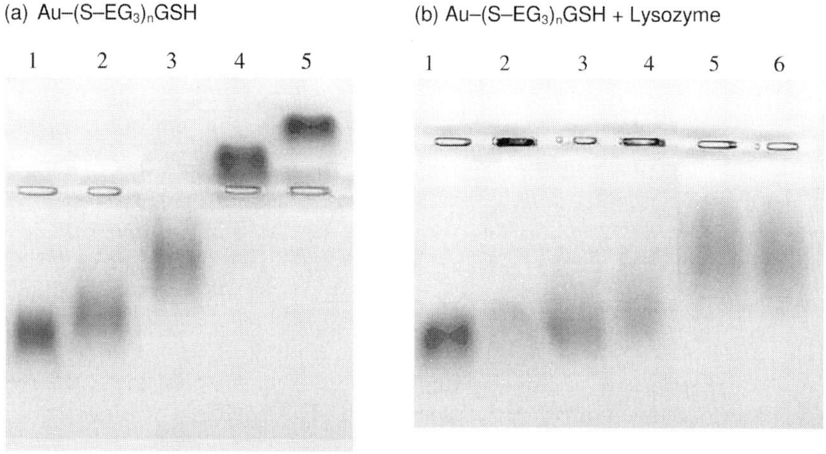

Fig. 4.12. (a) Gel electrophoresis image illustrating the migration of $(EG_3{-}S{-})$/GSH mixed monolayer protected nanoparticles as a function of feeding ratio of $[EG_3{-}SH]/[GSH]$. A 4% agarose gel was used and run at 90 V for 40 min. Lanes 1–4 are $Au(-S-EG_3)_{nfr}GSH$ with $n = 1$, 4, 14, and 19, respectively. Lane 5 is the pure $Au{-}S{-}EG_3$ nanoparticle. In all cases, 10 μL of Au particles at concentration of 50 μM were loaded onto the gel. (b) Gel electrophoresis image of the nanoparticles from Fig. 4.12(a) bonded with lysozyme. A 1% agarose gel was used and run at 90 V for 20 min. Lanes 1, 3 and 5 are $Au(-S-EG_3)_{nfr}GSH$ with $n = 1$, 4, and 14, respectively. Lanes 2, 4, and 6 are the mixture of lysozyme and $Au(-S-EG_3)_{nfr}GSH$ with $n = 1$, 4, and 14, respectively. Protein binding reactions were carried out by mixing 7 μL of 50 μM Au nanoparticles with 7 μL of 1 mg mL^{-1} lysozyme solution for 10 min incubation time at room temperature. (Reprinted with the permission from Ref. [59], M. Zheng, X. Huang, *J. Am. Chem. Soc.* **2004**, 126, 12047–12054. © 2004 American Chemical Society.)

Lanes 2–5 are the same amount of $Au(-S-EG_3)_{nfr}GSH$ nanoparticles with $n = 4$, 14, 19, and pure $Au{-}S{-}EG_3$, respectively. The migration speed of $Au(-S-EG_3)_{nfr}GSH$ nanoparticles decreased with decreasing percentage of GSH on the nanoparticle surface. In the mixed monolayer of (EG3–S–)/GSH protected gold nanoparticles, the major contribution for nonspecific binding is from the electrostatic interaction introduced by GSH molecules. Therefore, a positively charged protein lysozyme is a very good indicator for testing the nonspecific binding. Binding results for $Au{-}(S{-}EG_3)_nGSH$ nanoparticles are shown in Fig. 4.12(b). Lanes 1, 3, and 5 are $Au(-S-EG_3)_{nfr}GSH$ nanoparticles with $n = 1$, 4, and 14, respectively. Lanes 2, 4, and 6 are the same amount of $Au(-S-EG_3)_{nfr}GSH$ nanoparticles with $n = 1$, 4, and 14, respectively, mixed with lysozyme. When the molar feeding percentage of GSH is less than 20%, $(EG_3{-}S{-})$/GSH mixed monolayer protected nanoparticles have negligible binding with lysozyme. In this example, the ratio of $(EG_3{-}S{-})$/GSH on the nanoparticle surface was not measured and is unknown.

The GSH molecule on the $Au(-S-EG_3)_nGSH$ particle is a natural substrate for the enzyme glutathione-S-transferase (GST). The GST–GSH binding pair thus provides an opportunity to demonstrate the specific binding between nanoparticles

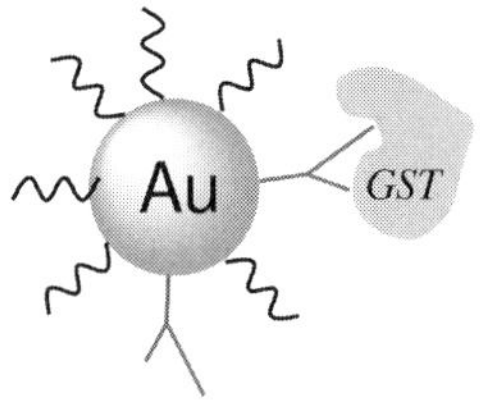

Fig. 4.13. Schematic of specific binding of GST protein to Au(–S–EG_3)$_n$GSH particles.

and proteins under more common biological conditions (Fig. 4.13). From the nonspecific binding tests for Au(–S–EG_3)$_{nfr}$GSH (Fig. 4.12) we saw negligible binding with lysozyme when the nanoparticle [EG3–SH]/[GSH] feeding ratio is at 4. Nanoparticles with feeding ratios of 9 and 14 were chosen for specific interaction with GST protein. Figure 4.14 demonstrates that neither Au(–S–EG_3)$_{9fr}$GSH nor Au(–S–EG_3)$_{14fr}$GSH bound to lysozyme (lanes 2 and 5, respectively), while both particles migrated faster (lanes 3 and 6) after incubation with GST protein, indicating their specific interaction with GST. The faster migration of the Au(–S–EG_3)$_{nfr}$GSH/GST complex is, presumably, due to the negative charge of the GST protein (pI 6.2) in the pH 8 gel running buffer (TBE).

In summary, gel electrophoresis of the nanoparticles has been used to identify the optimum feeding ratio of a capture ligand and EG_3–SH at which the nanoparticle enables maximum specific binding with a biological target without the interference of nonspecific interactions. This approach could be easily applied to other nanoparticles protected with a mixed monolayer of an ethylene glycol molecule and a ligand.

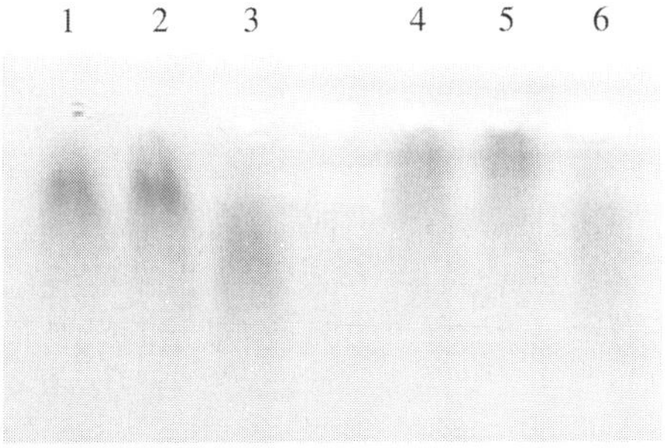

Fig. 4.14. Gel electrophoresis image illustrating specific binding of Au(–S–EG_3)$_{nfr}$GSH ($n = 9$ and 14) with GST protein. A 0.8% agarose gel was used and run at 90 V for 20 min. Gold particles were suspended in H_2O with a concentration of ~50 μM. Lane 1 is 10 μL of Au(–S–EG_3)$_{9fr}$GSH; lanes 2 and 3 are the same amount of Au particles incubated with 1 μL of lysozyme (10 mg mL^{-1} in water) and 5 μL of GST (0.5 mg mL^{-1} in water), respectively. Lanes 4–6 are identical to lanes 1–3, except that Au(–S–EG_3)$_{14fr}$GSH was used. (Reprinted with the permission from Ref. [59], M. Zheng, X. Huang, *J. Am. Chem. Soc.* **2004**, 126, 12047–12054. © 2004 American Chemical Society.)

4.6 Biological Applications

Water-soluble Au NPs have numerous applications in biology, medicine, catalysis, electronics, and optics. Here, we briefly review current efforts towards biological applications, which can be divided into subjects relating to nucleic acids, proteins, and cells and viruses.

4.6.1 Nucleic Acids

Mirkin et al. first demonstrated the Au NP color change from red to blue when two complementary strands of DNA on two different Au NPs hybridize to form a NP aggregate [49]. Mirkin et al. further discovered that the Au NP aggregate could be converted back into individual Au NPs by heating the NP aggregate to dehybridize DNA, and that this was a reversible process in solution [65]. When a multilayer of Au NPs was formed on a glass substrate by hybridization of DNA attached on the NPs, a sharp response of plasma resonance intensity to temperature was observed [66]. Based on these fundamental discoveries, Reichert et al. developed a chip-based optical detection of DNA through hybridization of the surface-immobilized capture probe oligonucleotide and the target probe attached on Au NPs [67]. Storhoff et al. developed an easy "spot-and-read" colorimetric detection method for highly sensitive DNA detection [68]. Mirkin et al., furthermore, developed a multiplexed detection of DNA targets in a microchip format with the detection limit as low as 20 femtomolar [56]. Such a high detection sensitivity was achieved by applying a thin Ag coating to the surface of DNA hybridized Au NPs and then using surface-enhanced Raman spectroscopy (SERS) as the detection tool. By developing a magnetically-induced solid-state electrochemical detection method instead of SERS, Wang et al. achieved a DNA detection limit at the level of ~1.2 fmol [69]. Another DNA detection method utilizes the ability of Au NP to quench fluorescence, which happens when a Au NP (2–3 nm) is in relatively close contact with a fluorophore (1–2 nm range), due to non-radioactive energy transfer from the excited fluorophore to Au NP [70]. This method employs a single stranded DNA with one end attached to an Au NP and the other end to a fluorophore to form a constrained loop DNA structure. When the DNA molecule on the Au NP hybridizes with a target ssDNA, the probe DNA loop on the Au NP opens and the fluorophore lights up. Based on this method, researchers have developed single-mismatch detection for oligonucleotides [70, 71]. Using DNA hybridization, Au NPs have also been assembled on the surface of carbon nanotubes [72].

4.6.2 Proteins

Unlike DNA, which is very hydrophilic and negatively charged, proteins are much more complicated. They can be either hydrophobic or hydrophilic, with either positive or negative charge. In addition, nonspecific binding can be a serious issue. Unsurprisingly, therefore, applications of Au NPs with proteins have been far less developed than with DNA. However, several published papers deal with the interactions between nanoparticles and proteins, and applications in protein detection [73, 74], enzyme inhibition [75, 76], biosensor [77–79], nano-domain structure control [80, 81], and control of the nonspecific interaction of nanoparticles with proteins [59]. The interaction between Au NPs and proteins has been studied extensively. Examples include controlling the orientation of cytochrome *c* on Au NPs [82] and maintaining the enzymatic activity of fungal protease on Au NPs [83]. For protein detection, Thanh et al. [74] used antigen-coated Au NPs to detect antibodies by measuring the Au NP plasmon resonance shift induced by the aggregation of Au NPs. The detection limit could reach 1 μg mL^{-1}. Mirkin et al. [77] used DNA hybridization to attach antigens to Au NPs and to then detect antibodies by a colorimetric scanner with a detection limit of ~20 nM. This group also capped oligonucleotide-Raman dye conjugated molecules on Au NPs, attached antigens through hybridization, and then detected antibodies by using SERS [78]. Mirkin's methods are suited for the detection of multiple proteins. In a different approach, Willner et al. [79] developed an amplified optical detection of thrombin by using the binding between aptamer attached Au NPs and adsorbed thrombin on aptamer functionalized surface (detection limit at 2 nM). In the area of enzyme inhibition, Rotello et al. have developed anionically functionalized, amphiphilic Au NPs to efficiently inhibit chymotrypsin through electrostatic interaction [75, 76]. They further demonstrated that Au NPs functionalized with alkanethiol-tetra(ethylene glycol) acetic acid bind to chymotrypsin, and the enzyme on the Au NP surface retains its activity and exhibits pronounced substrate chemoselectivity [84]. To build controlled Au NP structured materials, functionalized double stranded DNA has been used as a template to assemble protein attached Au NPs through the interaction between biotin bound on DNA and streptavidin on Au NP [80]. Enzymes, such as bacterial DNA methyltransferases could be used to manipulate the structure of DNA molecules linked with Au NPs, thus resulting in control of the distance between Au NPs [81]. In a biosensor application, Lu et al. demonstrated a colorimetric lead biosensor by using DNAzyme-directed assembly of Au NPs [85, 86]. The unique features of this method are its high speed (~10 min) and high sensitivity (~100 nM for Pb^{+2}).

4.6.3
Cells and Virus

Functionalized Au NPs have many attractive properties. They are nanometer in size, and may have various functional ligands on the surface. These special properties provide them with many possible modes of interaction with biological cells, such as specific binding to the cell membrane and penetration through the membrane to interact with biological molecules inside a cell or virus. For example, carbohydrate-functionalized Au NPs have been developed to explore their multivalent interactions with cell membrane surfaces, such as lectins [87]. These studies could have potential applications in lectin detection, control of cell fertilization, proliferation, viral infection, and inflammatory response. Dragnea et al. incorporated citrate-protected Au NPs inside brome mosaic virus and used them as a spectroscopic marker that could open up new opportunities for *in vivo* monitoring of viral capsid transitions [88].

Acknowledgments

We thank Dr David Londono, for the SAXS measurements, and Ms Ellen D. Semke for her contribution in protein purification.

References

1 M.-C. Daniel, D. Astruc, Gold nanoparticles: assembly, supramolecular chemistry, quantum-size-related properties, and applications toward biology, catalysis, and nanotechnology. *Chem. Rev.* **2004**, *104*, 293–346.

2 M. G. Warner, J. E. Hutchison in *Synthesis, Functionalization and Surface Treatment of Nanoparticles* (Ed. M.-I. Baraton), American Scientific Publishers: Stevenson Ranch, California, **2003**, Chapter 5, p. 67.

3 U. Kreibig, M. Vollmer, *Optical Properties of Metal Clusters*; Springer Series in Material Science, No. 25; Springer-Verlag: Berlin, **1995**, pp 187–201.

4 K. Moteshare, D. C. Myles, Molecular recognition in membrane mimics: A fluorescence probe. *J. Am. Chem. Soc.* **1994**, *116*, 7413–7414.

5 C. A. Mirkin, T. A. Taton, Materials chemistry: Semiconductors meet biology. *Nature* **2000**, *405*, 626–627.

6 M. Sastry, N. Lala, V. Patil, S. P. Chavan, A. G. Chittiboyina, Optical absorption study of the biotin-avidin interaction on colloidal silver and gold particles. *Langmuir* **1998**, *14*, 4138–4142.

7 D. Fitzmaurice, S. Connolly, Programmed assembly of gold nanocrystals in aqueous solution. *Adv. Mater.* **1999**, *11*, 1202–1205.

8 S. Mann, W. Shenton, M. Li, S. Connolly, D. Fitzmaurice, Biologically programmed nanoparticle assembly. *Adv. Mater.* **2000**, *12*, 147–150.

9 D. A. Handley in *Colloid Gold: Principles, Methods, and Applications*, (Ed. M. A. Hayat), Academic Press, Inc.: San Diego, California, **1989**, Volume 1, Chapter 2.

10 M. G. Warner, J. E. Hutchison in *Synthesis, Functionalization and Surface Treatment of Nanoparticles* (Ed. M.-I. Baraton), American Scientific Publishers, 2003, Chapter 5, p. 71.

11 F. Cariati, L. Naldini, Trianionoeptakis(triarylphosphine) undecagold cluster compounds. *Inorg. Chim. Acta* **1971**, *5*, 172.

12 M. Brust, M. Walker, D. Bethell, D. J. Schiffrin, R. Whyman, Synthesis of thiol-derivatised gold nanoparticles in a two-phase liquid–liquid system. *J. Chem. Soc., Chem. Commun.* **1994**, 801–802.

13 M. Brust, J. Fink, D. Bethell, D. J. Schiffrin, C. J. Kiely, Synthesis and reactions of functionalised gold nanoparticles. *J. Chem. Soc., Chem. Commun.* **1995**, 1655–1656.

14 T. G. Schaaff, G. K. Knight, M. N. Shafigullin, R. F. Borkman, R. L. Whetten, Isolation and selected properties of a 10.4 kDa gold:glutathione cluster compound. *J. Phys. Chem. B* **1998**, *102*, 10643.

15 A. C. Templeton, D. E. Cliffel, R. W. Murray, Redox and fluorophore

functionalization of water-soluble, tiopronin-protected gold clusters. *J. Am. Chem. Soc.* **1999**, *121*, 7081.

16 T. G. Schaaff, M. N. Shafigullin, J. T. Khoury, I. Vezmar, R. L. Whetten, W. Cullen, P. N. First, C. Gutierrez-Wing, J. Ascensio, M. Jose-Yacaman, Isolation of smaller nanocrystal Au molecules: robust quantum effects in optical spectra. *J. Phys. Chem. B* **1997**, *101*, 7885–7891.

17 A. C. Templeton, W. P. Wuelfing, R. W. Murray, Monolayer-protected cluster molecules. *Acc. Chem. Res.* **2000**, *33*, 27–36.

18 E. E. Foos, A. W. Snow, M. E. Twigg, M. G. Ancona, Thiol-terminated di-, tri-, and tetraethylene oxide functionalized gold nanoparticles: A water-soluble, charge-neutral cluster. *Chem. Mater.* **2002**, *14*, 2401.

19 M. Bartz, J. Kuther, G. Nelles, N. Weber, R. Seshadri, W. J. Tremel, Monothiols derived from glycols as agents for stabilizing gold colloids in water: synthesis, self-assembly and use as crystallization templates. *J. Mater. Chem.* **1999**, *9*, 1121.

20 M. Zheng, F. Davidson, X. Huang, Ethylene glycol monolayer protected nanoparticles for eliminating nonspecific binding with biological molecules. *J. Am. Chem. Soc.* **2003**, *125*, 7790–7791.

21 M. Zheng, Z. Li, X. Huang, Ethylene glycol monolayer protected nanoparticles: synthesis, characterization, and interactions with biological molecules. *Langmuir* **2004**, *20*, 4226–4235.

22 A. K. Kanaras, F. S. Kamounah, K. Schaumburg, C. J. Kiely, M. Brust, Thioalkylated tetraethylene glycol: a new ligand for water soluble monolayer protected gold clusters. *Chem. Commun.* **2002**, 2294–2295.

23 A. C. Templeton, S. Chen, S. M. Gross, R. M. Murray, Water-soluble, isolable gold clusters protected by tiopronin and coenzyme A monolayers. *Langmuir* **1999**, *15*, 66 76.

24 D. E. Cliffel, F. P. Zamborini, S. M. Gross, R. W. Murray, Mercaptoammonium-monolayer-protected, water-soluble gold, silver, and palladium clusters. *Langmuir* **2000**, *16*, 9699–9702.

25 X.-M. Li, V. Paraschiv, J. Huskens, D. N. Reinhoudt, Sulfonic acid-functionalized gold nanoparticles: A colloid-bound catalyst for soft lithographic application on self-assembled monolayers. *J. Am. Chem. Soc.* **2003**, *125*, 4279–4284.

26 K. Naka, H. Itoh, Y. Tampo, Y. Chujo, Effect of gold nanoparticles as a support for the oligomerization of L-cysteine in an aqueous solution. *Langmuir* **2003**, *19*, 5546–5549.

27 S. Chen, K. Kimura, Synthesis and characterization of carboxylate-modified gold nanoparticle powders dispersible in water. *Langmuir* **1999**, *15*, 1075–1082.

28 H. Yao, O. Momozawa, T. Hamatani, K. Kimura, Stepwise size-selective extraction of carboxylate-modified gold nanoparticles from an aqueous suspension into toluene with tetraoctylammonium cations. *Chem. Mater.* **2001**, *13*, 4692–4697.

29 Y. Negishi, T. Tsukuda, One-pot preparation of subnanometer-sized gold clusters via reduction and stabilization by *meso*-2,3-dimercaptosuccinic acid. *J. Am. Chem. Soc.* **2003**, *125*, 4046–4047.

30 K. Naka, H. Itoh, Y. Tampo, Y. Chujo, Effect of gold nanoparticles as a support for the oligomerization of L-cysteine in an aqueous solution. *Langmuir* **2003**, *19*, 5546–5549.

31 W. P. Wuelfing, S. M. Gross, D. T. Miles, R. W. Murray, Nanometer gold clusters protected by surface-bound monolayers of thiolated poly(ethylene glycol) polymer electrolyte. *J. Am. Chem. Soc.* **1998**, *120*, 12696–12967.

32 H. Otsuka, Y. Akiyama, Y. Nagasaki, K. Kataoka, Quantitative and reversible lectin-induced association of gold nanoparticles modified with α-lactosyl-ω-mercapto-poly(ethylene glycol). *J. Am. Chem. Soc.* **2001**, *123*, 8226–8230.

33 J. M. de la Fuente, A. G. Barrientos, T. C. Rojas, J. Rojo, J. Canada, A. Fernandez, S. Penades, Gold glyconanoparticles as water-soluble polyvalent models to study carbohydrate interactions. *Angew. Chem. Int. Ed.* **2001**, *40*, 2257–2261.

34 A. G. Barrientos, J. M. De la Fuente, T. C. Rojas, J. Rojo, A. Fernandez, S. Penades, Gold glyconanoparticles: synthetic polyvalent ligands mimicking glycocalyx-like surfaces as tools for glycobiological studies. *Chem. Eur. J.* **2003**, *9*, 1909–1921.

35 C.-C. Lin, Y.-C. Yeh, C.-Y. Yang, C.-L. Chen, G.-F. Chen, C.-C. Chen, Y.-C. Wu, Selective binding of mannose-encapsulated gold nanoparticles to type 1 Pili in *Escherichia coli*. *J. Am. Chem. Soc.* **2002**, *124*, 3508–3509.

36 C.-C. Lin, Y.-C. Yeh, C.-Y. Yang, C.-L. Chen, G.-F. Chen, C.-C. Chen, Y.-C. Wu, Quantitative analysis of multivalent interactions of carbohydrate-encapsulated gold nanoparticles with concanavalin A. *Chem. Commun.* **2003**, 2920–2921.

37 B. Nolting, J.-J. Yu, G.-Y. Liu, S.-J. Cho, S. Kauzlarich, and J. Gervay-Hague, Synthesis of gold glyconanoparticles and biological evaluation of recombinant Gp120 interactions. *Langmuir* **2003**, *19*, 6465–6473.

38 G. Schmid, N. Kelin, I. Korste, U. Kreibig, D. Schoenauer, Large transition metal clusters – VI. Ligand exchange reactions on $Au_{55}(PPh_3)_{12}Cl_6$ – the formation of a water soluble Au_{55} cluster. *Polyhedron* **1988**, *7*, 605–608.

39 M. J. Hostetler, S. J. Green, J. J. Stokes, R. W. Murray, Monolayers in three dimensions: synthesis and electrochemistry of functionalized alkanethiolate-stabilized gold cluster compounds. *J. Am. Chem. Soc.* **1996**, *118*, 4212–4213.

40 D. T. Miles, R. W. Murray, Redox and double-layer charging of phenothiazine functionalized monolayer-protected clusters. *Anal. Chem.* **2001**, *73*, 921–929.

41 S. Chen, Nanoparticle assemblies: "rectified" quantized charging in aqueous media. *J. Am. Chem. Soc.* **2000**, *122*, 7420–7421.

42 S. Chen, R. Pei, Ion-induced rectification of nanoparticle quantized capacitance charging in aqueous solutions. *J. Am. Chem. Soc.* **2001**, *123*, 10607–10615.

43 F. P. Zamborini, M. C. Leopold, J. F. Hicks, P. J. Kulesza, M. A. Malik, R. W. Murray, Electron hopping conductivity and vapor sensing properties of flexible network polymer films of metal nanoparticles. *J. Am. Chem. Soc.* **2002**, *124*, 8958–8964.

44 T. Gu, T. Ye, J. D. Simon, J. K. Whitesell, M. A. Fox, Subpicosecond transient dynamics in gold nanoparticles encapsulated by a fluorophore-terminated monolayer. *J. Phys. Chem. B* **2003**, *107*, 1765–1771.

45 T. Huang, R. W. Murray, Quenching of $[Ru(bpy)_3]^{2+}$ fluorescence by binding to Au nanoparticles. *Langmuir* **2002**, *18*, 7077–7081.

46 K. K. Sandhu, C. M. McIntosh, J. M. Simard, S. W. Smith, V. M. Rotello, Gold nanoparticle-mediated transfection of mammalian cells. *Bioconj. Chem.* **2002**, *13*, 3–6.

47 G. Wang, J. Zhang, R. W. Murray, DNA binding of an ethidium intercalator attached to a monolayer-protected gold cluster. *Anal. Chem.* **2002**, *74*, 4320–4327.

48 J. F. Hicks, Y. Seok-Shon, R. W. Murray, Layer-by-layer growth of polymer/nanoparticle films containing monolayer-protected gold clusters. *Langmuir* **2002**, *18*, 2288–2294.

49 C. A. Mirkin, R. L. Letsinger, R. C. Mucic, J. J. Storhoff, *Nature* **1996**, *382*, 607–611.

50 A. P. Alivisatos, K. P. Johnsson, X. Peng, T. E. Wilson, C. J. Loweth, M. P. Bruchez Jr., P. G. Schultz, Organization of 'nanocrystal molecules' using DNA. *Nature* **1996**, *382*, 609–611.

51 G. Wang, J. Zhang, R. W. Murray, DNA binding of an ethidium intercalator attached to a monolayer-

protected gold cluster. *Anal. Chem.* **2002**, *74*(17), 4320–4327.

52 M. Sastry, M. Rao, K. N. Ganesh, Electrostatic assembly of nanoparticles and biomacromolecules. *Acc. Chem. Res.* **2002**, *35*, 847–855.

53 C. M. Niemeyer, W. Burger, J. Peplies, Covalent DNA-streptavidin conjugates as building blocks for novel biometallic nanostructures. *Angew. Chem. Int. Ed.* **1998**, *37*, 2265–2268.

54 C. M. Niemeyer, M. Adler, S. Gao, L. Chi, Supramolecular nanocircles consisting of streptavidin and DNA. *Angew. Chem. Int. Ed.* **2000**, *39*, 3056–3059.

55 C. M. Niemeyer, Bioorganic applications of semisynthetic DNA-protein conjugates. *Chem. Eur. J.* **2001**, *7*, 3189–3195.

56 Y. Cao, R. Jin, C. A. Mirkin, Nanoparticles with Raman spectroscopic fingerprints for DNA and RNA detection. *Science* **2002**, *297*, 1536–1540.

57 C. J. Loweth, W. B. Caldwell, X. Peng, A. P. Alivisatos, P. G. Schultz, DNA-based assembly of gold nanocrystals. *Angew. Chem., Int. Ed. Engl.* **1999**, *38*, 1808–1812.

58 J. Nam, S. Park, C. A. Mirkin, Bio-barcodes based on oligonucleotide-modified nanoparticles. *J. Am. Chem. Soc.* **2002**, *124*, 3820–3821.

59 M. Zheng, X. Huang, Nanoparticles comprising a mixed monolayer for specific bindings with biomolecules. *J. Am. Chem. Soc.* **2004**, *126*, 12047–12054.

60 X. Huang, M. Zheng, *US Pat.* **2004**, 0115345 A1.

61 S. A. Wolfe, L. Nekludova, C. O. Pabo, DNA Recognition by Cys_2His_2 zinc finger proteins. *Annu. Rev. Biophys. Biomol. Struct.* **2000**, *29*, 183–212.

62 J. C. Venter et al, The sequence of the human genome. *Science* **2001**, *291*, 1304–1351.

63 N. P. Pavletich, C. O. Pabo, Zinc finger-DNA recognition: crystal structure of a Zif268-DNA complex at 2.8 Å. *Science* **1991**, *252*, 809–817.

64 J. S. Kim, C. O. Pabo, Getting a handhold on DNA: design of poly-zinc finger proteins with femotomolar dissociation constants. *Proc. Natl. Acad. Sci. U.S.A.* **1998**, *95*, 2812–2817.

65 J. J. Storhoff, A. A. Lazarides, R. C. Mucic, C. A. Mirkin, R. L. Letsinger, G. C. Schatz, What controls the optical properties of DNA-linked gold nanoparticle assemblies. *J. Am. Chem. Soc.* **2000**, *122*, 4640–4650.

66 T. A. Taton, R. C. Mucic, C. A. Mirkin, R. L. Letsinger, The DNA-mediated formation of supramolecular mono- and multilayered nanoparticle structures. *J. Am. Chem. Soc.* **2000**, *122*, 6305–6306.

67 J. Reichert, A. Csaki, J. M. Kohler, W. Fritzsche, Chip-based optical detection of DNA hybridization by means of nanobead labeling. *Anal. Chem.* **2000**, *72*, 6025–6029.

68 J. J. Storhoff, A. D. Lucas, V. Garimella, Y. P. Bao, U. R. Muller, Homogeneous detection of unamplified genomic DNA sequences based on colorimetric scatter of gold nanoparticle probes. *Nature Biotechnol.* **2004**, *22*, 883–887.

69 J. Wang, D. Xu, R. Polski, Magnetically-induced solid-state electrochemical detection of DNA hybridization. *J. Am. Chem. Soc.* **2002**, *124*, 4208–4209.

70 B. Dubertret, M. Calame, A. J. Libchaber, Single-mismatch detection using gold-quenched fluorescent oligonucleotides. *Nat. Biotechnol.* **2001**, *19*, 365–370.

71 D. J. Maxwell, J. R. Taylor, S. Nie, Self-assembled nanoparticle probes for recognition and detection of biomolecules. *J. Am. Chem. Soc.* **2002**, *124*, 9606–9612.

72 B. J. Taft, A. D. Lazareck, G. D. Withey, A. Yin, J. M. Xu, S. O. Kelley, Site-specific assembly of DNA and appended cargo on arrayed carbon nanotubes. *J. Am. Chem. Soc.* **2004**, *126*, 12750–12751.

73 W. Shenton, S. A. Davis, S. Mann, Directed self-assembly of nanoparticles into macroscopic materials using antibody-antigen

recognition. *Adv. Mater.* **1999**, *11*, 449–452.

74 N. T. K. Thanh, Z. Rosenzweig, Development of an aggregation-based immunoassay for anti-protein A using gold nanoparticles. *Anal. Chem.* **2002**, *74*, 1624–1628.

75 N. O. Fischer, C. M. McIntosh, J. M. Simard, V. M. Rotello, Inhibition of chymotrypsin through surface binding using nanoparticle-based receptors. *Proc. Natl. Acad. Sci. U.S.A.* **2002**, *99*, 5018–5023.

76 N. O. Fischer, A. Verma, C. M. Goodman, J. M. Simard, V. M. Rotello, Reversible "irreversible" inhibition of chymotrypsin using nanoparticle receptors. *J. Am. Chem. Soc.* **2003**, *125*(44), 13387–13391.

77 J.-M. Nam, S.-J. Park, C. A. Mirkin, Bio-barcodes based on oligonucleotide-modified nanoparticles. *J. Am. Chem. Soc.* **2002**, *124*, 3820–3821.

78 Y. C. Cao, R. Jin, J.-M. Nam, C. S. Thaxton, C. A. Mirkin, Raman dye-labeled nanoparticle probes for proteins. *J. Am. Chem. Soc.* **2003**, *125*, 14676–14677.

79 V. Pavlov, Y. Xiao, B. Shlyahovsky, I. Willner, Aptamer-functionalized Au nanoparticles for the amplified optical detection of thrombin. *J. Am. Chem. Soc.* **2004**, *126*, 11768–11769.

80 H. Li, S. H. Park, J. H. Reif, T. H. LaBean, H. Yan, DNA-templated self-assembly of protein and nanoparticle linear arrays. *J. Am. Chem. Soc.* **2004**, *126*, 418–419.

81 C. S. Yun, G. A. Khitrov, D. E. Vergona, N. O. Reich, G. F. Strouse, Enzymatic manipulation of DNA-nanomaterial constructs. *J. Am. Chem. Soc.* **2002**, *124*, 7644–7645.

82 C. D. Keating, K. M. Kovaleski, M. J. Natan, Protein:colloid conjugates for surface enhanced Raman scattering: stability and control of protein orientation. *J. Phys. Chem. B* **1998**, *102*, 9404–9413.

83 A. Gole, C. Dash, C. Soman, S. R. Sainkar, M. Rao, M. Sastry, On the preparation, characterization, and enzymatic activity of fungal protease-gold colloid bioconjugates. *Bioconj. Chem.* **2001**, *12*, 684–690.

84 R. Hong, T. Emrick, V. M. Rotello, Monolayer-controlled substrate selectivity using noncovalent enzyme-nanoparticle conjugates. *J. Am. Chem. Soc.* **2004**, *126*, 13572–13573.

85 J. Liu, Y. Lu, A colorimetric lead biosensor using DNAzyme-directed assembly of gold nanoparticles. *J. Am. Chem. Soc.* **2003**, *125*, 6642–6643.

86 J. Liu, Y. Lu, Accelerated color change of gold nanoparticles assembled by DNAzymes for simple and fast colorimetric Pb^{2+} detection. *J. Am. Chem. Soc.* **2004**, *126*, 12298–12305.

87 D. C. Hone, A. H. Haines, D. A. Russell, Rapid, quantitative colorimetric detection of a lectin using mannose-stabilized gold nanoparticles. *Langmuir* **2003**, *19*, 7141–7144.

88 B. Dragnea, C. Chen, E.-S. Kwak, B. Stein, C. C. Kao, Gold nanoparticles as spectroscopic enhancers for in vitro studies on single viruses. *J. Am. Chem. Soc.* **2003**, *125*, 6374–6375.

5 Biofunctionalization of Phospholipid Polymer Nanoparticles

Junji Watanabe, Jongwon Park, Tomomi Ito, Madoka Takai, and Kazuhiko Ishihara

5.1 Introduction

Recently, our interest in biomaterials has shifted to nanobiomaterials, which is integrated with nanofabrication. Nano-scaled fabrication is based on molecular assemblies such as micelles, self-assembled monolayers, and supramolecular compounds [1–8]. Also, many kinds of nano-scaled devices, such as bio-chips and nanoparticles, have been proposed and designed [9–17]. Nano-scaled chemistry and nanofabrication focus on chemical reactions and sensing. The most fascinating phenomena, chemical reactions, are created in a nano-scaled world, but are never carried out on an ordinary scale. In these nano-scaled devices, the biointerface property is the dominant factor in providing excellent performance. To enhance biofunctionalization it is most important for the nano-scaled device to suppress non-specific protein adsorption since the surface is exposed to many biological components; blood, serum, and cells. Few researchers have understood the importance of materials in the design of biointerfaces and bioconjugations on the nanoscale [18–21]. This chapter summarizes newly engineered materials using bioinspired phospholipid polymer chemistry for biofunctionalization, with particular focus on phospholipid polymer nanoparticles for molecular diagnosis. Phospholipid polymers are available in numerous situations for specific biomaterials [22–25], and could function as a molecular machine [26–28]. Ishihara et al. proposed a fundamental concept for the synthesis of phospholipid polymers in the early 1990s [29, 30]. Now, we easily purchase many kinds of products containing phospholipid polymer – cosmetics, eye care products, textile goods, and fine chemicals for advanced bioreactions – which were designed through collaborations between Professor Ishihara and industrial companies. This is typical process and development – from laboratory materials to commercial products. The developed phospholipid polymer synthesis has been recognized world-wide, and much work has been reported subsequently (see Ref. [31] for an excellent review). Further research into nanofabrication may well provide us with a better "quality of life" –

Nanotechnologies for the Life Sciences Vol. 1
Biofunctionalization of Nanomaterials. Edited by Challa S. S. R. Kumar

ISBN: 3-527-31381-8

perhaps especially when the design of biomaterials is based on phospholipid polymers.

5.2
Nanofabrication for Biomedical Applications

Nanoparticles are a good substrate for bioconjugation. They have (a) a relatively high specific surface area, (b) good dispersivity in aqueous media, and (c) can be combined with nano-processed bio-chips. These characteristics can be used in a wide variety of applications, e.g. medical diagnosis, drug delivery carriers for targeting, micro-total analysis systems, and biosensors [32–35]. The most important factor in improving the nanoparticles is the enhancement of specificity to the target biomolecule such as antigen, substrate, and DNA (i.e. selectivity), and the suppression of non-specific interactions (sensitivity). Thus, bioinspired phospholipid polymers are key materials in the research on and development of nanoparticles.

5.2.1
Nano-scaled Processing

Nanoparticles are a promising architecture for analyzing chemical species and providing a dynamic response. Many kinds of nanoparticles with unique structures have been prepared; Mori et al. have reported hybrid nanoparticles composed of a polymer shell with a silica core [36–38]. The polymer shell was carefully designed by the use of atom transfer radical polymerization, forming a hyperbranched structure. The nanoparticles showed reversible pH-induced complexations in a polyelectrolyte. Nanoparticles based on silica can be designed with unique structures, for easy dissolution by hydrogen fluoride. Kamata et al. have fabricated a core-shell spherical colloid with a hollow interior [39]. The hollow colloid provides a small container, in which a gold particle was trapped. The colloid particle, with its movable core, resembles a bell. The nanoparticles reported above could not be applied as advanced biomedical materials in their present form. However, suitable preparative techniques for biofunctionalization should soon be available.

Vertegel et al. have examined the size effect on the stabilization of immobilized enzyme by using silica nanoparticles (particle size 4–100 nm) [40]. Their report is impressive and important in terms of expressing biofunctions effectively. For enzyme immobilization, stronger protein–particle interactions exist on larger nanoparticles, resulting in multipoint immobilizations. The immobilized enzymes show less enzymatic activity. Akashi et al. have synthesized directly core-corona nanoparticles (one-pot preparation), which consist of a hydrophobic core and hydrophilic corona, by using water-soluble macromonomers [41, 42]. The key item is the water-soluble macromonomer; a typical example was reported using a methacrylate monomer containing a methoxy-terminated poly(ethylene glycol) side chain. The water-soluble segment was enriched spontaneously at the interface between the hydrophobic core and water, thus stabilizing the interfacial energy. The preparative conditions are easily changeable to prepare many kinds of nanoparticles with core-corona morphology. Recently, lectin-conjugated nanoparticles have been prepared for the purpose of detecting the HIV virus [42]. From human serum, the virus is easily captured, and the nanoparticles formed in a precipitation. Caldwell et al. evaluated surface coverage by the immobilization of biomolecules; in particular, oligonucleotides were attached to polystyrene-based nanoparticles [43]. A number of the attached oligonucleotides were evaluated using the sedimentation field flow fractionation technique (a type of chromatography). This characterization technique is a powerful tool for estimating surface conditions: a number of functional groups, active linkage for bioconjugation, immobilized proteins, and binding target molecules in each step.

5.2.2
Key Materials for Nanofabrication

We have proposed recently the assembly of phospholipids polar group on nanoparticles. Nanoparticles are generally unstable as colloid particles in aqueous media. A hydrophilic moiety and ionic groups are incorporated onto the surface to prepare the interface. One unusual interface is the cell membrane, which is composed of phospholipid molecules, glycoproteins, and channel-forming proteins. It provides not only division between the cytoplasm and the outer environment but also allows communication via antenna molecules and channels. Ishihara et al. have designed and synthesized a novel functional monomer with a phospholipid polar group, 2-methacryloyloxyethyl phosphorylcholine (MPC, Fig. 5.1), in order to fabricate the cell membrane structure as a biointerface [29–31]. MPC (methacrylate derivative) easily polymerized with any kind of acrylate and methacrylate monomers by conventional radical, living radical, and atom transfer radical polymerizations [44–47]. Finely designed polymers with phospholipid polar groups were easily prepared by these polymerization techniques. The phospholipid polymer could form the cell membrane-like interface using coating, polymer blending, and polymer graft techniques [48–53]. A typical phospholipid polymer is copolymerized with *n*-butyl methacrylate (BMA); the phospholipid polymer-coated surface is illustrated in Fig. 5.2. The phospholipid polymer provided a very bio-inert interface; in particular, a non-specific interactive biointerface was obtained on diverse materials, and many biomedical devices have been developed using phospholipid polymer technology [22–25]. The stability of the phospholipid polymer-modified enzyme was also significantly prolonged in comparison with the native enzyme [26–28]. Furthermore,

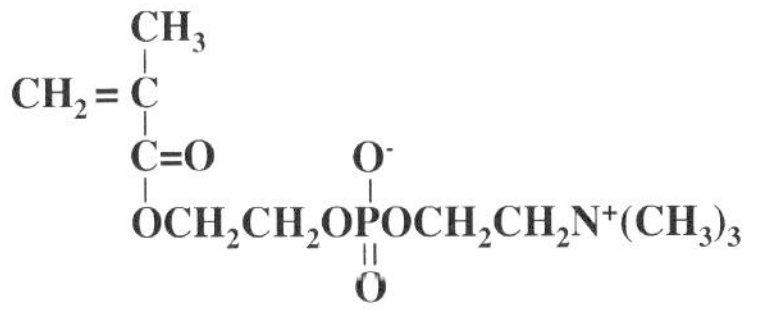

Fig. 5.1. Chemical structure of 2-methacryloyloxyethyl phosphorylcholine (MPC).

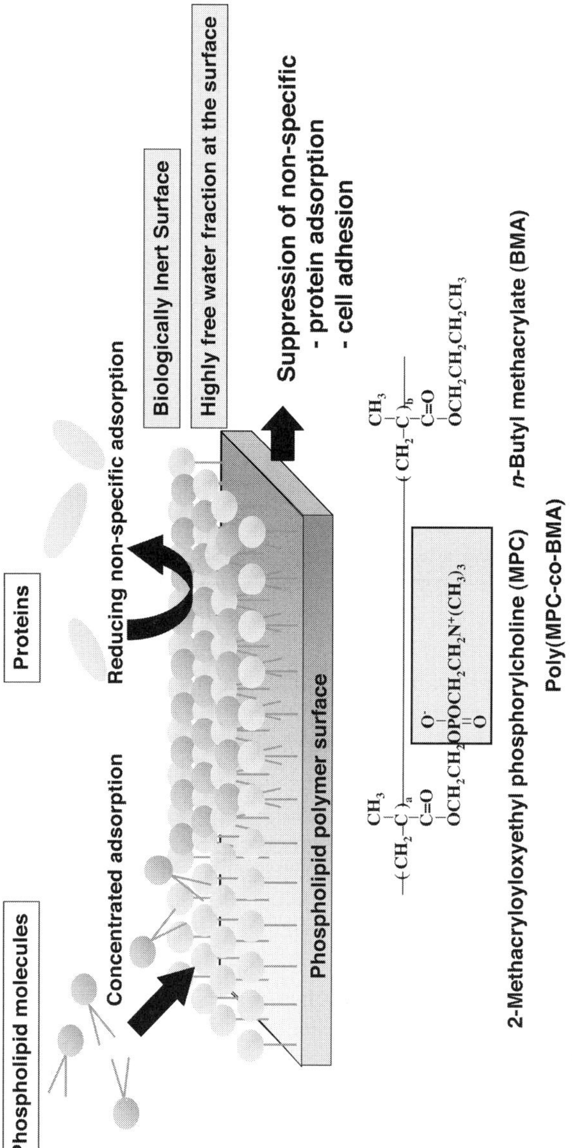

Fig. 5.2. Schematic illustration of bioinert properties on phospholipid polymer surfaces by poly(MPC-*co*-BMA).

the phospholipid polymer spontaneously formed nano-structured aggregations, indicating amphiphilic and surfactant-like properties [54]. Employment of a polymer-based biomimetic surface is a promising approach to prepare nano-scaled devices for biofunctionalization.

5.3
Design of Bioconjugate Nanoparticles

Bioconjugate nanoparticles have contributed to the development of advanced biomedical research. Nano-scaled materials are both available and very interesting. The most favorable characteristics of the nanoparticles are their ability to form fine, stable dispersions in aqueous media, the ease in which immobilized biomolecules can be located, and their relatively large surface area.

5.3.1
Bioconjugate Phospholipid Polymer

The phospholipid polymer was designed for bioconjugation with biomolecules such as proteins, peptides, and DNA. We have synthesized a functional monomer – a *p*-nitrophenyloxycarbonyl poly(oxyethylene) methacrylate (MEONP) – having an active ester linkage for bioconjugation [55]. MPC, MEONP, *n*-butyl methacrylate (BMA) were copolymerized to prepare the bioconjugate phospholipid polymer (PMBN, Fig. 5.3) by a conventional radical polymerization technique with 2,2′-azobisisobutyronitrile as an initiator. This polymer serves two functions – suppression of non-specific adsorption from the human body and the connection of biomolecules via an active ester group. Table 5.1 shows typical synthetic results. Two kinds of the phospholipid polymers were prepared with regards to solubility in water. The MPC unit is highly hydrophilic, so the solubility was changeable by MPC unit composition. Below 30 mol% of MPC unit, the phospholipid polymer could not dissolve in water but did so in ethanol. The water-insoluble polymer provided a stable biointerface for capillary electrophoresis [56]. A bioconjugate phospholipid polymer having 40 mol% of MPC could easily dissolve in water; 2 mol% of active ester groups were incorporated.

5.3.2
Solution Properties by Fluorescence Probe

The fluorescence probe sodium 1-anilinonaphthalene-8-sulfonate (ANS) is used as an indicator for the estimation of polarity in hydrophobic environments, showing a maximum fluorescence at 515 nm (λ_{EM}) in water and 475 nm (λ_{EM}) in *n*-butyl alcohol [excitation at 370 nm (λ_{EX})]. The maximum fluorescence wavelength depended on various environmental conditions. For example, it is possible to estimate micro-environment factors such as change in higher-ordered conformation in proteins. Generally, amphiphilic polymers spontaneously aggregate in an aqueous media.

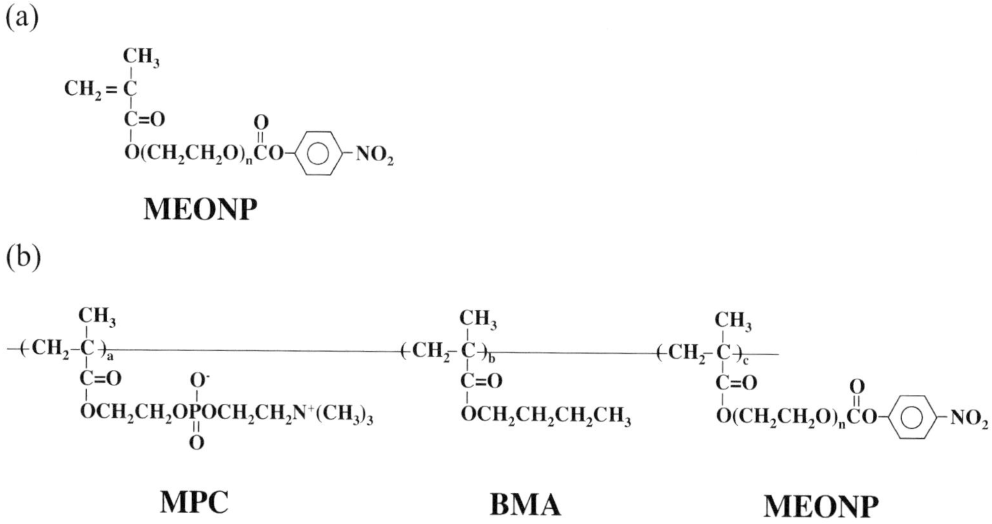

Fig. 5.3. Chemical structure of active ester monomer (MEONP) formed using *p*-nitrophenyl chloroformate (a) and the bioconjugate phospholipid polymer (PMBN) (b) derived from the copolymerization of MPC, BMA and MEONP. The average number of oxyethylene units was 4.5.

We evaluated the change in the maximum fluorescence wavelength by ANS. Figure 5.4 indicates that the maximum wavelength shifted upon increasing the polymer concentration. Above 0.1 mg mL^{-1} of polymer, the wavelength was below 480 nm, indicating that the ANS molecule is trapped in lower polarity. The change in maximum wavelength showed that the phospholipid polymer spontaneously formed aggregates, indicating that it could form hydrophobic domains in a water

Tab. 5.1. Synthetic results of bioconjugate phospholipid polymers.

	Monomer unit composition (mol%)		*Time (h)*	*Yield (%)*	M_W[b]	*Solubility in water*[c]
	In feed	*In copolymer*[a]				
	MPC/BMA/MEONP	*MPC/BMA/MEONP*				
PMBN30	30/65/5	27/61/12	6	–	3.8×10^4	–
PMBN40	40/55/5	36/62/2	3	77	6.2×10^4	++

[Monomer] = 1.0 mol L^{-1}, [AIBN] = 10 mmol L^{-1}
Reaction temperature 60 °C.
Precipitated by Diethyl ether/chloroform (8:2).
[a] Determined by ^1H NMR.
[b] Determined by GPC in water/methanol (3:7), PEO standard.
[c] Solubility described as soluble (++) and insoluble (–).

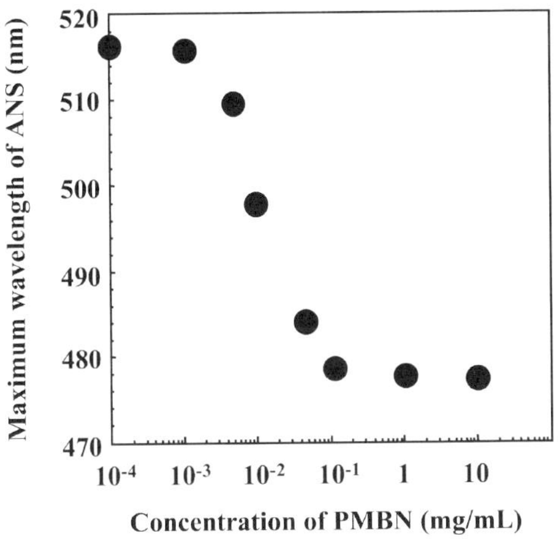

Fig. 5.4. Change in maximum fluorescence wavelength caused by phospholipid polymer aggregation ($\lambda_{EX} = 370$ nm).

environment. Therefore, phase-separated organic solvent containing polymer as core materials of the nanoparticles was stably dispersed in the phospholipid polymer aqueous solution as an emulsion, and the interface on the emulsion covered with the phospholipid polymer was then prepared. The ANS test confirmed that the phospholipid polymer aggregated in water above a concentration of 0.1 mg mL^{-1}, and could therefore be employed as an emulsifier and a surface modifier for nanoparticles.

5.3.3
Bioconjugate Nanoparticles

Bioconjugate nanoparticles have been prepared by solvent evaporation methods for the systematic design of core materials – polystyrene (PS) as a conventional polymer and poly(L-lactic acid) (PLA) as a biodegradable polymer. According to the molecular design of the bioconjugate phospholipid polymer, the hydrophobic chains, *n*-butyl groups, were considered to penetrate on the surface of nanoparticles. The phospholipid polar groups and active ester groups, which formed domains, were concentrated at the nanoparticle surface to stabilize the interface, and the *p*-nitrophenyl ester groups can freely conjugate with biomolecules (Fig. 5.5). In this section, we examine whether the characteristics of nanoparticles would alter by changing the core materials. As core polymer materials, PLA and PS were used to prepare PMBN/PLA or PMBN/PS nanoparticles by a solvent evaporation technique in aqueous medium [55, 57, 58]. In this process, the PMBN was utilized as an emulsifier, and the polymer concentration regulated the average diameter of the nanoparticles. The diameter decreased with increasing initial concentration of PMBN. Typical preparative concentrations of PMBN, PLA, and PS were 1.0, 10

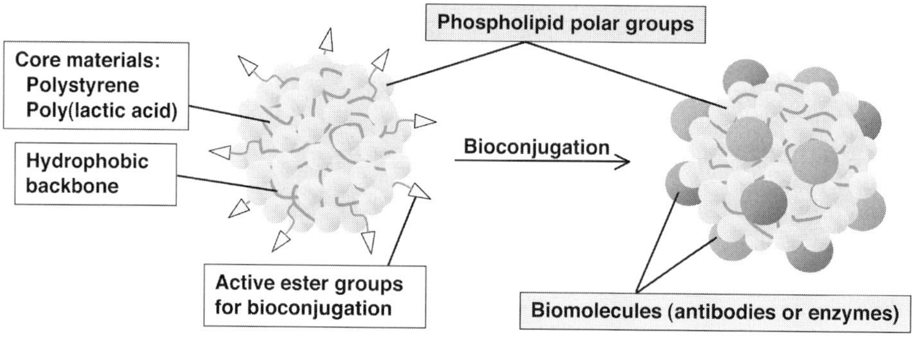

Fig. 5.5. Schematic illustration of bioconjugate phospholipid polymer nanoparticles.

and 10 mg mL^{-1}, respectively. The surface of the nanoparticles was characterized by X-ray photoelectron spectroscopy (XPS), surface ζ-potential, dynamic light scattering (DLS), scanning electron microscopy (SEM), and determination of active ester groups.

5.3.4
Surface Elemental Analysis by X-ray Photoelectron Spectroscopy

Surface analysis of the PMBN/PLA nanoparticles was carried out with XPS to estimate the phospholipid polar groups on the surface. Figure 5.6 shows the XPS spectra of C_{1s}, O_{1s}, N_{1s}, and P_{2p} on the surface of the PMBN nanoparticles. From the XPS analysis, O–C–O and C=O peaks from the phospholipid polymer were observed at 287.0 and 289.0 eV, respectively. Furthermore, a small broad peak attributed to an aromatic group based on the *p*-nitrophenyl ester group was also observed at 291.5 eV. Additionally, N_{1s} and P_{2p} peaks attributed to choline methyl (403.0 eV) and phosphate ester (134.0 eV) were observed. Moreover, the PMBN/PS nanoparticle was also characterized (Fig. 5.6). These results strongly indicated that the interface on the PMBN/PLA and PMBN/PS nanoparticles was covered with phospholipid polar groups and *p*-nitrophenyl ester groups.

5.3.5
Surface ζ-Potential on Nanoparticles

As an alternative characterization, surface ζ-potential was measured to estimate the coverage of the bioconjugate phospholipid polymer. The phospholipid polar group contains a quaternary choline methyl group (cation) and a phosphate ester group (anion). Their ions form an intramolecular ion pair; therefore, their charge is neutralized [59]. If the nanoparticles were covered with phospholipid polymers, the ζ-potential on the surface would be roughly 0 mV. That is why the ζ-potential was

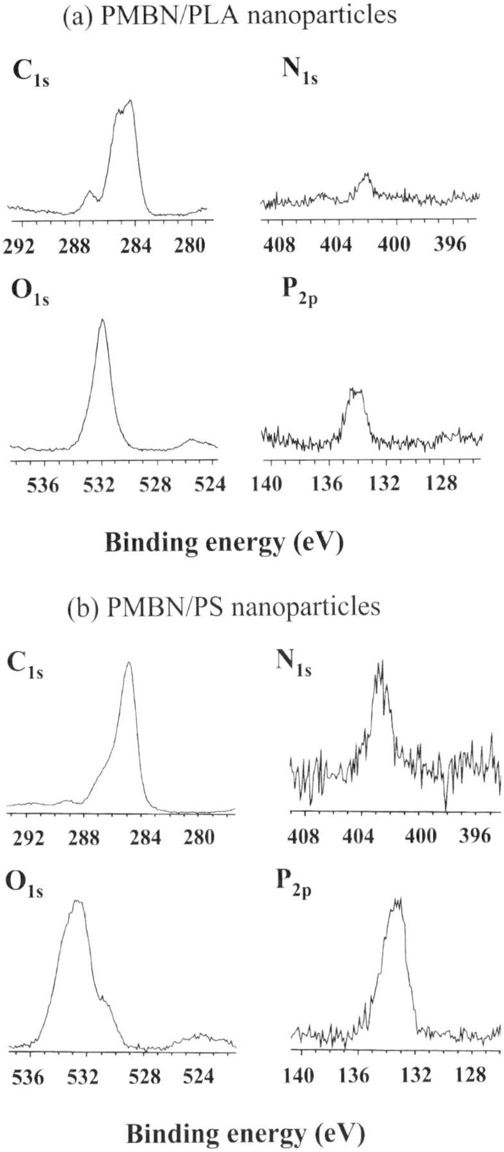

Fig. 5.6. X-ray photoelectron spectra of PMBN/PLA nanoparticles (a) and PMBN/PS nanoparticles (b).

measured for the phospholipid polymer coverage. The ζ-potential of the PMBN/PLA and PMBN/PS nanoparticles were -2.1 ± 3 mV and -2.3 ± 2 mV, respectively. The obtained ζ-potential is almost the same ratio and roughly 0 mV, as we expected. Farokhzad et al. reported a bioconjugate polymer nanoparticle composed of aptamers for targeting drug delivery to prostate cancer cells. The polymer used was PLA-*block*-poly(ethylene glycol) (PEG) with a terminal carboxylic group (PLA-PEG-COOH) [60]. According to the report, the ζ-potential of the PLA-PEG-COOH was -50 ± 3 mV, and of the PLA bare particle was -24 ± 5 mV. This indicates that the surface potential was significantly shifted to a more negative charge than the unmodified PLA nanoparticles, as a result of surface modification. Veronesi et al. reported that vanilloid (VR1) receptors on the cell membrane were activated by membrane depolarization, which is induced by charged polystyrene nanoparticles [61]. The acid-sensitive ionic channels could be activated by the electrostatic charge carried on chemically modified particles: neutral polystyrene nanoparticles (particle size: 750 nm), negative polystyrene nanoparticles (having carboxyl groups) (particle size: 860 nm), and positive polystyrene nanoparticles (having diamino groups) (particle size: 850 nm). The ζ-potential of each nanoparticle was −55 (neutral), −88 (carboxyl), and −23 (diamino) mV, respectively. From their reports, the nanoparticles showed a negative charge to maintain stability by electrostatic repulsion. For nanoparticles covered with the phospholipid polymer, the surface charge was nearly neutral, because it formed intramolecular ion pairs in phosphorylcholine groups. From the ζ-potential results, the phosphorylcholine groups were assembled on the nanoparticles.

5.3.6
Particle Size by Dynamic Light Scattering and Morphology by Scanning Electron Microscope

The particle size and size distribution of phospholipid polymer nanoparticles have been determined by dynamic light scattering measurements (DLS). The concentration of PMBN/PLA and PMBN/PS nanoparticles was 2.5 mg mL^{-1}. The size distribution of the nanoparticles is shown in Fig. 5.7. The particle size of PMBN/PLA was 270 ± 100 nm, and that of PMBN/PS was 320 ± 100 nm. It is considered that these two particles have almost the same diameter with monodispersity. The miscibility between the phospholipid polymer and core polymer materials was slightly different; the PLA core is a little superior to the PS core material. Monodispersed nanoparticles were easily, and in large quantities, prepared by an emulsion technique.

The particle size of the phospholipid polymer nanoparticles was observed using a scanning electron microscope (SEM). Figure 5.7 shows SEM pictures of the nanoparticles. From this result, the size of the PMBN/PLA and PMBN/PS nanoparticle were seen to be approximately similar, showing good agreement with the DLS measurement. Particle morphology was quite good, with a spherical form. Generally, the nanoparticle was utilized up to 100 μg mL^{-1}. Bioreactions were carried out in a 96-well multiplate, providing a maximum volume of 300 μL. To prepare nanoparticles in large quantities (mg scale), several kinds of bioreaction and biofunctionalizations can be fully designed at a laboratory level. With our emulsion technique, preparative conditions can easily be scaled-up, and the nanoparticles can then be produced on an industrial scale.

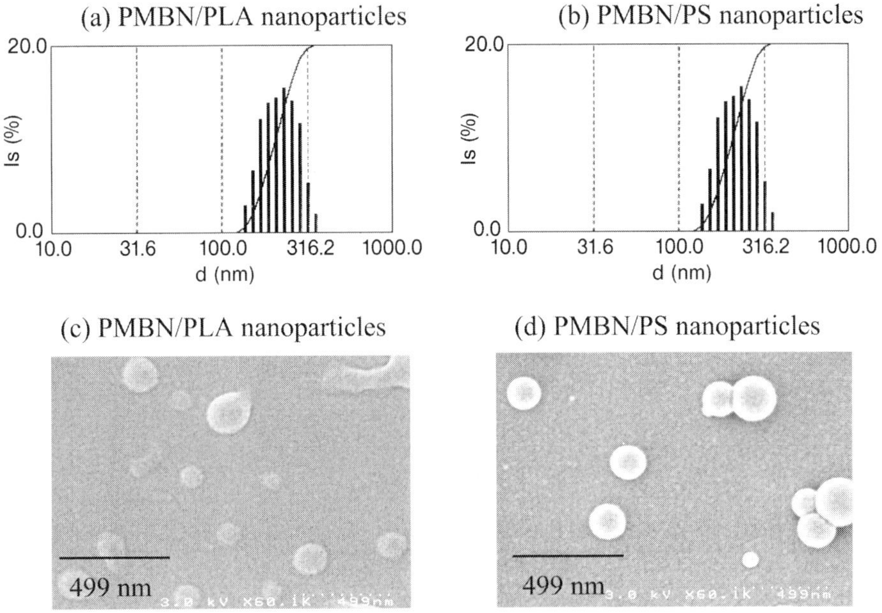

Fig. 5.7. Size distribution by dynamic light scattering of PMBN/PLA (a) and PMBN/PS (b) nanoparticles, and scanning electron microscope pictures of PMBN/PLA (c) and PMBN/PS (d) nanoparticles.

5.3.7 Determination of Active Ester Groups on Nanoparticles

Biomolecules can be quite easily immobilized on phospholipid polymer nanoparticles. A protein-bound amino group could, for example, couple to the ester groups on the polymer under physiological conditions, producing *p*-nitrophenol as a leaving group (Fig. 5.8). The bioconjugate reaction is accelerated under weak alkaline conditions. The conversion is easily estimated by the released *p*-nitrophenol. To quantify the active ester groups on the phospholipid polymer nanoparticles, NaOH aqueous solution (0.1 mol L^{-1}) was added to each suspension of PMBN/PLA and PMBN/PS for complete hydrolysis of the active ester groups. The released *p*-nitrophenol was detected by UV measurement at 400 nm. The molar extinction coefficient of the *p*-nitrophenol was calculated as $\varepsilon_{400} = 1.8 \times 10^4$ L mol^{-1} cm^{-1}. Figure 5.9 shows the change in UV spectra of PMBN/PLA nanoparticles after and before hydrolysis. From this result, the active ester groups on the PMBN/PLA nanoparticles were estimated as 1.0×10^{-9} mol (mg-nanoparticle)$^{-1}$. Thus, an active ester group exists on the PMBN/PLA nanoparticles, and the amount of such groups on PMBN/PS nanoparticles was roughly the same as on PMBN/PLA nanoparticles. The *p*-nitrophenyl ester groups, which could connect with the amino

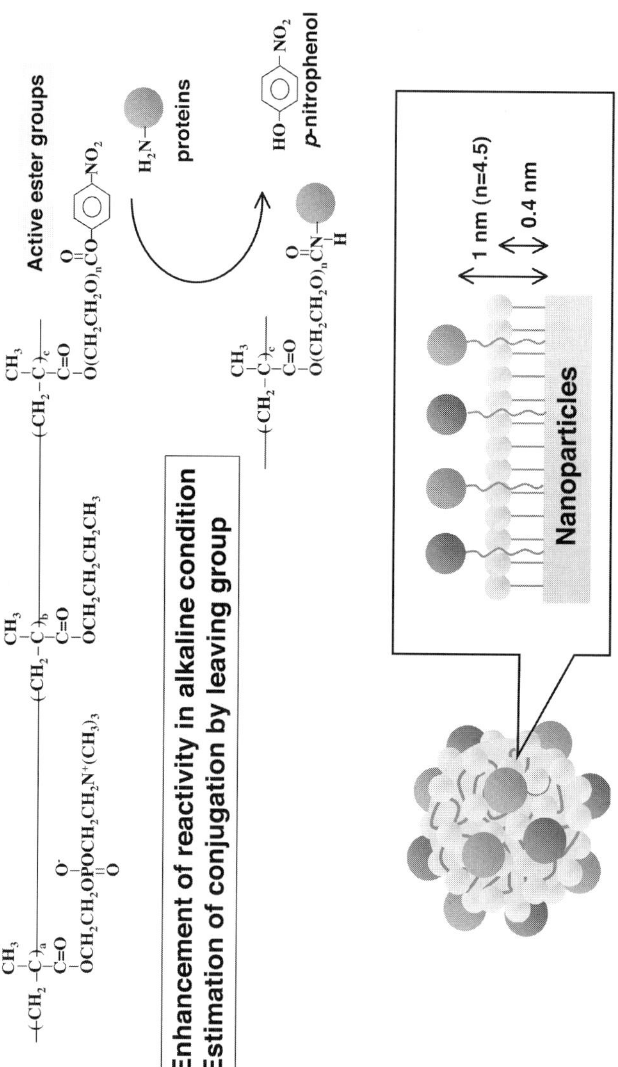

Fig. 5.8. Schematic illustration of bioconjugation on phospholipid polymer nanoparticles.

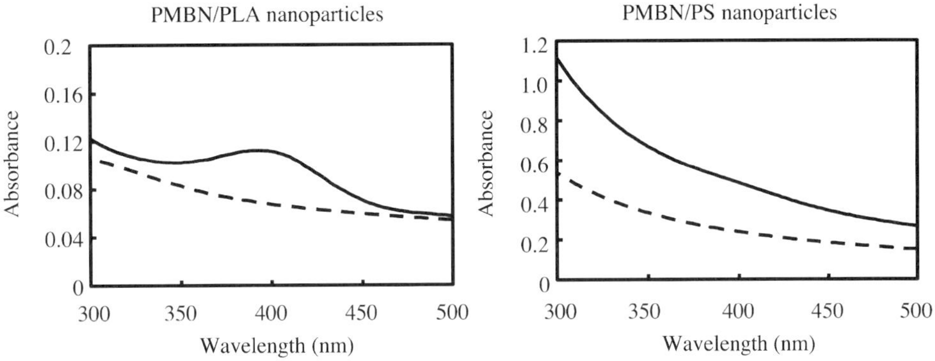

Fig. 5.9. UV spectra of *p*-nitrophenol (abs. 400 nm) before (dashed line) and after (solid line) hydrolysis of PMBN/PLA or PMBN/PS nanoparticles in 0.1 M NaOH aqueous solution.

groups on the proteins, were at the surface of the nanoparticles. Therefore, the interface of the PMBN/PLA and PMBN/PS nanoparticles was covered with active ester groups as well as phospholipid polar groups.

5.4 Biofunction on Nanoparticles

One biofunctional enzyme reaction has been evaluated on phospholipid polymer nanoparticles. In addition, a sequential enzymatic reaction has also been designed. The most favorable characteristic is the local concentration of enzyme on the nanoparticles. An increase in this local concentration is effective for valuable and rare biomolecules.

5.4.1 Design of Sequential Enzymatic Reaction

We have recently proposed a novel signal amplified diagnosis system using a sequential enzymatic reaction on nanoparticles. The nanoparticles are composed of a phospholipid polymer with active ester groups and polystyrene core. The amplified signal was evaluated by using choline oxidase and peroxidase, which were co-immobilized onto the nanoparticles. The choline oxidase reacts with choline chloride, producing hydrogen peroxide that is used as a substrate in the next enzymatic reaction by peroxidase. In this sequential reaction, the amount of tetramethylbenzidine is evaluated by change in absorbance, for the single enzymatic reaction (peroxidase) and/or sequential enzymatic reaction (choline oxidase and peroxidase) (see below for more details).

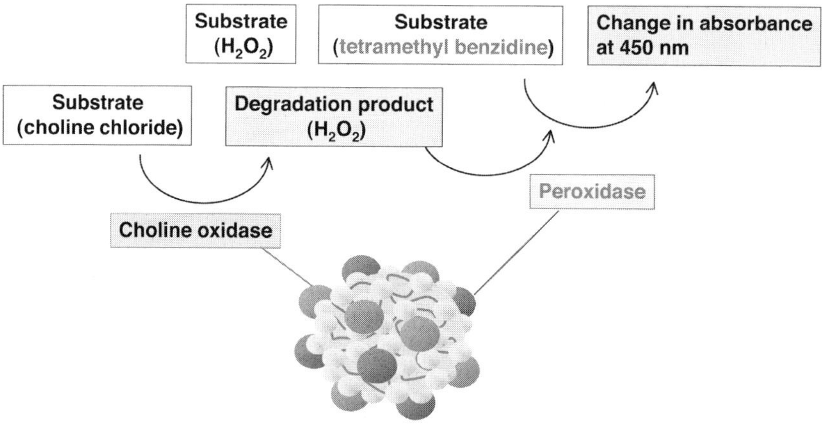

Fig. 5.10. Scheme of sequential enzymatic reactions via degradation product.

5.4.2
Amplified Signal on Nanoparticles

The active ester group on the nanoparticles is labile to the primary amino group, affording a carbamate linkage for bioconjugation. We have already estimated the conversion of the active ester linkage; 40% of the active ester linkage was converted by a reaction with proteins [58]. Two kinds of enzymes, choline oxidase and peroxidase, were co-immobilized onto the surface, and the sequential enzymatic reaction was then evaluated. The combination of the enzymes displayed communication via the degradation product (hydrogen peroxide) (Fig. 5.10). As a substrate, choline chloride (Cho), tetramethylbenzidine (TMBZ), and hydrogen peroxide (H_2O_2) were used. The Cho was oxidized by the choline oxidase, and H_2O_2 was newly produced as a degradation product. The produced H_2O_2 was used for the next enzymatic reaction; the oxidation of TMBZ by peroxidase. The H_2O_2, which was originally added to the media, could also be used as substrate.

Two kinds of protocol regarding the enzymatic reaction were examined: (a) TMBZ and H_2O_2 were added to the suspension and (b) Cho was added to the suspension with TMBZ and H_2O_2 (TMBZ/Cho). With protocol (a), only the enzymatic activity of the peroxidase was evaluated. However, newly produced H_2O_2 would enhance the sequential enzymatic reaction [protocol (b)]. The result of the enzymatic reaction was evaluated by the change in absorbance at 450 nm (Fig. 5.11). Enzymatic reaction on the nanoparticles was significantly greater than that of a simple enzyme solution, when TMBZ was added as the substrate. The total amount of enzymes in the enzyme solution was larger than that of the immobilized enzyme on the nanoparticles, because the concentration of the enzymes in the solution was the same as the feed concentration for the preparation of the enzyme-immobilized nanoparticles. Taking the total amount of the enzyme concentration into account, choline oxidase and peroxidase were considered to be locally concentrated on the particle surface in comparison with the solution.

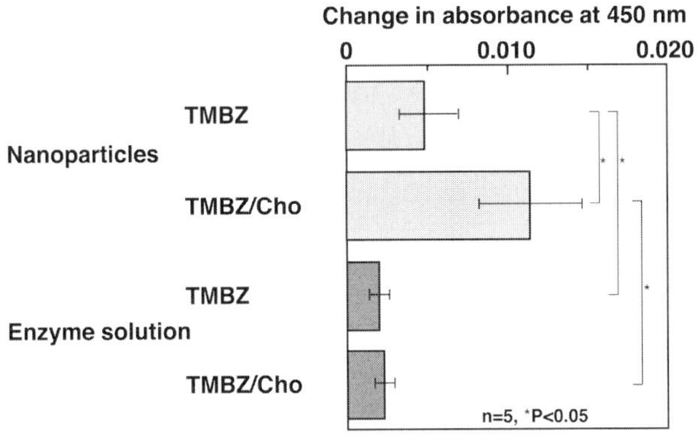

Fig. 5.11. Characterization of enzymatic reaction by changing substrate addition.

The sequential enzymatic reaction was also compared. The change in absorbance increased with addition of TMBZ/Cho, which was twice as large as that of the addition of only TMBZ. The increased enzymatic activity was considered to be based on choline oxidase, and the produced H_2O_2 was effectively free to move to its binding site at the substrate. Initially, sufficient H_2O_2 was added to the media to promote the enzymatic reaction; therefore, the increased enzymatic reaction was caused by H_2O_2 newly produced by choline oxidase. With nanoparticles, the enzymes, choline oxidase and peroxidase, were closely immobilized onto the nanoparticles; therefore, the diffusion pathway of the produced H_2O_2 was significantly shorter than that in solution. Thus, the produced H_2O_2 was differed from the originally added H_2O_2, which needed a long pathway to react with the peroxidase. Conversely, no significant difference in the enzyme solution was observed between the single reaction (TMBZ) and the sequential reaction (TMBZ/Cho). This indicated that the reaction with peroxidase proceeded through a single reaction, even if Cho was added to the media.

5.5 Application for Molecular Diagnosis

Recently, molecular diagnosis using bioconjugate nanoparticles has focused on the biomedical field. The obtained S/N ratio (signal/noise) generally decreased due to non-specific protein adsorption under physiological conditions. In this section we introduce a hyper-sensitive C-reactive protein detection system using the phospholipid polymer nanoparticles.

5.5.1 Example of C-reactive Protein Detection Using Nanoparticles

The C reactive protein (CRP) is synthesized by the liver in response to interleukin 6 and is well known as one of the classical acute-phase reactants and as a marker of inflammation. For some time, the measurement of CRP concentration has been used as a clinical bio-marker for monitoring autoimmune diseases and infectious processes, such as rheumatoid arthritis. It has recently been suggested that a marker of inflammation, along with serum cholesterol, are critical components in the development and progression of atherosclerosis [62, 63]. However, the prospect of using CRP as a predictor of future vascular risks faced a large obstacle because existing conventional assay methods were neither sensitive enough to detect very low-levels of CRP in serum nor concerned about problems of non-specific protein adsorption and denaturation of conjugated biomolecules [64, 65]. Among conventional analytical methods, immunoassay, which uses the specific affinity of antigen–antibody, has been considered as a useful technique for clinical analyses and medical diagnostics [66]. Major progress in the use of immunoassay principles occurred with the development of several fundamental techniques [67]. Among several methods, immunoagglutination using colloidal particles has been widely used because of its rapid, simple, and inexpensive properties [68, 69]. There have been many innovations in diagnostics since microsphere agglutination was first used in medical diagnosis as agglutination-based tests in the late 1950s [70]. Although various types of colloidal particles (e.g., latex, gold, sol, and polymeric particles) have been introduced to immobilize the biorecognition element (e.g., antibody, DNA, etc.) for immunoagglutination, the latex particle, prepared by emulsion polymerizations, has been widely used in the diagnostics of various infections and to detect biomarkers or some chemical compounds in biological fluids [71]. However, several problems need to be addressed to produce a sensitive and reliable immunoassay. For example, for medical diagnostics such as CRP detection, latex particles suffered from non-specific binding, which originated from plasma proteins in serum, because of its highly hydrophobic surface. Also, the immobilized biomolecule became denatured and inactivated when it was physically adsorbed on the latex particle surface despite several advantages of immunoagglutination. These findings reduced the sensitivity, and thus the reliability, of the diagnostics. To address these challenges, we prepared novel nanoparticles as immunoagglutination substrates based on our phospholipid polymer that had already solved existing problems.

The nanoparticles were prepared by the solvent evaporation technique under the systematic design of PMBN/PLA. According to the molecular design of PMBN, the PMBN chains, particularly *n*-butyl group, were considered to miscibly interpenetrate on the surface of PLA particle. The MPC domains were arranged at the surface owing to hydrophilicity, and then the *p*-nitrophenyl ester groups, which can be conjugated with biomolecules, were also freely arranged toward the outside. Monodispersion of the PMBN/PLA ($d = 205 \pm 43$ nm) measured by DLS was confirmed by field emission scanning electron microscopy (FE-SEM) [Fig. 5.12(a)]. Additionally, the ζ-potential of PMBN/PLA (-5.6 mV by electrophoresis light scattering measurement) indicated a slightly negatively charged surface. Biocomponents, including the plasma proteins, commonly have a slightly negative charge. Therefore, PMBN/PLA with a large negative ζ-potential must suffer from non-specific protein binding when it is used as an immunosensing tool. MPC-PNP was ex-

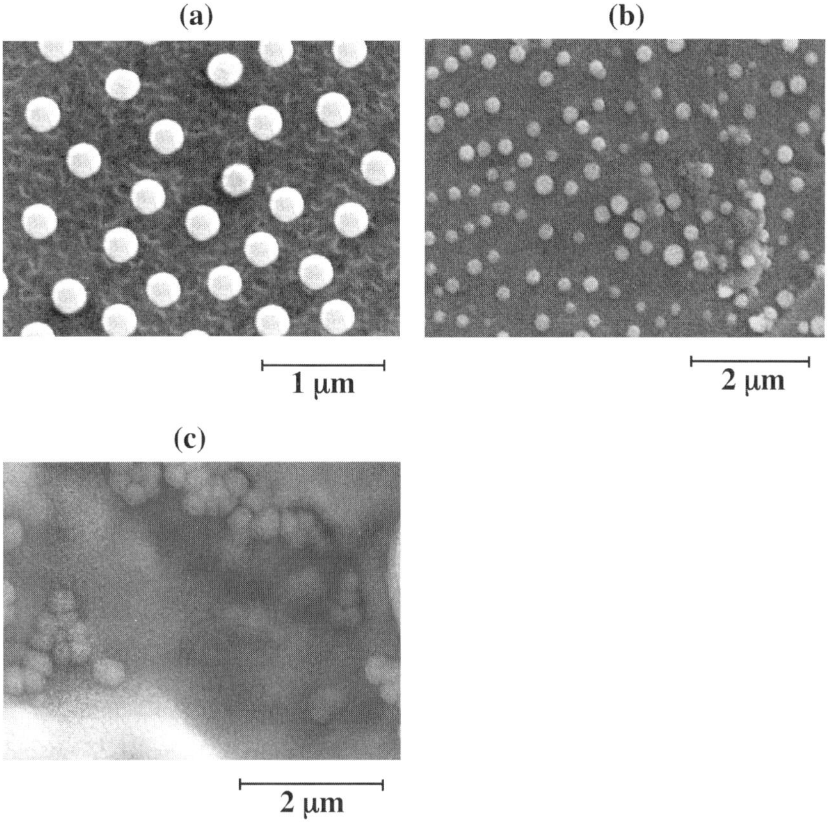

Fig. 5.12. SEM observations of anti-CRP antibody-immobilized PMBN/PLA nanoparticles: magnified view (a), normal view (b) and agglutination by antigen (c).

pected to show biocompatibility against non-specific binding of the plasma proteins with a slightly negatively charged surface, caused by arrangement of phosphorylcholine groups that were regarded as important to reduce protein adsorption, on PMBN/PLA.

PMBN/PLA can bind with biomolecules such as antibodies because it has *p*-nitrophenyl ester groups on its surface. Through a condensation reaction between amino groups of the antibody and *p*-nitrophenyl ester groups, the anti-CRP monoclonal antibody was immobilized on the MPC-PNP. For optimization, a fluorescent probe (Alexa Fluor 488, Molecular Probes, USA) labeled anti-CRP antibody was used to determine accurately the amount of antibody on PMBN/PLA. The immobilized amount of antibody was measured directly and calculated from the fluorescence intensity after immobilization. On the basis of experimental results, 100 $\mu g\ mL^{-1}$ of anti-CRP antibody was regarded as the optimal concentration for immobilization on PMBN/PLA. The remaining *p*-nitrophenyl ester groups on the surface were thoroughly blocked by 20 mM glycine. The ζ-potential of the PMBN/PLA (−25.3 mV) was further decreased after antibody immobilization because the antibody has a negative charge.

After preparation of the anti-CRP antibody immobilized PMBN/PLA, it was applied to detect serum-free CRP by the immunoagglutination method. Figure 5.12 also indicates FE-SEM photographs of the immunoagglutination at an initial state (b) and after aggregation (c). The immunoagglutination of PMBN/PLA was clearly successfully achieved by specific antigen–antibody binding. Following the confirmation of immunoagglutination, the dependency for serum-free CRP concentration was investigated with the anti-CRP antibody immobilized PMBN/PLA and commercially available polystyrene nanoparticles. The increase in optical density was investigated to evaluate the degree of immunoagglutination when agglutination occurred among particles. To avoid interference of light absorbance into antibody molecules, the optical density was measured at 570 nm when immunoagglutination was thoroughly performed for 90 min at 37 °C.

Figure 5.13 shows the calibration curves for serum-free CRP by PMBN/PLA and polystyrene nanoparticles. For PMBN/PLA, the calibration curve clearly had a linear correlation for serum-free CRP concentrations (from 0.01 to 10 mg dL^{-1}); polystyrene nanoparticles, however, had a limited linearity (from 0.1 to 10 mg dL^{-1}). The difference between the two calibration curves might be related to the resistance of protein adsorption on the surface of particles. With polystyrene nanoparticles, it could be that antigen–antibody binding did not occur and, instead, non-specific adsorption of CRP took place that affected the detection results. Overall, for polystyrene nanoparticles it was difficult to detect CRP at low concentrations although non-specific adsorption could be ignored at high concentrations because of the high response from antigen–antibody binding. Conversely, low concentrations

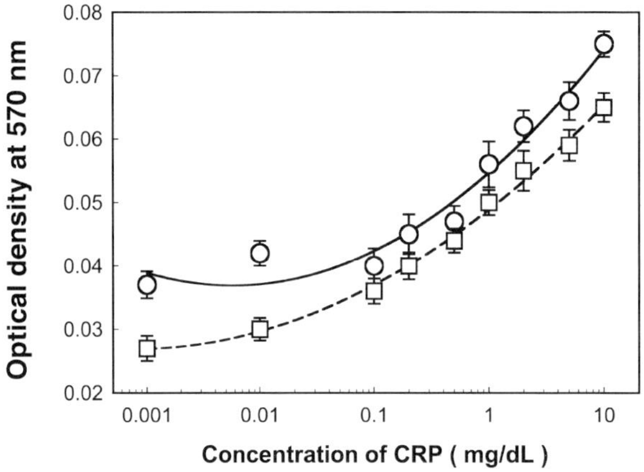

Fig. 5.13. Standard calibration curve for serum-free CRP obtained from the change in optical density at 570 nm when the immunoagglutination among anti-CRP antibody conjugated PMBN/PLA nanoparticles (□) and conventional polystyrene nanoparticles (○) was completed following each serum-free CRP injected.

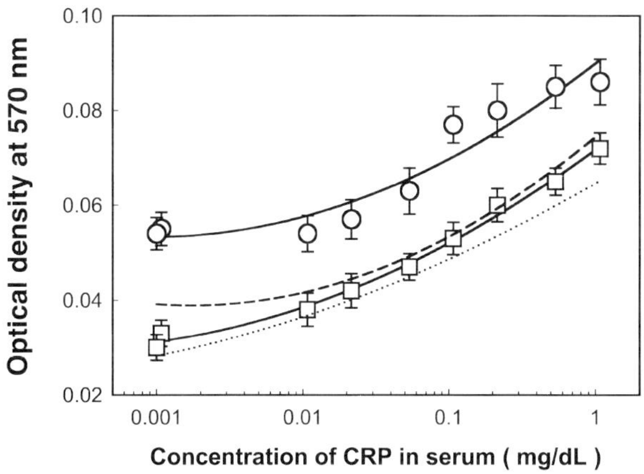

Fig. 5.14. Consideration of the regulating effect of non-specific binding from plasma proteins in human serum by comparing the calibration curves for serum-free CRP and CRP in serum; PMBN/PLA nanoparticles (□) and conventional polystyrene nanoparticles (○).

of CRP could be detected by PMBN/PLA because there were no problems with non-specific binding of CRP. From successfully obtained calibration curves, CRP detection was investigated with CRP in serum; the previous calibration curves in Fig. 5.13 were considered as standard calibration curves for CRP.

5.5.2 High-performance Diagnosis in Serum

Figure 5.14 indicates the change in optical density of serum-containing particles with CRP concentrations in serum. These were compared with standard calibration curves to consider non-specific binding from plasma proteins in serum. Adsorption of plasma proteins, such as BSA and γ-globulin, in serum on the particles might induce the agglutination of particles, and this non-specific agglutination would be a major problem for reliable CRP detection. As shown in Fig. 5.14, polystyrene nanoparticles gave a quite different standard curve because non-specific agglutination occurred, resulting in plasma protein adsorption. This phenomenon could also be explained by particle preparation parameters such as ionic strength and hydrophobicity. However, the calibration curve was almost identical when PMBN/PLA was used to detect the CRP in serum. Thus, non-specific binding of plasma proteins rarely occurred on the MPC-PNP, and highly sensitive and reliable CRP diagnostics could be obtained. Normally, the detection limit for CRP was below 0.06 mg dL^{-1} for medical diagnostics. Furthermore, with infants, much lower detection limits are required to detect CRP. The MPC-PNP fully satisfied the requirement for CRP detection.

To determine their thermal stability, anti-CRP antibody immobilized PMBN/PLA

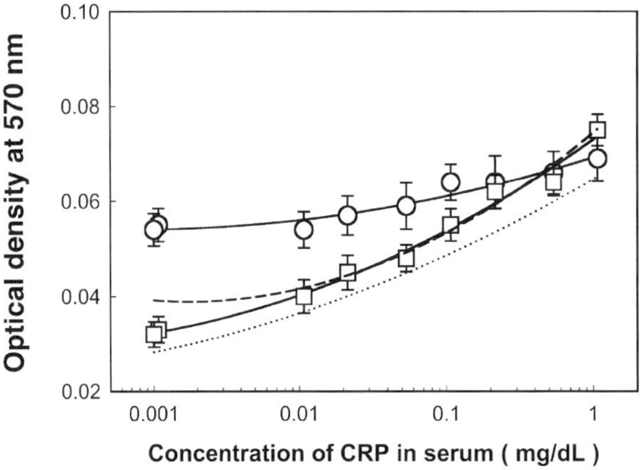

Fig. 5.15. Remaining immunologic activities of conjugated anti-CRP antibody on PMBN/PLA nanoparticles and conventional polystyrene NP; the calibration curves for serum-free CRP were obtained after 2 h storage 55 °C; PMBN/PLA nanoparticles (□) and conventional polystyrene nanoparticles (○).

and polystyrene nanoparticles were stored at 55 °C for 2 h, and were then used to detect serum-free CRP under the same conditions as for the determination of the standard calibration curves. Figure 5.15 shows the calibration curve for serum-free CRP obtained after this treatment. From the figure, the calibration curve of the PMBN/PLA was almost the same as the standard curve. However, the polystyrene nanoparticles gave a very different curve, indicating that anti-CRP antibody immobilized on polystyrene nanoparticles was denatured by the high temperature treatment and almost lost its selectivity for CRP. However, for PMBN/PLA, the immobilized antibody was clearly not influenced by the increase in temperature.

The resistance of protein adsorption and suppression of antibody denaturation on PMBN/PLA might be related to the hydration state of the phosphorylcholine groups. The following concept is generally accepted when considering protein adsorption on a polymer substrate [72]. Water molecules bind to the hydrophobic part of the polymer through van der Waals forces. These bound water molecules cause protein adsorption by hydrophobic interaction. When a protein molecule is adsorbed on a polymer surface, the water molecules between proteins and the polymer need to be replaced. This phenomenon induces a much stronger interaction with a change in the denaturation of the proteins. If the water at the surface is in a similar state to bulk water, the protein does not need to release bound water molecules even if the protein molecules are in contact with the surface. Under the hypothesis concerning the effect of water states, our group has previously analyzed the water state of hydrated MPC polymers, and recognized that the water state on the MPC polymer surface is naturally maintained [73, 74]. For PMBN/PLA, this hypothesis can also be used to explain several experimental results because its suron an alkylated surface. *Macromolecules* **2000**, *33*, 4205–4212.

5 Tegoulia, V. A., Cooper, S. L., Leukocyte adhesion on model surfaces under flow: effects of surface chemistry, protein adsorption, and shear rate. *J. Biomed. Mater. Res.* **2000**, *50*, 291–301.

6 Choi, H. S., Ooya, T., Sasaki, S., Yui, N., Ohya, Y., Nakai, T., Ouchi, T., Preparation and characterization of polypseudorotaxanes based on biodegradable poly(L-lactide)/poly(ethylene glycol) triblock copolymers. *Macromolecules* **2003**, *36*, 9313–9318.

7 Yui, N. (Ed.), *Supramolecular Design for Biological Applications*, CRC Press, Boca Raton, FL, **2000**.

8 Yui, N., Mrsny, R. J., Park, K., *Reflexive Polymers and Hydrogels: Understanding and Designing Fast Responsive Polymeric Systems*, CRC Press, Boca Raton, FL, **2004**.

9 Goodrich, T. T., Lee, H. J., Corn, R. M., Direct detection of genomic DNA by enzymatically amplified SPR imaging measurements of RNA microarrays. *J. Am. Chem. Soc.* **2004**, *126*, 4086–4087.

10 Liu, R. H., Yang, J., Lenigk, R., Bonanno, J., Grodzinski, P., Self-contained, fully integrated biochip for sample preparation, polymerase chain reaction amplification, and DNA microarray detection. *Anal. Chem.* **2004**, *76*, 1824–1831.

11 Siontorou, C. G., Nikolelis, D. P., Tarus, B., Dumbrava, J., Krull, U. J., DNA biosensor based on self-assembled bilayer lipid membranes for the detection of hydrazines. *Electroanalysis* **1998**, *10*, 691–694.

12 Oki, A., Adachi, S., Takamura, Y., Ishihara, K., Ogawa, H., Ogawa, Y., Ichiki, T., Horiike, Y., Electro-osmosis injection of blood serum into biocompatible microcapillary chip fabricated on quartz plate. *Electrophoresis* **2001**, *22*, 341–347.

13 Shimizu, N., Sugimoto, K., Tang, J., Nishi, T., Sato, I., Hiramoto, M., Aizawa, S., Hatakeyama, M., Ohba, R., Hatori, H., Yoshikawa, T., Suzuki, F., Oomori, A., Tanaka, H., Kawaguchi, H., Watanabe, H., Handa, H., High-performance affinity beads for identifying drug receptors. *Nat. Biotechnol.* **2000**, *18*, 877–881.

14 Serizawa, T., Hamada, K.-I., Akashi, M., Polymerization within a molecular-scale stereoregular template. *Nature* **2004**, *429*, 52–55.

15 Nam, J.-M., Thaxton, C. S., Mirkin, C. A., Nanoparticle-based bio-bar codes for the ultrasensitive detection of proteins. *Science* **2003**, *301*, 1884–1886.

16 Boal, A. K., Ilhan, F., DeRouchey, J. E., Thurn-Albrecht, T., Russell, T. P., Rotello, V. M., Self-assembly of nanoparticles into structured spherical and network aggregates. *Nature* **2000**, *404*, 746–748.

17 Oliva, A. g., Cruz, H. J., Rosa, C. C., Immunosensors for diagnostics. *Sensors Update* **2001**, *9*, 283–312.

18 Siegers, C., Biesalski, M., Haag, R., Self-assembled monolayers of dendritic polyglycerol derivatives on gold that resist the adsorption of proteins. *Chem. Eur. J.* **2004**, *10*, 2831–2838.

19 Sigal, G. B., Mrksich, M., Whitesides, G. M., Effect of surface wettability on the adsorption of proteins and detergents. *J. Am. Chem. Soc.* **1998**, *120*, 3464–3473.

20 Jenkins, S. H., Heineman, W. R., Halsall, H. B., Extending the detection limit of solid-phase electrochemical enzyme immunoassay to the attomole level. *Anal. Biochem.* **1988**, *168*, 292–297.

21 Ishihara, K., Bioinspired phospholipid polymer biomaterials for making high perfomance artificial organs. *Sci. Technol. Adv. Mater.* **2000**, *1*, 131–138.

22 Moro, T., Takatori, Y., Ishihara, K., Konno, T., Takigawa, Y., Matsushita, T., Chung, U.-I., Nakamura, K., Kawaguchi, H., Surface grafting of artificial joints with a biocompatible polymer for preventing periprosthetic osteolysis. *Nat. Mater.* **2004**, *3*, 829–836.

23 Yoneyama, T., Sugihara, K.-I.,

face was successfully covered with MPC units. Furthermore, as additional proof of the hypothesis, the colloidal stability of the PMBN/PLA was also explained. Generally, colloidal stability can be achieved in two ways: (a) the particles can be given an electric charge (either positive or negative) and if all have the same charge they will repel one another more or less strongly when they approach; (b) the particles can be coated with an adsorbed layer of some material (say a polymer), which itself prevents their close approach. Although the PMBN/PLA did not correspond to either situation it has good colloidal stability – as indicated in the FE-SEM picture for initial colloidal states [Fig. 5.12(a)]. On the basis of our hypothesis, it was strongly solvated with water molecules, and polar groups like bound water molecules resist coagulation among the PMBN/PLA nanoparticles.

5.6 Conclusions

Nanofabrication is a promising technique that opens up a new scientific field, integrating biochemistry, bioscience, material science, polymer chemistry, and nano-scaled processing. Under the nano-scale environment, surface properties (biointerface) are dominant factors and, thereby, regulate biofunctions. In particular, non-specific protein adsorption is a typical phenomenon in nanofabrication. A series of phospholipid polymers are good candidates for nanofabrication involving biofunctionalization.

Acknowledgments

Part of this study, which was carried out by the authors, was financially supported by the Industrial Technology Research Grant Program (03A23011a) from the New Energy and Industrial Technology Development Organization (NEDO) of Japan and the Scientific Research Fund (16650098) from the Japanese Society for the Promotion of Science.

References

1 Harada, A., Kataoka, K., Chain length recognition: core-shell supramolecular assembly from oppositely charged block copolymers. *Science* **1999**, *283*, 65–67.
2 Akiyoshi, K., Kang, E.-C., Kurumada, S., Sunamoto, J., Principi, T., Winnik, F. M., Controlled association of amphiphilic polymers in water; thermosensitive nanopariticles formed by self-assembly of hydrophobically modified pullulan and poly(N-isopropylacrylamides). *Macromolecules* **2000**, *33*, 3244–3249.
3 Yatvin, M. B., Kreutz, W., Horwitz, B. A., Shinitzky, M., pH-Sensitive liposome: possible clinical implications. *Science* **1980**, *210*, 1253–1255.
4 Orban, J. M., Faucher, K. M., Dluhy, R. A., Chaikof, E. L., Cytomimetic biomaterials. 4. In-situ photopolymerization of phospholipids

Ishihara, K., Iwasaki, Y., Nakabayashi, N., The vascular prosthesis without pseudointima prepared by antithrombogenic phospholipid polymer. *Biomaterials* **2002**, *23*, 1455–1459.

24 Ishihara, K., Iwasaki, Y., Nojiri, C., Phospholipid polymer biomaterials for making ventricular assist devices. *J. Congestive Heart Failure Circulatory Support* **2001**, *1*, 265–270.

25 Konno, T., Watanabe, J., Ishihara, K., Enhanced solubility of paclitaxel using water-soluble and biocompatible 2-methacryloyloxyethyl phosphorylcholine polymers. *J. Biomed. Mater. Res.* **2003**, *65A*, 210–215.

26 Miyamoto, D., Watanabe, J., Ishihara, K., Effect of water-soluble phospholipid polymers conjugated with papain on the enzymatic stability. *Biomaterials* **2004**, *25*, 71–76.

27 Miyamoto, D., Watanabe, J., Ishihara, K., Highly-stabilized papain conjugated with water-soluble phospholipid polymer chain having a reacting terminal group. *J. Appl. Polym. Sci.* **2004**, *91*, 827–832.

28 Miyamoto, D., Watanabe, J., Ishihara, K., Molecular design of reactive amphiphilic phospholipid polymer for bioconjugation with an enzyme. *J. Appl. Polym. Sci.* **2005**, *95*, 615–622.

29 Ishihara, K., Ueda, T., Nakabayashi, N., Preparation of phospholipid polymers and their properties as hydrogel membrane. *Polym. J.* **1990**, *23*, 355–360.

30 Ishihara, K., Oshida, H., Endo, Y., Ueda, T., Watanabe, A., Nakabayashi, N., Hemocompatibility of human whole blood on polymers with a phospholipid polar group and its mechanism. *J. Biomed. Mater. Res.* **1992**, *26*, 1543–1552.

31 Watanabe, J., Ishihara, K., Biointerface, bioconjugation, and biomatrix based on bioinspired phospholipid polymers, in *Handbook of Nanostructured Biomaterials and Their Applications*, Ed. by H. S. Nalwa, American Scientific Publishers, CA, **2005**, 129–165.

32 Stiriba, S.-E., Frey, H., Haag, R., Dendritic polymers in biomedical applications: from potential to clinical use in diagnostics and therapy. *Angew. Chem. Int. Ed.* **2002**, *41*, 1329–1334.

33 Sato, K., Hosokawa, K., Maeda, M., Rapid aggregation of gold nanoparticles induced by non-cross-linking DNA hybridization. *J. Am. Chem. Soc.* **2003**, *125*, 8102–8103.

34 Tabuchi, M., Ueda, M., Kaji, N., Yamasaki, Y., Nagasaki, Y., Yoshikawa, K., Kataoka, K., Baba, Y., Nano-spheres for DNA separation chips. *Nat. Biotechnol.* **2004**, *22*, 337–340.

35 Mucic, R. C., Storhoff, J. J., Mirkin, C. A., Letsinger, L., DNA-directed synthesis of binary nanoparticle network materials. *J. Am. Chem. Soc.* **1998**, *120*, 12674–12675.

36 Mori, H., Seng, D. C., Zhang, M., Müller, A. H. E., Hybrid nanoparticles with hyperbranched polymer shells via self-condensing atom transfer radical polymerization from silica surfaces. *Langmuir* **2002**, *18*, 3682–3693.

37 Mori, H., Seng, D. C., Lechner, H., Zhang, M., Müller, A. H. E., Synthesis and characterization of branched polyelectrolytes. 1. Preparation of hyperbranched poly(acrylic acid) via self-condensing atom transfer radical copolymerization. *Macromolecules* **2002**, *35*, 9270–9281.

38 Mori, H., Müller, A. H. E., Klee, J. E., Intelligent colloidal hybrids via reversible pH-induced complexation of polyelectrolyte and silica nanoparticles. *J. Am. Chem. Soc.* **2003**, *125*, 3712–3713.

39 Kamata, K., Lu, Y., Xia, Y., Synthesis and characterization of monodispersed core-shell spherical colloids with movable cores. *J. Am. Chem. Soc.* **2003**, *125*, 2384–2385.

40 Vertegel, A. A., Siegel, R. W., Dordick, J. S., Silica nanoparticle size influences the structure and enzymatic activity of adsorbed lysozyme. *Langmuir* **2004**, *20*, 6800–6807.

41 Akagi, T., Kawamura, M., Ueno, M.,

Hiraishi, K., Adachi, M., Serizawa, T., Akashi, M., Baba, M., Immunization with inactivated HIV-1-capturing nanospheres induces a significant HIV-1-specific vaginal antibody response in mice. *J. Med. Virol.* **2003**, *69*, 163–172.

42 Kaneko, T., Shimomai, S., Miyazaki, M., Baba, M., Akashi, M., IgG responses to itranasal immunization with cholera toxin-immobilized polymeric nanospheres in mice. *J. Biomater. Sci. Polym. Edn.* **2004**, *15*, 661–669.

43 Andersson, M., Elihn, K., Fromell, K., Caldwell, K. D., Surface attachment of nanoparticles using oligonucleotides. *Colloids Surf. B: Biointerfaces* **2004**, *34*, 165–171.

44 Inoue, Y., Watanabe, J., Takai, M., Ishihara, K., Surface characteristics of block-type copolymer composed of semi-fluorinated and phospholipid segments synthesized by living radical polymerization. *J. Biomater. Sci. Polym. Edn.* **2004**, *15*, 1153–1166.

45 Inoue, Y., Watanabe, J., Ishihara, K., Dynamic motion of phosphorylcholine groups at the surface of poly(2-methacryloyloxyethyl phosphorylcholine-random-2,2,2-trifluoroethyl methacrylate). *J. Colloid Interface Sci.* **2004**, *274*, 465–471.

46 Feng, W., Brash, J., Zhu, S., Atom-transfer radical grafting polymerization of 2-methacryloyloxyethyl phosphorylcholine from silicon wafer surfaces. *J. Polym. Sci. Part A: Polym. Chem.* **2004**, *42*, 2931–2942.

47 Inoue, Y., Watanabe, J., Takai, M., Ishihara, K., Regulation of nano-surface properties by finely synthesized fluorinated phosphorylcholine polymers. *Trans. Mater. Res. Soc. Jpn.* **2004**, *29*, 181–184.

48 Ishihara, K., Ishikawa, E., Iwasaki, Y., Nakabayashi, N., Inhibition of cell adhesion on the substrate by coating with 2-methacryloyloxyethyl phosphorylcholine polymers. *J. Biomater. Sci. Polym. Edn.* **1999**, *10*, 1047–1061.

49 Ishihara, K., Fukumoto, K., Iwasaki, Y., Nakabayashi, N., Modification of polysulfone with phospholipid polymer for improvement of the blood compatibility. Part 1. Surface characterization. *Biomaterials* **1999**, *20*, 1545–1551.

50 Ogawa, R., Iwasaki, Y., Ishihara, K., Thermal properties and processability of elastmeric polymer alloy composed of segmented polyurethane and phospholipid polymer. *J. Biomed. Mater. Res.* **2002**, *62*, 214–221.

51 Ye, S. H., Watanabe, J., Iwasaki, Y., Ishihara, K., Novel cellulose acetate membrane blended with phospholipid polymer for hemocompatible filtration system. *J. Membr. Sci.* **2002**, *210*, 411–421.

52 Iwasaki, Y., Nakabayashi, N., Ishihara, K., Preservation of platelet function on 2-methacryloyloxyethyl phosphorylcholine graft polymer compared to various water-soluble graft polymers. *J. Biomed. Mater. Res.* **2001**, *57*, 74–79.

53 Furuzono, T., Ishihara, K., Nakabayashi, N., Tamada, Y., Chemical modification of silk fibroin with 2-methacryloyloxyethyl phosphorylcholine I. Graft-polymerization onto fabric using ammonium persulfate and interaction between fabric and platelets. *J. Appl. Polym. Sci.* **1999**, *73*, 2541–2544.

54 Ishihara, K., Iwasaki, Y., Nakabayashi, N., Polymeric lipid nanosphere constituted of poly(2-methacryloyloxyethyl phosphorylcholine-co-n-butyl methacrylate). *Polym. J.* **1999**, *31*, 1231–1236.

55 Konno, T., Watanabe, J., Ishihara, K., Conjugation of enzymes on polymer nanoparticles covered with phosphorylcholine groups. *Biomacromolecules* **2004**, *5*, 342–347.

56 Takei, K., Konno, T., Watanabe, J., Ishihara, K., Regulation of enzyme-substrate complexation by phospholipid polymer conjugates for cell engineering. *Biomacromolecules* **2004**, *5*, 858–862.

57 Park, J.-W., Kurosawa, S., Watanabe, J., Ishihara, K., Evaluation of novel 2-methacryloyloxyethyl phosphorylcholine (MPC) polymeric nanoparticles for immunoassay of C-reactive

protein detection. *Anal. Chem.* **2004**, *76*, 2649–2655.
58 Watanabe, J., Ishihara, K., Highly efficient sequential enzymatic reaction on bio-conjugate phospholipid polymer nanoparticles. *Kobunshi Ronbunsyu* **2004**, *61*, 547–554.
59 Kiritoshi, Y., Ishihara, K., Preparation of cross-linked poly(2-methacryloyloxyethyl phosphorylcholine) gel and its strange swelling behavior in water/ethanol mixture. *J. Biomater. Sci. Polym. Edn.* **2002**, *13*, 213–224.
60 Farokhzad, O. C., Jon, S., Khademhosseini, A., Tran, T.-N. T., Lavan, D. A., Langer, R., Nanoparticle-aptamer bioconjugates: a new approach for targeting prostate cancer cells. *Cancer Res.* **2004**, *64*, 7668–7672.
61 Veronesi, B., Wei, G., Zeng, J.-Q., Oortgiesen, M., Electrostatic charge activates inflammatory vanilloid (VR1) receptors. *Neuro Toxicol.* **2003**, *24*, 463–473.
62 Whicher, J., Biasucci, L., Rifai, N., The acute phase response and atherosclerosis. *Clin. Chem. Lab. Med.* **1999**, *37*, 495–503.
63 Pentikanen, M. O., Oorni, K., Ala-Korpela, M., Kovanen, P. T., Trigger of atherosclerosis and inflammation in the arterial intima. *J. Intern. Med.* **2000**, *247*, 359–370.
64 Ridker, P. M., Cushman, M., Stampfer, M. J., Tracy, R. P., Hennekens, C. H., Plasma concentration of C-reactive protein and risk of developing peripheral vascular disease. *Circulation* **1998**, *97*, 425–428.
65 Haverkate, F., Thompson, S. G., Pyke, S. D. M., Gallimore, J. R., Pepys, M. B., Production of C-reactive protein and risk of coronary events in stable and unstable angina. *Lancet* **1997**, *349*, 462–466.
66 Diamandis, E. P., Analytical methodology for immunoassays and DNA hybridization assays-current status and selected systems. *Clin. Chim. Acta* **1990**, *194*, 19–50.
67 Aceti, A., Pennica, A., Teggi, A., Grilli, A., Caferro, M., Celestino, D., Leri, O., Sebastiani, A., De Rosa, F., The serological diagnosis of human hydatid disease by time-resolved fluoroimmunoassay. *J. Infect.* **1991**, *22*, 135–141.
68 Molina-Bolivar, J. A., Galisteo-Gonzalez, F., Hidalgo-Alvarez, R., Fractal aggregates induced by antigen-antibody interaction. *Langmuir* **2001**, *17*, 2514–2520.
69 Velev, O. D., Kaler, E. W., In situ assembly of colloidal particles into miniaturized biosensors. *Langmuir* **1999**, *15*, 3693–3698.
70 Bundy, J., Fenselau, C., Lectin-based affinity capture for MALDI-MS analysis of bacteria. *Anal. Chem.* **1999**, *71*, 1460–1463.
71 Perez-Amodio, S., Holownia, P., Davey, C. L., Price, C. P. Effect of the ionic environment, charge, and particle surface chemistry for enhancing a latex homogeneous immunoassay of C-reactive protein. *Anal. Chem.* **2001**, *73*, 3417–3425.
72 Lu, D. R., Lee, S. J., Park, K., Calculation of solvation interaction energies for protein adsorption on polymer surfaces. *J. Biomater. Sci. Polym. Edn.* **1991**, *3*, 127–147.
73 Kitano, H., Sudo, K., Ichikawa, K., Ide, M., Ishihara, K., Raman spectroscopic study on the surface of water in aqueous polyelectrolyte solutions. *J. Phys. Chem. B* **2002**, *104*, 10425–10429.
74 Kitano, H., Imai, M., Mori, T., Ide, G., Yokoyama, Y., Ishihara, K., Structure of water in the vicinity of phospholipid analogue copolymers as studied by vibrational spectroscopy. *Langmuir* **2003**, *19*, 10260–10266.

6
Biofunctionalization of Metallic Nanoparticles and Microarrays for Biomolecular Detection

Grit Festag, Uwe Klenz, Thomas Henkel, Andrea Csáki, and Wolfgang Fritzsche

6.1
Introduction

Characterization of molecular interactions represents a core technology for today's biomedical research. The specific binding of bioactive compounds to certain pathogens, the discovery of novel pathways in the cell, or the early detection of low numbers of disease-related molecules are examples of the wide application of biomolecular detection. With the ongoing elucidation of the molecular bases for life processes, a further demand for testing the presence and, eventually, the quantity of molecules of interest is expected. One interesting development is the field of point-of-care (POC) diagnostics that describes the application of biomolecular detection outside the dedicated laboratory and near the patient, such as in the medical practice. Other applications with similar technical requirements are, for example, the testing for toxic organisms in food processing factories or the detection of pathogens in air conditioning systems. This set of applications requires a highly robust technology, both regarding a minimized maintenance and stability against users not trained as laboratory personnel. It includes a signal that is easily transformed into results, without the need for user input or extended processing. The decentralized character of this approach asks for cost-efficiency of detection equipment that has to be provided in large quantity. The resulting need for miniaturization is matched by the general development towards minimal sample liquid volume. Although sample holders with several thousands of detection sites have been described already for gene expression chips, typical analytical questions for POC diagnostics will be limited to a handful of parallel tests. Moreover, the highly-developed fluorescence readers needed for the readout of expression chips are hardly suitable for POC applications due to their high costs and complicated detection setup.

What measurement principles are best suited for this novel field in bioanalytics? The demonstration of DNA-conjugated metal nanoparticles [1, 2] was the starting point for a novel family of detection techniques based on these particles. These particles allowed for various elegant detection schemes with sensitivities comparable or even better than for fluorescence-based assays. Surprisingly, the – in comparison

Nanotechnologies for the Life Sciences Vol. 1
Biofunctionalization of Nanomaterials. Edited by Challa S. S. R. Kumar

ISBN: 3-527-31381-8

to fluorescent dyes – large mass of the particles does not interfere with the specificity of the binding of the conjugated molecules. In certain applications they even enhance the specificity compared with fluorescence assays [3].

This chapter describes the application of biofunctionalized nanoparticles for biomolecular detections. The first section describes application aspects, including typical assay formats, array fabrication, and the numerous detection schemes established. The most important types of nanoparticles (regarding their composition) are introduced in Section 6.2.1. The following section describes the synthesis of metal particles. Particle biofunctionalization represents the key step for an integration of the nanoparticles into biological assays. The various bioconjugation approaches regarding gold nanoparticles are introduced in Section 6.2.3.1 for DNA and Section 6.2.3.2 for proteins. Other metal nanoparticles follow in Section 6.2.3.3. Section 6.2.4 gives the outlook for further applications of bioconjugated particles.

Although biofunctionalized particles are important for assays, substrates modified with capture molecules are often required to realize chip-based detection with its potential for miniaturization as well as parallelization. Such substrates usually exhibit self-assembled monolayers to bind the capture molecules (Section 6.3.1.1). For a typical system, optimization, regarding blocking of undesired unspecific interactions, is required (Section 6.3.1.2). Beside molecular layers, nanoporous gels provide another interesting option for efficient binding of capture molecules (Section 6.3.2). This chapter concludes with an outlook (Section 6.4) that forecasts future developments.

6.1.1
Applications

Nanotechnologies extend the limits of molecular diagnostics to the nanoscale and offer a broad spectrum of potential applications in molecular diagnostics, as summarized by Jain [4]. Beside technologies such as nanowires or nanopores, we will focus on nanoparticle technologies using, especially, gold nanoparticles as labels for biomolecule probes.

A typical assay in biomolecular detection probes the presence of target molecules by using capture molecules that are complementary to the targets. These capture molecules bind the target, and this binding is detected using labels that are either attached to the targets (e.g. by PCR in the case of DNA or RNA) or added by another binding molecule in a kind of sandwich assay (Fig. 6.1). Capture probes attached to solid substrates are easily incubated and washed. Moreover, by using separate binding spots for various capture probes, the assay can be multiplexed with only minimal sample volume requirement.

6.1.2
Array Fabrication

The need for analytical methods that can deal with many probes, and, ideally, analyze all of them together, led to the development of so-called microarrays or bio-

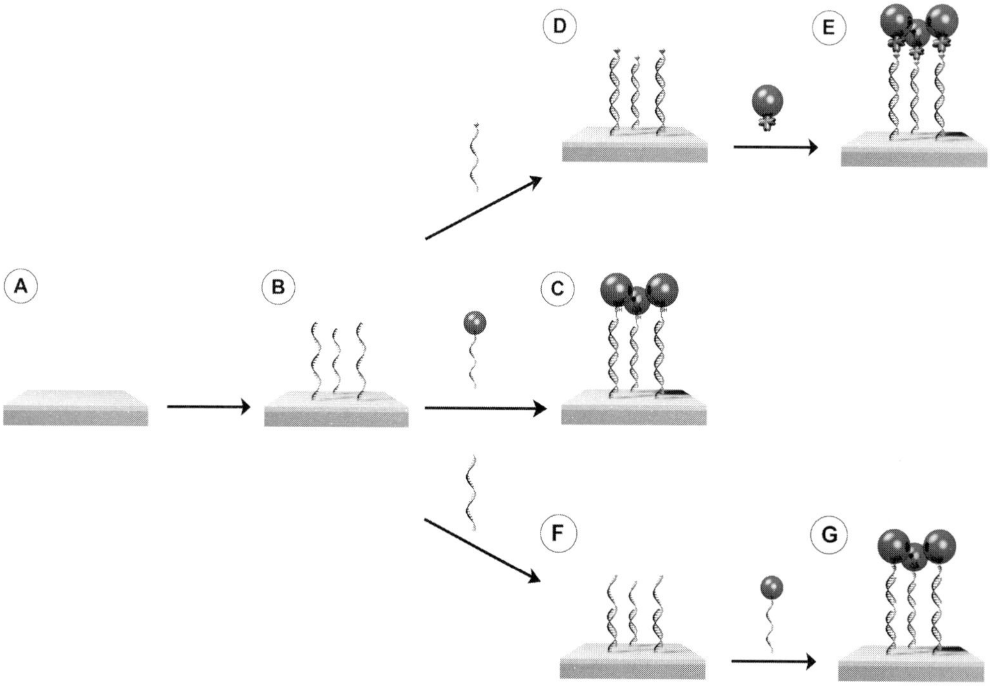

Fig. 6.1. Microarray-based, sequence-specific DNA detection with gold nanoparticle labels. (A) Solid substrate, functionalized for binding of capture probes. (B) Covalent attachment of capture-oligonucleotides. (C)–(E) For the direct detection scheme, the target probes have to be labeled prior to hybridization. (C) Hybridization of DNA target strands labeled with gold nanoparticles or (D) biotin molecules. (E) Labeling of the biotin-tagged targets with streptavidin-modified nanoparticles. (F) In the indirect approach (sandwich), the unlabeled target strands are hybridized to the capture strands first, (G) followed by an additional hybridization with labeled DNA probes.

chips, which enable massive parallel mining of biological data, multiplexing, and automation in a miniaturized format [5]. The particular strength of array analysis results from the highly redundant measurement of many parallel biomolecular hybridization or recognition events, which leads to an extraordinary level of assay validation [6, 7].

DNA microarrays can be fabricated by two strategies. In the first approach, the on-chip (*in situ*) synthesis of capture oligonucleotides at defined places provides high yields of capture probes that are consistent over the surface of the support. It permits combinatorial strategies for the fabrication of large oligonucleotide arrays. In the second strategy, an off-line approach in which pre-synthesized oligonucleotides have been deposited onto the substrate (*ex situ*), available in most biology laboratories, enables assessment of the capture probes before they are attached to the surface. Deposition is also the method of choice for long sequences as PCR products. When many arrays are needed with the same probes, deposition may be more economical than *in situ* synthesis.

6.1.3 Detection Methods

Different applications of metal nanoparticles for biomolecular detection are favored by their multi-purpose possibility of signal development.

The most common characterization techniques of metal nanoparticles are high-resolution transmission electron microscopy (HRTEM) as well as scanning tunneling microscopy (STM), atomic force microscopy (AFM), small-angle X-ray scattering, and X-ray diffraction [8]. For paralleled assays in microarray format, electrical/electrochemical and optical methods are preferred, such as optical absorbance as well as optical scattering, surface plasmon resonance (SPR) imaging, and surface-enhanced Raman spectroscopy (SERS).

6.1.3.1 Optical Absorbance

Imaging the optical absorbance of surface-bound particles is probably the simplest method for analyzing nanoparticle-labeled DNA at surfaces. The extinction coefficient of metal nanoparticles can exceed those of organic dyes by many orders of magnitude, which has been explained by the collective resonance of conduction electrons in the metal (surface plasmon resonance, SPR, [9–11]). An important enabling step for DNA labeling by nanoparticles was the development of a method in 1996 that allowed the direct oligonucleotide modification of gold nanoparticles [1, 2]. This enabled a simple optical characterization by monitoring a color change during hybridization events of two complementary DNA–nanoparticle complexes in solution. Solutions of gold nanoparticle aggregates with interparticle distances larger than the average particle size appear red. But when biomolecular recognition events lead to significantly decreased interparticle spacings the solution turns blue, which is detectable in a spectral shift. The dependency on interparticle spacing was also used in colorimetric, heterogeneous biomolecule detection schemes on thin-layer chromatography plates [12]. By using solid supports the color differentiation was enhanced; this is attributable to increased aggregation of the pre-organized DNA-linked nanoparticles upon drying the solution on the support, which also prevented samples (heated above the DNA dissociation temperature) from rehybridizing. Thus, a permanent record of the test could be obtained. Furthermore, gold nanoparticle-labeled probes exhibited characteristic, exceptionally sharp "melting transitions" compared with those of fluorophore-labeled targets, which allows the discrimination of even small DNA sequence defects. By aligning the oligonucleotides in a "tail-to-tail" [13] rather than "head-to-tail" fashion on the nanoparticles the sensitivity could be further improved, and it was even possible to distinguish target sequences with single nucleotide polymorphisms from the fully complementary target. The altered melting profiles yielded a selectivity that was over three times higher than that observed for fluorophore-labeled targets [3]. The absorbance signal of the surface-bound gold nanoparticles could be further amplified by autocatalytic deposition of silver metal [14]. Such silver enhancement leads to a growth of the gold nanoparticles (Fig. 6.2) and makes the nanoparticle based assays readable by simple flatbed scanners. The sensitivity of this scanomet-

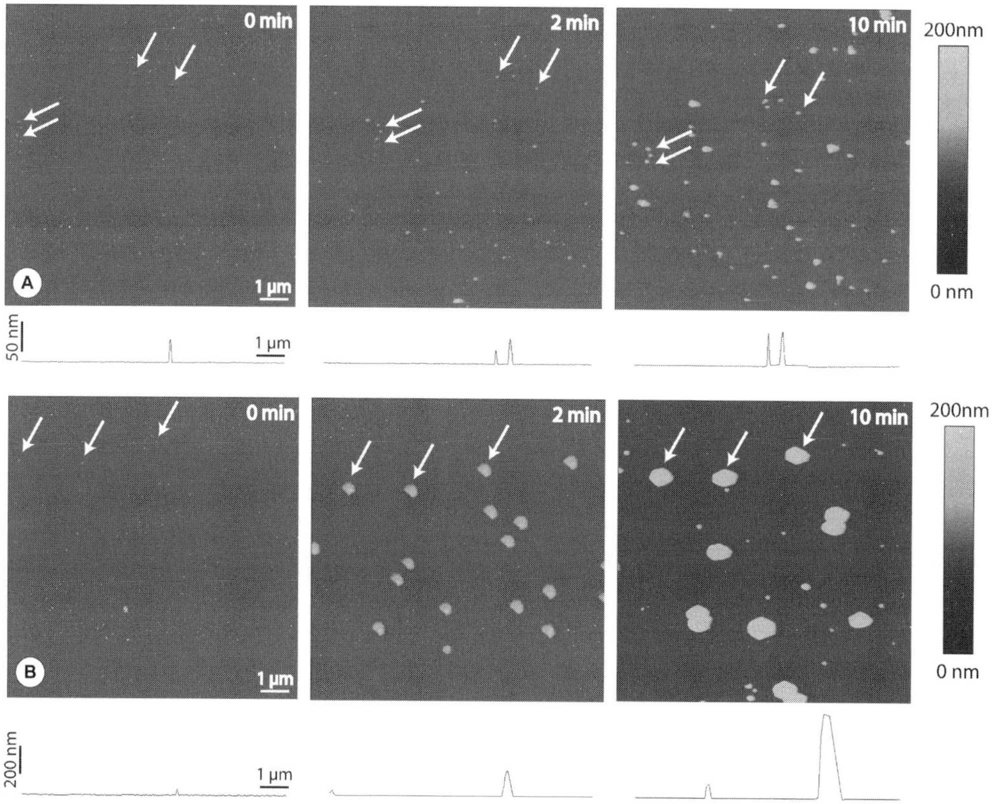

Fig. 6.2. Metal enhancement of gold nanoparticles by a stepwise electroless deposition of silver. Atomic force microscopy (AFM) images and their corresponding section analyses show the growth of single 30 nm-sized gold nanoparticles after 0, 2 and 10 min enhancement time, as examples. For orientation, selected particles are marked by arrows through the experiments. (A) Slowly growing particles by a homemade silver acetate/hydroquinone silver enhancement solution (average height of 31, 38 and 48 nm, respectively). (B) Fast growing particles by means of a commercial silver enhancement kit (Silver Enhancement Solution^{TM}, British Biocell) (31, 130, and 442 nm, respectively).

ric array detection exceeds that of analogous fluorophore systems by two orders of magnitude (50 fM vs. 5 pM, respectively) [3].

Microstructured biochips were introduced in this field to monitor the binding of nanoparticle-labeled target DNA to arrayed capture DNA probes by both reflected and transmitted light [15]. Moreover, the authors found that the intensity of reflected light directly relates to the number of bound particles and to the concentration of hybridizable targets in solution.

Beside the large extinction coefficient there is a just as huge scattering coefficient that enables extremely sensitive imaging and quantification of nanoparticle-tagged biomolecules by scattered light. This was shown for selenium nanoparticle–antibody conjugates that – bound to biotinylated target DNA – could be imaged by scattering light in an evanescent field [16]. The use of an internally reflecting waveguide allows for measurement of real-time binding or melting of a light-scattering label of a DNA array.

As well as for the optical absorbance, the spectrum and intensity strongly depends on the size, shape, and material composition of the nanoparticles. Thus, the use of different-sized gold nanoparticles as scattering labels results in different colors of scattered light, e.g. green-scattering 50 nm and orange-scattering 100 nm particles [17].

Li and Rothberg introduced a completely different approach by designing – in combination with gold nanoparticles – a novel fluorescent assay for DNA hybridization based on the electrostatic properties of DNA without the need for probe or surface modification [18]. The fluorescence of single-stranded dye-tagged DNA was efficiently quenched when the DNA probes had bound to gold nanoparticles, whereas double stranded DNA refused to adsorb to the particles (Section 6.2.3.1). Hence, these hybridization events could be measured indirectly as fluorescence signals.

6.1.3.2 **SPR Imaging**

In the past decade, SPR methods have contributed significantly to the sensing and quantification of biomolecule interactions; four emerging application areas have been identified: food analysis, proteomics, immunogenicity, and drug discovery [19]. SPR biosensors enable the measurement of analyte binding to immobilized biomolecules without using labels. The first SPR biosensor, introduced by Biocore AB in 1990, can detect protein–protein interactions and, moreover, was combined with miniaturized flow systems for efficient sample delivery to the sensor surface. Since it was possible to reproducibly self-assemble gold nanoparticles from solution onto glass surfaces – functionalized with amine or thiol groups – new SPR biosensors were developed that enable label-free optical detection in a chip-based format [20]. In a typical SPR spectroscopy setup a laser beam is aimed at the back of a substrate. Although even subtle changes in the refractive index at the surface of the substrate result in changes of its resonant reflection angle, nanoparticles bound to the sensed analytes increase the shifts in deflection angles, leading to a considerably elevated detection sensitivity [21].

6.1.3.3 **Raman Scattering**

The enhancement of optical signals by metal nanoparticles is also exploited at detection by Raman scattering [22, 23]. Especially, silver and gold nanoparticles are extremely effective at enhancing the scattering signal from adsorbed, Raman-active molecules. Thus, it was possible to detect different DNA target molecules by the use of DNA probes simultaneously labeled with both Raman-active ligands and nanoparticles by Raman spectroscopy [24]. The microarray format included capture DNA strands immobilized on a chip and, thereafter, incubated with target probes. Gold nanoparticles modified with Cy3-labeled, alkylthiol-capped oligonucleotides were used to monitor the presence of specific target DNA strands.

Initially, the nanoparticle probes were not visible to the naked eye, and no Raman signal was detectable. The authors assumed a lack of electromagnetic-field enhancement for the nanoparticles due to the large nanoparticle spacings compared with closely spaced gold nanoparticles that were shown to give a surface-enhanced Raman scattering (SERS) enhancement [25]. But, in contrast to the undeveloped particles, silver enhancement of the bound DNA-nanoparticle probes resulted in the growth of an Ag layer around each Cy3-labeld nanoparticle probe, thereby leading to large Raman scattering enhancements with an unoptimized detection limit of 20 fM target concentration.

6.1.3.4 Electrical Detection

In addition to these versatile optical detection schemes metal nanoparticles offer the possibility for an electrical readout. Owing to their conductivity, it seems self-evident to use them as a conductive bridge between two electrical leads. This can be used in DNA detection schemes by immobilizing capture oligonucleotides in a gap between two electrodes and a subsequent labeling with gold nanoparticles. Möller et al. were able to hybridize complementary, gold-nanoparticle-tagged oligonucleotides to the surface-bound capture DNA between two microstructured electrodes [26]. An additional silver enhancement step makes the bound nanoparticles grow and come into contact, thereby bridging the gap. The resulting drop of resistance was measured by an integrated measurement system consisting of a 'DNA chip reader' with an embedded PC [27] (Fig. 6.3). The microstructured chip had 42 1 μm-wide electrode gaps, each independently accessible and simultaneously read out. The system is transportable, autonomously working and therefore also suitable for readout outside the laboratory. It could detect 5 pM of target DNA concentration. Park et al. have described a similar resistive system with which they could detect target DNA down to 500 fM as well as single-nucleotide polymorphisms with a selectivity of up to 10^5:1 without a thermal-stringency wash [28].

By depositing biofunctionalized nanoparticles on electrode arrays Campas et al. were recently able to measure the hybridization efficiency by amperometry [29]. They achieved significant differences in current density between complementary and mutated oligonucleotide sequences. Similarly, electrodeposition of enzyme-modified colloidal gold on electrodes provided a proof-of-principle concept for enzymatic multisensors.

6.1.3.5 Electrochemical Detection

Other approaches used colloidal gold labels in novel, sensitive electrochemical sensors [30]. After oxidative gold metal dissolution under acidic conditions the resulting aqueous metal ions were detected by anodic stripping voltammetry (ASV). Dequaire et al. used disposable carbon-based electrodes and evaluated the method for a noncompetitive heterogeneous immunoassay of an immunoglobulin G with a detection limit of 3 pM [30]. In addition, ASV has been assigned to an electrochemical DNA detection method [31]. The combination of sensitive gold(III) determination at screen-printed microband electrodes with the large number of gold(III) ions released from each gold particle allowed detection of as low as 5 pM amplified

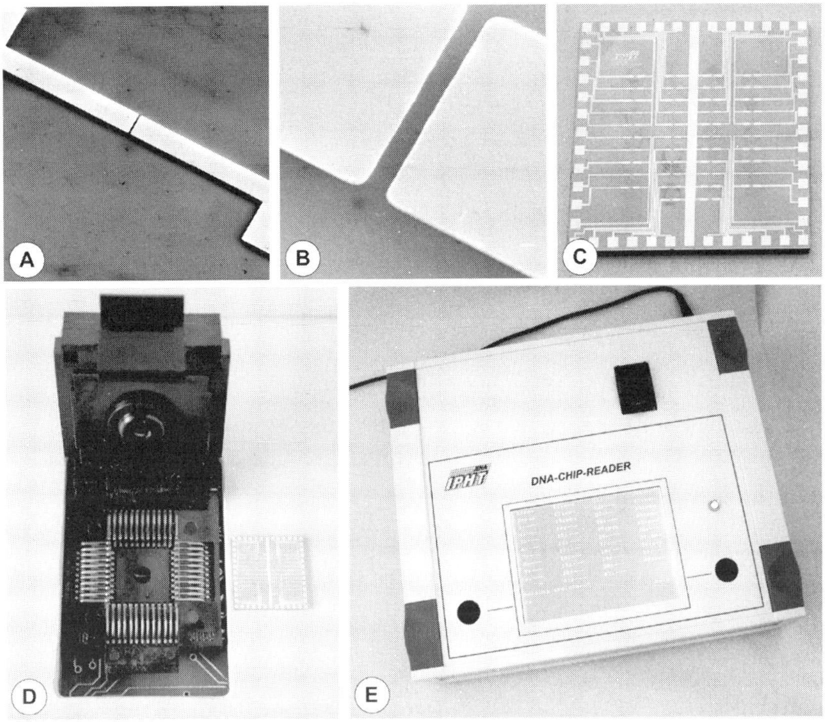

Fig. 6.3. Electrical detection of gold nanoparticle-labeled DNA. DNA strands ('captures') that bind the molecules of interest ('targets') are immobilized between micro-structured electrode gaps on a chip. If any complementary target DNA is present, the target molecules, labeled with gold nano-particles, will bind and form the starting point of subsequent metal enhancement steps. The resulting metal layer is detected by a significant drop in electrical resistivity between the electrodes. (A) Gold electrodes 10 μm wide were used to create gaps. (B) The zoom visualizes the details of one of the 1 μm gaps on the silicon oxide substrate. (C) Overview showing the half-inch chip. (D) DNA chip socket of the paralleled readout system. (E) The portable DNA chip reader. (Modified after Ref. [27].)

DNA fragment. Both an advanced magnetic processing technique and a deposition of gold onto the immobilized gold labels increased the sensitivity of the system by forcing DNA duplex isolation and increasing the number of gold atoms for the oxidation, respectively [32]. The use of different nanoparticles (PbS, CdS, ZnS) with different redox potentials enabled Wang et al. to establish a multilabel system, where every nanoparticle species encodes a different DNA sequence and can be selectively identified by ASV [33]. Using voltammetry makes the integration of a higher number of probes on one substrate problematic. Although Ozsoz et al. did not address the question of microarray formats, their use of differential pulse voltammetry would be appropriate for direct simultaneous detection of many nanoparticle probes at arrayed microelectrodes [34].

6.1.3.6 Gravimetric

Beside their advantageous optical and electrical properties, metal nanoparticles have a high specific mass that can be exploited in detection schemes based on gravimetric principles, as has been shown for both quartz-crystal-microbalances (QCMs) and oscillating microcantilevers. Extremely small mass changes at the oscillating surface cause characteristic changes in the frequency of nanomechanical resonator detectors.

Okahata et al. even reported binding kinetics of a protein to double stranded DNA immobilized on a QCM [35]. Metallic nanoparticles also enhance the sensitivity of gravimetric DNA sensors, up to a picomolar range, when using them as DNA labels [36]. A further increase, up to femtomolar sensitivities, was obtained either by hybridizing a second layer of nanoparticles to the first one [37] or by additional gold deposition on the nanoparticle labels [38].

Conversely, cantilever-based optical deflection assays were able to discriminate DNA single-nucleotide mismatches even without the need for external labeling. In these approaches the microcantilevers were functionalized with capture molecules. A subsequent biomolecule recognition reaction could be detected due to the induced deflection of the cantilever [39]. While hybridization of complementary target oligonucleotides resulted in net positive deflection, targets containing one or two internal mismatches caused net negative deflection. According to Thundat and colleagues, this cantilever approach can be adapted to high-throughput array formats providing distinct positive/negative signals for an easy interpretation of DNA hybridization. Moreover, Gimzewski and co-workers extended these oligonucleotide hybridization assays on individual cantilevers to cantilevers in an array [40]. The differential deflection of the cantilevers provided true molecular recognition signals despite the nonspecific responses of individual cantilevers. Beside the detection of oligonucleotide hybridization, the general applicability to biomolecular processes was demonstrated by monitoring molecular recognition between proteins as well.

6.2
Nanoparticles and their Biofunctionalization

Colloidal nanoparticles differ from bulk material due to their large surface-to-volume ratio. Since inorganic nanoparticles show interesting – strongly size-dependent – optical, electrical, magnetic, and/or electrochemical properties, they offer many opportunities in biological applications. Some of these will be described subsequently. Reference [41] reviews the different physical characteristics of metal nanoparticles and their implementation in assays.

The intense optical absorption of metal colloids is due to the collective electronic (or plasmon) resonance and is defined by the nanoparticle material, size, and geometry. Consequently, not only the size but also their shape plays an important role.

6.2.1
Types of Nanoparticles used for Biomolecular Detection

6.2.1.1 Metal Nanoparticles

Metal nanoparticles are dispersions of a solid phase in a liquid phase, mostly as metal colloids with dimensions of nm to μm (Au [42], Ag [43], [44], Pt [45], Pa [46], Cu, Fe, and Hg [47]). The most important metal particles are gold and silver sols synthesized from metal salts. Gold particles are composed of a starting atom surrounded by a defined quantity of gold-atoms, magic numbers corresponding to the formula $[10n^2 + 2]$ [8, 48], where n is the number of layers in the particle. The minimum size of these colloid particles is 13 atoms. Such particles are close to icosahedrons or dodecahedrons [49], approximating to spheres with increasing diameter.

6.2.1.2 Core/Shell Particles

Metal core/shell nanoparticles also have interesting optical properties. Heterogenic bimetallic nanoparticles exhibit two plasmon resonances, appropriate to the electronic bands of the pure elements (of both the core and the shell metal phases) [49]. The optical properties of such nanoparticles are explained by the Mie theory for cladded particles [50, 51]. Compared with heterogeneous species, homogenous bimetallic nanoparticles, synthesized, for example, by alloying under laser irradiation, exhibit only one surface plasmon peak, which lies between the absorption bands of the pure metals [49]. Bimetallic (mostly heterogeneous) nanoparticles also play an important role in biomolecular detection when Raman-active ligands are used [24].

Furthermore, pure metal nanoparticles have some disadvantages concerning their chemical stability or when used in different solvents. To prevent particle coalescence, colloids can be coated with a dielectric shell, e.g. a silica shell. Liz-Marzán et al. have used silane coupling agents as surface primers to make the particle surface vitreophilic, followed by self-assembly of a hydrated silica monolayer [43]. Thus, the resulting silica surface enables the same bioconjugation strategies as for silica nanoparticles. This has been summarized recently by Drake et al. [52].

After surface modification the inert metal core/dielectric shell nanoparticles could be transferred into practically any solvent. The thickness of the optically transparent silica layer could be determined in a controlled way. Varying the silica shell thickness and the refractive index of the surrounding solvent allowed control over the dispersions' optical properties. For example, the intensity of the plasmon bands of such nanoparticles depends on the shell thickness. With increasing silica shell thickness, up to a defined size, the intensity of the plasmon band increased and, simultaneously, the absorption peak shifted to longer wavelengths (redshift) due to the increased local refractive index around the particles. However, above the defined layer thickness of 80 nm scattering becomes significant, resulting in a strong increase in absorbance at shorter wavelengths (blue-shift), which is similar to the properties of gold-free silica particles. The same results were caused by (bio-)polymeric adsorption onto the metal particle surface. The polymeric shell also changed the geometric and dielectric parameters of the particles [53]. Moreover, the dependence of variations in extinction and light scattering spectra on the gold core diameter, the shell refractive index and thickness could adequately be described by the dipole approximation of the Mie theory.

Another type of nanoparticle composite consists of a metal shell encapsulating a dielectric core [54]. The optical properties of such monodisperse silica nanoparticles (so-called Stöber particles [55]) can be influenced by covering the particles with a thin, uniform metallic shell. Keeping the size of the dielectric core constant, the optical absorption shift is relatively sensitive to the shell thickness. Assuming a constant core/shell size ratio it depends on the absolute size whether the particles absorb or scatter light [56]. Implementation of such nanoshells in living tissue and application of near-infrared light can photothermally destroy the labeled cells [57].

6.2.1.3 Magnetic Nanoparticles

Magnetic nanoparticles are mostly compounds with iron oxides (Fe_3O_4/magnetite and γ-Fe_2O_3/maghemite) and are, therefore, not pure metal particles. However, they are mentioned here because they are also powerful, versatile nanoscaled tools in biology and medicine. There are two types of magnetic particles: (1) so-called magnetic beads containing nm-sized iron oxide particles surrounded by a polymer-silica matrix and (2) pure metal oxide particles in the nm-range (real nanoparticles, strictly speaking). Suspensions of small ferrimagnetic single-domain iron oxide particles are called ferrofluids and can be used for medical applications if biocompatible. Functionalization of these magnetic beads or nanoparticles, respectively, enables the binding of protein or DNA and, therefore, their application in biomolecular detection and their potential use in medical diagnostics and therapies, e.g. in thermal tumor treatment (magnetic hyperthermia [58]) where only biocompatible magnetic nanoparticles are usable. For many diagnostic applications both magnetic beads and nanoparticles are usable. Thus, they are employed as contrast agents in magnetic resonance imaging (MRI) as well as in detecting biomolecular binding events by means of magnetic sensors. Magnetoresistive detection methods exploit the fact that an applied magnetic field, e.g. due to magnetic particles attached to the sensor, causes a shift in electric resistivity [59–62]. Additionally, the magnetic separation of biomolecules attached to magnetic beads is a standard laboratory method. Thus, Ho et al. employed antibody-presenting magnetic nanoparticles as effective affinity probes for selectively concentrating traces of target bacteria from sample solutions [63].

6.2.1.4 Quantum Dots

Quantum dots are nanocrystals of cadmium chalcogenides (CdS, CdSe, CdTe), in the range of 200–10 000 atoms, that exhibit strongly size-dependent optical and electrical properties [64]. Irradiated with low-energy light of a broad, continuous excitation spectrum, semiconductor nanocrystals have a narrow, tunable emission spectrum, and, moreover, they are photochemically stable and therefore complementary, and in some cases perhaps even superior, to conventional fluorophores [65]. But, dependent on their size, the photoluminescence signal can consist of the entire spectrum of visible light. This enables the excitation of different sizes of quantum dots at the same time and makes them suitable as luminescent probes for labeling of biological systems [4, 66, 67].

6.2.2
Synthesis of Gold (Silver) Nanoparticles

The method used most for the synthesis of gold (as well as other metal) nanoparticles is the reduction of metal salts by different reducing agents (organic acids [68], substituted ammonias [68, 69], formaldehyde [70], hydrogen peroxide, phosphorus [71], gases, protecting agents [72, 73], and electrical fields [74]. Gold colloids are mostly synthesized by the reduction of gold(III) salts, and, among these, the citrate reduction of $HAuCl_4$ is the most common procedure [68], where sodium citrate acts both as a nucleating and reducing agent [47]. Initially, the citrate is oxidized to acetone dicarboxylic acid [49]. In the following step, gold ions become atoms by forming an intermediate complex and, thereafter, nucleation islands. The smallest island is composed of 13 gold atoms [75]. Further metal ions are reduced on the surface of such nucleation centers to give larger particles. The particle size (12–147 nm) is determined by the quantity of citrate ions [76]. The resulting polycrystalline, nearly spherical particles are polydispersed, showing a relatively uniform shape and homogeneous size distribution (standard deviations of 10–15%, depending on the particle diameter).

The stability of the citrate-reduced colloids is determined by the concentration of salt ions in the solution. A dielectric shell of charged ions keeps the particles apart, therefore stabilizing the solution against aggregation. Small changes in reaction conditions can make this shell partially unprotected, resulting in an irreversible coagulation of the colloid solution. By using different ligands during or after the synthesis the particles can be sterically stabilized (Section 6.2.3).

Another approach to synthesizing metal (gold) nanoparticles is the Brust–Schiffrin method, involving the phase transfer of a tetrachloroaurate complex from aqueous to organic solution, followed by reduction with sodium borohydride in the presence of a thiol-stabilizing ligand [72, 73, 77]. The resulting particles are smaller (1–3.5 nm) and more monodispersed than the citrate colloids.

Size control of gold nanoparticles by the use of different stabilizing agents depends on the ligand type and its properties [78]. For alkane thiol ligands the molar ratio of aurate to thiol influences the average particle size [79]. By using a multivalent alkane thiol stabilizer Yonezawa et al. obtained smaller, more monodisperse gold nanoparticles than with conventional monoalkanethiols, thereby enabling systematic size control with atomic precision [80].

6.2.3
Biofunctionalization

Colloidal metal particles can be modified either during or after particle synthesis. Similar to the formation of self-assembled monolayers (SAMs) on planar surfaces

(Section 6.3.1.1) the post-synthetic coupling of biomolecules to the particle surface occurs in various steps. First, the biomolecules bind through electrostatic interactions by displacing the surrounding citrate ions. Thereafter, a chemical bond between the ligand and the particle follows, e.g. a thiol-gold coupling.

6.2.3.1 Modification of Gold Nanoparticles with Oligonucleotides/DNA

Oligonucleotides can be attached to metal nanoparticles in different ways. Since the resulting DNA-nanoparticle conjugates differ in oligonucleotide surface densities, the availability for hybridization to targets, and in the tendency to nonspecifically bind to surfaces, the attachment chemistry impacts significantly on their use in heterogeneous detection schemes [81]. Bioconjugate chemistry has been studied most intensively for gold nanoparticles. As they provide the simplest, most stable conjugation chemistry for oligonucleotides, we will focus on the biofunctionalization of colloidal gold (Fig. 6.4).

Thiol, Di-, Trisulfide Nuzzo et al. have shown that gold surfaces can be easily functionalized by free thiols and disulfides [82, 83]. Their adsorption studies of methanethiol and dimethyl disulfide showed a strong binding of both adsorbates to gold surfaces, with the bonding of disulfide being greatly favored, probably due to dissociation of the disulfide bond to give a stable surface thiolate. However, these oligonucleotide–gold conjugates lose activity as hybridization probes when soaked in solutions containing thiols, which displace the derivatized oligonucleotide from the gold surface. To overcome this drawback Letsinger et al. described a new steroid-cyclic disulfide anchoring group for binding oligonucleotides to gold surfaces [84]. The resulting nanoparticle conjugates kept their hybridization activity and were much more resistant to attack by a thiol than conventional gold conjugates that contain alkyl mono-thiol or acyclic disulfide linkers. The same authors subsequently reported that oligonucleotides connected to gold through three sulfur groups were even more stable than these dithiane conjugates, stabilizing gold particles even larger than 30 nm in diameter [85].

Gold nanoparticles are usually linked to oligonucleotides by a thiol at the 5′ or 3′ end of the oligonucleotide, leaving the nucleotides unobstructed for hybridization to their complements. However, dependent on oligonucleotide content, length, and coverage, DNA tends to adsorb nonspecifically to gold surfaces through the nucleotides, inhibiting hybridization [86, 87]. To prevent DNA surface adsorption, mixed monolayers of the thiol-derivatized probe and a spacer-thiol have been explored. On planar surfaces, mercaptohexanol (MCH) can orient the DNA perpendicularly and facilitate hybridization by displacing the non-covalent and nonspecific adsorption of thiolated DNA [88–90]. Park et al. considered MCH concentration and reaction time as a key to controlling the conformation changes of oligonucleotides attached to gold nanoparticles [91]. With increasing MCH concentration (1 μM–1 mM) the electrophoresis mobility of the Au-DNA conjugates slightly decreased towards those of gold nanoparticles without DNA attached, but stabilized by BPS [bis(*p*-sulfonatophenyl)phenylphosphine dihydrate, dipotassium salt]. This result points to a stepwise loss of surface-bound oligonucleotides, which suggests that

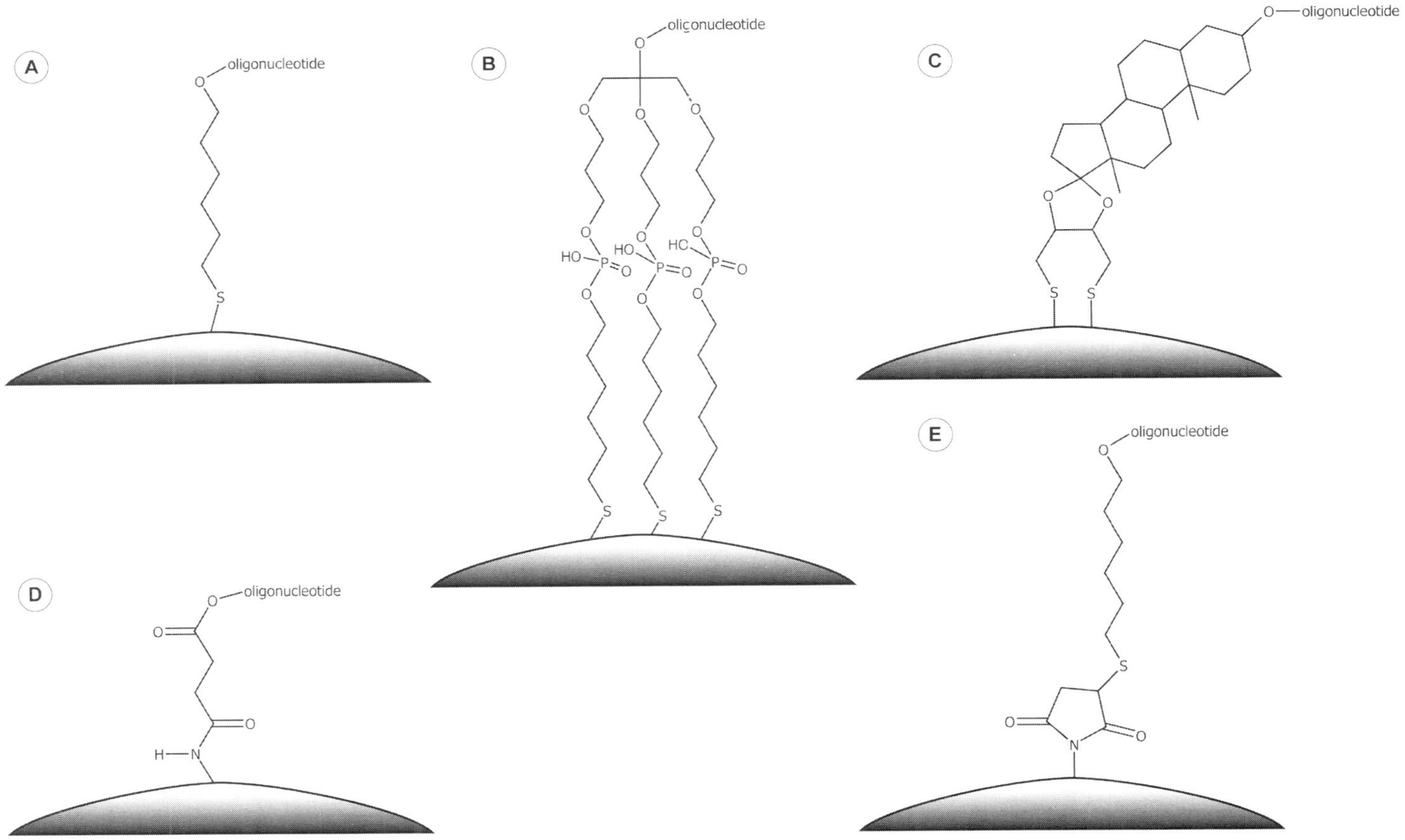

Fig. 6.4. Scheme of the covalent attachment of oligonucleotides to gold nanoparticles by different linker groups: (A) alkyl-thiol, (B) multiple-thiol anchor, (C) steroid disulfide, (D) amine/succinimide, and (E) maleimide.

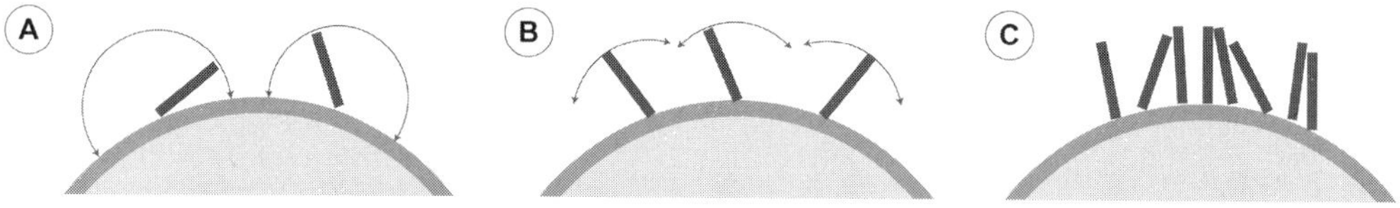

Fig. 6.5. Formation of oligonucleotide layers on gold nanoparticle surfaces. The conformation depends on the DNA molecule density on the surface. (A) At very low surface coverage, no steric interactions occur between strands on the surface. (B) For higher molecule densities, collisions will occur between the ends of neighboring oligonucleotides, restricting the possible strand orientations and forcing the DNA strands to "stand up". (C) As surface coverage increases, the oligonucleotides approach their theoretical limit of a densely packed monolayer of "standing up" DNA strands. (Modified after Ref. [92].)

reaction with concentrated MCH displaces the DNA molecules from the nanoparticle surface. Changes in effective size (D_{eff}) of the Au-DNA conjugates were quantified by the Ferguson plot method. The obtained drop in D_{eff} confirmed the loss of surface-bound oligonucleotides with higher MCH concentrations (>0.1 mM). However, MCH led to an increased hybridization capacity, presumably due to better availability of the oligonucleotides to base pairing. In addition, Rant et al. characterized the conformation of oligonucleotide layers on Au surfaces by fluorescence investigation [92] (Fig. 6.5).

Although thiols and mercaptoalkyl residues can be incorporated into DNA simply by adding the suitable phosphoramidite modifier through solid-phase DNA synthesis [93], thiol- or disulfide-modified DNA is commercially available.

Other Coupling Strategies (Phosphine, Maleimide, Amine/Succinimide, Lysine) In 1969, McPartlin et al. were the first to describe very small gold clusters that were passivated by organic groups (phosphines). This undecagold contains a gold core of 11 atoms, with the gold atoms on the surface attached covalently to phosphine groups [94]. By altering the organic groups the clusters were made water soluble [95] and derivatized to link to proteins [96–98]. Larger gold clusters were subsequently developed, showing better visibility at high magnification by transmission electron microscopy (TEM) and increased enhancement with silver [98]. These 1.4 nm-sized gold nanoparticles (Au_{55}) are commercially available bearing a single activated functional group (Nanogold™, Nanoprobes Inc.). They have been reacted with proteins or appropriately modified oligonucleotides to form 1:1 nanoparticle:biomolecule conjugates. Using a maleimide group or an *N*-hydroxysuccinimide, the gold clusters can react specifically with thiols or amino groups, respectively [100]. Thus, Au_{55} clusters passivated with a phosphine ligand shell, which is functionalized with a single reactive maleimide group, were used to prepare DNA–gold conjugates from disulfide-modified and thiolated oligonucleotides [101, 102].

As well as thiolated oligonucleotides, Ozsoz et al. used amino-modified oligonucleotide probes to covalently attach to gold nanoparticles bearing carboxy-groups [34]. After modifying the gold colloids with L-cysteine, standard activation methods converted the carboxylic acids into succinimide esters, which allow the formation of a peptide bond with amino-modified DNA.

DNA–nanoparticle conjugates are also an interesting alternative "bottom-up" fabrication technology to produce nanowires using long DNA molecules as templates. Due to the relatively poor intrinsic electric conductivity of DNA, metallization is required and can be achieved by nanoparticles. An *ex situ* approach uses the electrostatic interaction between positively charged particles and the negatively charged DNA phosphate backbone to attach lysine-capped gold colloidal particles to DNA double-helices [103, 104]. However, Harnack et al. discovered that negatively charged tris(hydroxymethyl)phosphine (THP)-capped gold nanoparticles also bind densely to DNA [105]. Although the binding mechanisms of THP-gold nanoparticles to DNA, and the factors controlling the binding efficiency, were still unclear, the authors expected hydrogen-bonding interactions to be important since each THP ligand provides three hydroxyl groups that can serve as either OH donors or O acceptors. Cooperative, THP-gold conjugates preferably adsorb to hydrophilic areas such as DNA molecules.

Supporting these observations, but in contrast to conventional wisdom, Li and Rothberg also showed that single stranded DNA (ss-DNA) adsorbed on negatively charged gold nanoparticles whereas double stranded oligonucleotides (ds-DNA) did not [106]. They attributed these different electrostatic propensities to the flexible structure of ss-DNA. Single strands can uncoil sufficiently to expose their bases so that attractive Van der Waals forces cause sticking to the gold. However, the duplex structure of ds-DNA does not permit the uncoiling needed to expose the bases. Hence, repulsion between the negatively charged phosphate backbone and the adsorbed citrate ions dominates so that ds-DNA will not adsorb. Moreover, they demonstrated that the adsorption rate of ss-DNA to gold nanoparticles is length and temperature dependent [107] and, additionally, can effectively stabilize the gold colloid against salt-induced aggregation. Exploiting these observations, they designed a simple, fast colorimetric hybridization assay that does not require functionalization of the gold, the probe or the target DNA, but was able to easily detect single base mismatches.

6.2.3.2 **Modification of Gold Nanoparticles with Proteins**

Proteins bind to gold colloids for three main reasons: sulfur bonding (cysteine and methionine), charge (lysine), and hydrophobic attraction (tryptophan) (Fig. 6.6). Generally, this conjugation is irreversible, but long-term storage at high pH or in a buffer containing surfactant may cause some proteins to dissociate.

Initially, the coupling of gold nanoparticles to proteins was used to visualize cellular structures by electron microscopy because of the high electric densities [108], as shown for antibodies and lectin [109, 110]. More recently, Ho et al. reported a method for fabricating biofunctionalized nanoparticles by attaching human immunoglobulin (IgG) on their surfaces through either electrostatic or covalent binding [63]. By selective binding of these IgG-presenting gold nanoparticles to bacterial cell walls they were able to study the interactions between IgG and pathogens by transmission electron microscopy.

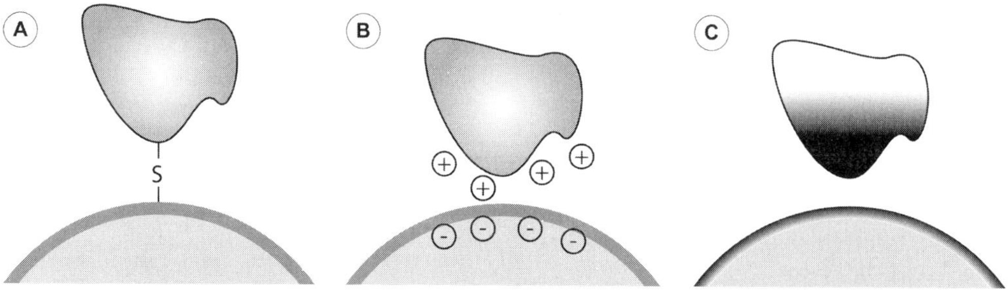

Fig. 6.6. Schematic summary of functionalization approaches of proteins to gold nanoparticles. Proteins bind to the particle surface by (A) sulfur bonding, (B) charge interactions, and/or (C) hydrophobic attractions (white: hydrophilic, black: hydrophobic regions), dependent on the amino acids exposed to the particle surface.

The first nanoparticle labeling of genomic nucleic acids was applied using the biotin/streptavidin biorecognition reaction [111].

Studying the association of proteins onto gold particles at various protein concentrations yield typical saturation curves [14]. The number of bound molecules depends on the molar concentration of the protein free in solution, the number of possible adsorption sites and inversely correlates with the equilibrium constant for dissociation of protein from particles. The applicability of Scatchard analysis to the formation of protein–gold complexes indicates a finite number of adsorption sites, leading to saturation, which is best explained by assuming a monomolecular shell of protein around the particles.

In the past, colloidal gold–protein complexes were used extensively in immunocytochemistry as secondary reagents for the localization of antigens. Horisberger et al. examined the adsorption of protein A onto 11.2 nm-sized gold nanoparticles, regarding the process and extent of the adsorption, the optimal conditions of preparation, and the stability of such gold–protein complexes [112]. The adsorption isotherm was independent of pH at low protein coverage. However, in the presence of a large excess of protein A, the highest coverage was obtained at pH 5.1, the isoelectric point of the protein. Furthermore, the extent of protein association onto gold particles also varied with the different protein coverage and decreased with increasing coverage. The obtained complexes were stable under storage at low but not at high protein coverage (up to 12 and 26 molecules adsorbed per particle, respectively). Beside use in immunoassays by coupling antibodies to colloidal gold, the streptavidin–biotin system [113] offers further possible applications (for a review see Ref. [114]). The tetravalent protein streptavidin can bind the small biomolecule biotin with high sensitivity and affinity. Thus, streptavidin-functionalized nanoparticles can be coupled easily to other molecules modified by biotin. By attaching biotinylated oligonucleotides to streptavidin-functionalized particles, DNA–nanoparticle conjugates have been formed [115], enlarging the recognition capacity of streptavidin by a highly specific binding site for the complementary DNA sequence. This offers the opportunity to detect DNA-DNA hybridization events by gold nanoparticles. Furthermore, Niemeyer and Ceyhan have described a DNA-directed functionalization of colloidal gold with protein [116]. Thereby, oligonucleotide-modified gold nanoparticles were coupled to complementary DNA–streptavidin conjugates, which also have been functionalized with biotinylated antibodies. The bioactivity of the resulting protein–gold conjugates was proved in an immunoassay.

Recently, Levy et al. have demonstrated a general approach to the synthesis of extremely stable gold nanoparticles using a pentapeptide ligand [117]. Based on protein folding considerations, the basic design principle aimed at a ligand that can readily attach to the surface of the gold particle and form a well-packed passivation layer with a hydrophilic terminus. The resulting pentapeptide thiol capping ligand was able to convert citrate-stabilized gold nanoparticles into stable, water-soluble nanoparticles with chemical properties comparable to those of proteins. The stability of different particle preparations conferred by ligands of various peptide sequences has been evaluated by exposing the particles to increasing salt concentrations until precipitation occurred. This stability depended on the ligand length, hydrophobicity, and charge.

In contrast to bioconjugation after nanoparticle synthesis, direct conjugation methods eliminate the need for intermediate stabilizing agents or dense passivation that minimizes the free surface area for interactions with the desired adsorbates and often tends to aggregation with even mild processing. Burt et al. were able to produce water-soluble gold nanoparticles less than 2 nm in diameter directly conjugated to bovine serum albumin (BSA) protein without application of high temperature or high pressure. They obtained a near-quantitative yield of well-dispersed, protein-conjugated gold nanoparticles that remain stable indefinitely in solution under ambient conditions [118].

6.2.3.3 Biofunctionalization of other Metal Nanoparticles

Oligonucleotides have been less successfully attached to nanoparticles made from materials other than gold (such as Ag, Cu, Pd, Pt), probably because of the weaker bond energies between sulfur and the other metals. Thiols possibly bound to these surfaces are readily displaced by oxidants or other competing ligands (including the DNA bases). A thin gold shell grown around metal cores of different materials and shapes can improve biomolecule attachment, retaining the characteristics of the core material, as shown for core-shell Ag/Au nanoparticles by Mirkin's group [115].

6.2.4 Biological Applications of Gold Nanoparticles

Due to their binding specificity as well as their large variety of functional groups, biomolecules (nucleic acids, proteins) are able to offer new opportunities for the functionalization of nanoparticles. Furthermore, efforts have been made to combine the intrinsic opportunities of proteins, c.g. optical, catalytic, mechanical or switchable properties, with the specific features of nanoparticles.

Gold nanoparticle-oligonucleotide-conjugates are of great interest since complementary DNA base pairing makes them specifically addressable. This can be used for biomolecular detection schemes as well as for organizing supramolecular nanostructures. It also offers versatile applications in the field of biosensors, disease diagnosis, gene expression, and molecular nanotechnology [8]. There are two pioneering strategies for the functionalization of gold nanoparticles with oligonucleotides. In 1996, Mirkin et al. used short DNA molecules as a linker between 13 nm-sized particles, resulting in macroscopic assemblies. The DNA attached to the gold nanoparticles remained accessible to hybridization with complementary DNA in a sequence-specific but reversible manner [1]. Conversely, DNA can be used as a template to bind small gold nanoparticles on a single oligonucleotide strand [2]. Furthermore, there are other strategies for forming supramolecular aggregates, e.g. semi-synthetic conjugates by self-assembly of nucleic acids, inorganic nanoparticles, and proteins such as streptavidin [119].

6.3 Substrates and their Biofunctionalization

Oligonucleotides and other biomolecules cannot be coupled directly to the surface silanol groups of silicon oxide or glass substrates. Therefore, the surface must be functionalized with a group that can be used either to initiate oligonucleotide synthesis or to which the pre-synthesized capture oligonucleotides can be attached. In principle, there are two means of obtaining substrates that can bind biomolecular capture probes: (1) nearly monomolecular thin films and (2) nanoporous gels (Fig. 6.7). The first method provides binding sites two-dimensionally, whereas the latter ones form 3D arrangements. The advantage of impermeable, monomolecular binding layers over nanoporous membranes/gels is that there is no need for diffusion into pores, i.e. capture and target molecules can access the probes immediately. This enhances the rate of capture probe immobilization as well as hybridization/binding rates, especially for extended molecules and/or labels that would be influenced by steric hindrance. However, 3D nanoporous gels yield a

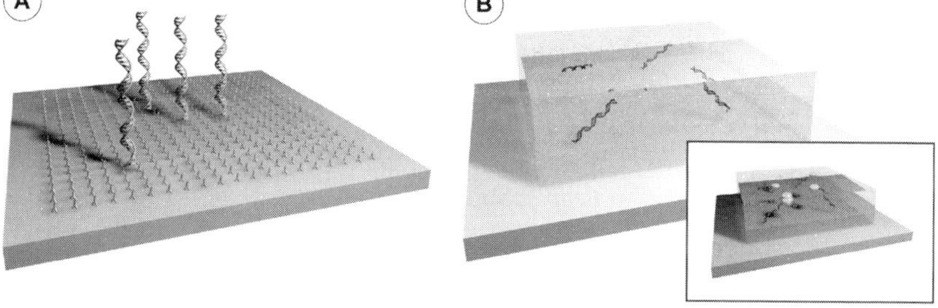

Fig. 6.7. Strategies of substrate biofunctionalization: (A) functional planar interfaces and (B) microscaled reaction volumes (nanoporous hydrogels). Inset: nanoparticle-labeled oligonucleotide strands immobilized in the gel.

largely enhanced surface area and, therefore, a higher capacity for binding of capture and target probes, leading to enhanced signal levels.

6.3.1 Molecular Thin Films

6.3.1.1 Self-assembly Monolayers

Adsorption of organic thin-films enables the biofunctionalization of planar surfaces. Typical approaches are either Langmuir–Blodgett (LB) techniques or a spontaneous organization of molecules into stable, well-defined structures (self-assembly). Self-assembled monolayers (SAMs) are widely used, highly ordered monomolecular films that spontaneously form on surfaces by chemisorption. These 2D monolayers consist of oriented molecules containing a head group that is reactive towards the surface. The alkyl chain usually influences the physicochemical properties and stabilizes the SAM by intermolecular interactions, whereas the tail groups define the binding properties of the layer to further possible ligands. Compared with the similar LB films, in SAMs the ligand covalently binds to the surface, resulting in a very strong bonding. Several systems give SAMs, e.g. organosulfur compounds on metal surfaces or carboxy groups on metal oxides [120, 121].

Exposure of gold surfaces to alkane-thiol solutions leads to the self-assembly of these molecules. The resulting organic ultrathin film can be monitored by surface plasmon resonance spectroscopy (SPRS). Peterlinz and Georgiadis introduced a novel two-color SPR method, with which they obtained both film thickness and film dielectric constant and studied the chain length- and concentration-dependent kinetics of film formation in different solvents. Self-assembly in ethanol consists of three distinct kinetics steps, whereas the formation in heptane can be described with a single-step Langmuir adsorption model [122]. In ethanol, the results were most consistent with a film formation mechanism involving adsorption of both chemisorbed and physisorbed molecules. Expanding their SPRS studies the authors examined the formation kinetics for a two-component monolayer film containing thiol-modified single strand DNA (ssDNA including a hexamethylene linker) as well as mercaptohexanol [123]. After adsorbing HS-C6-ssDNA, exposure to an aqueous solution of mercaptohexanol results in a very rapid mercaptohexanol adsorption followed by a slow desorption of HS-C6-ssDNA. The final coverage of thiol-tethered DNA with mercaptohexanol diluent was estimated as 5.2×10^{12} HS-C6-ssDNA cm^{-2}. This corresponds to coverage densities described elsewhere [124–126]. Coverage versus time data calculated from the two-color SPR best fitted those of a model that accounts for adsorption, desorption, and diffusion (ADD) of the adsorbate, although this model predicts a saturation coverage of 1×10^{14} molecules cm^{-2}. The adsorption and hybridization kinetics of surface-bound thiolated ssDNA hybridized to fully complementary ssDNA were remarkably similar for these two different interfacial binding processes. The occurrence of sequence-specific hybridization was confirmed by SPRS melting studies. The amount of surface-immobilized duplexes differed only slightly from that for the same duplexes in free solution. A hybridization coverage of about one-third of that for the adsorption accounts for a loss of some adsorbed HS-C_6-ssDNA during rinsing and mercaptohexanol-mediated desorption as well as for the hybridization efficiency.

The effect of DNA length and the presence of a thiol anchoring group on the assembly of oligonucleotides at gold surfaces was investigated by Steel et al. [127]. The thiol-anchoring group strongly enhanced oligonucleotide immobilization. Adsorbed thiol-ssDNA oligonucleotides shorter than 24 bases tended to organize in an end-tethered configuration, for which the surface coverage is largely independent of oligonucleotide length. However, for strands longer than 24 bases, the surface coverage starts to decrease considerably with probe length, presumably corresponding to a less ordered arrangement of DNA chains. Furthermore, Shchepinov et al. investigated the influence of steric factors on the hybridization of nucleic acids to oligonucleotide arrays [128]. They used spacer molecules to reduce steric interference of the support on the hybridization behavior of immobilized oligonucleotides. The optimal spacer length was determined to be at least 40 atoms, resulting in up to a 150-fold increased hybridization yields. Beyond this, steric hindrance can also be a problem if the surface-bound oligonucleotides are too close to each other. The highest hybridization yields were given for surfaces containing about 50% of the maximum oligonucleotide concentration. A further important factor influencing the hybridization efficiency is the base composition of the reacting oligonucleotides, owing to the lower stability of A:T versus G:C pairs. Southern et al. described the mechanism of duplex formation as a process that starts with the formation of a transient nucleation complex from the interaction of very few base pairs [129]. Mismatches close to the centre of an oligonucleotide have a strongly destabilizing effect on the duplex, whereas mismatches at the end are less destabilizing and thus more difficult to discriminate.

However, organosilicon derivatives on silicon oxide and glass are the most important for biological applications – and therefore we will focus on these.

Since all the standard surface modifications require silanol groups, the absolute number and relative distribution of surface hydroxyl (silanol) groups is important [130]. By varying the concentration of silanol groups it is possible to substantially change the properties of such a surface. Zhuravlev has studied the surface concentration of hydroxyl groups (silanol number α_{OH}) for a large variety of amorphous silicas [131]. By using the deuterio-exchange method with mass spectrometric analysis he estimated a silanol number of about 5.0 OH groups per nm^{-2} (corresponding to 5×10^{14} cm^{-2}), independent of the origin and structural characteristics of the fully hydroxylated surfaces, and considered the value as a physicochemical constant. However, preliminary vacuum treatment within the range from 200 to 1100 °C significantly decreased the concentration of hydroxyl groups ($\alpha_{OH} < 0.15$), pointing to strong dehydroxylation of the surface.

Furthermore, the coating morphology, including silane layer thickness, density, and the orientation of the surface molecules, strongly depends on the amount of water the solvent contains [130]. Once the surface offers functional groups for subsequent biomolecule coupling, there are different strategies for covalent attachment of DNA (or proteins) to glass surfaces to build microarrays, as described in Ref. [132]. To enable molecular interactions with other biomolecules (e.g. hybrid-

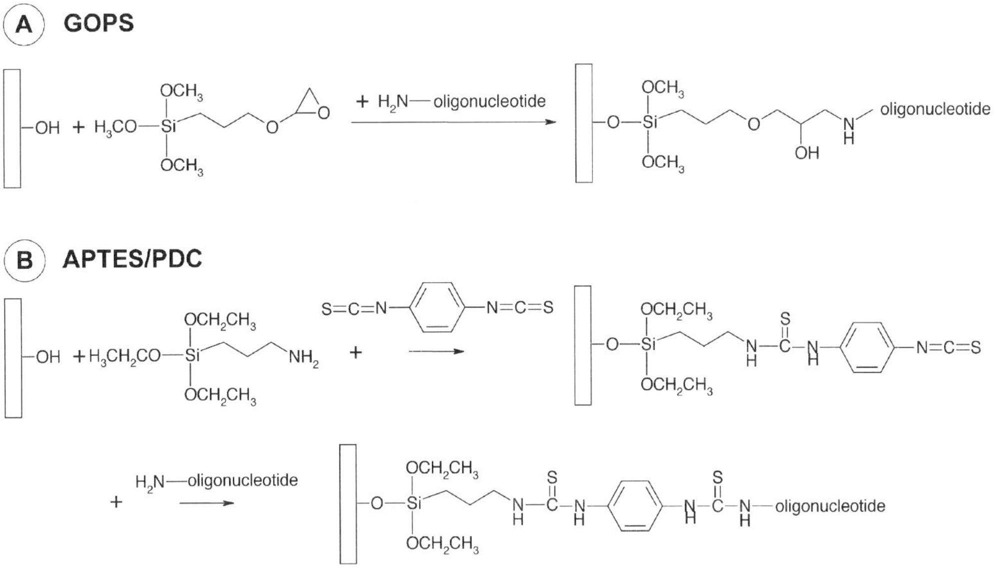

Fig. 6.8. Surface modification with silanes for DNA attachment. (A) Direct binding of amino-modified DNA by epoxy-groups of 3-glycidoxypropyltrimethoxysilane (GOPS). (B) Amino-attachment chemistry of 3-aminopropyltriethoxysilane (APTES). The binding of amino-modified oligonucleotides works indirectly by the bifunctional crosslinker 1,4-phenylenediisothiocyanate (PDC) [135].

ization) the immobilized capture probes should be fixed at their extremities. Therefore amino- or carboxy-modified DNA molecules are normally used, requiring adequate functionalized substrate surfaces. Consolandi et al. have described two robust procedures for oligonucleotide microarray preparation, including glass functionalization with appropriate silanes (Fig. 6.8), a coating step using polymers, and a surface activation step to allow for the attachment of amino-modified oligonucleotides [133]. These chemical platforms showed an overall high loading capacity and availability to hybridization against targets, a good uniformity, resistance to consecutive probing/stripping cycles, and the possibility of performing enzymatic reactions.

Recently, Martin-Palma et al. have presented a novel biofunctionalization technique for the deposition of amine groups on different surfaces [134]. The proposed activation method induced amino-group fixation on the surface of materials ranging from semiconductors to metals and insulating materials. The reactivity of the functionalized surfaces could be determined by using a fluorescent reagent that specifically reacts with amine groups.

6.3.1.2 **Optimization of Gold Nanoparticle-based Microarrays for DNA Detection**

However, substrate modification with silanes (as a prerequisite for capture DNA binding) often leads to inhomogeneous surfaces and/or non-specific binding of the labeled DNA. For that reason, Fritzsche and co-workers examined different cleaning strategies as a prerequisite for substrate functionalization, characterizing two different surface modification methods with silanes so as to provide functional groups for covalent attachment of amino-modified DNA [135]. To reduce non-specific binding of gold-tagged DNA molecules, different blocking strategies were examined, especially those for nanoparticle labeling. The two examined silanes differed in their DNA binding homogeneity, maximum signal intensities, and sensitivity. Non-specific gold binding could be blocked by treatment in 3% bovine serum albumin (BSA). Another approach to characterizing surface modification methods by silanes employed atomic force microscopy (AFM) [136]. After silanization of the silicon oxide substrate, parts of the surface were covered by an elastomeric mask and then treated with oxygen plasma, leading to damage of the silane layer. AFM characterization of the surface (Fig. 6.9) revealed a height difference of ~1.8 nm, which can be attributed to the thickness of the silane layer.

6.3.2
Nanoporous Gels

As well as glass or silicon surfaces, organic polymers offer another interesting option for the immobilization of nanoparticles. A higher loading capacity can be obtained by using thick layers consisting of a 3D network.

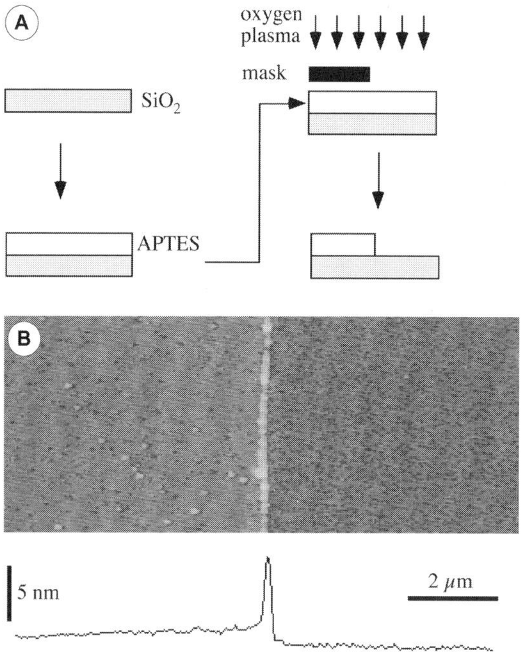

Fig. 6.9. DNA immobilization using APTES surfaces. A step in an APTES surface to measure the layer thickness was fabricated as follows: (A) parts of the silanized surface were covered by an elastomeric mask and thereby protected against damage by subsequent oxygen plasma. (B) The resulting step of about 1.8 nm is visible in the scanning force micrograph and represents the height of the silane layer. (Modified after Ref. [136] with permission of Oxford University Press.)

Since the first introduction of solid-phase synthesis on an organic polymer support (2% crosslinked polystyrene [137]), new biomaterials with polyethylene backbone structures have been developed. These materials are characterized by improved hydrophilic/hydrophobic properties as well as a good biocompatibility. Another important feature of these polymers is the resistance to standard solvents and their good swelling properties [138].

In addition to other applications the polymers can be used as beads for combinatorial synthesis resins such as Tentagel™ [139, 140], polyethylene glycol–polystyrol (PEG-PS) [139] and polyethylene glycol–polyacrylamide copolymers (PEGA) [141]. Furthermore, polymers suitable for solid-phase synthesis have been micropatterned by spinning-on the pure monomers without functionalization, followed by light-induced polymerization [142]. More recently, Amirgoulova et al. described polymer coatings based on PEG for the study of immobilized biomolecules [143]. The crosslinked, star-polymer derived surfaces not only allowed reversible protein unfolding and refolding but also interacted negligibly with the immobilized proteins.

While preparing the polymer, bacteria cells [144] as well as proteins [145, 146] can be enclosed for different microfluidic reactors and for biochemical reactions, respectively. Although in these processes the enzymes and cells were non-covalently bound at the matrix of the polymer, they were restrained/prevented sterically from leaving the gel.

Bieber and co-workers were able to immobilize *Salmonella* antibodies in a 3D polymer network based on acrylamide derivates and polyethylene linkers [147]. To extend this strategy the applied polyethylene glycol diacrylates and bisacrylated bis-diamino polyethylene glycols ($M_r = 4000, 6000$, and 8000) were functionalized by using hydroxy acrylate. Thus it was possible to bind biomolecules covalently instead of simply enclosing them in the polymer. Additionally, both the network structure (e.g. width of the meshes) and the functionality of the synthesized polymer could be adapted by an adjustable crosslinking reaction and the specific loading with functional groups, respectively. The resulting loading capacity of these spaces of biorecognition reactions were up to 1000× higher than those of plain 2D surfaces.

Before their immobilization by covalent binding in the nanoporous gel the biomolecules should be tested for their ability to penetrate coats of different hydrogels. A simple possibility is to use gel electrophoresis primarily employed for the separation and purification of DNA and proteins [148] (Fig. 6.10).

The investigated gels were loaded with a protein standard mixture and treated with sodium dodecyl sulfate (SDS), which binds to the amide groups in the protein. Thus, the protein becomes negatively charged, in dependency of the length of its amino acid chain. Application of an electric field forces the molecules through the gel with different electrophoretic mobility due to their different electric charge, which is proportional to the size of the molecule. Higher polymer concentrations and smaller monomers yield a 3D network with tighter meshes. Larger molecules are, therefore, unable to penetrate into the gel.

In addition to the immobilization of biomolecules on functionalized surfaces, 10 μm-thin coats of functionalized spots of polyethylene glycol-based polymers

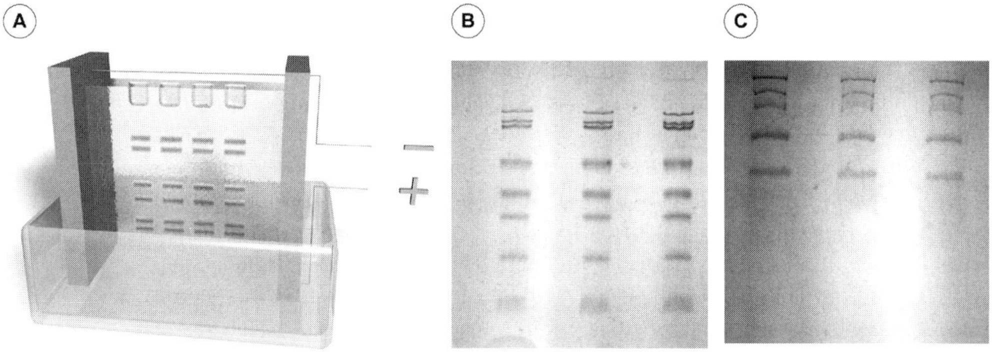

Fig. 6.10. (A) Electrophoresis is a rapid method for separating biomolecules according to their charge and molecular size/weight. When exposed to an electric field, biomolecules in the electrophoresis gel move towards one of the electrodes in a manner that depends on the molecule's charge and molecular size and on the size of the gel pores/meshes. Thereby, sodium dodecyl sulfate (SDS) gel electrophoresis is a rapid qualifying and quantifying method for proteins that can be separated only by their molecular weights. SDS binds to hydrophobic domains of proteins, masking their individual charge differences. SDS–protein complexes have a negative charge and can be size-separated since the resulting charge of the complex is proportional to the molecular weight of the protein. During separation, SDS–protein complexes are attracted to the anode and separated by enforcement through the porous gel structure, which allows small proteins to move very fast, whereas larger molecules show a significant decelerated mobility. (B) This principle can be utilized to characterize the pore size of nanoporous gels. A mixture of proteins of known size and mass (116.0, 66.2, 45.0, 35.0, 25.0, 18.0, and 14.4 kDa) was driven by an applied electric field into two different gels. A standard 12% polyacryl amide gel (A) leads to certain mobility and a complete separation of the mixture. (C) Under similar conditions regarding voltage and time, a 12% poly (bisacryl polyethylenglycol$_{4000}$) gel shows significantly different results: The proteins move much more slowly, and fewer bands are observed. This is because molecules above a certain threshold size become stuck in the gel, resulting in a band consisting of the remaining larger molecules.

(0.5–2 mm in diameter) have been prepared on glass substrates. These functionalized arrays are easy to use and suitable for commercial spotting systems. After activation of the glass supports and their modification with acrylsilane the monomer solution, containing a photo-initiator, was coated. To generate the spots ultraviolet radiation was applied through a mask, leading to polymerization at the exposed areas. At the non-exposed areas, unreacted monomer solution was rinsed off after polymerization had finished. Thereby, the loading of the hydrogel is influenced by the ratio of the different functional groups in the monomer solution. In subsequent steps the prepared hydroxy-functionalized spots were transformed into carboxylic acids and active esters, which can react with amino-modified, fluorescence-labeled DNA. Finally, the oligonucleotides are bound covalently at the polymer matrix and are then qualitatively and quantitatively detectible by the fluorescent group (Fig. 6.11).

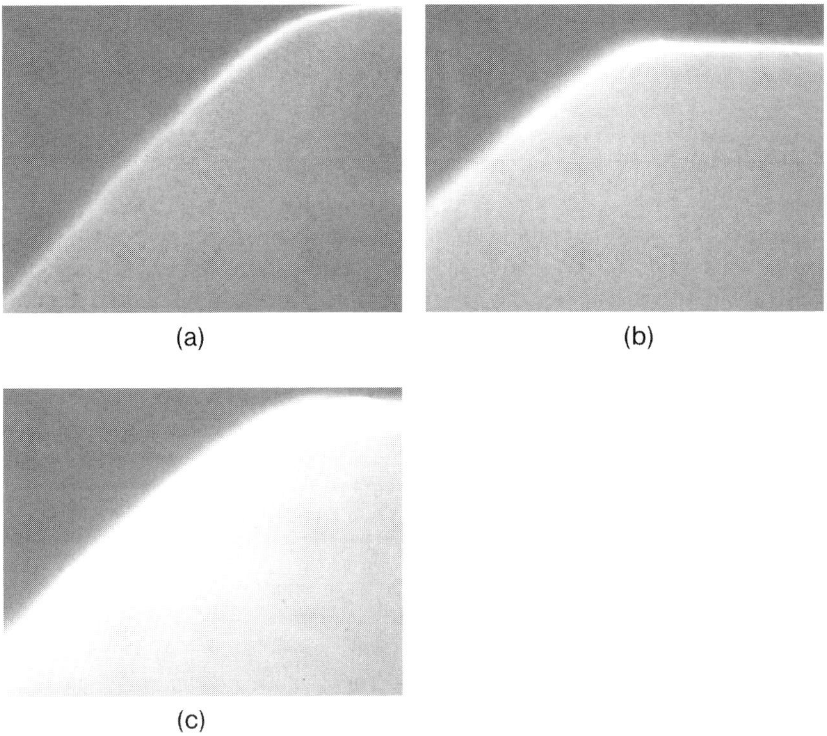

Fig. 6.11. Binding of fluorescence-labeled DNA molecules in a nanoporous hydrogel demonstrated by fluorescence microscopy. The gels were prepared with different hydroxy acrylate concentrations, (a) 0, (b) 1 and (c) 10 mM, leading to different concentrations of hydroxy groups in the gel network and, therefore, different binding capacity of the biomolecule/DNA loading. The area-related loading capacity of these reaction spaces is up to 1000× higher than for plain 2D surfaces.

6.4 Outlook

The detection and characterization of bioactive molecules represents a field of great importance for various aspects of our daily life, such as health management, food quality control, forensic, or environmental protection. Further development aims to increase the sensitivity and specificity of the assays; other important parameters are the robustness of the methods and their mobility to enable measurements outside dedicated laboratories and at the point of application. Thin molecular layers on solid substrates with nanometer dimensions are a key component of promising approaches in this field. Further developments aim for even simpler readout schemes (as demonstrated by metal nanoparticle-based assays), label-free assays, and handheld instrumentation to realize visions such as point-of-care diagnostics.

References

1 Mirkin, C.A., et al., A DNA-based method for rationally assembling nanoparticles into macroscopic materials. *Nature*, **1996**, *382*(6592), 607–9.

2 Alivisatos, A.P., et al., Organization of 'nanocrystal molecules' using DNA. *Nature*, **1996**, *382*(6592), 609–11.

3 Taton, T.A., C.A. Mirkin, R.L. Letsinger, Scanometric DNA array detection with nanoparticle probes. *Science*, **2000**, *289*, 1757–1760.

4 Jain, K.K., Nanodiagnostics: application of nanotechnology in molecular diagnostics. *Expert Rev. Mol. Diagn.*, **2003**, *3*(2), 153–161.

5 Southern, E.M., DNA chips: analysing sequence by hybridization to oligonucleotides on a large scale. *Trends Genet.*, **1996**, *12*(3), 110–5.

6 Schena, M., et al., Microarrays: biotechnology's discovery platform for functional genomics. *Trends Biotechnol.*, **1998**, *16*(7), 301–6.

7 Niemeyer, C.M. and D. Blohm, DNA Microarrays. *Angew. Chem.*, **1999**, *111*(19), 3039–3043.

8 Daniel, M.C. and D. Astruc, Gold nanoparticles: assembly, supramolecular chemistry, quantum-size-related properties, and applications toward biology, catalysis, and nanotechnology. *Chem. Rev.*, **2004**, *104*(1), 293–346.

9 Kreibig, U. and M. Vollmer, *Optical Properties of Metal Clusters*, Series in Materials Science, Vol. *25*, **1995**, Springer, Berlin.

10 Yguerabide, J. and E.E. Yguerabide, Light-scattering submicroscopic particles as highly fluorescent analogs and their use as tracer labels in clinical and biological applications. I. Theory. *Anal. Biochem.*, **1998**, *262*(2), 137–156.

11 Yguerabide, J. and E.E. Yguerabide, Light-scattering submicroscopic particles as highly fluorescent analogs and their use as tracer labels in clinical and biological applications. II. Experimental characterization. *Anal. Biochem.*, **1998**, *262*(2), 157–176.

12 Elghanian, R., et al., Selective colorimetric detection of polynucleotides based on the distance-dependent optical properties of gold nanoparticles. *Science*, **1997**, *277*(5329), 1078–81.

13 Storhoff, J.J., et al., One pot colorimetric differentiation of polynucleotides with single base imperfections using gold nanoparticle probes. *J. Am. Chem. Soc.*, **1998**. *120*, 1959–1964.

14 Hacker, G.W. in *Colloidal Gold: Principles, Methods, and Applications*, M.H. Hayat, (Ed.), **1989**, Academic Press: New Jersey, p. 297–321.

15 Reichert, J., et al., Chip-based optical detection of DNA hybridization by means of nanobead labeling. *Anal. Chem.*, **2000**, *72*, 6025–6029.

16 Stimpson, D.I., et al., Real-time detection of DNA hybridization and melting on oligonucleotide arrays by using optical wave guides. *Proc. Natl. Acad. Sci. U.S.A.*, **1995**, *92*(14), 6379–83.

17 Taton, T.A., G. Lu, C.A. Mirkin, Two-color labeling of oligonucleotide arrays via size-selective scattering of nanoparticle probes. *J. Am. Chem. Soc.*, **2001**, *123*, 5164–5165.

18 Li, H. and L.J. Rothberg, DNA sequence detection using selective fluorescence quenching of tagged oligonucleotide probes by gold nanoparticles. *Anal. Chem.*, **2004**, *76*(18), 5414–7.

19 Karlsson, R., SPR for molecular interaction analysis: a review of emerging application areas. *J. Mol. Recognit.*, **2004**, *17*(3), 151–61.

20 Nath, N. and A. Chilkoti, A colorimetric gold nanoparticle sensor to interrogate biomolecular interactions in real time on a surface. *Anal. Chem.*, **2002**, *74*(3), 504–9.

21 Lyon, L.A., M.D. Musick, M.J. Natan, Colloidal Au-enhanced surface plasmon resonance immunosensing. *Anal. Chem.*, **1998**, *70*(24), 5177–83.

22 Creighton, J.A., Surface enhanced Raman scattering, in *Metal Colloids*,

R.K. Chang and T.E. Furtak (Eds.), **1982**, Plenum: New York. p. 315–338.

23 Freeman, R.G., et al., Self-assembled metal colloid monolayers: an approach to SERS substrates. *Science*, **1995**, *267*, 1629–1632.

24 Cao, Y.W., R. Jin, C.A. Mirkin, Nanoparticles with Raman spectroscopic fingerprints for DNA and RNA detection. *Science*, **2002**, *297*, 1536–1540.

25 Musick, M.D.K., C.D. Keefe, H. Melinda, M.J. Natan, Stepwise construction of conductive Au colloid multilayers from solution. *Chem. Mater.*, **1997**, *9*, 1499–1501.

26 Möller, R., et al., Electrical classification of the concentration of bioconjugated metal colloids after surface adsorption and silver enhancement. *Langmuir*, **2001**, *17*, 5426–5430.

27 Urban, M., R. Möller, W. Fritzsche, A paralleled readout system for an electrical DNA-hybridization assay based on a microstructured electrode array. *Rev. Sci. Instrum.*, **2003**, *74*, 1077–1081.

28 Park, S.J., T.A. Taton, C.A. Mirkin, Array-based electrical detection of DNA with nanoparticle probes. *Science*, **2002**, *295*(5559), 1503–6.

29 Campas, M. and K. Ioannis, Strategy for the development of sensor platforms for multi-analysis. *Int. J. Environ. Anal. Chem.*, **2004**, *84*(11), 799–807.

30 Dequaire, M., C. Degrand, B. Limoges, An electrochemical metalloimmunoassay based on a colloidal gold label. *Anal. Chem.*, **2000**, *72*(22), 5521–8.

31 Authier, L., C. Grossiord, P. Brossier, Gold nanoparticle-based quantitative electrochemical detection of amplified human cytomegalovirus DNA using disposable microband electrodes. *Anal. Chem.*, **2001**, *73*(18), 4450–6.

32 Wang, J., et al., Metal nanoparticle-based electrochemical stripping potentiometric detection of DNA hybridization. *Anal. Chem.*, **2001**, *73*(22), 5576–81.

33 Wang, J., G. Liu, A. Merkoci, Electrochemical coding technology for simultaneous detection of multiple DNA targets. *J. Am. Chem. Soc.*, **2003**, *125*(11), 3214–5.

34 Ozsoz, M., et al., Electrochemical genosensor based on colloidal gold nanoparticles for the detection of Factor V Leiden mutation using disposable pencil graphite electrodes. *Anal. Chem.*, **2003**, *75*(9), 2181–7.

35 Okahata, Y., et al., Quantitative detection of binding of PCNA protein to DNA strands on a 27 MHz quartz-crystal microbalance. *Nucleic Acids Symp. Ser.*, **2000**, (44), 243–4.

36 Zhou, X.C., S.J. O'Shea, S.F.Y. Li, Amplified microgravimetric gene sensor using Au nanoparticle modified oligonucleotides. *Chem. Commun.*, **2000**, 953–954.

37 Patolsky, F., et al., Dendritic amplification of DNA analysis by oligonucleotide-functionalized Au-nanoparticles. *Chem. Commun.*, **2000**, 1025–1026.

38 Weizmann, Y., F. Patolsky, I. Willner, Amplified detection of DNA and analysis of single-base mismatches by the catalyzed deposition of gold on Au-nanoparticles. *Analyst*, **2001**, *126*(9), 1502–4.

39 Hansen, K.M., et al., Cantilever-based optical deflection assay for discrimination of DNA single-nucleotide mismatches. *Anal. Chem.*, **2001**, *73*(7), 1567–71.

40 Fritz, J., et al., Translating biomolecular recognition into nanomechanics. *Science*, **2000**, *288*(5464), 316–8.

41 Fritzsche, W. and T.A. Taton, Metal nanoparticles as labels for heterogeneous, chip-based DNA detection. *Nanotechnology*, **2003**, *14*, R63–R73.

42 Brust, M., et al., Synthesis and reactions of functionalized gold nanoparticles. *J. Chem. Soc., Chem. Commun.*, **1995**, 1655–1656.

43 Liz-Marzán, L.M., M. Giersig, P. Mulvaney, Synthesis of nanosized gold-silica core-shell particles. *Langmuir*, **1996**, *12*(18), 4329–4335.

44 Lee, P.C. and D. Meisel, Adsorption and surface-enhanced Raman of dyes on silver and gold sols. *J. Phys. Chem.*, **1982**, *86*, 3391–3395.
45 Turkevich, J., R.S. Miner, L. Babenkova, Further studies on the synthesis of finely divided platinum. *J. Phys. Chem.*, **1986**, *90*(20), 4765–4767.
46 Turkevich, J. and G. Kim, Palladium: Preparation and catalytic properties of uniform size. *Science*, **1970**, *169*, 873–879.
47 Kuyper, A.C., The oxidation of citric acid. *J. Am. Chem. Soc.*, **1933**, *55*(4), 1722–1727.
48 Wetten, R.L., et al., *Adv. Mater.*, **1996**, *8*, 428.
49 Abid, J.P., Laser induced synthesis and non linear optical properties of metal nanoparticles, in *Laboratorie d'Electrochimie*, **2003**, Ecole Polytechnique Federale de Lausanne: Lausanne.
50 Mie, G., Beiträge zur Optik trüber Medien speziell kolloidaler Metallösungen. *Ann. Physik*, **1908**, *25*, 377–445.
51 Debye, P., Der Lichtdruck auf Kugeln von beliebigem Material. *Ann. Phys.*, **1909**, *30*(57–136).
52 Drake, T.J., X.J. Zhao, W. Tan, Bioconjugated silica nanoparticles for bioanalytical applications, in *Nanobiotechnology*, Wiley-VCH: Weinheim, **2004**, p. 444–457.
53 Khlebtsov, N.G., et al., Two-layer model of colloidal gold bioconjugates and its application to the optimization of nanosensors. *Colloid J.*, **2003**, *65*(4), 508–518.
54 Westcott, S.L., et al., Formation and adsorption of clusters of gold nanoparticles onto functionalized silica nanoparticle surfaces. *Langmuir*, **1998**, *14*, 5396–5401.
55 Stöber, W., A. Fink, E. Bohn, Controlled growth of monodisperse silica spheres in the micron size range. *J. Colloid Interface Sci.*, **1968**, *26*(1), 62–69.
56 Halas, N., The optical properties of nanoshells. *Optics & Photonic News*, **2002**, 26–30.
57 Hirsch, L.R., et al., Nanoshell-mediated near-infrared thermal therapy of tumors under magnetic resonance guidance. *Proc. Natl. Acad. Sci. U.S.A.*, **2003**, *100*(23), 13549–54.
58 Hiergeist, R., et al., Application of magnetite ferrofluids for hyperthermia. *J. Magn. Magn. Mater.*, **1999**, *201*(1–3), 420–422.
59 Baselt, D.R., et al., A biosensor based on magnetoresistance technology. *Biosens. Bioelectron.*, **1998**, *13*(7–8), 731–9.
60 Edelstein, R.L., et al., The BARC biosensor applied to the detection of biological warfare agents. *Biosens. Bioelectron.*, **2000**, *14*(10–11), 805–13.
61 Gorschluter, A., et al., Electromagnetic base technology for extremely sensitive immunosensors and DNA-chips. *Biomed. Tech (Berl)*, **2002**, *47*(Suppl 1, Pt 1), 213–6.
62 Schotter, J., et al., A biochip based on magnetoresistive sensors. *IEEE Trans. Magn.*, **2002**, *38*(5), 3365–3367.
63 Ho, K.-C., et al., Using biofunctionalized nanoparticles to probe pathogenic bacteria. *Anal. Chem.*, **2004**, *76*(24), 7162–7168.
64 Alivisatos, A.P., Semiconductor clusters, nanocrystals, and quantum dots. *Science*, **1996**, *271*, 933–937.
65 Bruchez, M., Jr., et al., Semiconductor nanocrystals as fluorescent biological labels. *Science*, **1998**, *281*(5385), 2013–6.
66 Wu, X., et al., Immunofluorescent labeling of cancer marker Her2 and other cellular targets with semiconductor quantum dots. *Nat. Biotechnol.*, **2003**, *21*(1), 41–6.
67 Niemeyer, C.M., Functional hybrid devices of proteins and inorganic nanoparticles. *Angew. Chem. Int. Ed.*, **2003**, *42*(47), 5796–800.
68 Turkevich, J., P.L. Stevenson, J. Hiller, Nucleation and growth process in the synthesis of colloidal gold. *Discuss. Faraday Soc.*, **1951**, *11*, 55–75.
69 Gutbier, A., Beiträge zur Kenntnis anorganischer Kolloïde. *Z. Anorg. Chem.* (Now: *Z. Anorg. Allgem. Chem.*), **1902**, *32*(1), 347–356.
70 Zsigmondy, R.A., Zur erkenntnis des

kolloide gold. *Z. Elektrochem.*, **1889**, *4*, 546.

71 Roth, J., The preparation of protein A-gold complexes with 3 nm and 15 nm gold particles and their use in labelling multiple antigens on ultra-thin sections. *Histochem. J.*, **1982**, *14*(5), 791–801.

72 Schmid, G., et al., Au55[P(C6H5)3]12Cl6 – Ein Goldcluster ungewöhnlicher Größe. *Chem. Ber.*, **1981**, *114*, 3634–3642.

73 Brust, M., et al., Synthesis of thiol-derivatized gold nanoparticles in a two-phase liquid-liquid system. *J. Chem. Soc., Chem. Commun.*, **1994**, 801–802.

74 Ostwald, W., *Practical Colloid Chemistry*, **1924**, New York: Dutton.

75 Turkevich, J., Colloidal gold part I: Historical and preparative aspects, morphology and structure. *Gold Bull.*, **1985**, *18*, 86–91.

76 Frens, G., Controlled nucleation for the regulation of the particle size in monodisperse gold suspensions. *Nature*, **1973**, *241*, 20–22.

77 Schmid, G. and A. Lehnert, The complexation of gold colloids. *Angew. Chem., Int. Ed. Engl.*, **1989**, *28*(6), 780–781.

78 Giersig, M. and P. Mulvaney, Preparation of ordered colloid monolayers by electrophoretic deposition. *Langmuir*, **1993**, *9*(12), 3408–3413.

79 Hostetler, M.J., et al., Alkanethiolate gold cluster molecules with core diameters from 1.5 to 5.2 nm: Core and monolayer properties as a function of core size. *Langmuir*, **1998**, *14*(1), 17–30.

80 Yonezawa, T., K. Yasui, and N. Kmizuka, Controlled formation of smaller gold nanoparticles by the use of four-chained disulfide stabilizer. *Langmuir*, **2001**, *17*, 271–273.

81 Niemeyer, C.M., Nanoparticles, proteins, and nucleic acids: biotechnology meets materials science. *Angew. Chem. Int. Ed.*, **2001**, *40*(22), 4128–4158.

82 Nuzzo, R.G., B.R. Zegarski, L.H. Dubois, Fundamental studies of the chemisorption of organosulfur compounds on gold(111). Implications for molecular self-assembly on gold surfaces. *J. Am. Chem. Soc.*, **1987**, *109*(3), 733–740.

83 Nuzzo, R.G. and D.L. Allara, Adsoption of bifunctional organic disulfides on gold surfaces. *J. Am. Chem. Soc.*, **1983**, *105*, 4481–4483.

84 Letsinger, R.L., et al., Use of a steroid cyclic disulfide anchor in constructing gold nanoparticle-oligonucleotide conjugates. *Bioconj. Chem.*, **2000**, *11*(2), 289–91.

85 Li, Z., et al., Multiple thiol-anchor capped DNA-gold nanoparticle conjugates. *Nucleic Acids Res.*, **2002**, *30*(7), 1558–62.

86 Storhoff, J.J., et al., Sequence-dependent stability of DNA-modified gold nanoparticles. *Langmuir*, **2002**, *18*(17), 6666–6670.

87 Parak, W.J., et al., Conformation of oligonucleotides attached to gold nanocrystals probed by gel electrophoresis. *Nano Lett.*, **2003**, *3*(1), 33–36.

88 Herne, T.M. and M.J. Tarlov, Characterization of DNA probes immobilized on gold surfaces. *J. Am. Chem. Soc.*, **1997**, *119*, 8916–8920.

89 Levicky, R., et al., Using self-assembly to control the structure of DNA monolayers on gold: A neutron reflectivity study. *J. Am. Chem. Soc.*, **1998**, *120*, 9787–9792.

90 Mbindyo, J.K.N., et al., DNA-directed assembly of gold nanowires on complementary surfaces. *Adv. Mater.*, **2001**, *13*(4), 249–254.

91 Park, S., K.A. Brown, K. Hamad-Schifferli, Changes in olignucleotide conformation on nanoparticle surfaces by modification with mercapto-hexanol. *Nano Lett.*, **2004**, *4*(10), 1925–1929.

92 Rant, U., et al., Structural properties of oligonucleotide monolayers on gold surfaces probed by fluorescence investigations. *Langmuir*, **2004**, *20*(23), 10086–92.

93 Beaucage, S.L., Oligodeoxyribonucleotides synthesis. Phosphoramidite approach. *Methods Mol. Biol.*, **1993**, *20*, 33–61.

94 McPartlin, M., R. Mason, L. Malatesta, Novel cluster complexes of gold(0)-gold(I). *J. Chem. Soc., Chem. Commun.*, **1969**, 334.

95 Bartlett, P.A., B. Bauer, S.J. Singer, Synthesis of water-soluble undecagold cluster compounds of potential importance in electron microscopic and other studies of biological systems. *J. Am. Chem. Soc.*, **1978**, *100*(16), 5085–5089.

96 Reardon, J.E. and P.A. Frey, Synthesis of undecagold cluster molecules as biochemical labeling reagents. 1. Monoacyl and mono[N-(succinimidooxy)succinyl] undecagold clusters. *Biochemistry*, **1984**, *23*(17), 3849–56.

97 Safer, D., L. Bolinger, J.S. Leigh, Jr., Undecagold clusters for site-specific labeling of biological macromolecules: simplified preparation and model applications. *J. Inorg. Biochem.*, **1986**, *26*(2), 77–91.

98 Hainfeld, J.F., A small gold-conjugated antibody label: improved resolution for electron microscopy. *Science*, **1987**, *236*(4800), 450–3.

99 Hainfeld, J.F. and F.R. Furuya, A 1.4-nm gold cluster covalently attached to antibodies improves immunolabeling. *J. Histochem. Cytochem.*, **1992**, *40*(2), 177–84.

100 Hainfeld, J.F. and R.D. Powell, New frontiers in gold labeling. *J. Histochem. Cytochem.*, **2000**, *48*(4), 471–80.

101 Dubertret, B., M. Calame, A.J. Libchaber, Single-mismatch detection using gold-quenched fluorescent oligonucleotides. *Nat. Biotechnol.*, **2001**, *19*(4), 365–70.

102 Xiao, S., et al., Selfassembly of metallic nanoparticle arrays by DNA scaffolding. *J. Nanoparticle Res.*, **2002**, *4*, 313–317.

103 Kumar, A., et al., Linear superclusters of colloidal gold particles by electrostatic assembly on DNA templates. *Adv. Mater.*, **2001**, *13*(5), 341–344.

104 Sastry, M., et al., DNA-mediated electrostatic assembly of gold nanoparticles into linear arrays by a simple drop-coating procedure. *Appl. Phys. Lett.*, **2001**, *78*(19), 2943–2945.

105 Harnack, O., et al., Tris(hydroxymethyl)phosphine-capped gold particles templated by DNA as nanowire precursors. *Nano Lett.*, **2002**, *2*(9), 919–923.

106 Li, H. and L. Rothberg, Colorimetric detection of DNA sequences based on electrostatic interactions with unmodified gold nanoparticles. *Proc. Natl. Acad. Sci. U.S.A.*, **2004**, *101*(39), 14036–9.

107 Li, H., L.J. Rothberg, Label-free colorimetric detection of specific sequences in genomic DNA amplified by the polymerase chain reaction. *J. Am. Chem. Soc.*, **2004**, *126*(35), 10958–61.

108 Palade, G.E., Transport in quanta across the endothelium of blood capillaries. *Anat. Rec.*, **1960**, *136*, 254.

109 Faulk, W.P. and G.M. Taylor, An immunocolloid method for the electron microscope. *Immunochemistry*, **1971**, *8*, 1081.

110 Horisberger, M., J. Rosset, H. Bauer, Colloidal gold granules as markers for cell surface receptors in the scanning electron microscope. *Experientia*, **1975**, *31*, 1147.

111 Hiriyanna, K., et al., Electron microscopic visualization of sites of nascent DNA synthesis by streptavidin-gold binding to biotinylated nucleotides incorporated in vivo. *J. Cell Biol.*, **1988**, *107*(1), 33–44.

112 Horisberger, M. and M.F. Clerc, Labelling of colloidal gold with protein A. A quantitative study. *Histochemistry*, **1985**, *82*(3), 219–23.

113 Chaiet, L. and F.J. Wolf, The properties of streptavidin, a biotin-binding protein produced by Streptomycetes, *Arch. Biochem. Biophys.*, **1964**, *106*, 1–5.

114 Diamandis, E.P. and T.K. Christopoulos, The biotin-(strept)avidin system: principles and applications in biotechnology. *Clin. Chem.*, **1991**, *37*(5), 625–36.

115 Cao, Y., R. Jin, C.A. Mirkin, DNA-modified core-shell Ag/Au nanoparticles. *J. Am. Chem. Soc.*, **2001**, *123*(32), 7961–2.

116 Niemeyer, C.M. and B. Ceyhan,

DNA-directed functionalization of colloidal gold with proteins. *Angew. Chem. Int. Ed.*, **2001**, *40*(19), 3685–3688.

117 Levy, R., et al., Rational and combinatorial design of peptide capping ligands for gold nanoparticles. *J. Am. Chem. Soc.*, **2004**, *126*(32), 10076–84.

118 Burt, J.L., et al., Noble-metal nanoparticles directly conjugated to globular proteins. *Langmuir*, **2004**, *20*(26), 11778–83.

119 Niemeyer, C.M., Semi-synthetic DNA-protein conjugates: novel tools in analytics and nanobiotechnology. *Biochem. Soc. Trans.*, **2004**, *32*(Pt 1), 51–3.

120 Xia, Y. and G.M. Whitesides, Soft lithography. *Angew. Chem. Int. Ed.*, **1998**, *37*, 550–575.

121 Ulman, A., Formation and structure of self-assembled monolayers. *Chem. Rev.*, **1996**, *96*(4), 1533–1554.

122 Peterlinz, K.A. and R.M. Georgiadis, In situ kinetics of self-assembly by surface plasmon resonance spectroscopy. *Langmuir*, **1996**, *12*, 4731–4740.

123 Georgiadis, R.M., K.A. Peterlinz, A.W. Peterson, Quantitative measurements and modelling of kinetics in nucleic acid monolayer films using SPR spectroscopy. *J. Am. Chem. Soc.*, **2000**, *122*(13), 3166–3173.

124 Reichert, J., Herstellung und Charakterisierung lateral mikrostrukturierter molekularer monofilme auf silicium- und glas-chipoberflächen für die anwendung in bio-chips. **2003**, Friedrich Schiller Universität Jena: Jena.

125 Steel, A.B., T.M. Herne, M.J. Tarlov, Electrochemical quantitation of DNA immobilized on gold. *Anal. Chem.*, **1998**, *70*(22), 4670–7.

126 O'Donnell-Maloney, M.J. and D.P. Little, Microfabrication and array technologies for DNA sequencing and diagnostics. *Genet. Anal.*, **1996**, *13*(6), 151–7.

127 Steel, A.B., et al., Immobilization of nucleic acids at solid surfaces: effect of oligonucleotide length on layer assembly. *Biophys. J.*, **2000**, *79*(2), 975–81.

128 Shchepinov, M.S., S.C. Case-Green, E.M. Southern, Steric factors influencing hybridisation of nucleic acids to oligonucleotide arrays. *Nucleic Acids Res.*, **1997**, *25*(6), 1155–61.

129 Southern, E., K. Mir, M. Shchepinov, Molecular interactions on microarrays. *Nat. Genet.*, **1999**, *21*(1 Suppl), 5–9.

130 Van Der Voort, P. and E.F. Vasant, Silylation of the silica surface. A review. *J. Liq. Chromatogr. Relat. Technol.*, **1996**, *19*(17&18), 2723–2752.

131 Zhuravlev, L.T., Concentration of hydroxyl groups on the surface of amorphous silicas. *Langmuir*, **1987**, *3*, 316–318.

132 Zammatteo, N., et al., Comparison between different strategies of covalent attachment of DNA to glass surfaces to build DNA microarrays. *Anal. Biochem.*, **2000**, *280*(1), 143–50.

133 Consolandi, C., et al., Two efficient polymeric chemical platforms for oligonucleotide microarray preparation. *Nucleosides Nucleotides Nucleic Acids*, **2002**, *21*(8–9), 561–80.

134 Martin-Palma, R.J., et al., Surface biofunctionalization of materials by amine groups. *J. Mater. Res.*, **2004**, *19*(8), 2415–2420.

135 Festag, G., et al., Optimization of gold nanoparticle-based DNA detection for microarrays. *J. Fluoresc.*, **2005**, *15*(2), 161–170.

136 Möller, R., et al., DNA probes on chip surfaces studied by scanning force microscopy using specific binding of colloidal gold. *Nucleic Acids Res.*, **2000**, *28*(20e91), 1–5.

137 Merrifield, B., Solid phase synthesis. *J. Am. Chem. Soc.*, **1963**, *85*(14), 2149–2154.

138 Meldal, M., PEGA: A flow stable polyethylene glycol dimethyl acrylamide copolymer for solid phase synthesis. *Tetrahedron Lett.*, **1992**, *33*(21), 3077–3080.

139 Bayer and Rapp, New polymer supports for solid-liquid-phase peptide peptide sysnthesis in *Chemistry of Peptides and Proteins*. Vol. 3, **1986**,

Walter de Gryter & Co., Berlin, pp. 3–8.

140 Barany, G., et al., Biopolymer syntheses on novel polyethylene glycol-polystyrene (PEG-PS) graft supports. *Peptides: Chemistry and Biology*, J.A. Smith and J.E. Revier (Eds.), **1992**, Escom: Leiden, 603–604.

141 Renil, M., et al., PEGA support for combinatorial peptide synthesis and solid-phase enzymatic library assay. *J. Peptide Sci.*, **1998**, *4*, 195–210.

142 Revzin, A., et al., Fabrication of poly(ethylene glycol) hydrogel microstructures using photolithography. *Langmuir*, **2001**, *17*, 5440–5447.

143 Amirgoulova, E.V., et al., Biofunctionalized polymer surfaces exhibiting minimal interaction towards immobilized proteins. *ChemPhysChem*, **2004**, *5*(4), 552–5.

144 Heo, J., et al., A microfluidic bioreactor based on hydrogel-enrapped E. coli: Cell viability, lysis and intracellular enzyme reactions. *Anal. Chem.*, **2003**, *75*(1), 22–26.

145 Zhang, W., G.H. Seong, R.M. Crooks, Hydrogel-based microreactors as a functional component of microfluidic systems. *Anal. Chem.*, **2002**, *74*(18), 4647–4652.

146 Demers, N., et al., Immobilization of native and poly(ethylene glycol)-treated ('PEGylated') bovine serum amine oxidase into biocompatible hydrogel. *Biotechnol. Appl. Biochem.*, **2001**, *33*, 201–207.

147 Bieber, I., et al., Antibody arrays on micropatterned surfaces and in three-dimensional gel structures for detection of Salmonella isolates. *Biotest Bull.*, **2002**, 6, 235–342.

148 Lämmli, U., Cleavage of structural proteins during assembly of the head of bacterio-phage T4. *Nature*, **1970**, *227*, 680–685.

7
Conjugation of Nanomaterials with Proteins

Mohammed J. Meziani, Yi Lin, and Ya-Ping Sun

7.1
Introduction

The coupling of biomolecular entities and materials at the nanoscale has the potential to revolutionize many fields of science and technology, potentially having a significant impact on current biomedical technologies, nanoelectronics, and related areas [1–9]. Because nanoparticles and biomolecules typically have the same nanometer length scale, they are natural companions in hybrid systems. The availability of various nanostructures, such as semiconductor and metal particles and carbon nanotubes, with controlled properties at the nanoscale makes them extremely attractive candidates for use in biotechnological systems. These nanostructures possess strongly size-dependent optical, electrical, magnetic, and electrochemical properties [1–9]. In addition, simple modifications of these nanostructures, e.g. to their surface layer for enhanced aqueous solubility, biocompatibility or biorecognition, make them better suited for integration.

In the early stages, nucleic acids were preferentially investigated in the functionalization of nanostructures because they are more readily available by synthetic chemical means and more adaptable than proteins [10, 11]. Recently, significant progress has been made in extending the adaptability of nanostructures with proteins [1, 2, 12–22]. Proteins are involved in almost all biological processes and are employed in a wide range of forms because of their excellent functional specificity. Protein-based nanostructures are expected to offer some additional advantages and play a key role in the development of multifunctional materials and devices for bionanotechnological applications [1, 2, 12–22]. For example, nanostructures provide numerous complementary systems with a wide range of free energies of association. Also, methods for working with these systems are known from standard procedures in biochemistry and molecular immunology. Indeed, protein recognition chemistry has been widely applied in diagnostic testing. Future investigations are predicted to focus on the generation of altered protein building blocks for the self-assembly of novel biological reaction compartments using today's powerful techniques of molecular biology. Mutagenesis and protein engineering will allow the design of recombinant proteins that have optimized recognition capabilities for

Nanotechnologies for the Life Sciences Vol. 1
Biofunctionalization of Nanomaterials. Edited by Challa S. S. R. Kumar

ISBN: 3-527-31381-8

the assembly of distinctively shaped superstructures and have appropriate amino acid residues for the effective nucleation of organic and inorganic nanomaterials [1].

The conjugation of nanomaterials with proteins is a very broad field, especially in the light of recent advances in the development of various nanomaterials. In this chapter, we focus on nanomaterials based on nanoscale semiconductors and metals and on carbon nanotubes. Other significant classes of nanomaterials not covered here include polymeric nanoparticles and related nanostructures [23–27], fullerenes and derivatives [28–33] etc., which are by no means less important. Despite our interest in these other classes [34–39], it is probably better to cover them elsewhere. In the present chapter, we first provide an overview of current and emerging approaches in the coupling of metal and semiconductor nanostructures with proteins and their assemblies in different architectures. We then report recent achievements in the use of supercritical fluid processing technology as an alternative process. We also highlight recent successes in the conjugation of carbon nanotubes with proteins and the mechanistic issues involved with nanotube–protein interactions. Finally, we brief summarize the challenges and perspectives in this interdisciplinary field.

7.2 Coupling of Inorganic Nanoparticles with Proteins

7.2.1 Chemical Functionalization Methods

Wet-chemical preparation of conjugated nanoparticles involves mixing a protein with modified nanoparticles in solution. The modification of nanoparticles prior to mixing is usually by chemical functionalization with a linker. Here, the linker serves three functions: (1) it converts the hydrophobic nanoparticles into hydrophilic species to enable them to be transferred into aqueous solution, (2) to stabilize the nanoparticles to avoid their uncontrolled particle growth or agglomeration and (3) it has to recognize the protein (Fig. 7.1). The linker has to be chosen carefully for every nanoparticle material. The functional coupling groups in proteins are either available in the native form or incorporated by chemical means or by genetic engineering.

Figure 7.1 shows examples of chemical interactions used for the coupling of nanoparticles with protein molecules. Coupling to the particle surface is frequently preformed through citrate, thiol, and phosphane groups [1, 2]. With a labile capping layer, such as citrate, proteins can be linked directly with a metal particle by exchange reactions with stronger binding ligand. This method has been applied in the coating of colloidal gold with thiol-containing proteins, such as immunoglobulins (IgG) and serum albumins, which have cysteine residues that are accessible for heterogeneous interphase coupling [40, 41]. Gold and silver nanoparticles stabilized by citrate ligand have been functionalized with IgG molecules at a high pH,

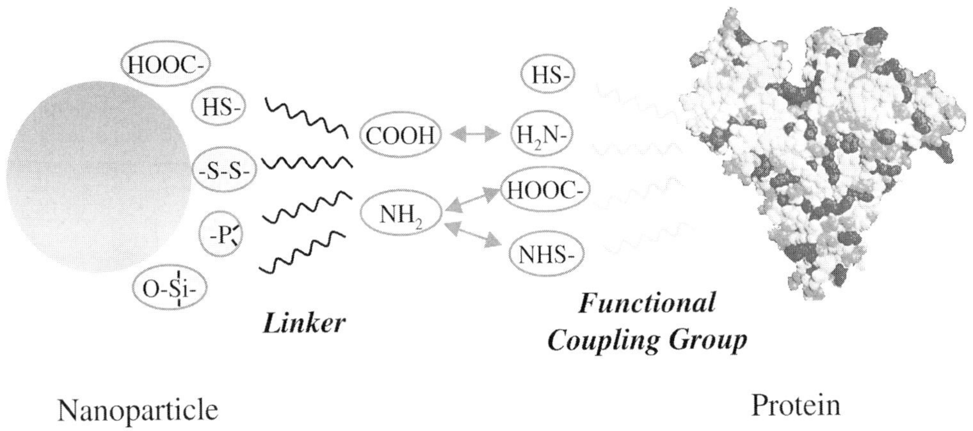

Fig. 7.1. Schematic representation of functional groups used to couple nanoparticles with protein species.

slightly above the isoelectric point of the citrate ligand [40]. Coupling was carried out by an effective binding between the negatively charged citrate groups of the colloids and the positively charged amino acid side chains of the protein. Other kinds of proteins were similarly coupled through electrostatic interactions [42–47], e.g., the directed adsorption of heme-containing redox enzymes at citrate-stabilized silver nanoparticles [42–44]. In a different approach, nanoparticles were also coupled to proteins by using linkers based on thiols or disulfides and phosphane ligands, which possess terminal carboxy, amino, and maleimide groups [48, 49]. Here the coupling is achieved by means of carbodiimide-mediated esterification and amidation or reaction with thiol groups. This strategy was routinely used for histological purposes by coupling proteins with well-defined 0.8 nm undecagold nanoclusters stabilized with arylphosphanes [48]. Cyclic disulfide linkers for coupling showed a better affinity to nanoparticles, and these conjugates are more stable towards ligand exchange than those prepared with a single thiol group or acyclic disulfide units. The high stability is probably a result of attaching the ligands to the nanoparticles through two sulfur atoms. These disulfide linkers have been used in generating gold nanoparticle–oligonucleotide conjugates as probes for recognizing specific sequences in DNA segments and as building blocks for assembling novel structures and materials [50].

The above-mentioned ligands have also been exploited to impart biocompatibility and bioactive functionalities to semiconductor nanoparticles through surface modification with biomolecules [10, 11, 16, 51–58]. There has been significant progress in the understanding of specificity and binding capabilities of proteins toward nanoscale semiconductor particles. [10, 11, 16, 51–64]. Globular protein bovine serum albumin (BSA) has been one of the widely used proteins. For example, BSA was used to form a bioconjugate with luminescent CdTe, CdS and CdSe nanoparticles, often referred to as quantum dots (QDs) [56, 61]. Such QDs are characterized by broad excitation and size-tunable photoluminescence spectra with narrow emission bandwidths that span the visible spectrum, allowing simultaneous excitation of several particle sizes at a single wavelength. They also have exceptional photochemical stability and relatively high quantum yields when used as luminescent probes in biological labeling [17–22]. Mamedova et al. [56] generated bioconjugates of BSA protein with cysteine-capped 2 nm-sized CdTe nanoparticles by using glutaric dialdehyde as a crosslinking agent. Such conjugation was reported to increase the luminescence intensities of the CdTe nanoparticles, which was attributed to the possible presence of resonance energy transfer from the tryptophan moieties in BSA to the CdTe nanoparticles. In a different study by Willard et al. [61] CdSe-ZnS core/shell particles of ~3 nm were coated by chemisorption to biotinylated BSA, which was specifically attached to tetramethylrhodamine-labeled streptavidin (Sav-TMR) (Fig. 7.2). In this conjugate, the TMR fluorescence caused by fluorescence resonance energy transfer (FRET) from the QD donors to the TMR acceptors was enhanced. In separate work, the same CdSe-ZnS core/shell nanoparticles, stabilized by dihydrolipoic acid ligands, were also coated with a recombinant variant of maltose-binding protein (MBP) containing a pentahistidine segment at its C-terminus and a single Cy3 fluorophore covalently attached to a distinct cysteine residue [62]. The binding sites of the approximately 10 MBP molecules per QD were occupied by β-cyclodextrin-Cy3.5 (β-CD-Cy3.5) conjugates. Also within these defined conjugates, the protein-bound Cy3 served as a bridging acceptor/donor for energy transfer from the QD to the maltose-displaceable β-CD-Cy3.5.

In many other cases, however, a simple thiol bond to the particle surface was not sufficient to accomplish a permanent linkage. Instead, an equilibrium is established, with dynamic ligand exchange. To avoid this, a shell of silica is often grown on the particle by means of a sol–gel technique, and the linkage groups pointing outward are added as functionalized alkoxysilanes during the polycondensation process [17]. Recently, thiolated DNA has been linked to the surface of silanized CdSe/ZnS particles through a heterofunctional linker. On an ideally shaped surface, the number of linkage groups should be adjustable, and inert functional groups that determine the solubility and the surface potential of the particles should be added. The linkage groups of the ligands should adhere to the crystallite surface as much as possible, and the ligands should be covalently linked together to avoid exchange completely.

Two fascinating examples of coupling biomolecules with inorganic nanoparticles have been reported recently. One, by Ishii et al. [58], used a wrapping approach to encapsulate 2–4 nm-sized CdS particles within chaperonin proteins. The chaperonin proteins GroEL and *T.th* encapsulate denatured proteins inside a cylindrical cavity. After refolding, the encapsulated proteins are released by the action of ATP, which induces a conformational change in the chaperonin's cavity. These proteins are characterized by a cylindrical cavity with a diameter of 4.5 nm and a wall thickness of 4.6 nm. For complexation, a solution of 2–4 nm-sized CdS particles in dimethylformamide was mixed with an aqueous solution of the chaperonin proteins in Tris–HCl buffer. The characteristic photoluminescence of the CdS particles within the chaperonin–CdS nanoparticle complex lasted for an unusually

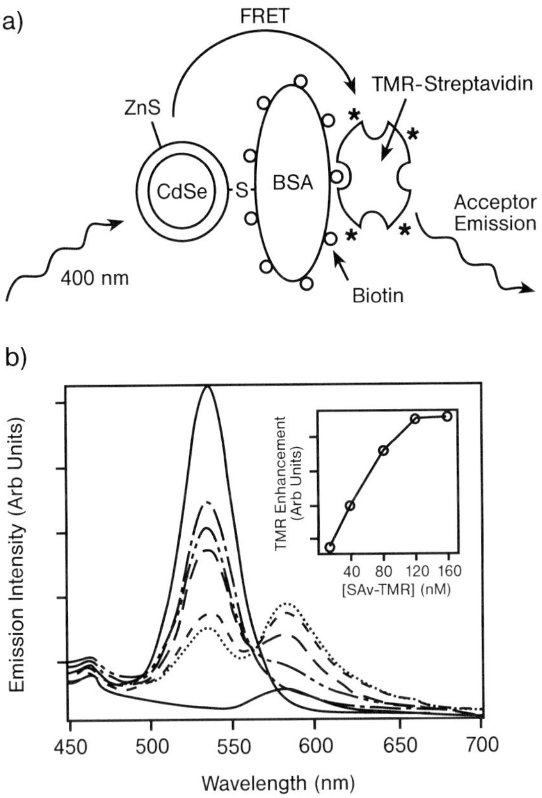

Fig. 7.2. (a) Scheme of a FRET system assembled by chemisorption of thiol-modified biotinylated BSA to CdSe (QD) and subsequent coupling of TMR-STV. (b) Fluorescence emission spectra from solutions containing ~15 nM QD-bBSA and 0 (–), 16 (–*θ*–), 40 (–*θθ*–), 80 (– – –), 120 (– – –), and 160 nM (*θθθ*) SAv-TMR. The lower solid curve is from a 160 nM SAv-TMR control. An excitation wavelength of 400 nm was used for all samples. Inset: enhanced TMR fluorescence intensity at 585 nm from QD-bBSA/SAv-TMR solutions as a function of SAv-TMR concentration. (From Ref. [61].)

long time (more than 400 days) in the presence of GroEL complexes; in the absence of GroEL, photoluminescence disappeared within 2 hours. The second example, reported by Willner and et al. [64], consisted of nanowiring redox enzymes with gold nanoparticles to enhance the routing of electrons from the enzymes to electrodes. An "electrical nanoplug" was obtained by assembling an Au nanoparticles (1.4 nm)–glucose oxidase (GOx) conjugate at the macroscopic Au electrode. The bridge between the macroscopic electrode and the gold nanoparticles consisted of dithiol spacer units. Investigation of the catalytic properties of the assembly by cyclic voltammetry revealed that glucose oxidation occurred with a unimolecular electron-transfer seven times higher than the electron transfer rate constant of native GOx with O_2.

While the use of surface-modified nanoparticles has been a typical route in preparing conjugates, the linker and chemical functionalization for the modification are added complications to an already sophisticated conjugate system. However, despite some obvious advantages, direct conjugation of biological species to inorganic nanoparticles has not been a common practice. This is probably a result of the generally incompatible experimental conditions required for biological species and for the formation and stabilization of nanoparticles. Some recent examples of direct coupling are highlighted below.

7.2.2
Protein-assisted Assemblies of Inorganic Nanoparticles

Self-assembly processes represent the state-of-the-art for organizing nanoscale objects into periodically ordered macroscopic materials. While this biomimetic process is not new, scientists have only recently begun to realize its potential for the artificial control of matter. This interesting class of nanomaterials provides exceptional potential for a wide variety of applications, including photonic and memory devices, two-dimensional (2D) arrays of magnetic nanoparticles [65–70]. Methods developed to produce these bulk-like hierarchical structures include biomimetic methods and amphiphile and colloidal templating, among others. In this section, we review only those approaches related to the use of proteins as crosslinkers, or as templates (assemblies and systems), in the organization and patterning of inorganic nanoparticles into two- and three-dimensional functional structures.

7.2.2.1 Crosslinking Route through Protein Recognition

Protein molecules can serve as crosslinkers because of their tremendous recognition capabilities. Their coupling to nanoparticles has generally been performed in three ways (Fig. 7.3): (a) nanoparticles are functionalized with individual recognition groups that are complementary; (b) particle-bound recognition groups are bridged through a bispecific linker molecule; and (c) a bispecific linker that directly recognizes the surfaces of the nanoparticles is used.

One protein system with highly specific recognition properties consists of antibodies and antigens, which are excellent candidate molecules for the programmed assembly of a wide range of nanoparticles in solution. Shenton et al. [40] first reported a strategy based on the surface attachment of either IgE or IgG antibodies followed by interparticle conjugation of gold and silver in the presence of bivalent antigens with appropriate double-headed functionalities (Fig. 7.3). The resulting structures were in the form of macroscopic filaments that consisted of a network of spatially separated Au and Ag nanoparticles. Similarly, streptavidin (STV)–biotin binding has been used to assemble nanocrystals in solution or onto a substrate. The STV–biotin interaction is considered the strongest ligand–receptor interaction currently known [12, 13]. Another great advantage of STV is its extreme chemical and thermal stability. Connolly and Fitzmaurice [13] used this approach to functionalize gold nanocrystals by chemisorption of a disulfide biotin analogue (DSBA), and then crosslinked by multi-site binding on subsequent addition of the

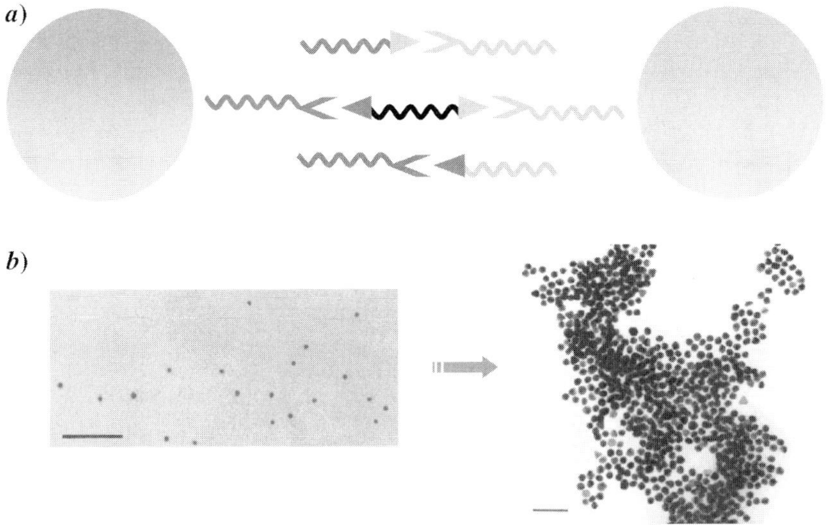

Fig. 7.3. (a) Scheme showing the approaches based on protein recognition systems for the assembly of nanoparticles in solution. (b) Example of TEM images showing colloidal Au/anti-dinetrophenyl DNP antibody conjugate before (left) and after (right) addition of DNP-DNP double-headed antigen. Scale bars 150 and 60 nm, respectively. (From Ref. [40].)

protein, streptavidin. The applicability of the STV–biotin system for generating supramolecular aggregates is also enhanced by the availability of various biotin analogues [71, 72] and recombinant STV mutants [73–77].

Today, with the power of biotechnological innovations, it is also possible to generate new proteins that can specifically recognize and grow inorganic "building blocks" (Fig. 7.4). This is a promising approach for selecting peptides that can recognize specific inorganic crystals and crystallographic orientations of nonbiological origin, including InP, GaAs, and Si [52], and can control II–VI (ZnS, CdS, CdSe, ZnSe, and PbS) semiconductor nanocrystal size, crystal structure, shape, and optical properties.

To identify the appropriate compatibilities and combinations of biological-inorganic materials, a combinatorial library of genetically engineered M13 bacteriophage was used to rapidly select peptides that could not only recognize but also control the growth of specific inorganic materials (Fig. 7.4). The phage display library is based on a combinatorial library of random peptides of a given length (e.g., 7 or 12 mers) that are fused to the pIII minor coat protein of the filamentous coliphage M13. Five copies of the fused random pIII coat protein are located on one end of the phage particle and account for 10–16 nm of the particle. Belcher and co-workers [52] used phage display to select peptide sequences with binding specificity for III–V semiconductor materials based on pIII minor coat protein expression. Brown [78] used repeating polypeptides displayed on the surface of the

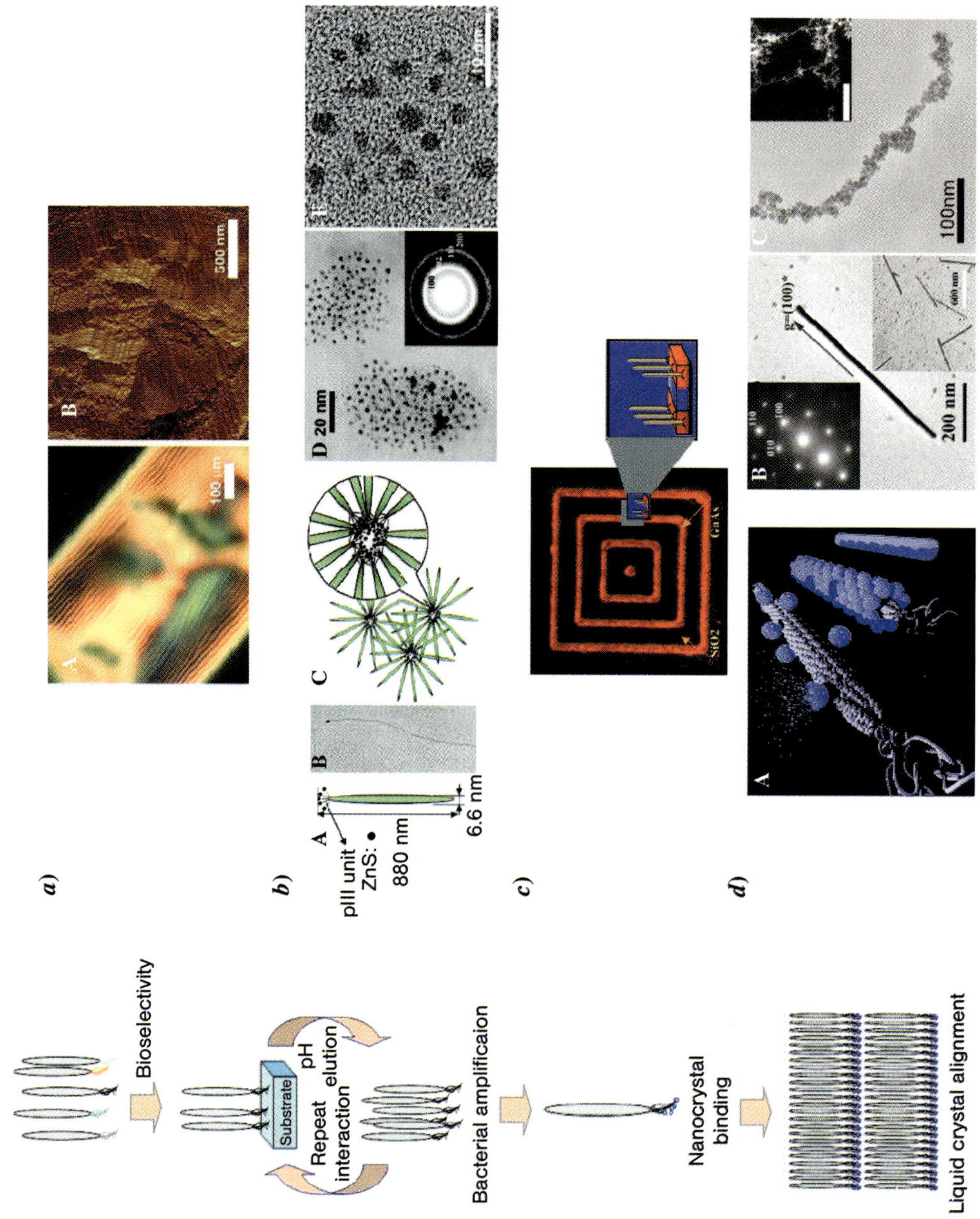
Bioselectivity
Substrate
Repeat interaction
pH elution
Bacterial amplificaion
Nanocrystal binding
Liquid crystal alignment
a)
A
100 μm
B
500 nm
b)
pIII unit
ZnS: •
880 nm
6.6 nm
A
B
C
D 20 nm
E
c)
SiO2
GaAs
d)
A
B
200 nm
C
100nm

bacterium *Escherichia coli* to bind selectively to metal particles. Selected viral-bound pIII peptides can also be used to nucleate II–VI materials for which they were selected [79]. Highly ordered composite material from genetically engineered M13 bacteriophage and ZnS nanocrystals has been generated by using a liquid crystal system (Fig. 7.4) [80–82]. The nucleating peptides have also been expressed in higher copy number along the protein VIII (pVIII) major protein coat of the virus, facilitating the organization of II–VI nanocrystals into highly ordered nanowires [83]. Recently, a virus-based scaffold produced through the self-assembly motifs employed by the M13 bacteriophage was used as a template for the synthesis of single-crystal ZnS, CdS, and freestanding chemically ordered CoPt and FePt nanowires, with the means of modifying substrate specificity through standard biological methods [84].

7.2.2.2 **Template-directed Approach**

An alternative approach to establish nanoparticle organization in supramolecular architectures involves the *in situ* formation of nanoparticles within preformed biological or biomimetic templates; in particular, those based on regular 2D lattices of bacterial cell surface proteins and hollow biomolecular compartments such as virus particles.

Crystalline bacterial cell surface layers (S-layers) are one of the most common outermost cell envelope components of a broad spectrum of bacteria and archaea. These S-layers are monomolecular arrays composed of a single protein or glycoprotein species and represent the simplest biological membranes developed during evolution. S-layer lattices exhibit either oblique, square or hexagonal lattice symmetry with unit cell dimensions in the range of 3–30 nm, and they are generally

Fig. 7.4. Left-hand side: scheme of the process used to generate nanocrystal alignment by the phage display method. Right-hand side: (a) Characterization of the liquid crystalline suspensions of A7 phage-ZnS nanocrystals (A7-ZnS) and cast film. (A) Characteristic fingerprint texture of the cholesteric phase of an A7-ZnS suspension (76 mg mL^{-1}). (B) AFM image of a cast film from an A7-ZnS suspension showing close-packed structures of the A7 phage particles. (b) (A) Scheme of the individual A7 phage and ZnS nanocrystals. (B) TEM image of an individual A7 phage and ZnS nanocrystals, stained with 2% uranyl acetate. (C) Schematic of the micelle-like structures, in which ZnS nanocrystal aggregates are surrounded by A7 phage. (D) The sample shows that 100 to 150 nanocrystals formed aggregates. (E) High-resolution TEM image of A7-ZnS suspension, showing lattice fringe images of wurtzite ZnS nanocrystals. (From Ref. [80].) (c) Phage recognition of semiconductor heterostructures; fluorescence images related to GaAs recognition by phage. (From Ref. [52].) (d) Visualization of the M13 bacteriophage and subsequent nanowire synthesis. (A) The nanowire synthesis scheme is visualized for the nucleation, ordering, and annealing of virus-particle assemblies. (B) Bright-field TEM image of an individual ZnS single-crystal nanowire formed after annealing. Inset, upper left: ED pattern along the [001] zone axis, showing a single-crystal wurtzite structure of the annealed ZnS nanowire. Inset, lower right: Low-magnification TEM image showing the monodisperse, isolated single-crystal nanowires. (C) TEM image of the unannealed CoPt nanoparticle-virus system. Inset: STEM image of the unannealed CoPt wires. (From Ref. [84].)

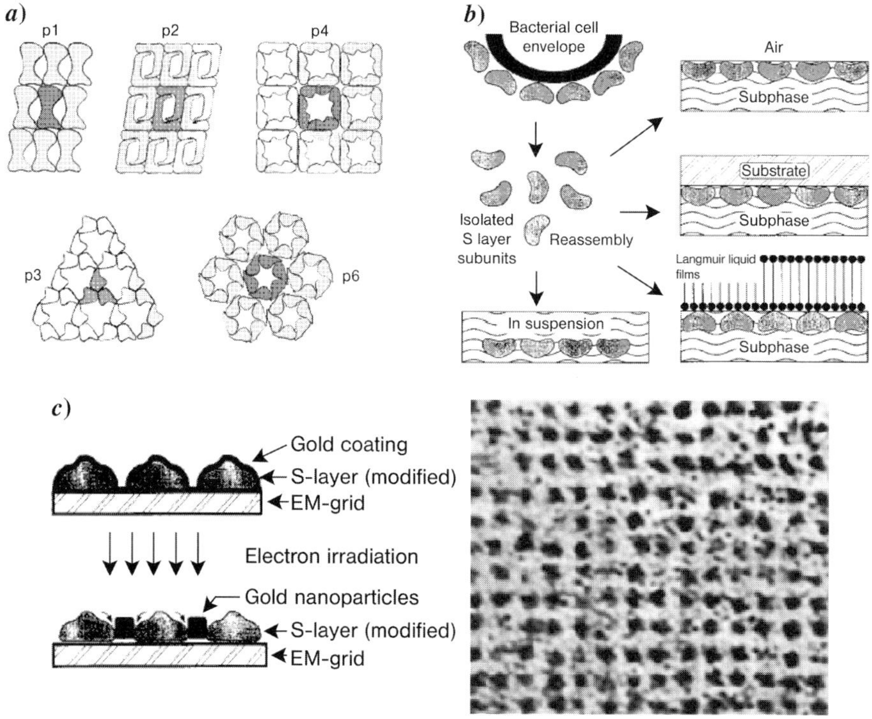

Fig. 7.5. (a) Different S-layer lattice types with oblique (p1, p2), square (p4), or hexagonal (p3, p6) symmetry. (b) Isolation of S-layer proteins from bacterial cells and their reassembly into crystalline arrays in suspension. (c) TEM image of gold nanoparticles prepared by using a square S-layer lattice. (From Ref. [85].)

5–10 nm thick and show pores of identical size (diameter, 2–8 nm) and morphology. The availability of these regular pores within the 2D protein crystal S-layers has allowed controlled nucleation of inorganic nanoparticles into ordered arrays (Fig. 7.5) [85].

Recently, it was demonstrated that S-layer proteins recrystallized on solid supports, or S-layer self-assembly products deposited on such supports, may be used to induce the formation of CdS particles [86] or gold nanoparticles [87, 88]. Inorganic superlattices of CdS with either oblique or square lattice symmetries were prepared by exposing self-assembled S-layer lattices to $CdCl_2$ solutions followed by slow reaction with H_2S. Precipitation of the inorganic phase was confined to the pores of the S-layers, with the result that CdS superlattices with prescribed symmetries were prepared. In a similar procedure, a square superlattice of uniform 4 to 5 nm-size gold particles with a 12.8 nm repeat distance was generated [87]. In this procedure, a square S-layer lattice chemically modified with thiol groups was exposed to tetrachloroauric(III) acid and then electronically irradiated through TEM.

The shape of the gold particles resembled the morphology of the pore region of the square S-layer lattice. Electron-diffraction patterns revealed that the gold nanoparticles failed to form a perfect lattice. These experiments were repeated with a broad range of metal salts, such as $PdCl_2$, $NiSO_4$, $KPtCl_6$, $Pb(NO_3)_2$, and $K_3Fe(CN)_6$ [89]. In general, the inner cavities of the protein layer serve as localized reservoirs of cations that are reduced *in situ* to metal clusters under the electron beam. These experiments clearly demonstrated that nanocrystal superlattices can be induced by S-layers as templates with a broad range of particle sizes (5–15 nm in diameter), interparticle spacings (up to 30 nm), and lattice symmetries (oblique, square or hexagonal).

Other processes dealing with the hollow protein compartments have also yielded fascinating results in the generation and assembly of nanoparticles (Fig. 7.6). For instance, the ferritin-like protein of the bacteria *Listeria innocua* [90] and the cowpea chlorotic mottle virus (CCMV) [91] furnished a suitable constrained reaction environment for the synthesis of monodisperse inorganic nanoparticles since they have hollow spherical supramolecular structures with internal cavity diameters of 5 and 18–24 nm, respectively. In both systems, the interior surfaces have regions of high charge density, which act as sites for synthetic mineral nucleation. Iron oxide particles of about 5 and 27 nm, respectively, were generated through incubation of these protein templates with iron(II) solutions at controlled pH and temperature followed by oxidation [90, 91]. The organization of these bioinorganic nanoparticles into network structures was also explored, e.g., through the coupling of biotin recognition groups to the ferritin and then conjugation in solution with streptavidin [14]. In other work, iron oxide nanoparticles of about 8 nm were also synthesized within the cavity of lumazine synthase protein [92].

Similarly, wild-type and recombinant tobacco mosaic virus (TMV) hollow cylinders have been used as templates to generate inorganic-organic nanotube composites by means of template mineralization [93–96]. The highly polar exterior surface of TMV has been used for surface mineralization of iron oxyhydroxides, CdS, PbS, and silica [95]. These materials form a thin coating over the virus nanorod, affording inorganic nanofibrils 20–30 nm in diameter and as long as 1 μm. Dujardin et al. [96] recently used TMV as a template for the alignment and controlled deposition of Pt, Au, and Ag nanoparticles. By varying the deposition conditions, they demonstrated that one can either specifically decorate the external surface with metallic nanoparticles via the chemical reduction of $[PtCl_6]_2-$ or $[AuCl_4]_2-$ or obtain constrained growth of Ag nanoparticles within the 4 nm internal channel present in the virus through the photochemical reduction of Ag salts. In principle, as suggested by these investigators, 1D arrays of a wide range of quantum dots should become accessible by engineering and templated mineralization of the internal and external surfaces of TMV tubules. Microtubules prepared by polymerization of the protein tubulin have also been utilized as templates for the synthesis of inorganic nanomaterials [97].

The above examples demonstrate that sophisticated nanostructured architectures can be designed when protein molecules and nanoparticles are combined. Future

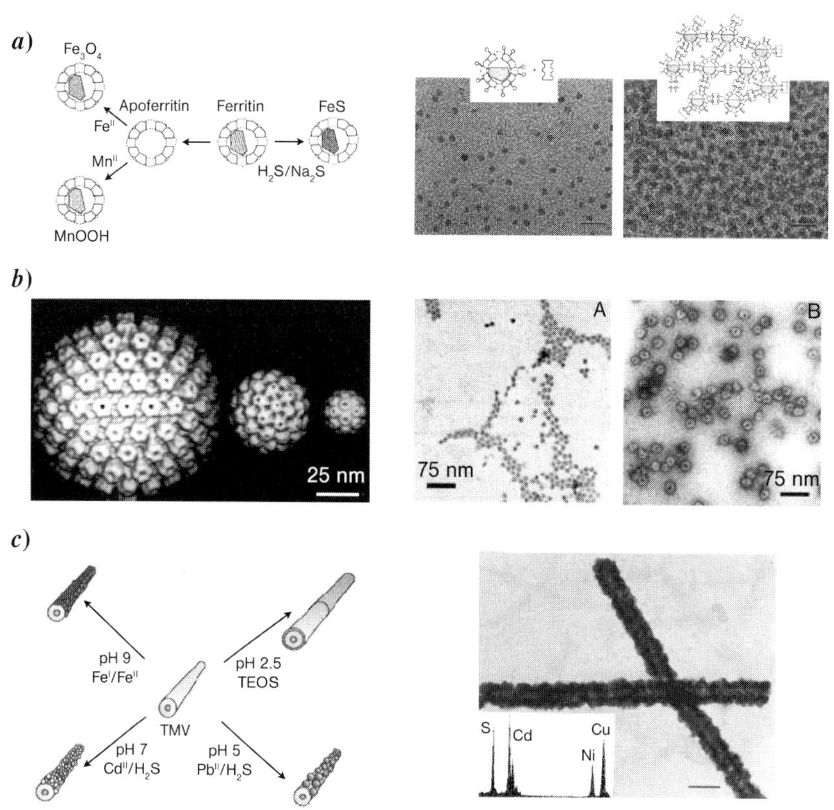

Fig. 7.6. (a) (left): Hollow protein cages used for the growth of inorganic nanoparticles; (right) schematic and TEM images showing biotin–streptavidin crosslinking of inorganic magnetic nanoparticles encapsulated within ferritin. (From Ref. [14].) (b) (left): Image reconstructions of spherical viruses with different diameters: equine herpes (100 nm), cauliflower mosaic (50 nm), and CCMV (26 nm). (right) TEM images of (A) assembled CCMV virions mineralized with cores of $(NH_4)_{10}H_2W_{12}O_{42}$ showing electron dense mineral particles and (B) negatively stained samples of mineralized CCMV, showing the presence of the protein coat surrounding each mineral particle. (From Ref. [54].) (c) (left): Synthesis of nanotube composites using TMV templates. (right) Example TEM image of CdS-mineralized TMV particles, scale bar 50 nm. (From Ref. [95].)

development in this field will benefit from the rapid advances being made in chemistry and protein technology. However, there is still a great demand for alternative methods to resolve typical problems that arise in the biofunctionalization of inorganic nanoparticles. In particular, harsh reaction conditions often lead to the degradation and inactivation of sensitive biological compounds, and to the formation of unstable bioconjugates because of ligand-exchange reactions that occur at the colloid surface. Among other limitations associated with these processes are excessive solvent use, disposal and trace residues, and multi-step operations.

7.2.3 Supercritical Fluid Methods

Supercritical fluid (SCF) technology in nanomaterial preparation and processing is one alternative method in the biofunctionalization of inorganic nanoparticles that shows great promise in addressing many of the challenges highlighted above. SCFs are solvents operating above their critical temperature and pressure. Among the most important properties of SCFs are their low and tunable densities, which can be easily varied from gas-like to liquid-like via a simple change in pressure at constant temperature. Numerous investigations have been conducted on SCFs [98–103]. Results have demonstrated their unique advantages as alternative media for both chemical reactions and materials processing. Example applications and related advantages are their use as environmentally benign solvents [98], the ability to selectively tune chemical reactions or processes [104–110], enhancement of reaction rates due to the low viscosities or high diffusivities in the fluids [109–110], the ability to solvate or precipitate solutes selectively [111], and the production of fine particles and fibers via rapidly expanding SCF solutions [112, 113].

Among the most widely investigated techniques for the processing of fine particles are SAS (Supercritical Anti-Solvent) [114–117] and RESS (Rapid Expansion of Supercritical Solutions) [118–123]. These techniques have comprehensively reviewed [102, 103]. Briefly, in RESS the solute is dissolved in a SCF, and then the solution is rapidly expanded through a small nozzle or orifice into a region of lower pressure [114, 118, 124, 125]. The rapid reduction in pressure (and thus, density) results in rapid precipitation of the solute. Experimentally, the supercritical solution can be generated either by heating and pressurizing a solution from room temperature or by continuously extracting the solute using an extraction column [125]. The RESS process is driven by a decrease in pressure, which can propagate at up to the speed of sound in the expansion nozzle. Because solubilities in SCFs can be up to a million times higher than those under ideal gas conditions, rapid expansion from supercritical pressure to ambient pressure results in extremely high supersaturation (and, consequently, homogeneous nucleation of the solute), leading to narrow size distributions in the products. Cosolvents, such as methanol or acetone, can be mixed with carbon dioxide (CO_2) to increase the solvating power in RESS.

Because some compounds in commonly used SCFs have low solubility, the SAS process was developed. In SAS precipitation, one or more solutes immiscible with SCF are dissolved in a conventional solvent that is miscible with SCF. The solution is then "mixed" with the SCF to precipitate the solute particles. This can be achieved by introducing the SCF into a batch of solution in a chamber or by spraying solution through a nozzle into an SCF-filled chamber. A variation of this process is to mix solution and SCF continuously in a co-current or a counter-current fashion. Other minor variations of this mode of operation of antisolvent process are the bases for several techniques now in use, including Precipitation with Compressed Antisolvent (PCA), Solution Enhanced-dispersion by Supercritical fluids (SEDS), and Aerosol Supercritical Extraction System (ASES) [126–128]. All these processes have been used to produce micron and submicron particles from various materials, including inorganics (metal, semiconductor), polymers, proteins, and other small organic molecules such as drugs [102, 103]. For example, several pharmaceutical compounds, such as lovastatin, stigmasterol, salicylic acid and theophylline, have been processed via RESS into micron- and sub-micron-sized particles [102]. Several reports have also considered using the RESS process for the direct formulation of drug:polymer systems by a co-precipitation strategy. The SAS process also produced micron-sized particles of proteins such as insulin, lysozyme and trypsin. Adding a polymer to the system as a carrier may furnish active protein-loaded microparticles.

Results from these experiments and others suggest that these processes generally produce micron- or submicron-sized particles [113, 129–132]. For nano-sized particles, Sun and co-workers [102, 103] made a simple but significant modification to the traditional RESS by using a liquid solvent or solution at the receiving end of the supercritical solution expansion, or the Rapid Expansion of a Supercritical Solution into a Liquid SOLVent (RESOLV). The RESOLV process produces exclusively nanoparticles from various materials [59, 60, 102, 103, 133–140]. For example, cadmium sulfide (CdS) nanoparticles of ~3 nm in average diameter have been prepared using RESOLV by rapidly expanding a supercritical ammonia solution of $Cd(NO_3)_2$ into a room-temperature aqueous or ethanol solution of Na_2S [133]. The nanoparticles so-produced could be prevented from aggregating by the presence of a polymeric or other protection agent in the receiving solution [133]. The same RESOLV process with a similar reaction scheme has been applied to the production of many other metal and semiconductor nanoparticles. These nanoparticles are all small, on average less than 10 nm in diameter, and are protected to form stable suspensions [59, 60, 102, 103, 133–138]. As recognized by Sun and co-workers [59, 60, 138], a unique feature of the RESOLV process for nanoparticle production is that it requires no nanoscale templating agents for nanoparticle formation because the templating effect is provided by the supercritical fluid rapid expansion process, thus offering a clean way to directly couple nanoparticles with biological species. For example, Sun and co-workers have demonstrated recently that the metal and semiconductor nanoparticles coated directly with natural protein species could be prepared in the RESOLV process [59, 60, 138]. Figure 7.7 shows a typical RESOLV apparatus for preparing protein-conjugated nanoparticles.

7.2.3.1 BSA-conjugated Silver Nanoparticles

An example use of RESOLV in the direct conjugation of nanoparticles with proteins is the coupling of nanoscale Ag with bovine serum albumin (BSA) [138]. Typically, a methanol solution of $AgNO_3$ was added to the syringe pump, followed by evaporation of the solvent methanol. The syringe pump was then filled with liquid ammonia. When pumped through the heating unit, the ammonia solution of $AgNO_3$ was heated and equilibrated at 160 °C before reaching the expansion nozzle. The supercritical solution was rapidly expanded via a 50 μm fused silica capillary nozzle into a room-temperature aqueous solution of N_2H_4 or $NaBH_4$. The system pressure was kept constant during the rapid expansion. BSA protein was in

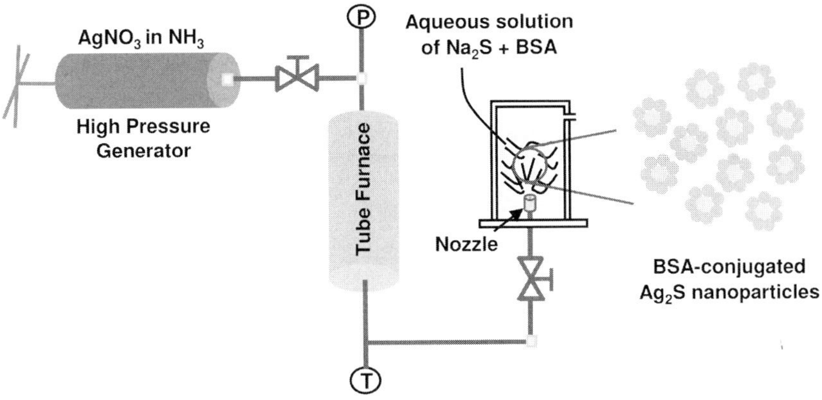

Fig. 7.7. Experimental setup for preparing protein-conjugated Ag_2S nanoparticles via RESOLV [60].

the aqueous receiving solution for direct conjugation with the Ag nanoparticles as they form in the rapid expansion process.

The BSA-conjugated Ag nanoparticles form a stable aqueous suspension that resembles a homogeneous solution. As shown in Fig. 7.8(a), the surface plasmon absorption band (~420 nm) of the Ag nanoparticles broadens upon protein conjugation, reflecting changes in nanoparticle surface properties due to interactions with the protein species. X-Ray powder diffraction analyses of the solid-state samples (Fig. 7.8a) confirmed the expected presence of nanoscale Ag (fcc) particles. Figure 7.8(b) shows the low and high-resolution TEM images of BSA-protected Ag nanoparticles with hydrazine reductions. The average particle size and size distribution standard deviation are 43 and 10 nm, respectively. These nanoparticles appear to be polycrystalline with multiple misaligned lattice fringes, suggesting that the BSA-protected Ag nanoparticles are probably agglomerated smaller nanoparticles. Gel electrophoresis, used to analyze the conformation of BSA protein conjugated to Ag nanoparticles, showed two bands corresponding to BSA monomer and dimer that were much weaker in the nanoparticle sample than in the blank BSA sample; most of the nanoparticle sample becomes stationary, appearing at the gel onset. These low mobility species are probably BSA-protected Ag nanoparticles.

The assembly of smaller Ag nanoparticles produced initially in RESOLV with chemical reduction is likely driven by protein aggregation to form larger, but relatively well-organized, structures of Ag nanoparticles (Fig. 7.8c).

7.2.3.2 BSA-conjugated Semiconductor Nanoparticles

BSA-conjugated Ag_2S and CdS nanoparticles have also been prepared via the RESOLV procedure [59, 60]. Similar experimental parameters were used to produce Ag_2S and luminescent CdS nanoparticles. Here, a supercritical ammonia solution of $AgNO_3$ or $Cd(NO_3)_2$ was used in the rapid expansion and a room-temperature aqueous solution of Na_2S (10 mg mL^{-1}) was at the receiving end. After rapid ex-

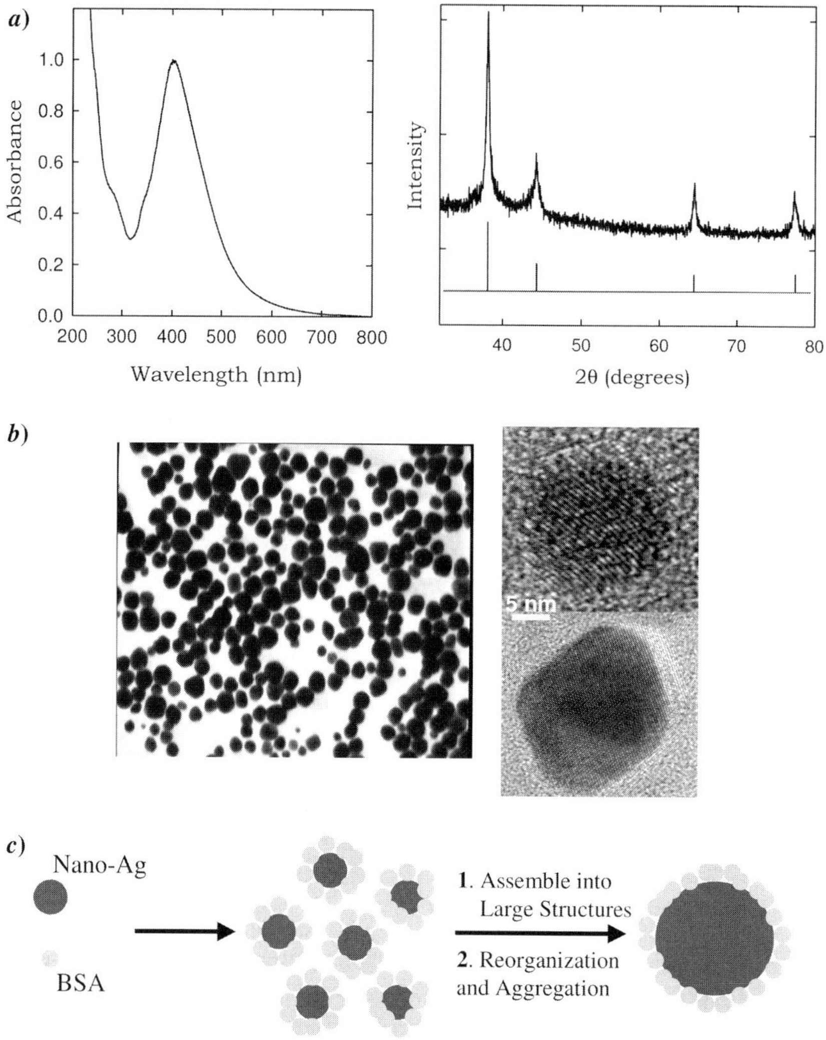

Fig. 7.8. (a) UV/Vis absorption spectrum (left) and X-ray powder diffraction pattern (right) of the BSA-conjugated Ag nanoparticles prepared via RESOLV. (b) TEM images of BSA-conjugated Ag nanoparticles. (c) Scheme illustrating the assembly of smaller protein-conjugated Ag nanoparticles into larger and organized structures, driven by protein aggregation. (From Ref. [138].)

pansion was complete, the ambient suspension of nanoparticles was transferred to membrane tubing with large pore sizes for dialysis to remove free BSA and other salts and reagents.

BSA-conjugated Ag_2S nanoparticles thus produced in RESOLV form a yellowish suspension without precipitation under ambient conditions. The UV/Vis absorption spectrum of the nanoparticle suspension is a structureless curve with gradu-

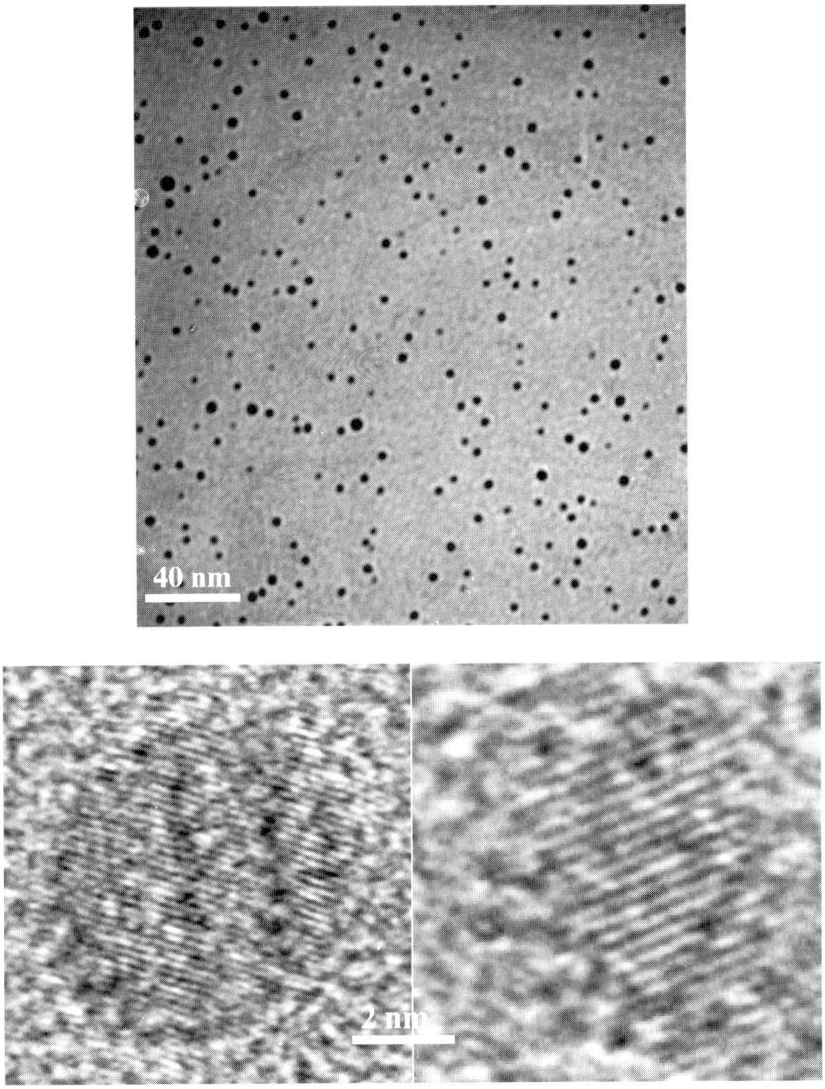

Fig. 7.9. TEM images of BSA-conjugated Ag_2S nanoparticles prepared via RESOLV and then dialysis. (From Ref. [60].)

ally increasing absorbance towards shorter wavelengths, indicating that these nanoparticles are quantum confined. According to TEM analyses (Fig. 7.9), the BSA-conjugated Ag_2S nanoparticles are well-dispersed, mostly single crystals, with an average particle size of 6.3 nm and a size distribution standard deviation of 1.6 nm.

Atomic force microscopy (AFM) results (Fig. 7.10) provide strong evidence for well-dispersed Ag_2S nanoparticles uniformly coated with BSA in a core/shell-like

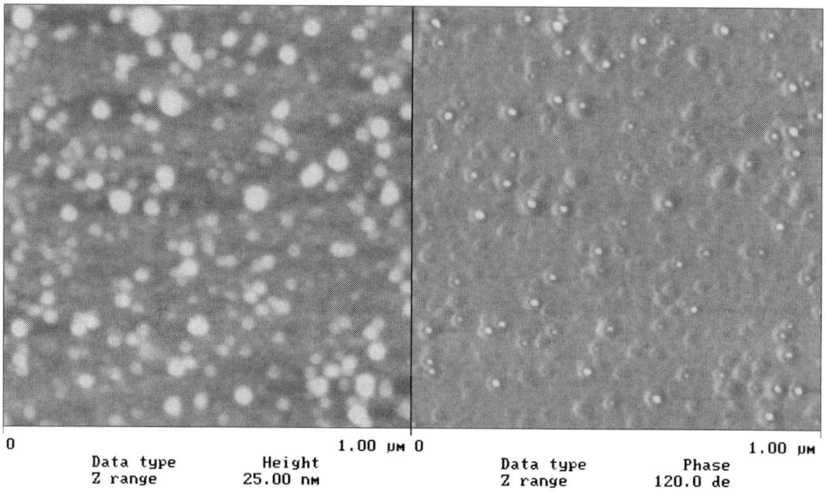

Fig. 7.10. Height (left) and phase (right) images from the AFM analysis of BSA-conjugated Ag_2S nanoparticles prepared via RESOLV and then dialysis. (From Ref. [60].)

arrangement, with overall circular features of 20–30 nm (the larger apparent particle size is due to the tip convolution effect [141]).

Similarly, a yellowish homogeneous suspension of BSA-conjugated CdS nanoparticles was obtained after dialysis. Apparently, interactions between BSA protein species and CdS nanoparticles are relatively strong to sustain the conjugation [59]. The UV/Vis absorption spectrum of the suspension exhibits a well-defined peak at 320 nm (Fig. 7.11a), indicating that the BSA-conjugated CdS nanoparticles are around 2–3 nm in diameter [142]. According to powder X-ray diffraction analysis, the nanoparticle sample is probably a mixture of cubic and hexagonal CdS. TEM results (Fig. 7.11b) show that the CdS nanoparticles are mostly single crystals with an average particle size of 2.9 nm and a size distribution standard deviation of 0.7 nm.

BSA protein species conjugated to the CdS nanoparticle surface have been visualized via AFM imaging (Fig. 7.12a). These images are dominated by circular features of around 20 nm in size, which are consistent with well-dispersed individual CdS nanoparticles that are each coated with BSA protein species in a core/shell-like arrangement [59]. The presence of BSA on the CdS nanoparticle surface is also made evident by the well-known affinity of the conjugate to the surface of nanoscale gold (Fig. 7.12b) [16, 143].

BSA-conjugated CdS nanoparticles produced via RESOLV have interesting luminescence properties (Fig. 7.13). The luminescence spectrum has a relatively narrow bandwidth close to the absorption onset with no surface defect emissions at long wavelengths. This is primarily the exciton emission associated with band-gap excitation [142]. The observed luminescence quantum yield is high, ~20% with

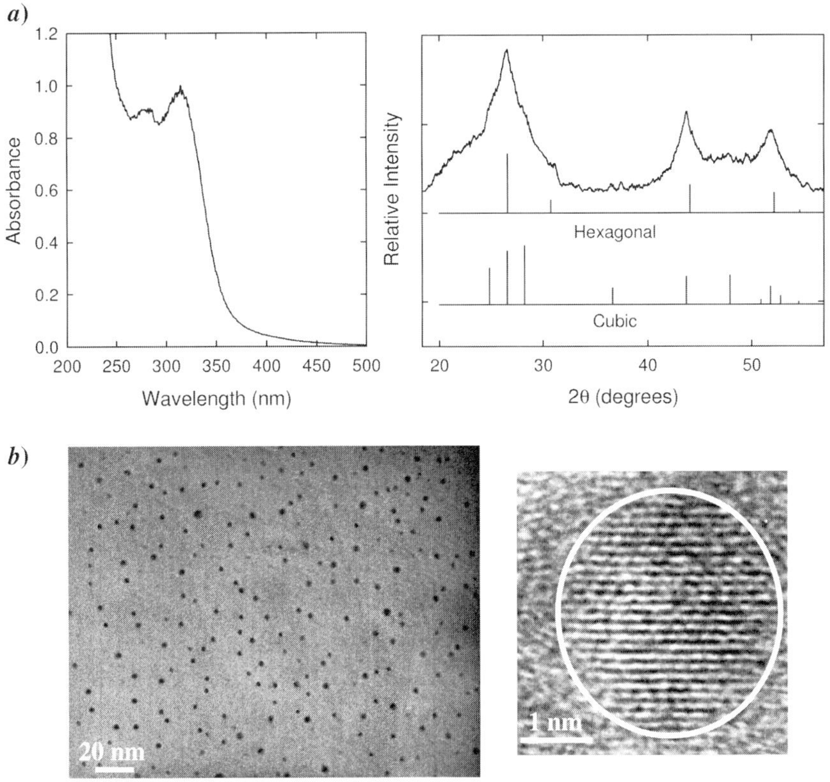

Fig. 7.11. (a) UV/Vis absorption spectrum (left) and X-ray powder diffraction pattern (right) of the BSA-conjugated CdS nanoparticles. (b) TEM images of the BSA-conjugated CdS nanoparticles. (From Ref. [59].)

reference to the fluorescence standard 9,10-diphenylanthracene, which is also consistent with substantial contributions from exciton emission [142]. The rapid expansion of supercritical ammonia solution may have a special passivation effect on the nanoparticle surface [133], suppressing the surface defect luminescence and enhancing the exciton emission from the CdS nanoparticle [133, 142, 144]. Conversely, the broad emission seen for CdS nanoparticles generated by other methods, such as those encapsulated in the micelles of sodium dioctyl sulfosuccinate (AOT) [145], is due primarily to energy trapping states associated with surface defects [142, 144, 145].

BSA protein species conjugated to the Ag_2S and CdS nanoparticles through the RESOLV process remain intact, according to the modified Lowry assay for total protein analysis [146–148]. BSA conjugation serves the dual purposes of stabilizing these nanoparticles to prevent agglomeration in aqueous suspension and introducing biocompatible functionalities into these nanoparticles for further biological interactions or couplings (e.g., antibody attachment).

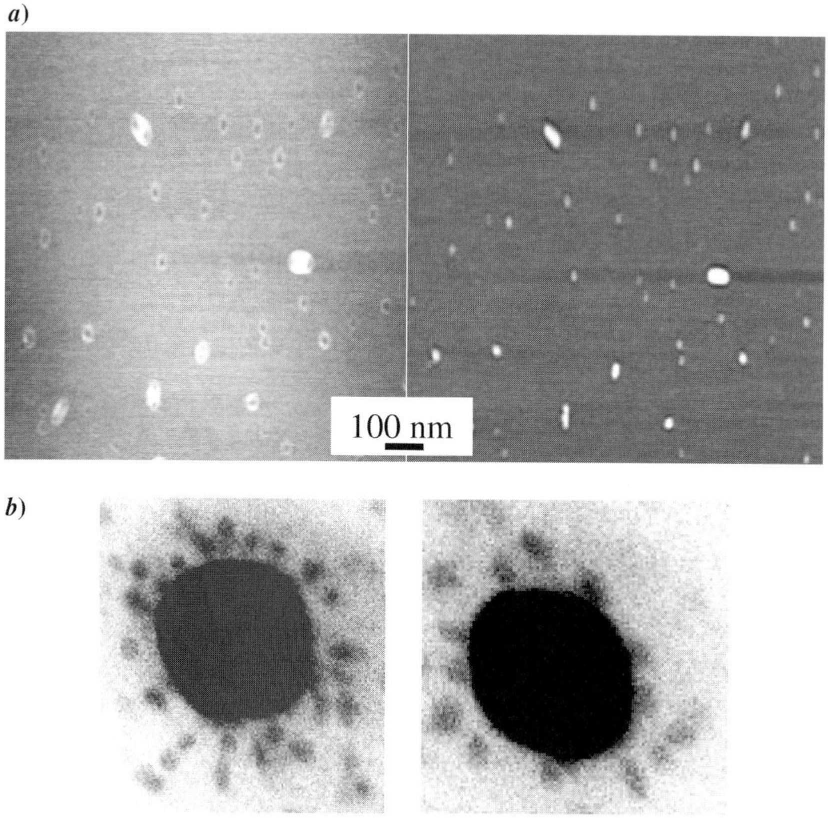

Fig. 7.12. (a) Height (left) and phase (right) images from the AFM analysis of BSA-conjugated CdS nanoparticles. (b) Scanning TEM (Z-contrast mode) image for the coating of colloidal gold by BSA-conjugated CdS nanoparticles. (From Ref. [59].)

Mechanistically, the relatively strong interactions between BSA and these semiconductor nanoparticles (strong enough to remain stable in dialysis) are worth noting. BSA protein contains 60 amino moieties in lysine residues, 26 arginine moieties in guanidino side chains, and also 17 disulfide bonds with one free thiol in cysteine residues [149]. These functionalities are probably responsible for the conjugation to these nanoparticles through thiolate linkages and/or weak covalent bonds with alkylamines [150–152].

7.2.3.3 Assembly and Disassembly of Nanoparticles through Protein Isomeric Conversion

Protein-conjugated semiconductor nanoparticles produced through the supercritical fluid processing method RESOLV can also be organized into supramolecular architectures by simply using isomeric conformations of proteins. For example,

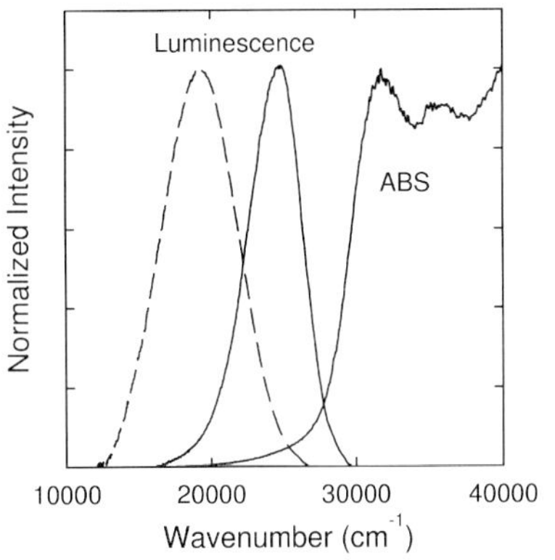

Fig. 7.13. Luminescence spectrum of BSA-conjugated CdS nanoparticles in a stable aqueous suspension (—) compared with that of the similarly sized CdS nanoparticles prepared and encapsulated in AOT micelles (– –). (From Ref. [59].)

Meziani et al. [60] have demonstrated the possibility of assembling and disassembling BSA-conjugated Ag_2S and CdS nanoparticles by adjusting solution pH. Under high pH conditions (pH ~ 12), BSA is expected to be in the aged form, in which the protein drastically expands and forms soluble aggregates through intermolecular disulfide exchanges [60]. Aggregation is reflected by the clustering of these nanoparticles, as observed in AFM images of the Ag_2S sample (Fig. 7.14). In these clusters, individual Ag_2S nanoparticles are still separated by protein species and protected from agglomeration into larger Ag_2S nanoparticles. At neutral

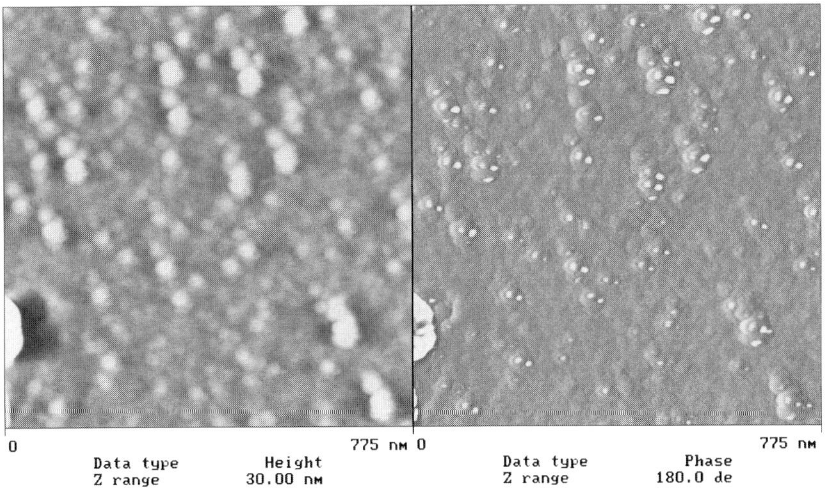

Fig. 7.14. AFM height (left) and phase (right) images of BSA-conjugated Ag_2S nanoparticles at high pH ~ 12. (From Ref. [60].)

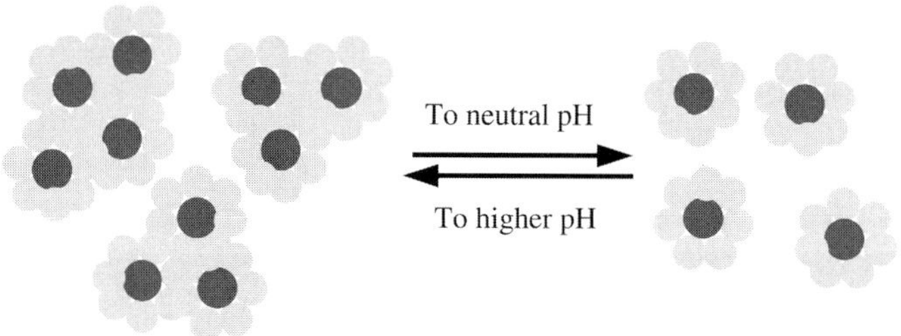

Fig. 7.15. Scheme illustrating the assembly and disassembly of BSA-conjugated semiconductor nanoparticles due to changes in BSA conformations at different solution pHs. (From Ref. [60].)

pH, the BSA protein coating the well-dispersed Ag_2S nanoparticles (Fig. 7.10) is predominantly in the native form. This pH-dependent assembly and disassembly of BSA-conjugated Ag_2S nanoparticles, driven by the isomeric conversion of the protein, is qualitatively reversible [60]. In the isomeric conversion, BSA protein is relatively unharmed at high pH and, for the most part, can return to its native configuration, thus making it possible to maintain the reversibility (Fig. 7.15).

In summary, the supercritical fluid processing method RESOLV can be used effectively as an alternative and unique way of producing clean, active protein-conjugated nanoparticles. Since the nanoparticle formation involves no templating agents in an aqueous environment, the method can enable direct conjugation of nanoparticles to proteins. These protein-conjugated nanoparticles are stable (without agglomeration and precipitation) in an aqueous suspension, and the protein species associated with the nanoparticles remain intact, and are amenable to further biofunctionalizations. The produced semiconductor nanoparticles, such as CdS, can have strongly luminescent features, which are particularly valuable in biosensor-related applications.

7.3
Coupling of Carbon Nanotubes and Proteins

Among various large-aspect-ratio nanomaterials, carbon nanotubes possess unique and rich physical and chemical properties because of the one-dimensional structural arrangement of a chemically versatile element [153–156]. Conceptually, carbon nanotubes may be formed by rolling graphene sheets into tubular structures – single-walled carbon nanotubes (SWNTs) from a single graphene layer and multiple-walled carbon nanotubes (MWNTs) from multiple layers [153]. The chiral vector for rolling-up ($\boldsymbol{C}_h = n\boldsymbol{a}_1 + m\boldsymbol{a}_2$), often referred as the chiral index (n, m), uniquely defines the diameter (d) and the chiral angle (θ) of the SWNT (Fig.

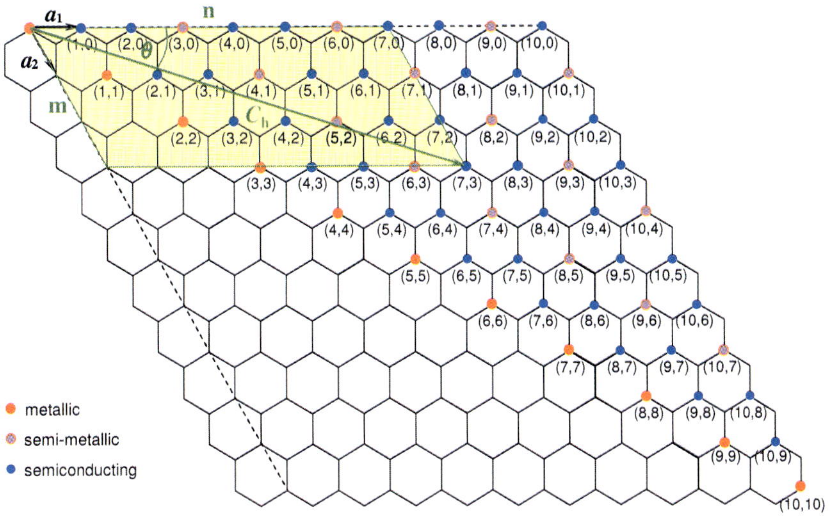

Fig. 7.16. Conceptual formation of carbon nanotubes by rolling up a graphene sheet.

7.16) [Eqs. (1) and (2), where a_{c-c} (~0.142 nm) is the nearest neighbor C–C distance].

$$d = \frac{\sqrt{3}a_{c-c}}{\pi}\sqrt{n^2 + nm + m^2} \tag{1}$$

$$\theta = \tan^{-1}[\sqrt{3}m/(2n + m)] \tag{2}$$

The chiral index also directly determines the electronic structure of the nanotube: metallic when $(n - m)/3$ is integer ("semi-metallic" if $n \neq m$) and otherwise semiconducting [154].

Biological applications of carbon nanotubes through their integration with bioactive molecules in particular have been investigated both in solution phase and in solid state [157–163]. For solution-phase applications, such as substance delivery [163–168], pathogen detection [169, 170], and other biomedical applications, the nanotubes should be dispersible or soluble in physiological environments. Thus, the aqueous solubilization of carbon nanotubes is essential [158, 159, 161–163], and has benefited enormously from recent developments in the chemical functionalization of nanotubes [171–175]. Examples of solid-state bioapplications of carbon nanotubes include scaffolds for cell growth [162, 176–178], biosensors and biocatalytic electrochemical devices [157, 160, 179], electromechanical devices [180], sharp scanning microscopy probes [181], etc.

Protein–carbon nanotube conjugates were among the earliest and most popular topics in multidisciplinary research efforts on the bioapplications of nanotubes. These conjugates may be formed either non-specifically or specifically (see below). Examples in various related applications are also reviewed below.

7.3.1
Non-specific Adsorption

Like other nanomaterials, carbon nanotubes have a high surface area, but with a surface of quantum-confined conjugated carbon networks. However, it was the nanometer-sized hollow interior of these tubular species that drew most initial attention, stimulating the imagination that they could be used as carriers to encapsulate and deliver bioactive species to selected targets [182–185]. As supportive evidence, some enzymes encapsulated in MWNTs seemed to retain their biocatalytic properties [183]. However, the encapsulate-and-deliver idea is still a matter of theory since there has been no report of the controlled release of these encapsulated species from nanotubes at any targeted site. Furthermore, problems with such encapsulation are far from resolved.

The early experiments on encapsulating proteins into nanotubes revealed that proteins were adsorbed on the MWNT exterior surface [185]. This phenomenon became widely known when Balavoine et al. [186] found that streptavidin and HupR readily adsorbed onto the MWNT surface, with the adsorbed proteins sometimes even forming helical array structures along the nanotube sidewall. Although the reproducibility for the ordered arrays was poor, these results suggested strongly that there are indeed competent noncovalent and non-specific interactions between carbon nanotubes and protein species.

Despite efforts to ensure the specific conjugation of carbon nanotubes and proteins (Section 7.3.2), several groups realized that non-specific interactions between these two entities are almost inevitable. Dai and co-workers [179, 187] reported that streptavidin, avidin, BSA, α-glucosidase, and staphylococcal A are adsorbable to SWNTs. Similarly, Azamian et al. [188] found that proteins with different isoelectric points, such as cytochrome *c* (pI $\sim$ 10.8) and ferritin (pI $\sim$ 4.6), exhibit similar affinity toward SWNTs (Fig. 7.17).

Since ferritin contains an iron core, Lin et al. [189] used it as a model protein to study protein–nanotube interactions in aqueous media via TEM. It was qualitatively but unambiguously demonstrated that non-specific interactions between ferritin and SWNTs were so significant that the nanotubes were solubilized in water as a result. In agreement with reports by Azamian et al. [188], the ferritin–nanotube conjugation via such non-specific interactions was quite similar to that in the presence of special reagents for covalent coupling during reaction. Despite the visual similarity, the non-specific conjugates were much less stable than covalent ones (Section 7.3.2) [189].

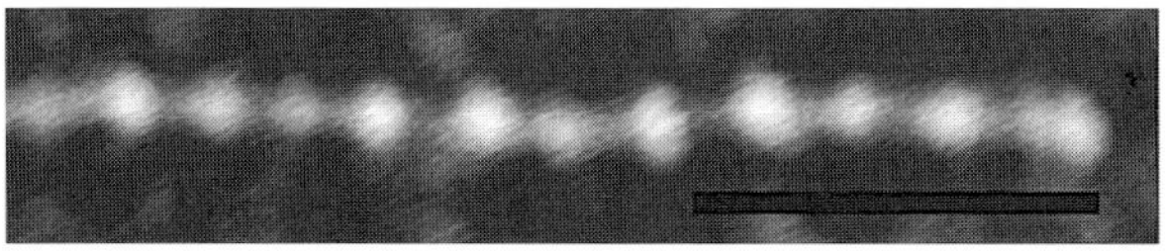

Fig. 7.17. AFM image of a cytochrome *c*–SWNT conjugate from non-specific adsorption. Scale bar = 90 nm. (From Ref. [188].)

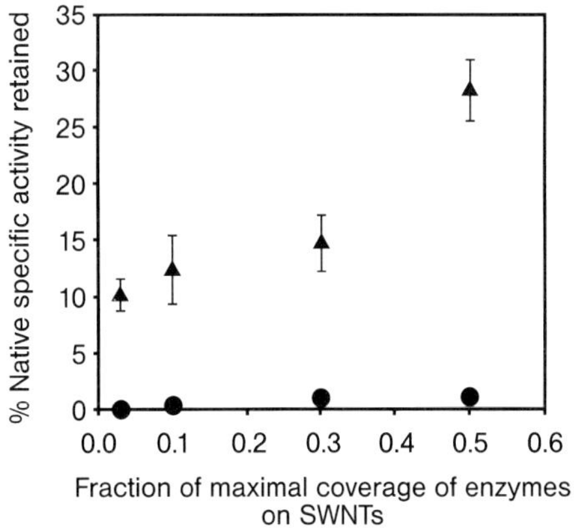

Fig. 7.18. Enzymatic activity retained as a function of surface coverage of enzymes on SWNTs: adsorbed SBP (▲) and adsorbed CT (●). Each point represents an average of a minimum of three separate experiments, with some points showing errors smaller than the symbol. Specific activities above half-maximal coverage could not be obtained because of leaching of the adsorbed enzyme during activity measurement. (From Ref. [191].)

Rege et al. [190] reported enhanced retention of the enzymatic activity of α-chymotrypsin (CT) embedded in polymer–SWNT composite films compared with those without nanotube fillers. They speculated that this could be a consequence of enzyme–nanotube hydrophobic interactions that slowed the leaching of enzymes from the films. However, other reported results contradict this conclusion. As recently reported by Karajanagi et al. [191], CT almost completely lost its enzymatic activity upon non-specific conjugation with SWNTs (Fig. 7.18), possibly due to its structure unfolding. These authors showed by AFM that the tertiary structures of CT molecules, upon adsorption onto SWNTs, changed significantly from those in solution phase. However, another enzyme, soybean peroxidase (SBP), retained its structure when adsorbed, which is consistent with the observed retention of a reasonable fraction of activity. Also consistent are quantitative FT-IR investigations, which demonstrated much more significant secondary structural changes of CT than SBP in both α-helix and β-sheet contents upon the enzyme–nanotube conjugation [191].

Microscopy techniques are widely used to visualize both aqueous soluble protein–nanotube conjugates and those on substrates. For the latter, other instrumental techniques are also used to obtain additional information. For example, quartz crystal microbalance (QCM) has been used to trace the protein adsorption event on a SWNT film that was evenly formed on a gold-coated QCM quartz crystal substrate [179]. The signal change marked the adsorption events on the film and scaled with the concentration of the protein solution for adsorption. The results obtained for adsorptions of various proteins on SWNTs are in reasonable agreement with microscopy observations. However, protein adsorption on the substrates could interfere in such evaluations unless the substrates are fully covered by a monolayer of nanotubes.

Protein adsorption on carbon nanotubes can also be detected electrochemically. In particular, solid-state field-effect transistor (FET) devices from semiconducting SWNTs have been envisioned for use as biosensors [160, 179, 192]. In principle, some small perturbation on the electronic structure of the semiconducting SWNT from the adsorption of even a trace amount of guest molecules may induce a detectable electrical response in the device characteristics [192–195]. Metallic SWNTs, however, are much less sensitive to changes in chemical environments. For example, the adsorption of cytochrome *c* (pI ~ 10.8) in a buffer solution onto a SWNT FET device was detected by measuring the device conductance change [196]. Consistent with microscopy results, the change in conductance was quantified to be from the adsorption of ~20 protein molecules per μm length of a semiconducting SWNT under the given experimental conditions. In fact, the detection limit of such FET devices is of the order of 100 pM of cytochrome *c*.

A consistent observation by different groups is that the conductance of the nanotubes decreases upon protein adsorption, regardless of the charge of the proteins at physiological pH. This is obviously not solely due to the electrostatic gating effect from charge injection from protein molecules to the p-type semiconducting SWNT [179, 196, 197]. Besteman et al. [197] proposed that such a conductance decrease (as a function of the liquid-gate voltage) could originate from the nanotube capacitance change upon the adsorption event, during which ion proximity to the nanotube is limited. However, vigorous debates continue on whether the device response is from the non-specific adsorption of proteins on nanotubes at all [198]. It has been argued that the adsorption of proteins with rather small charge (pI ~ 5–7) at the electrode–nanotube contacts contributes more to the detected conductance change than that along the nanotube sidewall [198]. Poly(ethylene glycol) (PEG) is a well-known protein-resistant material that is often used to protect surfaces from protein adsorption [199, 200]. By selectively applying a PEG layer onto the metal electrodes, these researchers showed that there was no detectable electronic response of the nanotube FET device to the adsorption events at protein concentrations of 100 nM [198] (Fig. 7.19). There was an exception, avidin, which is highly positively charged at neutral pH (pI ~ 10–11). This protein was capable of inducing a response even when the electrodes were protected, although the signals were much weaker than those from non-protected devices. As expected, when the nanotube surface was also protected via protein-resistant species, no device response could be detected with any of the proteins investigated.

Whatever the sensing mechanism might be in the FET devices upon protein–nanotube conjugation, the evidence is already overwhelming for non-specific adsorption of proteins onto carbon nanotubes. The mechanism for such conjugation, however, is complicated and subject to further investigation. The nanotube surface has been widely considered as being hydrophobic [201]. Thus, it has been suggested intuitively that the hydrophobic interactions between nanotubes and certain protein structural units play a significant role in the observed adsorption. For example, Karajanagi et al. [191] attributed the differences in changes in the structures and enzymatic activities of two enzymes (SBP and CT, *vide supra*) upon their adsorption on SWNTs to hydrophobic interactions. For SBP, there is a hydrophobic

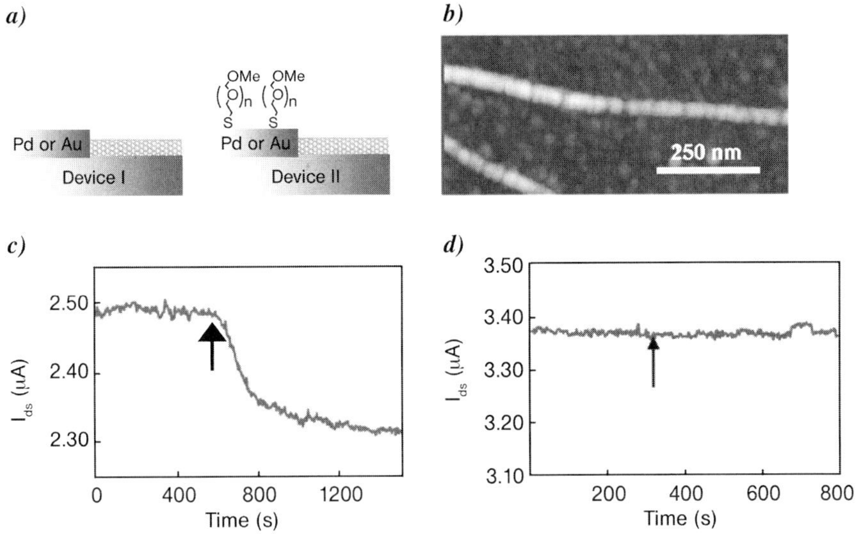

Fig. 7.19. (a) Configuration sketches of SWNT FET devices type I (unprotected Pd/Au electrodes) and type II (electrodes coated with a PEG self-assembled monolayer). (b) AFM image of a SWNT type II device after exposure to human chorionic gonadotropin (hCG). (c) Electrical data of type I device during exposure to hCG. (d) Electrical data of type II device during exposure to hCG. (From Ref. [198].)

"pocket" with 19 amino acid residues on the surface, distant from the enzymatic active sites in its tertiary structure, which may help the enzyme to retain a significant fraction of its activity. Conversely, CT does not contain a large hydrophobic cluster, which was speculated to be the cause for the loss of activity upon its adsorption onto SWNTs with significant secondary and tertiary structural changes [191]. Also consistent with the hydrophobic interaction scheme is the finding that the amphiphilicity of the large peptide species favors their binding with nanotubes in aqueous solution, similar to the surfactant effects [202]. Dieckmann and coworkers [203, 204] took advantage of a similar concept and designed an amphiphilic peptide with an α-helix secondary structure for the noncovalent aqueous solubilization of SWNTs (Fig. 7.20). However, one example is clearly inconsistent with the hydrophobic scheme. Fibrinogen, a well-known soluble plasma glycoprotein that is affinitive to many hydrophobic surfaces, was found to be inert to SWNTs. This might be due to the protein's large size (molecular weight $\sim$ 340 kDa) [187].

Among other possible mechanisms for non-specific protein–nanotube conjugation are electrostatic interactions and hydrogen bonding, especially when carbon nanotubes are pre-treated with oxidative acids. After such treatment, the nanotube surface usually becomes defective, with many oxygen-containing groups, such as carboxylic acids, hydroxyls, ketones, etc., at the defect sites [205–207]. These organic groups make electrostatic interactions and hydrogen bonding between nanotubes and certain surface residues of proteins quite plausible. Electrostatic interactions obviously do not dominate as several groups have shown that SWNTs are

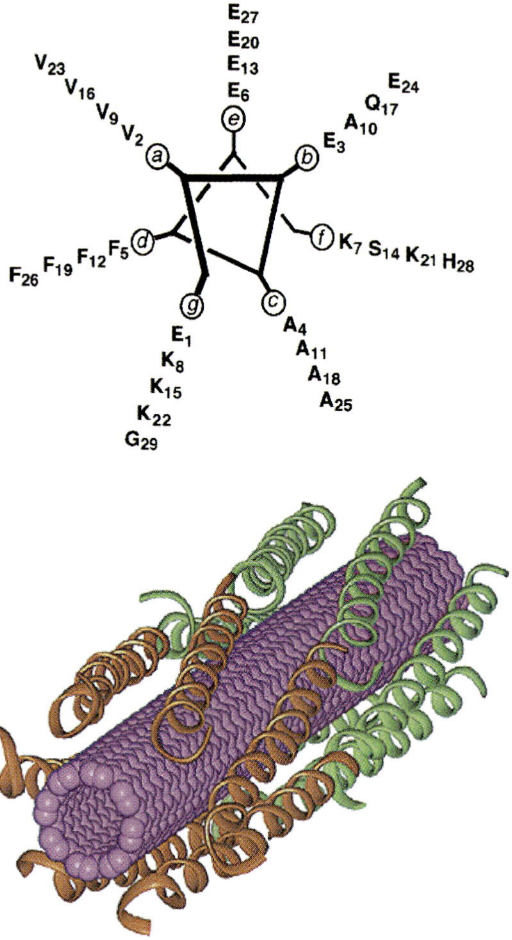

Fig. 7.20. Design of α-helix peptide (top) and a model sketch of the peptide–SWNT conjugate by noncovalent interaction (bottom). (From Ref. [203].)

attractive to both positively and negatively charged protein species in aqueous solutions [188] and at device level [179, 198] at physiological pH.

The increasing evidence for amino-affinity of semiconducting SWNT surfaces [194, 208–210] might also help to explain the above phenomenon, since most proteins under consideration contain lysine and/or arginine units that provide primary amino groups. For example, previous studies show that there is ~0.04 electron donation to a semiconducting SWNT per adsorbed amine [211]. From such a unit quantity of charge transfer, Bradley et al. [212] estimated that a significant portion of the threshold shift of the gate voltage in a nanotube FET device upon streptavidin adsorption is due to charge transfer from amino groups to the semiconducting SWNT. However, they also suspected that other residues, such as tryptophan and tyrosine, may play a secondary role in the charge transfer because they contain aromatic structures. Indeed, investigations conducted with a peptide library have found that the tryptophan residue, in particular, was affinitive towards the SWNT surface [202].

7.3.2
Specific Conjugation and Biorecognition

Specific conjugation of proteins and carbon nanotubes is opposite to non-specific conjugation. In the former, selected chemical reagents are used with known chemistry to link proteins to nanotubes in a more controllable fashion. Protein surface amino groups from residues, such as lysine, are widely involved in some of these specific conjugations. For example, nanotube-bound carboxylic acids, often generated from oxidative acid treatments, can be coupled with protein amines to form amide linkages (Scheme 7.1), which was extrapolated from chemistry developed previously for functionalizing carbon nanotubes with other polymeric and oligomeric molecules [171–175, 181, 213]. Various types of proteins, such as BSA, ferritin, and cytochrome *c*, have been conjugated to carbon nanotubes via this route [188, 189, 214, 215]. The reactions were often carried out in the presence of carbodiimide reagents, such as 1-ethyl-3-(3-dimethylaminopropyl)carbodiimide (EDAC), which are specific for the formation of amide linkages by converting carboxylic acids into more reactive intermediates toward coupling with amines. The carbodiimide-nanotube reaction has been referred to as the activation step and is sometimes assisted by sonication [213]. Many proteins also contain carboxylic acids, which may compete with those from nanotubes in the amidation reactions, resulting in possible protein self-aggregation. Thus, the activation step is better carried out in the absence of proteins so that excess carbodiimide molecules can be removed before the conjugation reaction. The addition of *N*-hydroxysuccinimide (NHS) after carbodiimide activation may further enhance the stability of the reactive intermediate, and thus be beneficial to the yields of the covalent protein–nanotube conjugates [215]. This and similar strategies have been used to functionalize carbon nanotubes with other biomolecules (such as nucleic acids and their analogs [216, 217]) under physiologically benign conditions.

Amide linkages between proteins and carbon nanotubes have also been reported to be formed in room-temperature ester-to-amide transformation reactions in aqueous solution (Scheme 7.1) – an even milder approach [218]. In the reaction, a water-soluble nanotube sample with ester-attached oligomeric PEG functionalities was placed in small-pore-size dialysis tubing with a protein (e.g. BSA). Although the PEG functionalities on the nanotubes might have resisted approaching proteins in aqueous solution, the final protein–nanotube conjugation obtained this way was in fact quite similar to that obtained by carbodiimide-activated coupling reactions [214]. The driving force for such a mild transformation, which overcomes the initial protein-resistivity of nanotube-bound PEG groups, likely comes from both the thermodynamic stability of the amide linkages (compared with ester

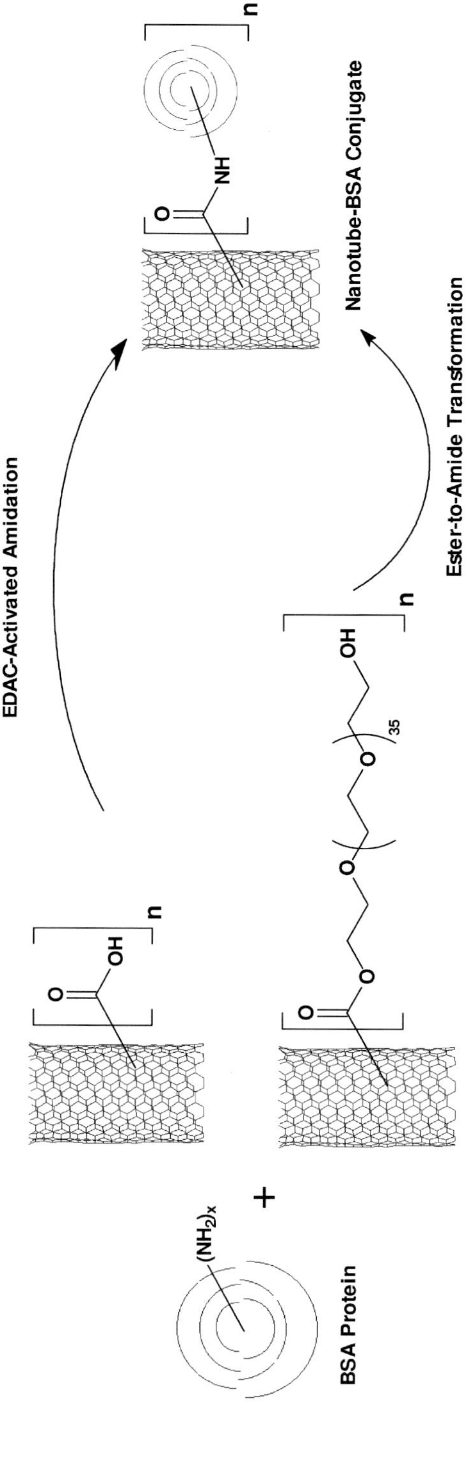

BSA Protein
$(NH_2)_x$
+
EDAC-Activated Amidation
Ester-to-Amide Transformation
Nanotube-BSA Conjugate
O
OH
NH
35
n

Scheme 7.1

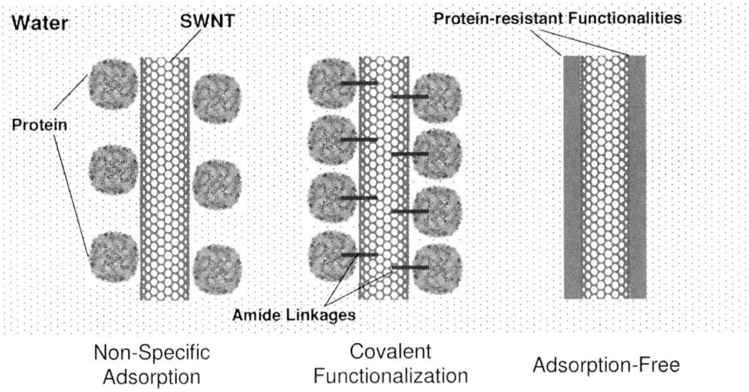

Scheme 7.2

ones) and the *in situ* removal of relatively small PEG molecules via dialysis. In addition, hardly any NMR signals from PEG moieties could be detected from the conjugates after the reaction, indicating the effectiveness of the method.

Covalent functionalization seems to facilitate the aqueous solubilization of SWNTs, resulting in enhanced yields of solubilized nanotubes compared with non-specific interactions under similar conditions [189]. Aqueous-soluble covalent protein–nanotube conjugates are also much more stable than non-specific conjugates. For example, as discussed in Section 7.3.1, water-soluble covalent ferritin-SWNT conjugates are much more stable in solution when subjected to long-period standing or vigorous dialysis conditions than non-specific ones. After dialysis, although there seemed to be some protein loss in the covalent conjugates, the protein–nanotube association was still much more pronounced than that in non-specific conjugates similarly dialyzed [189]. Probably, the non-specific adsorption contributes significantly to the initial approaching of proteins toward nanotubes during covalent conjugation. The formation of amide linkages then "locks" the proteins on the nanotube surface defect sites where carbodiimide-activated intermediates are present (Scheme 7.2) [159, 189].

Covalent water-soluble protein–nanotube conjugates have found some applications in bacterial detection. Elkin et al. [169] adsorbed anti-*Escherichia coli* polyclonal antibodies onto BSA-functionalized SWNTs in physiological solutions. The nanotube-bound antibodies efficiently captured *E. coli* O157:H7 in solution, which was demonstrated by both SEM (Fig. 7.21) and confocal microscopy. Because of the high surface area and one-dimensional flexible structure of SWNTs, such multi-copy antibody displays might be of enhanced pathogen detection sensitivity and could also potentially be used for decontamination of bacterial cells in complex matrices.

Another form of interaction of carbon nanotubes with cells is the translocation of nanotubes through the cell membranes – internalization. In a recent example, SWNTs were functionalized with biotin using a similar carbodiimide coupling

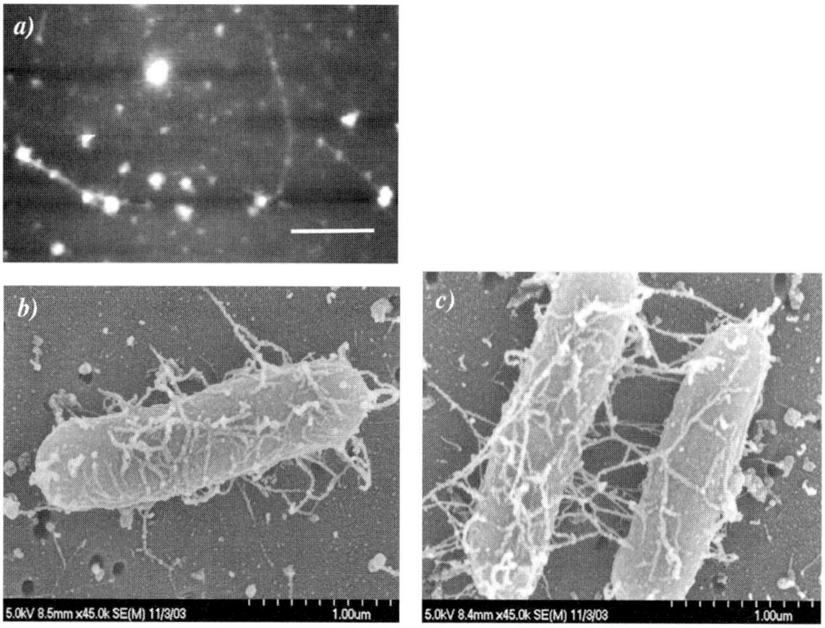

Fig. 7.21. (a) AFM image of a covalent BSA-SWNT conjugate sample. (b) and (c) SEM images showing the strong interactions of immuno-SWNTs (SWNT-BSA-antibody goat anti-*Escherichia coli* O157 conjugate) with pathogenic *E. coli* O157:H7 cells. (From Ref. [169].)

method, and then conjugated to streptavidin via selective biotin–streptavidin interactions [167]. While streptavidin proteins cannot enter cells by themselves, the water-soluble SWNT–biotin–streptavidin conjugates were able to internalize into many types of cells, such as human promyelocytic leukemia (HL60), Chinese hamster ovary, and 3T3 fibroblast cells (Fig. 7.22). Streptavidin alone did not show appreciable cytotoxicity to HL60 cells. However, the cytotoxicity of SWNT–biotin–streptavidin conjugates toward the same cell line was dose-dependent, which is consistent with protein internalization via nanotube carriers. SWNT–biotin–streptavidin internalization is probably accomplished through endocytosis, which could be blocked at 4 °C. Co-localization of SWNTs and endosomes formed during such endocytosis is direct evidence for internalization.

SWNTs functionalized by a peptide that mimics the function of G_S protein were able not only to penetrate human and murine fibroblast and keratinocytes cells membranes but also to translocate into the cell nucleus [161, 165]. The nanotube functionalization was covalent, but based on 1,3-dipolar addition of azomethine ylides onto the nanotube sidewalls [161, 164]. The functional group end-capped with amine was then modified with peptide sequences to obtain peptide–SWNT conjugates. Murine 3T3 fibroblast cells were still largely viable when the soluble

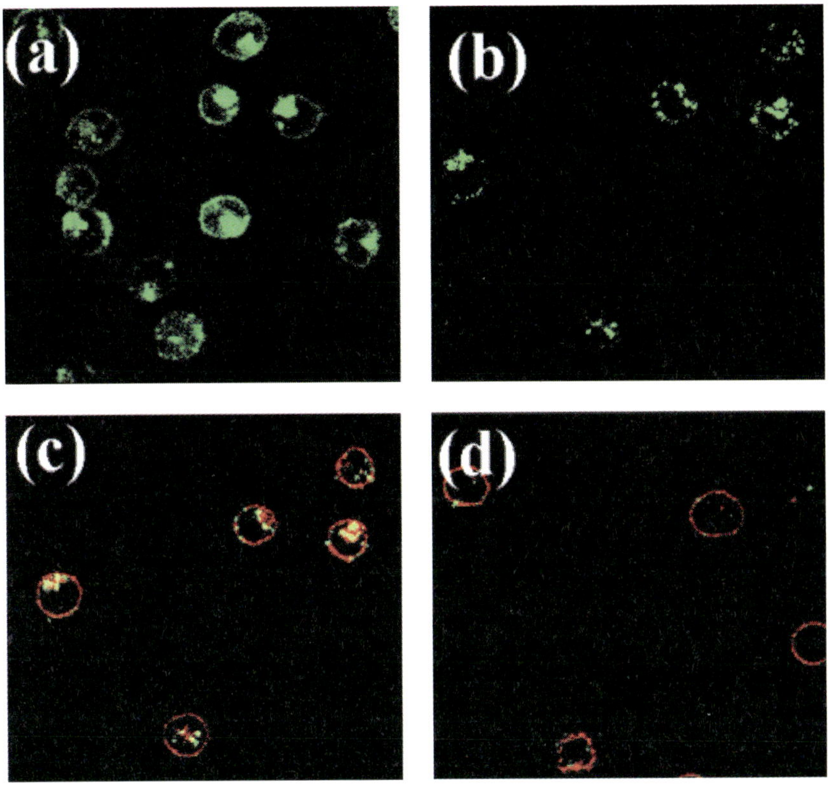

Fig. 7.22. Confocal images of HL60 cells after incubation in solutions of (a) a fluorescein-labeled SWNT sample; (b) a mixture of SWNT-biotin-fluoresceinated streptavidin conjugate (green) and the red endocytosis marker FM 4-64 at 37 °C (image showing fluorescence in the green region only); (c) same as (b) but with additional red fluorescence shown due to FM 4-64 stained endosomes; (d) same as (c) after incubation at 4 °C. (From Ref. [167].)

functionalized SWNT concentration was as high as 5 μM, but the nanotube solution quickly became toxic to these cells upon increasing the concentration by only twice as much. The uptake mechanism, however, is not due to endocytosis, since the internalization is temperature independent (the same at both 4 and 37 °C) [165]. Nevertheless, there are several other reports on the cell internalization of both non-functionalized carbon nanotubes and those functionalized with other bioactive species (such as nucleic acids) [166, 219, 220]. These reports discuss the cytotoxicity of carbon nanotubes [219] and their potential in bioimaging (via nanotube near-IR fluorescence) [220] and drug, vaccine, and gene delivery systems [164–168].

In addition to direct covalent methods, specific protein–nanotube conjugation can also be achieved through the use of a bifunctional molecule, with one end attaching to the protein and the other end to the nanotube. Chen et al. [221] reported the use of 1-pyrenebutanoic acid succinimidyl ester as a linker for indirect protein–SWNT conjugation. The pyrene moieties of the bifunctional molecules are proposed to interact noncovalently with the nanotube surface via "π–π" stacking, while the succinimides react with pendant amino groups on the protein to form amide linkages. This method was successfully applied to SWNTs at device level [197]. However, the necessity of using this linker molecule has never been seriously determined, especially considering the competitive non-specific interaction bindings from proteins themselves. In Chen et al.'s original control experiment [221], it was claimed that no binding was found between ferritin and SWNTs grown on a TEM grid without the presence of the linker molecule. This contradicts later observations by other workers, who consistently found that ferritins are actually very affinitive to SWNTs, even in aqueous solution [188, 189].

Although considered to be specific conjugation modes, neither direct covalent functionalization nor the usage of pyrene-succinimide bifunctional molecule could provide the selectivity for carbon nanotubes to bind one protein but repel another. One general prerequisite to obtaining such selectivity or biorecognition is efficient elimination of non-specific adsorption. Thus, the application of a protein-resistant layer (such as PEG) on the nanotubes prior to protein conjugation is essential. Shim et al. [187] first demonstrated such a possibility by adsorbing surfactant Triton X-100 and then PEG to SWNTs on silica surface. They proposed that the hydrophobic part of Triton molecule adsorbs onto SWNTs, while its hydrophilic tail facilitates subsequent adsorption of PEG, which alone hardly interacts with the nanotube surface. SWNT devices protected this way were resistant to streptavidin and other protein molecules. With biotin modification on adsorbed PEG, however, streptavidin efficiently coated the nanotube surface, which still repelled other proteins [187]. The well-known biotin–streptavidin interaction obviously accounts for such observed selectivity or biorecognition.

Although each Triton molecule contains an oligomeric ethylene glycol chain as its hydrophilic tail, a simple Triton coating is not sufficient to prevent non-specific adsorption of proteins on nanotubes [187]. Some other surfactants, such as Tween-20, which has dendritic PEG tails, protect the nanotubes much better, even without additional PEG adsorption. Such surfactant coating is quite useful for SWNTs on substrates in devices [179], but not so impressive in aqueous solutions [188]. In a report by Erlanger et al. [222], an anti-fullerene IgG monoclonal antibody was claimed to be specifically conjugated to SWNTs in the presence of Tween-20 in an aqueous environment. Although this antibody is known to be specific to fullerene C_{60}, the observed binding might simply be another example of non-specific adsorption. Further evidence is definitely required to prove whether the anti-fullerene antibody is truly selective toward SWNTs.

Nevertheless, biorecognition sites can be created similarly at the PEG end of Tween-20 surfactant molecules. For example, with biotin attachment to the dendritic PEG tails of Tween-20 prior to its adsorption on SWNT FET devices, no protein except streptavidin could be conjugated [179]. In another report, PEG was co-adsorbed onto SWNT devices with another functional polymer, polyethylene

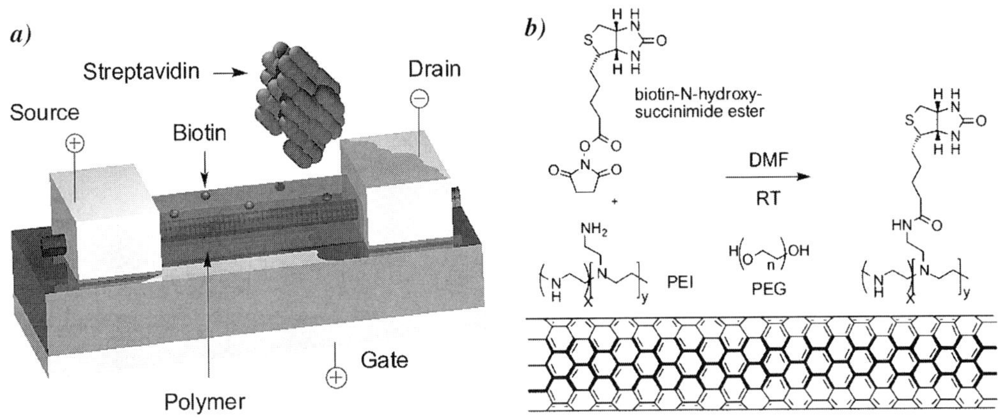

Fig. 7.23. (a) Schematic diagram illustrating a biotinylated SWNT-FET for streptavidin recognition. (b) Biotinylation of PEI on the nanotube surface, with co-adsorbed PEG. (From Ref. [223].)

imine (PEI), instead of surfactant molecules [223]. The pendant primary amine groups on PEI were available for subsequent biotin derivatization and, thus, streptavidin recognition (Fig. 7.23).

The protein-resistivity of PEG-coated SWNTs on substrates may be interfered with by the same PEG coating on substrates themselves [Fig. 7.24(a, b)]. The availability of highly water-soluble SWNTs with PEG functionalities [224, 225] provides an excellent opportunity to demonstrate unambiguously the protein-resistant function of the PEG layer on the nanotubes in aqueous solution. As Lin et al. [189] reported, PEG-functionalized SWNTs can totally repel ferritins in aqueous solution. As shown in the TEM image (Fig. 7.24c), ferritins surround the nanotubes, but obviously at a distance, which is due to the PEG functionalities. Other water-soluble SWNTs, such as those functionalized by poly(propionyl ethylenimine-*co*-ethylenimine) (PPEI-EI) [213, 226] or poly(vinyl alcohol) (PVA) [227], similarly repel proteins in aqueous solution [189]. The protein-resistance coupled with the water-solubility of these functionalized SWNTs could be important in their biomedical applications. Data from other PEG-containing materials suggest that such protein-resistant nanotubes may have reduced cytotoxicity and increased retention time in the circulatory system [228]. All of these hypotheses, however, remain to be verified.

In addition to the well-known biotin–streptavidin interaction, biorecognition may also be achieved through other biologically known supramolecular pairwise selective interactions, such as the antibody–antigen interaction, carbohydrate–lectin interaction, and others. For this purpose, the indirect but selective attachment of different types of proteins to carbon nanotubes can be achieved via initial nanotube functionalization with the corresponding counterpart species. For in-

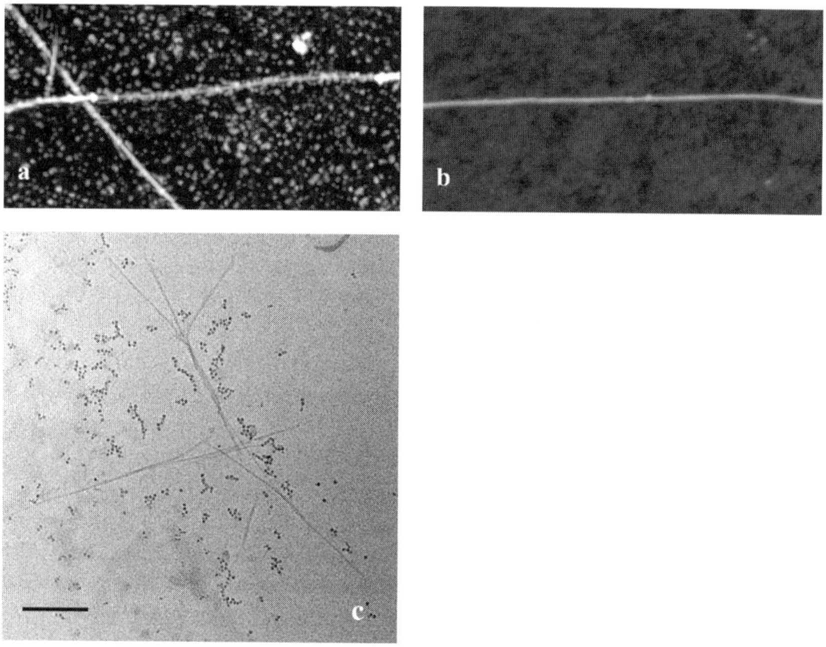

Fig. 7.24. (a) AFM image showing the non-specific binding of streptavidin on SWNTs as-grown on substrate. (b) AFM image showing that the non-specific binding was largely prevented by coating SWNTs with surfactant Triton X-100 followed by PEG. (From Ref. [187].) (c) TEM image showing that the non-specific binding of ferritin species to water-soluble SWNTs was completely prevented by the covalent PEG functionalities on SWNTs.

stance, an antigen named U1A was attached to Tween-20 molecules and adsorbed onto a SWNT FET device, which was then only responsive to the U1A's antibody counterpart, 10E3 [179]. SWNTs were also co-functionalized in a carbodiimide-activated reaction with an antibody and an enzyme, alkaline phosphatase (ALP), with the latter serving as the electrochemical tag [229]. Such conjugates have been used in combination with immunological magnetic beads for ultrasensitive immunosensing or antigen detection. The antigen was attached in a sandwich-like configuration to nanotube-bound and magnetic-bead-bound antibodies. The captured antigens were then separated magnetically. The electrochemical detection signals were enhanced by comparing multiple copies of enzymatic species on the nanotube surface to single enzyme tags. DNA sensing was achieved via a similar strategy, with selectivity coming from the complementary DNA sequence hybridization instead of antibody–antigen interactions [229].

A natural β-1,3-glucan, schizophyllan (SPG), was found to be able to noncovalently wrap around and solubilize SWNTs in water [230]. Using SPG with lactoside appendages, the carbohydrate-functionalized SWNTs can be conjugated to *Ricinus communis* agglutinin, a lactoside-specific lectin that is inert to other carbohydrates such as α-mannose and some other monosaccharides. In another example taking advantage of carbohydrate–lectin specific interactions, β-D-galactose-functionalized SWNTs could be crosslinked by a galactoside-specific lectin from the peanut *Arachis hypogaera*, forming interconnected networks [231].

Very recently, noncovalent functionalization of SWNTs by a mucin-mimic with α-*N*-acetylgalactosamine (α-GalNAc) moieties has been reported [232]. These sugar moieties could be recognized by *Helix pomatia* agglutinin (HPA), α-GalNAc's specific counterpart (Fig. 7.25). When HPA was plugged with free GalNAc, no binding occurred between the deactivated agglutinin and the α-mucin mimic-SWNT conjugate. Specificity was further demonstrated by a noncovalent conjugate sample of SWNTs with a similar mucin mimic but bearing sugar moieties of β-configuration. Again, no binding was found between HPA and the β-mucin mimic–SWNT conjugate.

In a similar strategy, Gu et al. [170] reported recently multivalent carbohydrate display on SWNTs for the detection of *E. coli* O157:H7, which took advantage of the selective interactions of the nanotube-bound sugar moieties (β-D-galactose) with the periplasmic galactose-binding proteins on the pathogen surface. The pathogen cells could be agglutinated by the β-D-galactose-functionalized SWNTs, while inert to those functionalized by either α-D-mannose or BSA protein [170].

Reconstitution of flavoenzymes was also used for enzyme–nanotube conjugation for the purpose of subsequent electronic sensing of a catalytic event via nanotube conductor arrays. As reported by Patolsky et al. [233], the glucose oxidase (GOx) cofactor, flavin adenine dinucleotide (FAD), was first functionalized covalently onto the SWNT array, which was formed by self-assembly on an Au substrate as the electrode. With the protection of SWNTs with PEG, apo-GOx proteins were then immobilized onto the SWNTs via apoenzyme-FAD reconstitution. The conversion of glucose into gluconic acid by the redox enzyme was found to be efficiently transferred to the Au electrode and was highly dependent upon the lengths of the nanotubes, which apparently serve as the pathway for electron transfer [233].

Since these supramolecular but selective interactions are well-known in biology, scientists in the bio-nano field are more inclined to use these interactions to conjugate proteins and nanomaterials, including carbon nanotubes, for biologically and biomedically significant purposes. Proteins conjugated this way probably retain their bioactive structures and functions. However, when proteins are conjugated to carbon nanotubes via other covalent or noncovalent pathways, their secondary and other advanced structures are largely unknown because of their close proximity to the nanotubes. This should be investigated, especially in the light of a recent valuable attempt by Karajanagi et al. [191] on the advanced structures of two enzymes (SBP vs. CT) upon adsorption on SWNTs. From that work, it seems that the secondary and tertiary structures of proteins could easily be affected when adsorbed onto carbon nanotubes. However, the structural and biofunctional alterations to each protein induced in the conjugation events will need to be carefully evaluated on a case-by-case basis before mechanistic details of the interactions

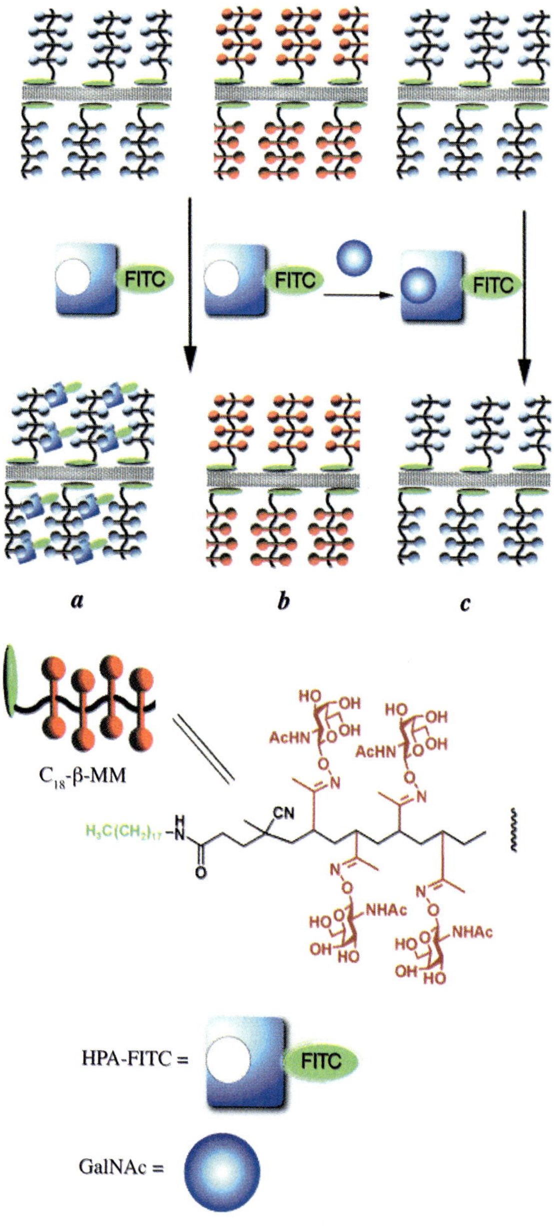

Fig. 7.25. Specific binding of HPA to α-mucin mimic-coated nanotubes: (a) specific binding of HPA to the surface of α-mucin mimic-SWNTs; (b) lack of binding of HPA to β-mucin mimic-SWNTs; and (c) inhibition of HPA binding by soluble GalNAc. (From Ref. [232].)

and any potential regulations for the changes in protein structures and biological functions are understood.

7.4 Conclusions and Perspectives

As described in this chapter, exciting progress has been made over the past few years in the coupling and assembly of proteins and nanostructured materials (metal, semiconductor and nanotubes). A typical route for preparing these conjugates involves mixing proteins with chemically modified nanomaterials. Protein molecules can also act as crosslinkers or as templates to build nanometer-sized supramolecular structures by self-assembly. The field continues to grow and contribute to new interdisciplinary areas concerned with the synthesis, self-assembly, and processing of organized matter. Despite the progress made, this field is still in its infancy, with many challenges ahead. For example, there is still great demand for alternative and selective coupling methods that allow the preparation of stable, clean, and stoichiometrically well-defined bioconjugate nanomaterials. In this regard, an interesting recent development is the use of supercritical fluid processing, wherein a protein can be attached directly to inorganic nanoparticles in an effective and clean fashion. Other areas where there is much to be learnt are the surface interaction and the interface between nanomaterials and proteins and the control of shape and physico-chemical properties of proteins by means of genetic engineering and bioconjugate chemistry.

Among the enormous challenges are how to design well-ordered structures and how to adapt them efficiently in the macroscopic world. Here, the electrostatic and topographic properties of biological macromolecules, such as bacterial superstructures and hollow protein compartments, still must be understood. Research effort on the discovery, selection and development of peptides from combinatorial peptide and protein libraries will also benefit this field. It will allow the production of even more suitable biological structures, since they can provide recombinant protein units that have optimized recognition capabilities for inorganic materials and their assemblies in distinctively shaped superstructures.

Further future investigations should also address the issues of the applications of these bioconjugate materials. Interdisciplinary research in this filed has great potential for discovering and producing advanced materials, which can then lead to novel devices for sensing, signal transduction, catalysis, and new biocompatible materials and interfaces desired for biomedical sciences and tissue engineering.

Acknowledgment

Financial support from NSF, NASA, Department of Energy, and the Center for Advanced Engineering Fibers and Films (NSF-ERC at Clemson University) is gratefully acknowledged.

References

1 Niemeyer, C. M., Nanoparticles, proteins, and nucleic acids: biotechnology meets materials science. *Angew. Chem. Int. Ed.* **2001**, *113* (22), 4128–4158; Functional hybrid devices of proteins and inorganic nanoparticles. *Angew. Chem. Int. Ed.* **2003**, *42* (47), 5796–5800.

2 Katz, E., I. Willner, Integrated nanoparticle-biomolecule hybrid systems: synthesis, properties, and applications. *Angew. Chem. Int. Ed.* **2004**, *43* (45), 6042–6108.

3 Katz, E., A. N. Shipway, I. Willner, Biomaterial-nanoparticle hybrid systems: Synthesis, properties and applications, in *Nanoparticles – From Theory to Applications*, (Ed.: G. Schmid), Wiley-VCH, Weinheim, 2003, 368–421.

4 Parak, W. J., D. Gerion, T. Pellegrino, D. Zanchet, C. Micheel, S. C. Williams, R. Boudreau, M. A. Le Gros, C. A. Larabell, A. P. Alivisatos, Biological applications of colloidal nanocrystals. *Nanotechnology* **2003**, *14* (7), R15–R27.

5 Csaki, A., G. Maubach, D. Born, J. Reichert, W. Fritzsche, DNA-based molecular nanotechnology. *Single Mol.* **2002**, *3* (5–6), 275–280.

6 Penn, S. G., L. Hey, M. J. Natan, Nanoparticles for bioanalysis. *Curr. Opin. Chem. Biol.* **2003**, *7* (5), 609–615.

7 West, J. L., N. J. Halas, Engineered nanomaterials for biophotonics applications: improving sensing, imaging, and therapeutics. *Annu. Rev. Biomed. Eng.* **2003**, *5*, 285–292.

8 Alivisatos, A. P. The use of nanocrystals in biological detection. *Nat. Biotechnol.* **2004**, *22*, 47–52.

9 Verma, A., V. M. Rotello. Surface recognition of biomacromolecules using nanoparticle receptors. *Chem. Commun.* **2005**, *3*, 303–312.

10 Storhoff, J. J., C. A. Mirkin, Programmed materials synthesis with DNA. *Chem. Rev.* **1999**, *99* (7), 1849–1862.

11 Mirkin, C. A. Programming the assembly of two- and three-dimensional architectures with DNA and nanoscale inorganic building blocks. *Inorg. Chem.* **2000**, *39* (11), 2258–2272.

12 Niemeyer, C. M., W. Bürger, J. Peplies, Covalent DNA – streptavidin conjugates as building blocks for novel biometallic nanostructures. *Angew. Chem. Int. Ed.* **1998**, *37* (16), 2265–2268.

13 Connolly, S., D. Fitzmaurice, Programmed assembly of gold nanocrystals in aqueous solution. *Adv. Mater.* **1999**, *11* (14), 1202–1205.

14 Li, M., K. W. K. Wong, S. Mann, Organization of inorganic nanoparticles using biotin-streptavidin connectors. *Chem. Mater.* **1999**, *11* (1), 23–26.

15 Niemeyer, C. M., B. Ceyhan, DNA-directed functionalization of colloidal gold with proteins. *Angew. Chem. Int. Ed.* **2001**, *40* (19), 3685–3688.

16 Kreuter, J. Nanoparticles – preparation and applications, in *Microcapsules and Nanoparticles in Medicine and Pharmacy*, (Ed.: M. Donbrow), CRC, Boca Raton, FL, **1992**, 125–148.

17 Bruchez, Jr., M., M. Moronne, P. Gin, S. Weiss, A. P. Alivisatos, Semiconductor nanocrystals as fluorescent biological labels. *Science* **1998**, *281* (5385), 2013–2015.

18 Chan, W. C. W., S. M. Nie, Quantum dot bioconjugates for ultrasensitive nonisotopic detection. *Science* **1998**, *281* (5385), 2016–2018.

19 Mattoussi, H., J. M. Mauro, E. R. Goldmann, G. P. Anderson, V. C. Sundar, F. V. Miculec, M. G. Bawendi, Self-assembly of CdSe-ZnS quantum dot bioconjugates using an engineered recombinant protein. *J. Am. Chem. Soc.* **2000**, *122* (49), 12142–12150.

20 Wu, X. Y., H. J. Liu, J. Q. Liu, K. N. Haley, J. A. Treadway, J. P. Larson, N. F. Ge, F. Peale, M. P. Bruchez, Immunofluorescent labeling of cancer marker Her2 and other cellular targets with semiconductor quantum dots. *Nat. Biotechnol.* **2003**, *21* (1), 41–46.

21 Jaiswal, J. K., H. Mattoussi, J. M. Mauro, S. M. Simon, Long-term multiple color imaging of live cells using quantum dot bioconjugates. *Nat. Biotechnol.* **2003**, *21* (1), 47–51.

22 Han, M. Y., X. H. Gao, J. Z. Su, S. M. Nie, Quantum-dot-tagged microbeads for multiplexed optical coding of biomolecules. *Nat. Biotechnol.* **2001**, *19* (7), 631–635.

23 Konno, T., J. Watanabe, K. Ishihara, Conjugation of enzymes on polymer nanoparticles covered with phosphorylcholine groups. *Biomacromolecules* **2004**, *5* (2), 342–347.

24 Qi, K., Q. Ma, E. E. Remsen, C. G. Jr. Clark, K. L. Wooley, Determination of the bioavailability of biotin conjugated onto shell cross-linked (SCK) nanoparticles. *J. Am. Chem. Soc.* **2004**, *126* (21), 6599–6607.

25 Soppimath, K. S., T. M. Aminabhavi, A. R. Kulkarni, W. E. Rudzinski, Biodegradable polymeric nanoparticles as drug delivery devices. *J. Controlled Release* **2001**, *70* (1–2), 1–20.

26 Sakuma, S., M. Hayashi, M. Akashi, Design of nanoparticles composed of graft copolymers for oral peptide delivery. *Adv. Drug Deliv. Rev.* **2001**, *47* (1), 21–37.

27 Takeuchi, H., H. Yamamoto, Y. Kawashima, Mucoadhesive nanoparticulate systems for peptide drug delivery. *Adv. Drug Deliv. Rev.* **2001**, *47* (1), 39–54.

28 Nednoor, P., M. Capaccio, V. G. Gavalas, M. S. Meier, J. E. Anthony, L. G. Bachas, Hybrid nanoparticles based on organized protein immobilization on fullerenes. *Bioconj. Chem.* **2004**, *15* (1), 12–15.

29 Hasobe, T., P. V. Kamat, V. Troiani, N. Solladie, T. K. Ahn, S. K. Kim, D. Kim, A. Kongkanand, S. Kuwabata, S. Fukuzumi, Enhancement of light-energy conversion efficiency by multi-porphyrin arrays of porphyrin-peptide oligomers with fullerene clusters. *J. Phys. Chem. B* **2005**, *109* (1), 19–23.

30 Nakamura, E., H. Isobe, Functionalized fullerenes in water. The first 10 years of their chemistry, biology, and nanoscience. *Acc. Chem. Res.* **2003**, *36* (11), 807–815.

31 Pantarotto, D., A. Bianco, F. Pellarini, A. Tossi, A. Giangaspero, I. Zelezetsky, J.-P. Briand, M. Prato, Solid-phase synthesis of fullerene-peptides. *J. Am. Chem. Soc.* **2002**, *124* (42), 12543–12549.

32 Murakami, H., R. Matsumoto, Y. Okusa, T. Sagara, M. Fujitsuka, O. Ito, N. Nakashima, Design, synthesis and photophysical properties of C-60-modified proteins. *J. Mater. Chem.* **2002**, *12* (7), 2026–2033.

33 Bosi, S., T. DaRos, G. Spalluto, M. Prato, Fullerene derivatives: an attractive tool for biological applications. *Eur. J. Medic. Chem.* **2003**, *38* (11–12), 913–923.

34 Fu, K. F., A. Kitaygorodskiy, Y.-P. Sun, Fullerene-centered macromolecules as unimolecular micellar structures. *Chem. Mater.* **2000**, *12* (8), 2073–2075.

35 Martin, R. B., K. F. Fu, H. P. Li, D. Cole, Y.-P. Sun, Interesting fluorescence properties of C-60-centered dendritic adduct with twelve symmetrically attached pyrenes. *Chem. Commun.* **2003**, *18*, 2368–2369.

36 Sun, Y.-P., G. E. Lawson, W. J. Huang, A. D. Wright, D. K. Moton, Preparation and characterization of highly water-soluble pendant fullerene polymers. *Macromolecules* **1999**, *32* (26), 8747–8752.

37 Taylor, S., L. Qu, A. Kitaygorodskiy, J. Teske, R. A. Latour, Y.-P. Sun, Synthesis and characterization of peptide-functionalized polymeric nanoparticles. *Biomacromolecules* **2004**, *5* (1), 245–248.

38 Qu, L., P. G. Luo, S. Taylor, Y. Lin, W. Huang, N. Anyadike, T.-R. J. Tzeng, F. Stutzenberger, R. A. Latour, Y.-P. Sun, Visualizing adhesion-induced agglutination of *Escherichia coli* with mannosylated nanoparticles. *J. Nanosci. Nanotechnol.* **2005**, *5* (2), 320–323.

39 Qu, L., L. Gu, H. Li, S. Taylor, T. Elkin, P. G. Luo, T.-R. J. Tzeng, X. Jiang, R. A. Latour, F. Stutzenberger, A. Williams, Y.-P. Sun,

Galactosylated polymeric nanoparticles: Synthesis and adhesion interactions with *Escherichia coli*. *J. Biomed. Nanotechnol.* **2005**, *1* (1), 61–67(7).

40 SHENTON, W., S. A. DAVIES, S. MANN, Directed self-assembly of nanoparticles into macroscopic materials using antibody-antigen recognition. *Adv. Mater.* **1999**, *11* (6), 449–452.

41 HAYAT, M. A. *Colloidal Gold: Principles, Methods, and Applications*, Academic Press, New York, **1989**.

42 KEATING, C. D., K. M. KOVALESKI, M. J. NATAN, Protein: colloid conjugates for surface enhanced Raman scattering: Stability and control of protein orientation. *J. Phys. Chem. B* **1998**, *102* (47), 9404–9413.

43 BRODERICK, J. B., M. J. NATAN, T. V. OHALLORAN, R. P. VAN DUYNE, Evidence for retention of biological-activity of a nonheme iron enzyme adsorbed on a silver colloid – a surface-enhanced resonance Raman-scattering study. *Biochemistry* **1993**, *32* (50), 13771–13776.

44 SCHULTZ, S., D. R. SMITH, J. J. MOCK, D. A. SCHULTZ, Single-target molecule detection with nonbleaching multicolor optical immunolabels. *Proc. Natl. Acad. Sci. U.S.A.* **2000**, *97* (3), 996–1001.

45 MACDONALD, I. D. G., W. E. SMITH, Orientation of cytochrome c adsorbed on a citrate-reduced silver colloid surface. *Langmuir* **1996**, *12* (3), 706–713.

46 ROSPENDOWSKI, B. N., K. KELLY, C. R. WOLF, W. E. SMITH, Surface-enhanced resonance Raman-scattering from cytochromes-P-450 adsorbed on citrate-reduced silver sols. *J. Am. Chem. Soc.* **1991**, *113* (4), 1217–1225.

47 BURT, J. L., C. GUTIERREZ-WING, M. MIKI-YOSHIDA, M. JOSE-YACAMAN, Noble-metal nanoparticles directly conjugated to globular proteins. *Langmuir* **2004**, *20* (26), 11778–11783.

48 SAFER, D., L. BOLINGER, J. S. LEIGH, Undecagold clusters for site-specific labeling of biological macromolecules – simplified preparation and model applications. *J. Inorg. Biochem.* **1986**, *26* (2), 77–91.

49 HAINFELD, J. F., F. R. FURUYA, A 1.4-nm gold cluster covalently attached to antibodies improves immunolabeling. *J. Histochem. Cytochem.* **1992**, *40* (2), 177–184.

50 LETSINGER, R. L., R. ELGHANIAN, G. VISWANADHAM, C. A. MIRKIN, Use of a steroid cyclic disulfide anchor in constructing gold nanoparticle-oligonucleotide conjugates. *Bioconj. Chem.* **2000**, *11* (2), 289–291.

51 DAMERON, C. T., R. N. REESE, R. K. MEHRA, A. R. KORTAN, P. J. CARROLL, M. L. STEIGERWALD, L. E. BRUS, D. R. WINGE, Biosynthesis of cadmium-sulfide quantum semiconductor crystallites. *Nature* **1989**, *338* (6216), 596–597.

52 WHALEY, S. R., D. S. ENGLISH, E. L. HU, P. F. BARBARA, A. M. BELCHER, Selection of peptides with semiconductor binding specificity for directed nanocrystal assembly. *Nature* **2000**, *405* (6787), 665–668.

53 HERMANSON, G. T. in *Bioconjugate Techniques*, Academic Press, New York, 1996.

54 DOUGLAS, T., M. YOUNG, Host-guest encapsulation of materials by assembled virus protein cages. *Nature* **1998**, *393* (6681), 152–155.

55 GESTWICKI, J. E., L. E. STRONG, L. L. KIESSLING, Visualization of single multivalent receptor-ligand complexes by transmission electron microscopy. *Angew. Chem. Int. Ed.* **2000**, *39* (24), 4567–4570.

56 MAMEDOVA, N. N., N. A. KOTOV, A. L. ROGACH, J. STUDER, Albumin-CdTe nanoparticle bioconjugates: preparation, structure, and interunit energy transfer with antenna effect. *Nano Lett.* **2001**, *1* (6), 281–286.

57 WANG, S. P., N. N. MAMEDOVA, N. A. KOTOV, W. CHEN, J. STUDER, Antigen/antibody immunocomplex from CdTe nanoparticle bioconjugates. *Nano Lett.* **2002**, *2* (8), 817–822.

58 ISHII, D., K. KINBARA, Y. ISHIDA, N. ISHII, M. OKOCHI, M. YOHDA, T. AIDA, Chaperonin-mediated stabilization and ATP-triggered release of semiconductor nanoparticles. *Nature* **2003**, *423* (6940), 628–632.

59 Meziani, M. J., P. Pathak, B. A. Harruff, R. Hurezeanu, Y.-P. Sun, Direct conjugation of semiconductor nanoparticles with proteins. *Langmuir* **2005**, *21* (5), 2008–2011.

60 Meziani, M. J., Y.-P. Sun, Protein-conjugated nanoparticles from rapid expansion of supercritical fluid solution into aqueous solution. *J. Am. Chem. Soc.* **2003**, *125* (26), 8015–8018.

61 Willard, D. M., L. L. Carillo, J. Jung, A. Van Orden, CdSe-ZnS quantum dots as resonance energy transfer donors in a model protein-protein binding assay. *Nano Lett.* **2001**, *1* (9), 469–474.

62 Medintz, I. L., A. R. Clapp, H. Mattoussi, E. R. Goldman, B. Fisher, J. M. Mauro, Self-assembled nanoscale biosensors based on quantum dot FRET donors. *Nat. Mater.* **2003**, *2* (9), 630–638.

63 Medintz, I. L., J. H. Konnert, A. R. Clapp, I. Stanish, M. E. Twigg, H. Mattoussi, J. M. Mauro, J. R. Deschamps, A fluorescence resonance energy transfer-derived structure of a quantum dot-protein bioconjugate nanoassembly. *Proc. Nat. Acad. Sci. U.S.A.* **2004**, *101* (26), 9612–9617.

64 Willner, I., E. Katz, Integration of layered redox proteins and conductive supports for bioelectronic applications. *Angew. Chem. Int. Ed.* **2000**, *39* (7), 1180–1218.

65 Zhong, Z. Y., B. Gates, Y. N. Xia, D. Qin, Soft lithographic approach to the fabrication of highly ordered 2D arrays of magnetic nanoparticles on the surfaces of silicon substrates. *Langmuir* **2000**, *16* (26), 10369–10375.

66 Zahn, M., Magnetic fluid and nanoparticle applications to nano-technology. *J. Nanoparticle Res.* **2001**, *3* (1), 73–78.

67 Shi, J., S. Gider, K. Babcock, D. D. Awschalom, Magnetic clusters in molecular beams, metals, and semiconductors. *Science* **1996**, *271* (5251), 937–941.

68 Lebreton, C., C. Vieu, A. Pépin, M. Mejias, F. Carcenac, Y. Jin, and H. Launois, Coulomb blockade effect through a 2D ordered array of Pd islands obtained by colloidal deposition. *Microelectron. Eng.* **1998**, *42*, 507–510.

69 Yoffe, A. D. Semiconductor quantum dots and related systems: electronic, optical, luminescence and related properties of low dimensional systems. *Adv. Phys.* **2001**, *50* (1), 1–208.

70 Kouwenhoven, L. P., D. G. Austing, S. Tarucha, Few-electron quantum dots. *Rep. Prog. Phys.* **2001**, *64* (6), 701–736.

71 Sinha, B. K., C. F. Chignell, The synthesis and use of spin-labeled analogs of biotin in the study of avidin. *Methods Enzymol.* **1979**, *62*, 295–308.

72 Piran, U., W. J. Riordan, Dissociation rate-constant of the biotin-streptavidin complex. *J. Immunol. Methods* **1990**, *133* (1), 141–143.

73 Sano, T., M. W. Pandori, X. M. Chen, C. L. Smith, C. R. Cantor, Recombinant core streptavidins – a minimum-sized core streptavidin has enhanced structural stability and higher accessibility to biotinylated macromolecules. *J. Biol. Chem.* **1995**, *270* (47), 28204–28209.

74 Sano, T., C. R. Cantor, Intersubunit contacts made by tryptophan-120 with biotin are essential for both strong biotin binding and biotin-induced tighter subunit association of streptavidin. *Proc. Natl. Acad. Sci. U.S.A.* **1995**, *92* (8), 3180–3184.

75 Reznik, G. O., S. Vajda, C. L. Smith, C. R. Cantor, T. Sano, Streptavidins with intersubunit crosslinks have enhanced stability. *Nat. Biotechnol.* **1996**, *14* (8), 1007–1011.

76 Schmidt, T. G. M., J. Koepke, R. Frank, A. Skerra, Molecular interaction between the Strep-tag affinity peptide and its cognate target, streptavidin. *J. Mol. Biol.* **1996**, *255* (5), 753–766.

77 Sano, T., S. Vajda, C. R. Cantor, Genetic engineering of streptavidin, a versatile affinity tag. *J. Chromatogr. B* **1998**, *715* (1), 85–91.

78 Brown, S. Engineered iron oxide-

adhesion mutants of the Escherichia-coli phage-lambda receptor. *Proc. Nat. Acad. Sci. U.S.A.* **1992**, *89* (18), 8651–8655.
79 Flynn, C. E., C. Mao, A. Hayhurst, J. L. Williams, G. Georgiou, B. Iverson, and A. M. Belcher, Synthesis and organization of nanoscale II–VI semiconductor materials using evolved peptide specificity and viral capsid assembly. *J. Mater. Chem.* **2003**, *13* (10), 2414–2421.
80 Lee, S.-W., C. Mao, C. E. Flynn, A. M. Belcher, Ordering of quantum dots using genetically engineered viruses. *Science* **2002**, *296* (5569), 892–895.
81 Lee, S.-W., B. M. Wood, A. M. Belcher, Chiral smectic C structures of virus-based films. *Langmuir* **2003**, *19* (5), 1592–1598.
82 Lee, S.-W., S.-K. Lee, A. M. Belcher, Virus-based alignment of inorganic, organic, and biological nanosized materials. *Adv. Mater.* **2003**, *15* (9), 689.
83 Mao, C. B., C. E. Flynn, A. Hayhurst, R. Y. Sweeney, J. Qi, J. Williams, G. Georgiou, B. Iverson, and A. M. Belcher, Viral assembly of oriented quantum dot nanowires. *Proc. Natl. Acad. Sci. U.S.A.* **2003**, *100* (12), 6946–6941.
84 Mao, C. B., D. J. Solis, B. D. Reiss, S. T. Kottmann, R. Y. Sweeney, A. Hayhurst, G. Georgiou, B. Iverson, and A. M. Belcher, Virus-based toolkit for the directed synthesis of magnetic and semiconducting nanowires. *Science* **2004**, *303* (5655), 213–217.
85 Sleytr, U. B., P. Messner, D. Pum, M. Sara, Crystalline bacterial cell surface layers (S layers): from supramolecular cell structure to biomimetics and nanotechnology. *Angew. Chem. Int. Ed.* **1999**, *38* (8), 1034–1054.
86 Shenton, W., D. Pum, U. B. Sleytr, S. Mann, Synthesis of cadmium sulphide superlattices using self-assembled bacterial S-layers. *Nature* **1997**, *389* (6651), 585–587.
87 Dieluweit, S., D. Pum, U. B. Sleytr, Formation of a gold superlattice on an S-layer with square lattice symmetry. *Supramol. Sci.* **1998**, *5* (1–2), 15–19.
88 Hall, S. R., W. Shenton, H. Engelhardt, S. Mann, Site-specific organization of gold nanoparticles by biomolecular templating. *Chem. Phys. Chem.* **2001**, *2* (3), 184–186.
89 Mertig, M., R. Kirsch, W. Pompe, H. Engelhardt, Fabrication of highly oriented nanocluster arrays by biomolecular templating. *Eur. Phys. J. D* **1999**, *9* (1–4), 45–48.
90 Allen, M., D. Willits, J. Mosolf, M. Young, T. Douglas, Protein cage constrained synthesis of ferrimagnetic iron oxide nanoparticles. *Adv. Mater.* **2002**, *14* (21), 1562–1565.
91 Douglas, T., E. Strable, D. Willits, A. Aitouchen, M. Libera, M. Young, Protein engineering of a viral cage for constrained nanomaterials synthesis. *Adv. Mater.* **2002**, *14* (6), 415–418.
92 Shenton, W., S. Mann, H. Cölfen, A. Bacher, M. Fischer, Synthesis of nanophase iron oxide in lumazine synthase capsids. *Angew. Chem. Int. Ed.* **2001**, *40* (2), 442–444.
93 Stryer, L. *Biochemistry*, Freeman, New York, 1988.
94 Stubbs, G. in *The Viruses.* (Eds.: A. Mc Pherson, F. Jurnak), Wiley, New York, 1984, Vol. 1, 149–202.
95 Shenton, W., T. Douglas, M. Young, G. Stubbs, S. Mann, Inorganic-organic nanotube composites from template mineralization of tobacco mosaic virus. *Adv. Mater.* **1999**, *11* (3), 253–256.
96 Dujardin, E., C. Peet, G. Stubbs, J. N. Culver, S. Mann, Organization of metallic nanoparticles using tobacco mosaic virus templates. *Nano Lett.* **2003**, *3* (3), 413–417.
97 Boal, A. K., T. J. Headley, R. G. Tissot, B. C. Bunker, Microtubule templated synthesis of inorganic nanomaterials. Biomolecular materials and interfaces. *Mater. Res. Soc. Symp. Proc.* **2004**, *823*, 3–8.
98 Shaw, R. W., T. B. Brill, A. A. Clifford, C. A. Eckert, E. U. Franck, Supercritical water – a

medium for chemistry. *Chem. Eng. News* **1991**, *69* (51), 26–39.

99 Savage, P. E., S. Gopalan, T. I. Mizan, C. J. Martino, E. E. Brock, Reactions at supercritical conditions – applications and fundamentals. *AIChE J.* **1995**, *41* (7), 1723–1778.

100 Clifford, T., K. Bartle, Chemical reactions in supercritical fluids. *Chem. Ind.* **1996**, *12*, 449–452.

101 Bunker, C. E., H. W. Rollins, Y.-P. Sun, Fundamental properties of supercritical fluids, in *Supercritical Fluid Technology in Materials Science and Engineering: Synthesis, Properties, and Applications.* (Ed.: Y.-P. Sun), Marcel Dekker, New York, 2002, 1–57.

102 Sun, Y.-P., H. W. Rollins, B. Jayasundera, M. J. Meziani, C. E. Bunker, Preparation and processing of nanoscale materials by supercritical fluid technology, in *Supercritical Fluid Technology in Materials Science and Engineering: Synthesis, Properties, and Applications.* (Ed.: Y.-P. Sun), Marcel Dekker, New York, 2002, 491–576.

103 Sun, Y.-P., M. J. Meziani, P. Pathak, L. W. Qu, Polymeric nanoparticles from rapid expansion of supercritical fluid solution. *Chem. Eur. J.* **2005**, *11*, 1366–1373.

104 Andrew, D., B. T. Des Islet, A. Margaritis, A. C. Weedon, Photo-fries rearrangement of naphthyl acetate in supercritical carbon-dioxide – chemical evidence for solvent-solute clustering. *J. Am. Chem. Soc.* **1995**, *117* (22), 6132–6133.

105 Hrnjez, B. J., A. J. Mehta, M. A. Fox, K. P. Johnston, Photodimerization of isophorone in supercritical trifluoromethane and carbon-dioxide. *J. Am. Chem. Soc.* **1989**, *111* (7), 2662–2666.

106 Kimura, Y., Y. Yoshimura, M. Nakahara, Chemical-reaction in medium density fluid – solvent density effects on the dimerization equilibrium of 2-methyl-2-nitrosopropane in carbon-dioxide. *J. Chem. Phys.* **1989**, *90* (10), 5679–5686.

107 Kimura, Y., Y. Yoshimura, Chemical-equilibrium in fluids from the gaseous to liquid states – solvent density dependence of the dimerization equilibrium of 2-methyl-2-nitrosopropane in carbon-dioxide, chlorotrifluoromethane, and trifluoromethane. *J. Chem. Phys.* **1992**, *96* (4), 3085–3091.

108 Weinstein, R. D., A. R. Renslo, R. L. Danheiser, J. G. Harris, J. W. Tester, Kinetic correlation of Diels-Alder reactions in supercritical carbon dioxide. *J. Phys. Chem.* **1996**, *100* (30), 12337–12341.

109 Isaacs, N. S., N. J. Keating, The rates of a Diels-Alder reaction in liquid and supercritical carbon dioxide. *J. Chem. Soc., Chem. Comm.* **1992**, 876–877.

110 Bunker, C. E., H. W. Rollins, J. R. Gord, Y.-P. Sun, Efficient photodimerization reaction of anthracene in supercritical carbon dioxide. *J. Org. Chem.* **1997**, *62* (21), 7324–7329.

111 Ksibi, H., P. Subra, Y. Garrabos, Formation of fine powders of caffeines by RESS. *Adv. Powder Technol.* **1995**, 6 (1), 25–33.

112 Subra, P., P. Testin, Powders elaboration in supercritical media: comparison with conventional routes. *Powder Technol.* **1999**, *103* (1), 2–9.

113 Weber, M., M. C. Thies, Understanding the RESS process, in *Supercritical Fluid Technology in Materials Science and Engineering: Synthesis, Properties, and Applications.* (Ed.: Y.-P. Sun), Marcel Dekker, New York, 2002, 387–437.

114 Debenedetti, P. G., J. W. Tom, X. Kwauk, S. D. Yeo, Rapid expansion of supercritical solutions (RESS) – fundamentals and applications. *Fluid Phase Equilib.* **1993**, *82*, 311–321.

115 Reverchon, E. Supercritical antisolvent precipitation of micro- and nano-particles. *J. Supercrit. Fluids* **1999**, *15* (1), 1–21.

116 Dixon, D. J., G. Lunabarcenas, K. P. Johnston, Microcellular microspheres and microballoons by precipitation with a vapor-liquid compressed fluid antisolvent. *Polymer* **1994**, *35* (18), 3998–4005.

117 Dixon, D. J., K. P. Johnston, R. A. Bodmeier, Polymeric materials formed by precipitation with a

compressed fluid antisolvent. *AIChE J.* **1993**, *39* (1), 127–139.

118 Tom, J. W., P. G. Debenedetti, Particle formation with supercritical fluids – a review. *J. Aerosol Sci.* **1991**, *22* (5), 555–584.

119 Krukonis, V. J. Supercritical fluids nucleation of difficult-to-comminute solids. *Paper at Annual Meeting AIChE*, San Francisco, November **1984**.

120 Matson, D. W., J. L. Fulton, R. D. Smith, Formation of fine particles in supercritical fluid micelle systems. *Mater. Lett.* **1987**, *6* (1–2), 31–33.

121 Matson, D. W., R. C. Petersen, R. D. Smith, Formation of silica powders from the rapid expansion of supercritical solutions. *Adv. Ceram. Mater.* **1986**, *1*, 242–246.

122 Matson, D. W., J. L. Fulton, R. C. Petersen, R. C. Smith, Rapid expansion of supercritical fluid solutions – solute formation of powders, thin-films, and fibers. *Ind. Eng. Chem. Res.* **1987**, *26* (11), 2298–2306.

123 Matson, D. W., R. C. Petersen, R. C. Smith, Production of powders and films by the rapid expansion of supercritical solutions. *J. Mater. Sci.* **1987**, *22* (6), 1919–1928.

124 Eckert, C. A., B. L. Knutson, P. G. Debenedetti, Supercritical fluids as solvents for chemical and materials processing. *Nature* **1996**, *383* (6598), 313–318.

125 McHugh, M. A., V. J. Krukonis, in *Supercritical Fluid Extraction: Principles and Practice*; 2 edn. Butterworth-Heinemann Series in Chemical Engineering, Butterworth-Heinemann, Stoneham, MA, 1994.

126 Jung, J., M. Perrut, Particle design using supercritical fluids: literature and patent survey. *J. Supercrit. Fluids* **2001**, *20* (3), 179–219.

127 York, P. Strategies for particle design using supercritical fluid technologies. *Pharm. Sci. Tech. Today* **1999**, *2* (11), 430–440.

128 Stanton, L. A., Dehghani, F., Foster, N. R. Improving drug delivery using polymers and supercritical fluid technology. *Aust. J. Chem.* **2002**, *55* (6–7), 443–447.

129 Mohamed, R. S., D. S. Halverson, P. G. Debenedetti, R. K. Prud'homme, Solids formation after the expansion of supercritical mixtures, in *Supercritical Fluid Science and Technology*, (Eds.: K. P. Johnston, J. M. L. Penninger), ACS symposium Series 406, Washington DC, 1989, 355–378.

130 Domingo, C., E. Berends, G. M. Van Rosmalen, Precipitation of ultrafine organic crystals from the rapid expansion of supercritical solutions over a capillary and a frit nozzle. *J. Supercrit. Fluids* **1997**, *10* (1), 39–55.

131 Kröber, H., U. Teipel, H. Krause, Manufacture of submicron particles via expansion of supercritical fluids. *Chem. Eng. Technol.* **2000**, *23* (9), 763–765.

132 Helfgen, B., M. Türk, K. Schaber, Theoretical and experimental investigations of the micronization of organic solids by rapid expansion of supercritical solutions. *Powder Technol.* **2000**, *110* (1–2), 22–28.

133 Sun, Y.-P., H. W. Rollins, Preparation of polymer-protected semiconductor nanoparticles through the rapid expansion of supercritical fluid solution. *Chem. Phys. Lett.* **1998**, *288* (2–4), 585–588.

134 Sun, Y.-P., H. W. Rollins, R. Guduru, Preparation of nickel, cobalt, and iron nanoparticles through the rapid expansion of supercritical fluid solution (RESS) and chemical reduction. *Chem. Mater.* **1999**, *11* (1), 7–9.

135 Sun, Y.-P., R. Guduru, F. Lin, T. Whiteside, Preparation of nanoscale semiconductors through the rapid expansion of supercritical solution (RESS) into liquid solution. *Ind. Eng. Chem. Res.* **2000**, *39* (12), 4663–4669.

136 Sun, Y.-P., P. Atorngitjawat, M. J. Meziani, Preparation of silver nanoparticles via rapid expansion of water in carbon dioxide microemulsion into reductant solution. *Langmuir* **2001**, *17* (19), 5707–5710.

137 Meziani, M. J., P. Pathak, L. F. Allard, Y.-P. Sun, Nanoparticle formation in rapid expansion of water-

in-carbon dioxide microemulsion into liquid solvent, in *Supercritical Carbon Dioxide Separations and Processes*, (Ed.: A. S. Gopalan, C. M. Wai, H. K. Jacobs), ACS Symposium Series 860, Washington DC, 2003, 309–323.

138 Meziani, M. J., H. W. Rollins, L. F. Allard, Y.-P. Sun, Protein-protected nanoparticles from rapid expansion of supercritical solution into aqueous solution. *J. Phys. Chem. B* **2002**, *106* (43), 11178–11182.

139 Meziani, M. J., P. Pathak, R. Hurezeanu, M. C. Thies, R. M. Enick, Y.-P. Sun, Supercritical-fluid processing technique for nanoscale polymer particles. *Angew. Chem. Int. Ed.* **2004**, *43* (6), 704–707.

140 Pathak, P., M. J. Meziani, T. Desai, Y.-P. Sun, Nanosizing drug particles in supercritical fluid processing. *J. Am. Chem. Soc.* **2004**, *126* (35), 10842–10843.

141 Waner, M. J., M. Gilchrist, M. Schindler, M. Dantus, Imaging the molecular dimensions and oligomerization of proteins at liquid/solid interfaces. *J. Phys. Chem. B* **1998**, *102* (9), 1649–1657.

142 Wang, Y. Photophysical and photochemical processes of semiconductor nanoclusters. *Adv. Photochem.* **1995**, *19*, 179.

143 Quaroni, L., G. Chumanov, Preparation of polymer-coated functionalized silver nanoparticles. *J. Am. Chem. Soc.* **1999**, *121* (45), 10642–10643.

144 Wang, Y., A. Suna, J. McHugh, E. F. Hilinski, P. A. Lucas, R. D. Johnson, Optical transient bleaching of quantum-confined CdS clusters – the effects of surface-trapped electron-hole pairs. *J. Chem. Phys.* **1990**, *92* (11), 6927–6939.

145 Harruff, B. A., C. E. Bunker, Spectral properties of AOT-protected CdS nanoparticles: quantum yield enhancement by photolysis. *Langmuir* **2003**, *19* (3), 893–897.

146 Lowry, O. H., N. J. Rosenbrough, A. L. Farr, R. J. Randall, Protein measurement with the folin phenol reagent. *J. Biol. Chem.* **1951**, *193*, 265–275.

147 Ohnishi, S. T., J. K. Barr, A simplified method of quantitating proteins using the biuret and phenol reagents. *Anal. Biochem.* **1978**, *86* (1), 193–200.

148 Peterson, G. L. Review of the Folin phenol protein quantitation method of Lowry, Rosebrough, Farr and Randall. *Anal. Biochem.* **1979**, *100* (2), 201–220.

149 Foster, J. F. in *Albumin Structure, Function and Uses*. (Eds.: V. M. Rosenoer, M. Oratz, M. A. Rothschild), Pergamon, Oxford, U.K., 1977, 53–84.

150 Sasaki, Y. C., K. Yasuda, Y. Suzuki, T. Ishibashi, I. Satoh, Y. Fujiki, S. Ishiwata, Two-dimensional arrangement of a functional protein by cysteine-gold interaction: Enzyme activity and characterization of a protein monolayer on a gold substrate. *Biophys. J.* **1997**, *72* (4), 1842–1848.

151 Brelle, M. C., J. Z. Zhang, L. Nguyen, R. K. Mehra, Synthesis and ultrafast study of cysteine- and glutathione-capped Ag_2S semiconductor colloidal nanoparticles. *J. Phys. Chem. A* **1999**, *103* (49), 10194–10201.

152 Leff, D. V., L. Brandt, J. R. Heath, Synthesis and characterization of hydrophobic, organically-soluble gold nanocrystals functionalized with primary amines. *Langmuir* **1996**, *12* (20), 4723–4730.

153 Dresselhaus, M. S., G. Dresselhaus, P. C. Eklund, *Science of Fullerenes and Carbon Nanotubes*, Academic Press, New York, 1996.

154 Ajayan, P. M., Nanotubes from carbon. *Chem. Rev.* **1999**, 99 (7), 1787–1800.

155 Special issue on carbon nanotubes. *Acc. Chem. Res.* **2002**, *35* (12).

156 Special issue on advances in carbon nanotubes. *MRS Bull.* **2004**, *29* (4).

157 Davis, J. J., K. S. Coleman, B. R. Azamian, C. B. Bagshaw, M. L. H. Green, Chemical and biochemical sensing with modified single walled carbon nanotubes. *Chem. Eur. J.* **2003**, 9 (16), 3732–3739.

158 Bianco, A., M. Prato, Can carbon

nanotubes be considered useful tools for biological applications? *Adv. Mater.* **2003**, *15* (20), 1765–1768.

159 LIN, Y., S. TAYLOR, H. LI, K. A. S. FERNANDO, L. QU, W. WANG, L. GU, B. ZHOU, Y.-P. SUN, Advances toward bioapplications of carbon nanotubes. *J. Mater. Chem.* **2004**, *14* (4), 527–541.

160 KATZ, E., I. WILLNER, Biomolecule-functionalized carbon nanotubes: Applications in nanobioelectronics. *ChemPhysChem* **2004**, *5* (8), 1084–1104.

161 BIANCO, A., K. KOSTARELOS, C. D. PARTIDOS, M. PRATO, Biomedical applications of functionalised carbon nanotubes. *Chem. Commun.* **2005**, (5), 571–577.

162 BEKYAROVA, E., Y. NI, E. B. MALARKEY, V. MONTANA, J. L. MCWILLIAMS, R. C. HADDON, V. PARPURA, Applications of carbon nanotubes in biotechnology and biomedicine. *J. Biomed. Nanotech.* **2005**, *1* (1), 3–17.

163 PASTORIN, G., K. KOSTARELOS, M. PRATO, A. BIANCO, Functionalized carbon nanotubes: Toward the delivery of therapeutic molecules. *J. Biomed. Nanotech.* **2005**, *1* (2), in press.

164 PANTAROTTO, D., C. D. PARTIDOS, J. HOEBEKE, F. BROWN, E. KRAMER, J.-P. BRIAND, S. MULLER, M. PRATO, A. BIANCO, Immunization with peptide-functionalized carbon nanotubes enhances virus-specific neutralizing antibody responses. *Chem. Biol.* **2003**, *10* (10), 961–966.

165 PANTAROTTO, D., J.-P. BRIAND, M. PRATO, A. BIANCO, Translocation of bioactive peptides across cell membranes by carbon nanotubes. *Chem. Commun.* **2004**, (1), 16–17.

166 PANTAROTTO, D., R. SINGH, D. MCCARTHY, M. ERHARDT, J.-P. BRIAND, M. PRATO, K. KOSTARELOS, A. BIANCO, Functionalized carbon nanotubes for plasmid DNA gene delivery. *Angew. Chem. Int. Ed.* **2004**, *43* (39), 5242–5246.

167 KAM, N. W. S., T. C. JESSOP, P. A. WENDER, H. DAI, Nanotube molecular transporters: Internalization of carbon nanotube-protein conjugates into mammalian cells. *J. Am. Chem. Soc.* **2004**, *126* (22), 6850–6851.

168 LU, Q., J. M. MOORE, G. HUANG, A. S. MOUNT, A. M. RAO, L. L. LARCOM, P. C. KE, RNA polymer translocation with single-walled carbon nanotubes. *Nano Lett.* **2004**, *4* (12), 2473–2477.

169 ELKIN, T., X. JIANG, S. TAYLOR, Y. LIN, L. GU, H. YANG, J. BROWN, S. COLLINS, Y.-P. SUN, Immuno-carbon nanotubes and recognition of pathogens. *ChemBioChem* **2005**, *6* (4), 640–643.

170 GU, L., T. ELKIN, X. JIANG, H. LI, Y. LIN, L. QU, T.-R. J. TZENG, R. JOSEPH, Y.-P. SUN, Single-walled carbon nanotubes displaying multivalent ligands for capturing pathogens. *Chem. Commun.* **2005**, (7), 874–876.

171 CHEN, J., M. A. HAMON, H. HU, Y. CHEN, A. M. RAO, P. C. EKLUND, R. C. HADDON, Solution properties of single-walled carbon nanotubes. *Science* **1998**, *282* (5386), 95–98.

172 HIRSCH, A. Functionalization of single-walled carbon nanotubes. *Angew. Chem. Int. Ed.* **2002**, *41* (11), 1853–1859.

173 BAHR, J. L., J. M. TOUR, Covalent chemistry of single-walled carbon nanotubes. *J. Mater. Chem.* **2002**, *12* (7), 1952–1958.

174 NIYOGI, S., M. A. HAMON, H. HU, B. ZHAO, P. BHOWMIK, R. SEN, M. E. ITKIS, R. C. HADDON, Chemistry of single-walled carbon nanotubes. *Acc. Chem. Res.* **2002**, *35* (12), 1105–1113.

175 SUN, Y.-P., K. FU, Y. LIN, W. HUANG, Functionalized carbon nanotubes: Properties and applications. *Acc. Chem. Res.* **2002**, *35* (12), 1096–1104.

176 MATTSON, M. P., R. C. HADDON, A. M. RAO, Molecular functionalization of carbon nanotubes and use as substrates for neuronal growth. *J. Mol. Neurosci.* **2000**, *14* (3), 175–182.

177 HU, H., Y. NI, V. MONTANA, R. C. HADDON, V. PARPURA, Chemically functionalized carbon nanotubes as substrates for neuronal growth. *Nano Lett.* **2004**, *4* (3), 507–511.

178 CORREA-DUARTE, M. A., N. WAGNER, J. ROJAS-CHAPANA, C. MORSCZECK, M. THIE, M. GIERSIG, Fabrication and

biocompatibility of carbon nanotube-based 3D networks as scaffolds for cell seeding and growth. *Nano Lett.* **2004**, *4* (11), 2233–2236.
179 Chen, R. J., S. Bangsaruntip, K. A. Drouvalakis, N. W. S. Kam, M. Shim, Y. Li, W. Kim, P. J. Utz, H. Dai, Noncovalent functionalization of carbon nanotubes for highly specific electronic biosensors. *Proc. Natl. Acad. Sci. U.S.A.* **2003**, *100* (9), 4984–4989.
180 Baughman, R. H., C. Cui, A. A. Zakhidov, Z. Iqbal, J. N. Barisci, G. M. Spinks, G. G. Wallace, A. Mazzoldi, D. De Rossi, A. G. Rinzler, O. Jaschinski, S. Roth, M. Kertesz, Carbon nanotube actuators. *Science* **1999**, *284* (5418), 1340–1344.
181 Wong, S. S., E. Joselevich, A. T. Woolley, C. C. Cheung, C. M. Lieber, Covalently functionalized nanotubes nanometre-sized probes in chemistry and biology. *Nature* **1998**, *394* (6688), 52–55.
182 Tsang, S. C., J. J. Davis, M. L. H. Green, H. A. O. Hill, Y. C. Leung, P. J. Sadler, Immobilization of small proteins in carbon nanotubes – High-resolution transmission electron-microscopy study and catalytic activity. *J. Chem. Soc., Chem. Commun.* **1995**, (17), 1803–1804.
183 Davis, J. J., M. L. H. Green, H. A. O. Hill, Y. C. Leung, P. J. Sadler, J. Sloan, A. V. Xavier, S. C. Tsang, The immobilisation of proteins in carbon nanotubes. *Inorg. Chim. Acta* **1997**, *272* (1–2), 261–266.
184 Tsang, S. C., Z. Guo, Y. K. Chen, M. L. H. Green, H. A. O. Hill, T. W. Hambley, P. J. Sadler, Immobilization of platinated and iodinated oligonucleotides on carbon nanotubes. *Angew. Chem. Int. Ed.* **1997**, *36* (20), 2198–2200.
185 Guo, Z., P. J. Sadler, S. C. Tsang, Immobilization and visualization of DNA and proteins on carbon nanotubes. *Adv. Mater.* **1998**, *10* (9), 701–703.
186 Balavoine, F., P. Schultz, C. Richard, V. Mallouh, T. W. Ebbesen, C. Mioskowski, Helical crystallization of proteins on carbon nanotubes: A first step towards the development of new biosensors. *Angew. Chem. Int. Ed.* **1999**, *38* (13/14), 1912–1915.
187 Shim, M., N. W. S. Kam, R. J. Chen, Y. Li, H. Dai, Functionalization of carbon nanotubes for biocompatibility and biomolecular recognition. *Nano Lett.* **2002**, *2* (4), 285–288.
188 Azamian, B. R., J. J. Davis, K. S. Coleman, C. B. Bagshaw, M. L. H. Green, Bioelectrochemical single-walled carbon nanotubes. *J. Am. Chem. Soc.* **2002**, *124* (43), 12664–12665.
189 Lin, Y., L. F. Allard, Y.-P. Sun, Protein-affinity of single-walled carbon nanotubes in water. *J. Phys. Chem. B* **2004**, *108* (12), 3760.
190 Rege, K., N. R. Raravikar, D.-Y. Kim, L. S. Schadler, P. M. Ajayan, J. S. Dordick, Enzyme-polymer-single walled carbon nanotube composites as biocatalytic films. *Nano Lett.* **2003**, *3* (6), 829–832.
191 Karajanagi, S. S., A. A. Vertegel, R. S. Kane, J. S. Dordick, Structure and function of enzymes adsorbed onto single-walled carbon nanotubes. *Langmuir* **2004**, *20* (26), 11594–11599.
192 Dai, H., Carbon nanotubes: Synthesis, integration, and properties. *Acc. Chem. Res.* **2002**, *35* (12), 1035–1044.
193 Tans, S. J., A. R. M. Verschueren, C. Dekker, Room temperature transistor based on a single carbon nanotube. *Nature* **1998**, *393* (6680), 49–52.
194 Kong, J., N. R. Franklin, C. Zhou, M. G. Chapline, S. Peng, K. Cho, H. Dai, Nanotube molecular wires as chemical sensors. *Science* **2000**, *287* (5453), 622–625.
195 Avouris, P. Carbon nanotube electronics and optoelectronics. *MRS Bull.* **2004**, *29* (6), 403–410.
196 Boussaad, S., N. J. Tao, R. Zhang, T. Hopson, L. A. Nagahara, *In situ* detection of cytochrome c adsorption with single walled carbon nanotube device. *Chem. Commun.* **2003**, (13), 1502–1503.
197 Besteman, K., J.-O. Lee, F. G. M. Wiertz, H. A. Heering, C. Dekker,

Enzyme-coated carbon nanotubes as single-molecule biosensors. *Nano Lett.* **2003**, *3* (6), 727–730.

198 Chen, R. J., H. C. Choi, S. Bangsaruntip, E. Yenilmez, X. Tang, Q. Wang, Y.-L. Chang, H. Dai, An investigation of the mechanisms of electronic sensing of protein adsorption on carbon nanotube devices. *J. Am. Chem. Soc.* **2004**, *126* (5), 1563–1568.

199 Sadana, A. Protein adsorption and inactivation on surfaces – Influence of heterogeneities. *Chem. Rev.* **1992**, *92* (8), 1799–1818.

200 Vermette, P., L. Meagher, Interactions of phospholipid- and poly(ethylene glycol)-modified surfaces with biological systems: Relation to physico-chemical properties and mechanisms. *Colloids Surf. B* **2003**, *28* (2–3), 153–198.

201 O'Connell, M. J., S. M. Bachilo, C. B. Huffman, V. C. Moore, M. S. Strano, E. H. Haroz, K. L. Rialon, P. J. Boul, W. H. Noon, C. Kittrell, J. Ma, R. H. Hauge, R. B. Weisman, R. E. Smalley, Band gap fluorescence from individual single-walled carbon nanotubes. *Science* **2002**, *297* (5581), 593–596.

202 Wang, S., E. S. Humphreys, S.-Y. Chung, D. F. Delduco, S. R. Lustig, H. Wang, K. N. Parker, N. W. Rizzo, S. Subramoney, Y.-M. Chiang, A. Jagota, Peptides with selective affinity for carbon nanotubes. *Nat. Mater.* **2003**, *2* (3), 196–200.

203 Dieckmann, G. R., A. B. Dalton, P. A. Johnson, J. Razal, J. Chen, G. M. Giordano, E. Munoz, I. H. Musselman, R. H. Baughman, R. K. Draper, Controlled assembly of carbon nanotubes by designed amphiphilic peptide helices. *J. Am. Chem. Soc.* **2003**, *125* (7), 1770–1777.

204 Zorbas, V., A. Ortiz-Acevedo, A. B. Dalton, M. M. Yoshida, G. R. Dieckmann, R. K. Draper, R. H. Baughman, M. Jose-Yacaman, I. H. Musselman, Preparation and characterization of individual peptide-wrapped single-walled carbon nanotubes. *J. Am. Chem. Soc.* **2004**, *126* (23), 7222–7227.

205 Liu, J., A. G. Rinzler, H. Dai, J. H. Hafner, R. K. Bradley, P. J. Boul, A. Lu, T. Iverson, K. Shelimov, C. B. Huffman, F. Rodriguez-Macias, Y. S. Shon, T. R. Lee, D. T. Colbert, R. E. Smalley, Fullerene pipes. *Science* **1998**, *280* (5367), 1253–1256.

206 Hu, H., P. Bhowmik, B. Zhao, M. A. Hamon, M. E. Itkis, R. C. Haddon, Determination of the acidic sites of purified single-walled carbon nanotubes by acid-base titration. *Chem. Phys. Lett.* **2001**, *345* (1–2), 25–28.

207 Mawhinney, D. B., V. Naumenko, A. Kuznetsova, J. T. Yates, J. Liu, R. E. Smalley, Surface defect site density on single walled carbon nanotubes by titration. *Chem. Phys. Lett.* **2000**, *324* (1–3), 213–216.

208 Kong, J., H. Dai, Full and modulated chemical gating of individual carbon nanotubes by organic amine compounds. *J. Phys. Chem. B* **2001**, *105* (15), 2890–2893.

209 Basiuk, E. V., V. A. Basiuk, J. G. Banuelos, J. M. Saniger-Blesa, V. A. Pokrovskiy, T. Y. Gromovoy, A. V. Mischanchuk, B. G. Mischanchuk, Interaction of oxidized single-walled carbon nanotubes with vaporous aliphatic amines. *J. Phys. Chem. B* **2002**, *106* (7), 1588–1597.

210 Chattopadhyay, D., I. Galeska, F. Papadimitrakopoulos, A route for bulk separation of semiconducting from metallic single-wall carbon nanotubes. *J. Am. Chem. Soc.* **2003**, *125* (11), 3370–3375.

211 Bradley, K., J.-C.-P. Gabriel, M. Briman, A. Star, G. Gruner, Charge transfer from ammonia physisorbed on nanotubes. *Phys. Rev. Lett.* **2003**, *91* (21), 218301.

212 Bradley, K., M. Briman, A. Star, G. Gruner, Charge transfer from adsorbed proteins. *Nano Lett.* **2004**, *4* (2), 253–256.

213 Huang, W., Y. Lin, S. Taylor, J. Gaillard, A. M. Rao, Y.-P. Sun, Sonication-assisted functionalization and solubilization of carbon

nanotubes. *Nano Lett.* **2002**, *2* (3), 231–234.

214 Huang, W., S. Taylor, K. Fu, Y. Lin, D. Zhang, T. W. Hanks, A. M. Rao, Y.-P. Sun, Attaching proteins to carbon nanotubes via diimide-activated amidation. *Nano Lett.* **2002**, *2* (4), 311–314.

215 Jiang, K., L. S. Schadler, R. W. Siegel, X. Zhang, H. Zhang, M. Terrones, Protein immobilization on carbon nanotubes via a two-step process of diimide-activated amidation. *J. Mater. Chem.* **2004**, *14* (1), 37–39.

216 Dwyer, C., M. Guthold, M. Falvo, S. Washburn, R. Superfine, D. Erie, DNA-functionalized single-walled carbon nanotubes. *Nanotechnology* **2002**, *13* (5), 601–604.

217 Williams, K. A., P. T. M. Veenhuizen, B. G. de la Torre, R. Eritja, C. Dekker, Carbon nanotubes with DNA recognition. *Nature* **2002**, *420* (6917), 761.

218 Fu, K., W. Huang, Y. Lin, D. Zhang, T. W. Hanks, A. M. Rao, Y.-P. Sun, Functionalization of carbon nanotubes with bovine serum albumin in homogeneous aqueous solution. *J. Nanosci. Nanotechnol.* **2002**, *2* (5), 457–461.

219 Monteiro-Riviere, N. A., R. J. Nemanich, A. O. Inman, Y. Y. Wang, J. E. Riviere, Multi-walled carbon nanotube interactions with human epidermal keratinocytes. *Toxicol. Lett.* **2005**, *155* (3), 377–384.

220 Cherukuri, P., S. Bachilo, S. H. Litovsky, R. B. Weisman, Near-infrared fluorescence microscopy of single-walled carbon nanotubes in phagocytic cells. *J. Am. Chem. Soc.* **2004**, *126* (48), 15638–15639.

221 Chen, R. J., Y. Zhang, D. Wang, H. Dai, Noncovalent sidewall functionalization of single-walled carbon nanotubes for protein immobilization. *J. Am. Chem. Soc.* **2001**, *123* (16), 3838–3839.

222 Erlanger, B. F., B.-X. Chen, M. Zhu, L. Brus, Binding of an anti-fullerene IgG monoclonal antibody to single wall carbon nanotubes. *Nano. Lett.* **2001**, *1* (9), 465–467.

223 Star, A., J. C. P. Gabriel, K. Bradley, G. Gruner, Electronic detection of specific protein binding using nanotube FET device. *Nano Lett.* **2003**, *3* (4), 459–463.

224 Huang, W., S. Fernando, L. F. Allard, Y.-P. Sun, Solubilization of single-walled carbon nanotubes with diamine-terminated oligomeric poly(ethylene glycol) in different functionalization reactions. *Nano Lett.* **2003**, *3* (4), 565–568.

225 Fernando, K. A. S., Y. Lin, Y.-P. Sun, High aqueous solubility of functionalized single-walled carbon nanotubes. *Langmuir* **2004**, *20* (11), 4777–4778.

226 Lin, Y., A. M. Rao, B. Sadanadan, E. A. Kenik, Y.-P. Sun, Functionalizing multiple-walled carbon nanotubes with aminopolymers. *J. Phys. Chem. B* **2002**, *106* (6), 1294–1298.

227 Lin, Y., B. Zhou, K. A. S. Fernando, P. Liu, L. F. Allard, Y.-P. Sun, Polymeric carbon nanocomposites from carbon nanotubes functionalized with matrix polymer. *Macromolecules* **2003**, *36* (19), 7199–7204.

228 Uhrich, K. E., S. M. Cannizzaro, R. S. Langer, K. M. Shakesheff, Polymeric systems for controlled drug release. *Chem. Rev.* **1999**, *99* (11), 3181–3198.

229 Wang, J., G. Liu, M. R. Jan, Ultrasensitive electrical biosensing of proteins and DNA: Carbon-nanotube derived amplification of the recognition and transduction events. *J. Am. Chem. Soc.* **2004**, *126* (10), 3010–3011.

230 Hasegawa, T., T. Fujisawa, M. Numata, M. Umeda, T. Matsumoto, T. Kimura, S. Okumura, K. Sakurai, S. Shinkai, Single-walled carbon nanotubes acquire a specific lectin-affinity through supramolecular wrapping with lactose-appended schizophyllan. *Chem. Commun.* **2004**, (19), 2150–2151.

231 Matsuura, K., K. Hayashi, N. Kimizuka, Lectin-mediated supramolecular junctions of galactose-derivatized single-walled carbon nanotubes. *Chem. Lett.* **2003**, *32* (3), 212–213.

232 Chen, X., G. S. Lee, A. Zettl, C. R. Bertozzi, Biomimetic engineering of carbon nanotubes by cell surface mucin mimics. *Angew. Chem. Int. Ed.* **2004**, *43* (45), 6112–6116.

233 Patolsky, F., Y. Weizmann, I. Willner, Long range electrical contacting of redox enzymes by SWCNT connectors. *Angew. Chem. Int. Ed.* **2004**, *43* (16), 2113–2117.

8
Stabilization and Functionalization of Metallic Nanoparticles: the Peptide Route

Raphaël Lévy and R. Christopher Doty

8.1
Introduction

Gold and silver nanoparticles have attracted a great deal of recent attention due to their potential use in a numerous applications such as biosensing, bottom-up assembly of nanodevices, and catalysis. The advantages of these particles include easy, non-toxic synthesis and chemical modification protocols, and outstanding optical properties that enable single-particle detection with no blinking or bleaching. Many of these applications depend crucially on the stabilization and functionalization of metal nanoparticles with adequate capping ligands.

This chapter begins with a discussion of aqueous synthesis protocols for different shapes and sizes of gold and silver nanoparticles, and various strategies to transfer nanoparticles synthesized in organic solvents into water. As the nanoparticle size increases, the dominant optical characteristic changes from fluorescence to absorbance to scattering. For each regime there is an optical technique capable of achieving single-particle detection. The role of Au nanoparticles in DNA sensing is discussed along with the use of DNA and proteins to assemble Au nanoparticles into discrete structures. Long-range ordering of Au nanoparticles on two-dimensional (2D) protein crystal templates is presented as an alternative assembly method. The chapter continues with a description of stabilization and functionalization of metallic nanoparticles using peptides. The concept of a peptide toolbox for bionanotechnology containing capping ligands, recognition and self-assembly motifs is introduced. The interaction of amino acids, peptides and proteins with gold and silver is briefly reviewed. Rational and combinatorial designs of peptides provide capping ligands to convert nanoparticles into protein-like materials. A major advantage of the peptide route is that stabilization and functionalization are achieved in a single step. A wide variety of functions can be easily transferred to the nanoparticles using peptides with extensions. Furthermore, their protein-like properties open up new possibilities to purify and handle nanoparticles and prepare conjugates with a defined number of recognition groups per particle. Finally, some remarkable properties of peptides that have not yet been used in the context of nanoparticles are presented.

Nanotechnologies for the Life Sciences Vol. 1
Biofunctionalization of Nanomaterials. Edited by Challa S. S. R. Kumar

ISBN: 3-527-31381-8

8.2
Metallic Nanoparticles – An Overview

8.2.1
Metallic Nanoparticles – Preparation

While fluorescence from semiconductor nanocrystals ranging from the UV to the near-IR is best achieved with particles less than 10 nm in diameter, sizes easily obtained by syntheses in organic solvents, metal nanocrystals need to be greater than 30 or 40 nm in diameter to take advantage of their light-scattering properties. This is too large for synthesis in organic solvents, but an aqueous synthesis utilizing sodium citrate as both reducing agent and electrostatic stabilizer can produce Au nanocrystals between 10 and 150 nm in diameter [1]. For reproducible, quantitative results, nanocrystals need to be monodisperse in both size and shape. Unfortunately, the citrate-reduction synthesis gives highly polydisperse results for nanocrystals greater than ca. 30 nm in diameter. Recent work using 12 nm citrate-stabilized Au nanocrystals as seeds for the growth of larger nanocrystals has allowed the synthesis of monodisperse, spherical nanocrystals, with diameters between 30 and 110 nm, and monodisperse, ellipsoidal nanorods of similar size [2, 3] (Fig. 8.1A).

Gold nanoparticles in the shape of rods, rectangles, cubes, triangles, hexagons, and branched structures can be synthesized in very high yield by varying the ratios of an interdependent mixture of small Au nanoparticle seeds, cetyltrimethylammonium bromide (CTAB), $HAuCl_4$, $AgNO_3$, and ascorbic acid [4–6] (Fig. 8.1B–D). For some shapes, especially rods, the presence of Ag^+ was essential for their synthesis in high yield. The precise role of the Ag ions is unknown, but it is believed that an interaction with the Br ions of CTAB affects either the surface of the Au nanoparticle or the shape of the CTAB template.

Although tremendous advances have been made in the synthesis of large, water-soluble Au nanocrystals, the same cannot be said for Ag nanocrystals. Silver oxidizes much more readily than Au, and the larger van der Waal's attraction between Ag spheres compared with Au spheres reduces the effectiveness of electrostatic repulsion as a method of stabilization. Thus far, this problem has been solved by depositing Au around the Ag nanocrystal, much like the seeded growth syntheses mentioned above, to reduce oxidation of the Ag surface. In monolayer and bilayer quantities, this does not affect the absorption or light-scattering properties of the original Ag core [7].

Silver nanoparticles have also been synthesized as rods, wires, and triangular prisms – the first two shapes by a very similar procedure to that used to obtain Au nanorods [8]. Silver nanoparticle seeds (4 nm diameter) were added to a growth solution containing $AgNO_3$, CTAB, and ascorbic acid. The pH was then increased with NaOH to enable the ascorbic acid to reduce the Ag ions. The ratio of nanoparticle seeds to Ag ions and the pH are key factors in determining whether rods or wires are produced. Nanorods can be synthesized reproducibly with aspect ratios between 2.5 and 15 for widths of 10 to 15 nm. Nanowires of similar width and up

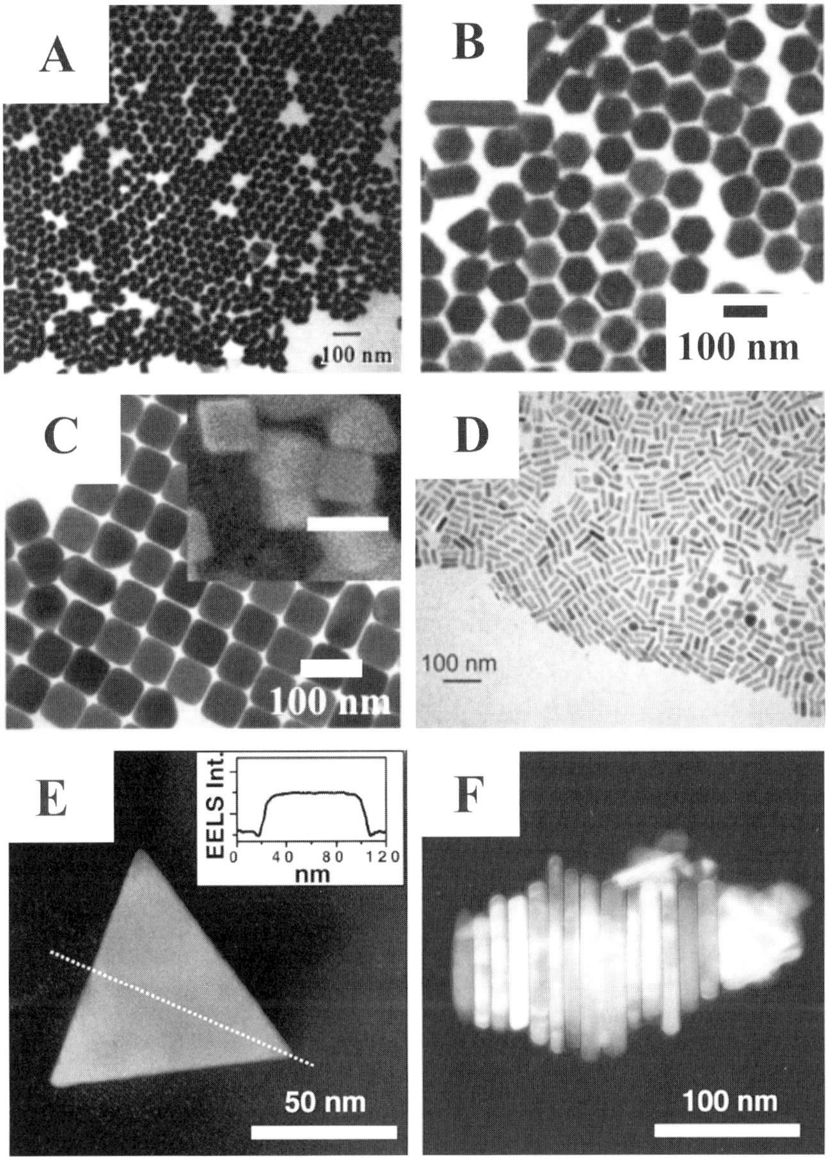

Fig. 8.1. Transmission electron microscope (TEM) images of (A) 37 nm Au spheres, (B) 70 nm Au hexagons, (C) 90 nm Au cubes, (D) 50 × 15 nm Au rods, and (E) and (F) 100 nm Ag prisms. The inset to (C) is a scanning electron microscope image showing the three-dimensional nature of the Au cubes. Inset to (E) is an electron energy loss spectroscopy scan, showing that the Ag prisms are flat on top and not shaped like pyramids. This is also displayed in (F), where several Ag prisms are stacked together. (A) reprinted with permission from [3]. Copyright (2001) by the American Chemical Society (ACS). (B) and (C) reprinted with permission from [6]. Copyright (2004) by the ACS. (D) reprinted with permission from [5]. Copyright (2004) by the ACS. (D) and (E) reprinted with permission from [9]. Copyright (2001) by the AAAS.

to 4 mm long have been produced. The many spherical Ag nanoparticles produced along with the nanorods and nanowires must be removed by centrifugation. Triangular prisms have been synthesized in very high yield by the photoinduced conversion of spherical Ag nanoparticles [9]. A solution containing 8 nm citrate-stabilized Ag nanoparticles and a particle stabilizing agent were irradiated with a 40 W fluorescent light for 3 days. The spherical nanoparticles were gradually converted into nanoprisms with an edge length of 100 nm [Fig. 8.1(E) and 8.1(F)].

In addition to synthesis in aqueous solutions, nanoparticles can be synthesized in organic solvents and transferred into the aqueous phase via ligand-exchange. Solubilization via ligand-exchange requires displacement of the hydrophobic molecule attached to the nanoparticle surface by a hydrophilic one, usually a carboxylic acid-terminated molecule [10, 11]. A particularly good example of this technique is the use of a thioalkylated monohydroxy tetraethylene glycol (PEG-OH) to transfer tetraoctylammonium bromide-stabilized Au nanoparticles from toluene to water [12]. These 5 to 8 nm particles displayed excellent stability between pH 0 and 14 and in 3.5 M NaCl. They also did not aggregate in the presence of proteins. The particles' extraordinary stability is due to the bifunctional nature of the PEG-OH capping ligand. The alkanethiol end forms a strong bond with the Au surface and a tight hydrophobic shell around the particle while the ethylene glycol end imparts water solubility and presents an uncharged surface to the aqueous environment. Gold nanoparticles have also been synthesized in the presence of PEG-OH [12]. These particles had diameters between 2 and 4 nm and displayed the same excellent stability as the larger nanoparticles produced by ligand-exchange. The efficiency of ligand exchange depends upon the relative bond strengths between the two molecules and the nanoparticle surface, and usually requires a large excess of the hydrophilic molecule in solution during the ligand exchange. Unfortunately, this requirement precludes direct attachment of some biological molecules that are not available, or are prohibitively expensive, in such large quantities, e.g. many peptides and proteins.

Another approach to making nanocrystals water-soluble is to encapsulate them in a layer of silica/siloxane via a surface silanization procedure [13, 14]. In subsequent crosslinking reactions, charged molecules can be incorporated into the shell to provide electrostatic stabilization to the water-soluble nanocrystals, or long-chained, hydrophilic molecules, such as polyethylene glycol, can be used to provide steric stabilization. The resulting silica shell has exposed amino, mercapto, and phosphate groups that can be used to further functionalize the nanocrystal surface. While the silica-encapsulated nanocrystals are very stable and do not aggregate in aqueous solution, gradual decomposition of the silica layer eventually leads to nanocrystal precipitation and limits the length of time they can be left in water.

8.2.2
Metallic Nanoparticles – Optical Properties

Almost every application of metallic nanoparticles takes advantage of their ability to strongly absorb and scatter light. This is because they possess a distinctive optical property known as surface plasmon resonance, which is effectively due to the collective oscillation of free electrons. For Ag and Au nanocrystals the wavelength at which this occurs is in the vicinity of 400 and 500 nm, respectively, and is a function of the nanocrystal size and composition, the molecules attached to the surface of the nanocrystal, and the surrounding medium. Many biological applications of metal nanocrystals will rely on their light scattering properties because scattered light can be detected thousands of times more sensitively than transmitted light [15, 16]. A solution of nanocrystals will scatter an incident beam of monochromatic light without changing its frequency, but when illuminated with an incident beam of white light, the wavelength at which the scattered light is a maximum is a function of particle size, shape, and composition (Fig. 8.2A and 8.2B). Through a combination of Ag and Au nanocrystals of different sizes, one can view scattered light of every color in the visible light spectrum (Fig. 8.2C). The particle size dependence of the wavelength of scattered light was predicted by Mie using classical electromagnetic theory [1, 17]. In the Rayleigh limit ($R < \lambda/20$, where R is the radius of the nanocrystal and λ is the wavelength of incident light) the wavelength of scattered light remains unchanged, while the intensity increases as R^6. For nanocrystals outside the Rayleigh limit, an increase in particle size broadens the scattering spectrum and shifts it to longer wavelengths. In general, the maximum intensity of light scattered from an Ag nanocrystal is at least 10× that of an Au nanocrystal of the same size, and the spectral shifts with regard to particle size are more pronounced. The scattering spectra are also affected by the refractive index of the medium containing the nanocrystals. Increasing the refractive index increases the intensity of scattered light and shifts it to longer wavelengths. The intensity of scattered light for Au nanocrystals is enhanced by an increase in the medium refractive index more so than Ag, but the spectra of Ag shift more than those of Au [15]. These effects are important experimentally, because raising the refractive index of the medium increases the signal-to-noise ratio of a particular measurement, by both increasing the scattering from the metal nanocrystals and decreasing the background scattering from dielectric materials. Light scattering from metal nanocrystals cannot be quenched, and the nanocrystals do not degrade under optical excitation like many molecular fluorophores, permitting time-dependent studies. In fact, the scattered light intensity of a 60 nm diameter Au nanocrystal is approximately equivalent to the fluorescent light intensity of 270 000 fluorescein molecules [15]. This allows the detection of a single particle using a simple optical microscope in dark-field mode. The main drawback of this detection strategy is the background scattering from the biological sample and from defects in microscope slides. This background cannot be removed by an emission filter in an experiment where the illumination and detection have to be at the same wavelength, but, as mentioned above, refractive index matching can be effective. To ensure that the detected light comes from a metallic particle, more sophisticated instrumentation is needed in which the scattered light is analyzed using a spectrometer coupled to the microscope or a tunable filter to recognize the characteristic scattering spectrum of the metallic nanoparticles.

While light absorption and scattering are practical detection methods for large

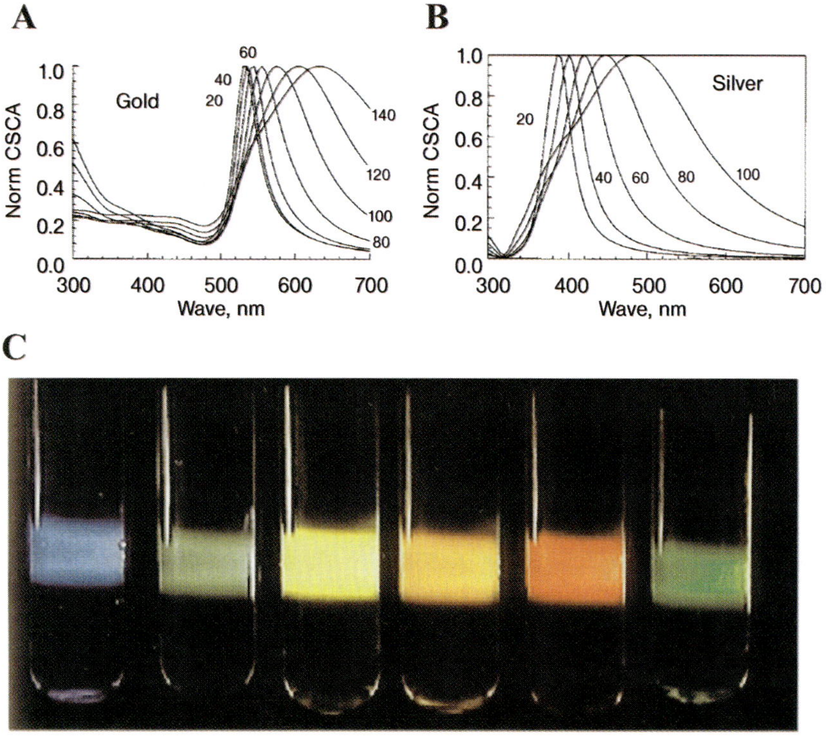

Fig. 8.2. Normalized scattering cross-sections as a function of wavelength for (A) gold and (B) silver nanoparticles of various sizes. (C) Light scattering from aqueous solutions of (from left to right) 40 nm Ag nanoparticles; 40, 78, 118, and 140 nm Au nanoparticles; and fluorescein illuminated by a single beam of white light. (Reprinted with permission from [15]. Copyright (1998) by Academic Press.)

metal nanoparticles, small (diameter < 5 nm) nanoparticles can be detected by light emission. Previous work has shown blue, red, and near-IR emission from water-soluble Au nanoparticles [18, 19]. The exact mechanism is unknown, but it is thought that relaxation of excited conduction electrons into sp- and d-band holes, intraband and interband, respectively, combined with surface effects from the ligand shell can explain the different light emission peaks. Although these nanoparticles show a million-fold enhancement in fluorescence quantum yield compared with bulk gold, the quantum yields (10^{-3}–10^{-5}) are still much lower than for organic fluorophores and semiconductor quantum dots. Recent work on nanodots, however, has further increased the quantum yield of Au one hundred-fold [20, 21]. An eight-atom cluster of Au stabilized by a poly(amidoamine) (PAMAM) dendrimer emits blue light ($\lambda_{max} = 450$ nm) with a quantum yield of $41 \pm 5\%$ [20]. Additional work on 5-, 13-, 23-, and 31-atom clusters extended the emission into the UV and the near-IR (Fig. 8.3), with a quantum yield of 70% for the five-atom, UV-emitting cluster [21]. The quantum yield decreases to 10% as the emission energy decreases from the UV to the near-IR, as a result of increased competition

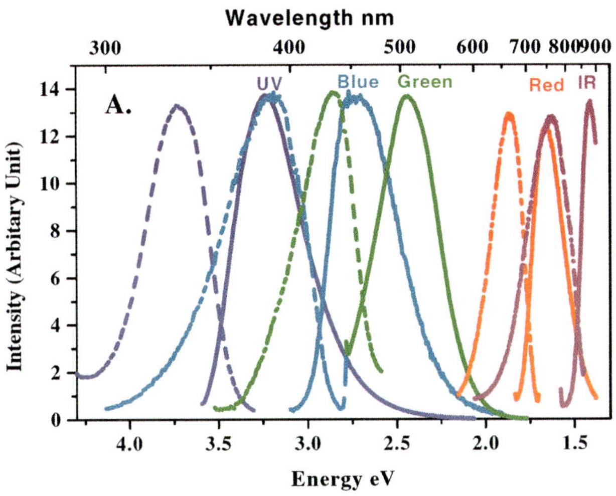

Fig. 8.3. Photoluminescence excitation (dashed lines) and emission (solid lines) spectra for Au nanodots with cluster sizes of 5, 8, 13, 23, and 31 atoms. The emission spectra redshift as cluster size increases. (Reprinted with permission from [21]. Copyright (2004) by American Physical Society (APS).)

from nonradiative pathways. The emission energy scales with the number of atoms, as predicted by a jellium model, indicating that the fluorescence is "proto-plasmonic" and arises from intraband transitions of the free electrons. The clusters are stable over long periods in water, can be stored as dry powders, and, unlike semiconductor quantum dots, their synthesis is easy and non-toxic. Their discrete excitation spectra, however, excludes their use in the single-excitation, multiplexed bioassays for which semiconductor quantum dots show so much promise. However, it does allow them to function as energy transfer pairs and long lifetime fluorescent labels for *in vivo* imaging.

In addition to Au nanodots, Dickson and co-workers have also produced fluorescent Ag nanodots [22, 23]. Silver ions were photoreduced in the presence of PAMAM dendrimers to produce two- to eight-atom clusters [22]. Single nanodot fluorescence was detected at between 530 and 650 nm. Photoluminescence beyond 600 nm was also seen from Ag nanodots formed by the chemical reduction of Ag ions in the presence of oligonucleotides [23]. Mass spectral analysis showed that the cluster size was between one and four Ag atoms. Chemical shifts in the NMR spectra of the cytosine bases suggest that base-specific interactions may play an important role in nanodot formation and that oligonucleotides with specific sequences may be able to control cluster stoichiometry. Unlike the Au nanodots discussed above, the photoluminescence of different-sized Ag nanodots can be excited by a single source, making them available for applications that require a degree of multiplexing.

Particles that are too small to be detected by light scattering and too big to fluoresce with any efficiency can be detected using a recently developed photothermal technique [24]. Called photothermal interference contrast, it relies on the increase in temperature around a metal nanoparticle when it absorbs laser light at the same frequency as its plasmon resonance. Changes in the temperature-dependent local index of refraction can be detected optically using a second laser beam. One benefit of this technique is that it does not detect non-absorbing scatterers. For instance, 10 and 80 nm Au particles were mixed with 300 nm latex spheres and spin-coated onto a substrate. As shown in Fig. 8.4(A), the 80 nm Au particles and 300 nm latex spheres were detected using differential interference contrast. Using the photothermal technique, only the 80 and 10 nm Au nanoparticles were detected (Fig. 8.4B and 8.4C). Nanoparticles as small as 2.5 nm have been optically detected using the photothermal detection system [24]. Another benefit of this technique is that organic and biological samples have a negligible photothermal background. This was shown in the visualization of individual 10 nm Au particles attached to membrane proteins of COS7 cells. By tilting the sample, 3D images of the Au nanoparticles were obtained [25]. Because absorption is used, there is no photobleaching, blinking, or saturation of the metal nanoparticles. One concern with this technique is that the temperature rise around the nanoparticles could interfere with the function of live biological samples. For a 10 nm particle, the temperature increase on the surface of the particle is estimated to be 15 K. This can be lowered by changing the laser power and the location of the laser beams in relation to the particles.

8.2.3
Metallic Nanoparticles – Applications

The uniformity of citrate-stabilized Au nanocrystals, the ease with which the citrate molecules can be displaced from the Au surface, and the unique optical properties of both individual and aggregated clusters of Au nanocrystals are all critical to successful utilization in biological applications. An area of early success was the attachment of thiol-terminated DNA oligonucleotides to Au nanocrystals, in which complementary strands of DNA were used to assemble both dimers and trimers and large, aggregated structures of nanocrystals [26, 27]. The nucleotide-induced aggregation caused a red to blue color change in the aqueous nanocrystal solution. This aggregation is reversible upon heating the solution above the melting temperature of the DNA [28]. In this way the absorbance of Au nanocrystals is used to detect DNA hybridization [29, 30]. A more solid-state approach to the detection of DNA hybridization is to immobilize a strand of DNA on a substrate and flow a solution of nanocrystals containing the complementary strand of DNA over the substrate [31, 32] (Fig. 8.5). The attachment of nanocrystals on the surface can be detected by light scattering. This technique offers greater sensitivity and can detect DNA in the femtomolar concentration range [31, 33].

Complementary strands of DNA can be attached to nanocrystals of different size, shape, and/or composition. In this way, large nanocrystals can be surrounded by small ones [34], metal nanocrystals can be surrounded by semiconductor ones [35], and vice-versa [36]. The challenge with this technique is to control the degree of nanocrystal ordering (Fig. 8.6). Ideally, one would form dimers, trimers, and

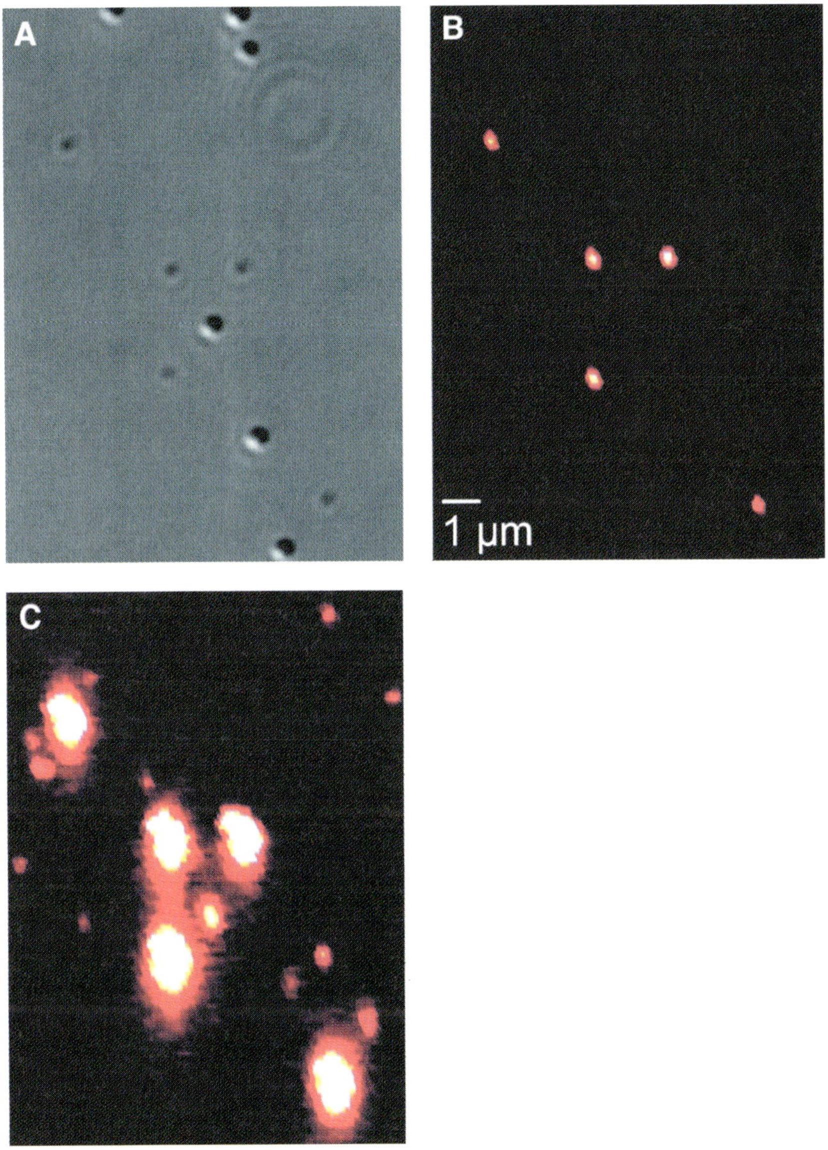

Fig. 8.4. (A) Differential interference contrast image of 10 and 80 nm Au particles with 300 nm latex particles. Only the 80 nm Au and 300 nm latex particles can be detected. (B) Photothermal image at low heating laser power shows the 80 nm Au particles but not the 300 nm latex particles. (C) Increasing the laser power brings the 10 nm Au particles into view. (Reprinted with permission from [24]. Copyright (2002) by AAAS.)

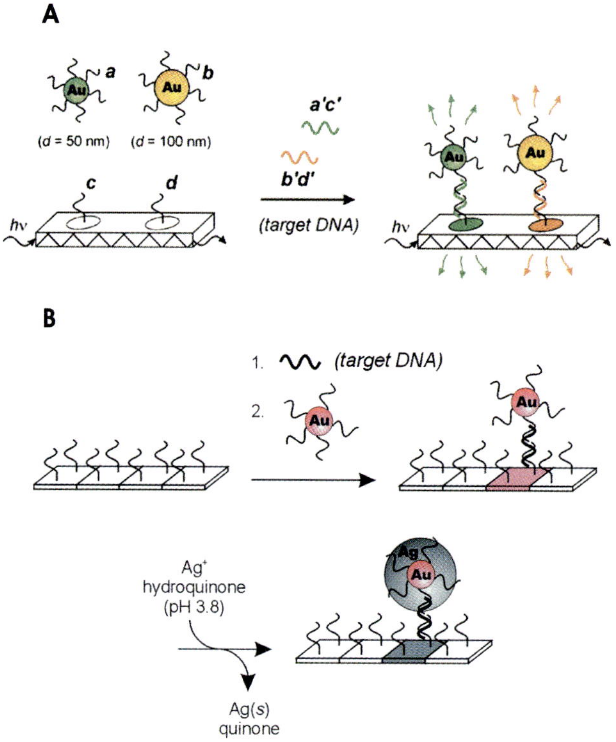

Fig. 8.5. Two different types of three component sandwich assays for oligonucleotide detection. (A) A two-color detection method taking advantage of the light scattering properties of different sized Au nanoparticles. (B) An extremely sensitive detection method in which silver atoms are reduced onto 13 nm Au particles to amplify the signal for detection by a flatbed scanner. (A) reprinted with permission from [32]. Copyright (2001) by ACS. (B) reprinted with permission from [31]. Copyright (2000) by AAAS.

other well-defined structures, such as monolayers and multilayers [37]. However, this requires precise control of the number of DNA molecules attached to the nanocrystal surface, and it is not currently possible to generate a solution of nanocrystals with only, and exactly, one (or two, or three, etc.) DNA molecule per nanocrystal. In a given solution there is a statistical distribution of desired capping ligands per nanocrystal. The challenge then is to separate the nanocrystals with one oligonucleotide from those with two, three, four, etc., which at present has only been consistently achieved by gel electrophoresis [36, 38, 39]. To achieve maximum resolution the nanocrystals should be size-monodisperse and homogeneous in charge, and the DNA molecules should have a mobility similar to that of the nanocrystals so that the attachment of only one or two oligonucleotides has a significant effect on the overall mobility through the gel. Besides being time-consuming and relatively inefficient, the pore size of the gel presents a serious limitation to the size of nanocrystals that can be separated.

In addition to using nanoparticles to detect biological molecules, biological mol-

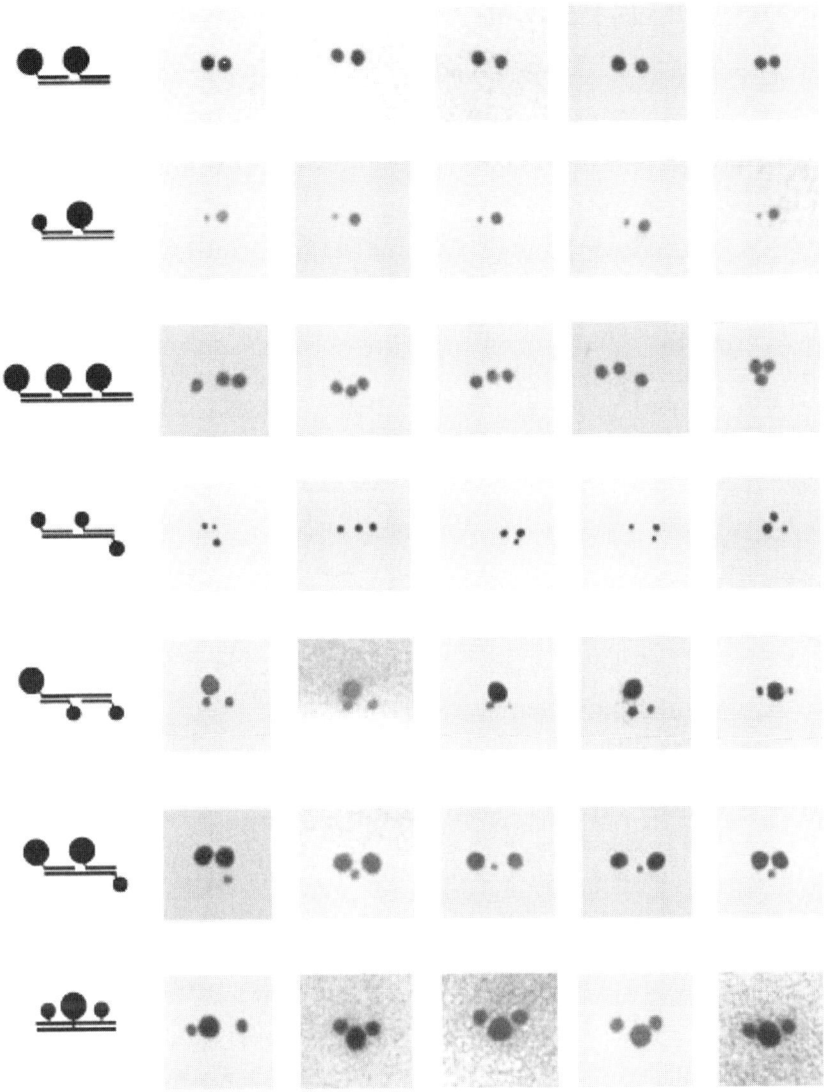

Fig. 8.6. TEM images of dimers and trimers of 5 and 10 nm Au nanoparticles linked by DNA. A schematic of the particular DNA-based assembly method is shown to the left of the TEM images. (Reprinted with permission from Ref. [37].)

ecules can be used to self-assemble nanoparticles into patterns that are not otherwise thermodynamically or kinetically favorable. As discussed in the previous section, DNA has been used to assemble dimers, trimers and much larger aggregated structures. Another potentially powerful, high-yield method for creating dimers, trimers, or chains of nanoparticles involves the use of solid-phase reactions on PS

Wang or HMPA-PEGA resins and Fmoc protecting groups [40]. This technique takes advantage of the low-density packing of functional groups, in this case lysine, on the resins. Thus, a 2.2 nm Au nanoparticle with a ligand shell consisting of equal parts octanethiolate and mercaptoundecanoic acid will react with only one lysine. Protection of the remaining carboxyl groups in the ligand shell with methylamine followed by cleavage of the resin bead leaves a single carboxylic acid on the nanoparticle available for further functionalization. Monofunctionalization was tested by dimerizing nanoparticles with ethylenediamine. The overall efficiency of this process is extremely low, however; only 3% and 15% of the nanoparticles remained after cleavage of the PS Wang and HMPA-PEGA resins, respectively. Of those remaining particles, around 60% formed dimers, with some forming higher-order clusters. To form chains of nanoparticles using this method, the efficiency needs to be much higher, but it is nonetheless a powerful method for monofunctionalizing nanoparticles.

A single biotinylated dextran molecule has been conjugated to 15 nm Au particles through careful consideration of the molecular weight of the aminodextran molecules and the surface area of the nanoparticles [41]. A 2000 kDa aminodextran was functionalized with pyridyldithio propionate to create the disulfide bonds, and biofunctionality was imparted by conjugation with biotin. The benefit of this technique is the stability imparted to the nanoparticle by coating it with one molecule capable of forming hundreds of thiol bonds rather than with hundreds of individual thiol-containing molecules. As proof of this the particles were run through a typical polymerase chain reaction protocol without loss of biological activity. This technique can be expanded beyond biotin to include haptens, antibodies, and oligonucleotides. The number and type of functional molecules per dextran can be altered as required for use in sensitive bioassays or programmed self-assembly.

In addition to the well-known biotin–streptavidin system, antibodies and antigens can be used to link nanoparticles together. Mann and co-workers have shown that Au nanoparticles stabilized by IgE and IgG antibodies assemble into 3D networks in the presence of bivalent antigens [42]. Macroscopic filaments with aspect ratios greater than 100 precipitated from solution when the conformational freedom of the bivalent hetero-antigen was increased by doubling the size of the spacer between its functional ends. They were also able to form bimetallic aggregates by mixing IgE-stabilized Au nanoparticles and IgG-stabilized Ag nanoparticles with a bivalent hetero-antigen. The feasibility of aggregation-based immunoassays has been demonstrated by Thanh and Rosenzweig [43]. At a comparable sensitivity to ELISA, the concentration of anti-protein A in serum samples was determined by following the aggregation of protein-A coated Au nanoparticles with a UV/Visible spectrophotometer.

Thus far, the aggregation-based techniques intended for the long-range assembly of ordered nanoparticle structures have resulted in large, disordered 3D clusters. A template-based method for precise positioning of nanoparticles using S-layer proteins is an interesting alternative [44, 45]. S-layer proteins are found on the surface of prokaryotic (e.g., bacteria) cells and can self-assemble into 2D structures on solid supports. Interestingly, for nanotechnology, the symmetry and lattice constants of

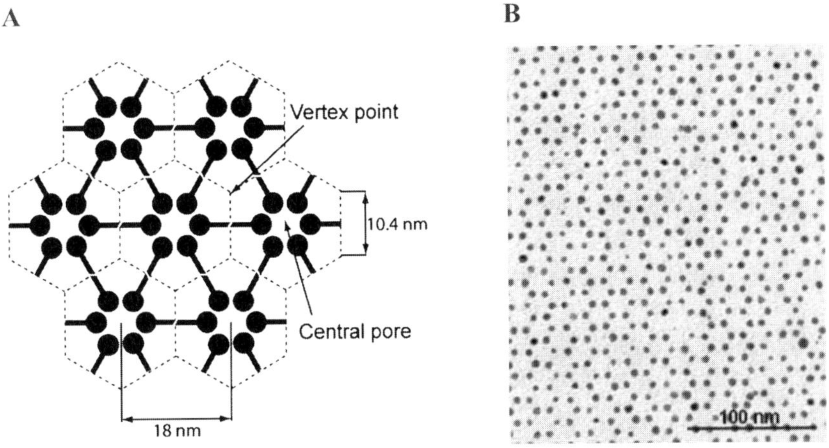

Fig. 8.7. (A) Schematic representation of the hexagonal ordering of S-layer proteins. Protein monomers arrange to form a central pore 2 nm in diameter and 18 nm apart. Vertex points are 10.4 nm apart. (B) TEM image of 5 nm citrate-stabilized Au nanoparticles on the hexagonally packed S-layer. Addition of 25 mM NaCl resulted in the long-range ordering shown. The interparticle spacing is 10 nm. (Reprinted with permission from [45]. Copyright (2004) by ACS.)

the self-assembled structure can be tailored, and the protein units contain identical central pores with diameters that can range between 2 and 6 nm. An S-layer protein investigated recently for long-range ordering of nanoparticles has hexagonal symmetry, a central pore size of 2 nm, and a lattice constant of 18 nm (Fig. 8.7A). Mann and co-workers found that negatively charged citrate-stabilized Au nanoparticles with a diameter of 5 nm formed long-range, ordered assemblies with hexagonal symmetry and a center-to-center distance of 18 nm [44]. The same was true of a solution of 10 nm citrate-stabilized Au particles, except that the particles that bound to the S-layer template were 8.0 nm. They also found that the 5 nm particles bound preferentially to the 9.7 nm particles when a solution containing a mixture of the two was placed on the protein template. Particles larger than the lattice constant of the template only bound randomly to the structure, as did smaller Au nanoparticles with a positive surface charge. While Mann and co-workers were unable to determine if the nanoparticles were located in the central pore of the S-layer protein units, Bergkvist et al. showed that the nanoparticles were in fact located at the vertex point of three protein units [45]. The center-to-center distance of 18 nm was maintained by nanoparticle adsorption to every other vertex point. Adding 25 mM NaCl during nanoparticle adsorption resulted in the occupation of every vertex point and a center-to-center distance of 10 nm [Fig. 8.7(B)]. Nanoparticle adsorption to the protein template is a result of electrostatic interactions between the negatively charged Au nanoparticles and positively charged residues of the S-layer protein, while interparticle separation is controlled by electrostatic repulsions between Au nanoparticles.

Metal nanoparticles could also be used as scaffolds for the self-assembly of enzymes and receptors. Still in its infancy, several proof of principle experiments have been published, mainly by the groups of Rotello and Scrimin [46]. The mobility of thiols on gold surfaces and the possibility to easily make mixed self-assembled monolayers presenting various chemical moieties are key ingredients in these studies. An early example demonstrated that flavin binding sites could be imprinted in a gold nanoparticle supported monolayer containing both hydrogen bonding and aromatic stacking elements [47]. More recently, dipeptide-functionalized nanoparticles with esterase-like activity have been prepared [48]. Confinement of the catalytic units in the monolayer drives a 300-fold enhancement of activity compared with the dispersed monomeric dipeptide, demonstrating the crucial role of cooperativity in these systems.

8.3 Stabilization and Functionalization of Metallic Nanoparticles – The Peptide Route

8.3.1 Peptides, Proteins and Nanoscale Science

Peptides are short sequences of amino acids linked by peptide bonds. When a sequence is longer than 30 α-amino acids, the molecule is generally called a protein or a polypeptide if it is a synthetic polymer. Proteins are biopolymers composed of the 20 natural α-amino acids. Essential components of life, they fulfill the roles of elastic material, enzymes, motors, signal transducers etc. Protein function arises from precisely defined folding of the polymer chain into a 3D structure. Whereas elaborate tasks are generally assumed by large proteins or complexes of proteins (3–100 nm), short sequences composed of less than ten α-amino acids are used by living organisms as highly specific recognition sequences (e.g., cellular localization sequences, enzyme substrate and ligand–receptor recognition sequences).

Understanding the relationship between the amino acid sequence of a protein and its structure is a major and fundamental field of research known as the folding problem. It has wide implications for drug development and discovery. One of the tests of this understanding is the ability to design from first principles unnatural sequences that fold according to predictions. This has been successfully achieved at the level of secondary structures (e.g. helix and beta-sheet) [49–51], while the *de novo* design of catalytic proteins is an emerging field (e.g., Kaplan and colleagues have reported the design of an O_2-dependent phenol oxidase whose structure, sequence, and activity have been designed from first principles [52]).

One of the challenges of nanotechnology is to create nanostructures capable of handling complex tasks. In the nanometer range, proteins are fairly clearly the most advanced devices known. Furthermore, molecular biology offers powerful tools to modify, adapt, purify and manipulate these natural devices. Therefore, two complementary approaches have been taken. The first seeks to modify existing proteins or viruses [53, 54] to solve technological problem on the nanoscale [55],

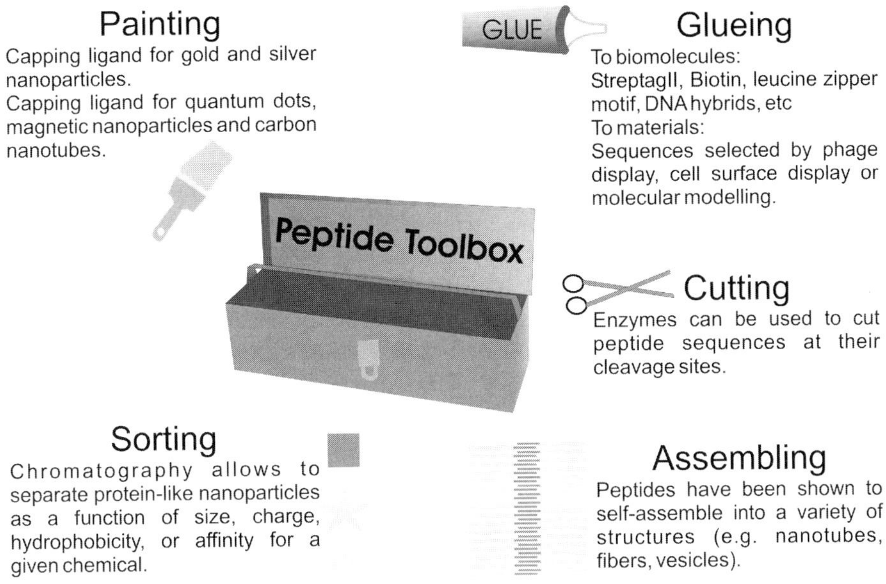

Fig. 8.8. Peptide toolbox for bionanotechnology.

whereas the second seeks to confer protein-like properties to artificial nanomaterials having useful physical properties (e.g., metallic nanoparticles, quantum dots and carbon nanotubes). In the following, we focus on protein-like metallic nanoparticles obtained using peptides as capping ligands.

8.3.2 Peptide Toolbox for Bionanotechnology

Peptides are a large family of commercially available molecules. The concept of a *peptide toolbox* is emerging from recent work. As illustrated in Fig. 8.8, this toolbox contains sequences that can achieve various tasks. Peptides can be used as a capping ligand to control the surface properties of nanomaterials. They offer various affinity pairs as well as binding motifs to synthetic materials. Enzymes can be used to cleave or modify peptide sequences at precisely defined sites. Most powerful biochemistry tools are intrinsically parts of the peptide toolbox and are readily available to handle and modify peptide-capped materials. This includes various chromatography techniques that allow nanomaterials to be separated on the basis of size, charge, hydrophobicity and affinity as well as various well-established bioconjugation reagents. Designed peptides can self-assemble into extended structures from micelles, fibers, and nanotubes to vesicles and hydrogels. The toolbox has only been superficially explored in the context of nanoparticles and their assemblies. Most importantly, peptide-capped nanoparticles may offer a path for integrating various properties into well-defined complex materials. Examples will be given to show that peptide properties can be readily transferred to metallic nanoparticles by using peptides as capping ligands.

8.3.3 Peptides as Capping Ligands

8.3.3.1 Interactions of Amino Acids with Noble Metals

To our knowledge, no systematic study of amino acid interactions with gold is available. However, thiols and amine groups are known to interact strongly with gold. For example, alkanethiol, mercapto- and amino-dextrans have been used as capping ligands for gold nanoparticles [56, 57]. Therefore, as expected, cysteine (thiol on its side chain) and lysine (primary amine on its side chain) do bind to gold nanoparticles [58].

Sastry and co-workers have published several studies on amino acid interactions with metallic nanoparticles (Ref. [59] gives a more complete review). Cysteine, [60] lysine [61] and tryptophan [62] were used as a capping ligand for silver or gold nanoparticles. Lysine-capped nanoparticles disperse in acidic aqueous solution, while aggregation attributed to hydrogen bonding occurs at neutral and basic pH [61]. In addition, water-dispersible gold nanoparticles have been synthesized by the spontaneous reduction of aqueous chloroaurate ions by tryptophan [62]. The same group has used isothermal titration calorimetry to characterize the pH-dependant binding of lysine and aspartic acid to gold nanoparticles [63]. Xu and colleagues have shown that lysine-capped nanoparticles can be assembled into suprastructures through peptide bond formation in the presence of a condensation agent [EDC, ethyl-3-(dimethylaminopropyl)carbodiimide] [64]. Modulation of the lysine to gold ratio allows the assembly of linear chains of nanoparticles [65]. Aggregation of nanoparticles has been seen upon addition of thiol-containing amino acids and peptides [66, 67].

Lysine residues on proteins play an important role in their adsorption onto gold. Xie and colleagues have characterized in detail the use of peptide–bovine serum albumin (BSA) conjugates as capping ligand for gold nanoparticles (BSA contains 59 lysines, of which up to 35 are thought to reside on its surface) [68]. BSA can also be used during the synthesis of gold nanoparticles, resulting in water-soluble sub-2 nm particles [69].

8.3.3.2 Peptides as Reducing Agent and Template in Metallic Nanoparticle Synthesis

Peptides were first used in noble metal nanoparticle synthesis in the seminal work of Schaaff and colleagues in 1998, where the tripeptide glutathione GSH was used to obtain 1.5 nm gold clusters encapsulated in a peptide layer. Synthesis involved the decomposition of polymeric Au(I)SG compounds [70]. Inspired by biological mechanisms for the reduction and mineralization of noble metals, Slocik and colleagues have used a histidine-rich peptide to mediate the formation of various metal, metal oxide and metal sulfide clusters [71, 72]. They have also shown that, in some cases, antibodies can recognize the peptide sequence immobilized on the particle surface. Djalali and colleagues reported that the same histidine-rich peptide immobilized on a heptane dicarboxylate nanowire template was able to control the nucleation and growth of monodisperse highly packed gold nanoclusters [73, 74]. This approach has been extended to the synthesis of continuous platinum nanowires using a slightly different peptide sequence [75]. Two-dimensional arrays of a self-assembled protein complex, chaperonin, have been used for the constrained synthesis of Ni-Pd and Co-Pd nanoparticles [76]. The sub-unit proteins were genetically engineered to expose a large number of histidines inside the solvent-accessible pore of the chaperonin and, hence, promote the binding of metal ions. Sequences selected by phage-display technology for their affinity to metallic surfaces have been used in silver and cobalt nanoparticle synthesis [77]. In an even more elaborate study, the same group has immobilized a silver-binding peptide in the inner cavity of the self-assembled cage protein ferritin [78]. Controlled growth of a silver nanocrystal within the cavity was observed in the presence of silver nitrate. This approach might be extended to other materials using other peptide templates.

8.3.3.3 Rational Design of a Peptide Capping Ligands for Gold Nanoparticles: CALNN

Based on protein folding considerations, we have recently designed a pentapeptide ligand, CALNN, that converts citrate-stabilized gold nanoparticles into extremely stable protein-like gold nanoparticles [79]. Soluble proteins are usually folded in such a way that their hydrophobic groups are located in the interior of the macromolecule, while charged and hydrophilic groups are exposed to water. The pentapeptide CALNN (Chart 8.1) was designed to mimic this architecture. The thiol group in the side chain of the N-terminal cysteine (C) can bind covalently to the gold surface. Alanine (A) and leucine (L) in positions 2 and 3 possess hydrophobic side chains and were chosen to promote the self-assembly of the peptide. Asparagine (N) in positions 4 and 5 is an uncharged, but hydrophilic amino acid due to the amide group on the side chain, and the C-terminal asparagine in position 5 bears a negative charge due to the terminal carboxylic group.

This design proved to be extremely successful at providing peptide-capped particles that are stable over a wide range of pH and ionic strength (up to 1 M NaCl for 13 nm gold nanoparticles at pH 7 and up to 4 M NaCl for 4 nm gold nanoparticles). Importantly, CALNN-capped nanoparticles can be manipulated like a robust protein, e.g., they can be freeze-dried and resuspended in water, purified by size-exclusion and ion-exchange chromatography.

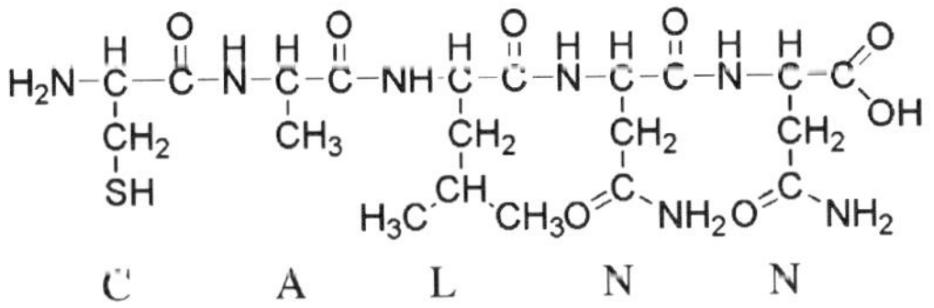

Chart 8.1. CALNN structure.

8.3.3.4 Combinatorial Exploration of Peptides as Capping Ligands: the CALNN Family

CALNN is one of 3 200 000 possible sequences of five natural amino acids, and the remarkable stability that it imparts to gold nanoparticles encouraged us to further investigate its structural basis. Thus, exactly like mutagenesis is used to identify the active domain of proteins, we studied the effect of systematic variations of peptide sequence on stability to achieve a better understanding of peptide capping ligands [79]. The variation criteria were the peptide length, N-terminal amino acid (first amino acid), which when cysteine is likely to be the anchor, the peptide core (second and third amino acids), and the peptide carboxyl terminus (fourth and fifth amino acids). A subset of these peptides induced immediate aggregation of the nanoparticle solution. A common feature of peptides in this subset was the presence of two groups having a strong affinity for gold (cysteine, lysine and arginine) at the two ends of the sequence. A striking example is NNLAC, the reverse sequence from CALNN that has the N-terminus amino group at the distal end from the cysteine and induces immediate aggregation, whereas CALNN is an excellent capping ligand. This exemplifies how subtle changes in peptide sequences can have a dramatic effect on performance as capping ligand.

The effect of the remaining peptides on the electrolyte-induced aggregation of gold nanoparticles was then systematically studied. Quantitative analysis of the experimental data corroborates the initial design criteria, establishing the need for a cysteine as an anchor to the gold nanoparticle, a clear correlation between peptide length and stability, and the need for interaction between adjacent peptide chains through hydrophobic interactions or hydrogen bonding. The balance between peptide charge and cohesive interaction also plays a major role.

8.3.3.5 Peptide-capped Silver Nanoparticles

Despite having superior light absorption and scattering properties, silver nanoparticles have not had the same impact as gold nanoparticles in applications that require work in aqueous environments. This is due primarily to a tendency to oxidize that leads to a complete loss of particle stability, most notably in acidic environments. Also, a higher van der Waals' interaction results in particle aggregation at lower ionic strengths than for Au nanoparticles – a problem for biological applications that take place in buffered saline solutions. All of these issues have been overcome through the use of the pentapeptide CALNN [80]. Addition of peptide to relatively unstable 15 nm citrate-stabilized Ag particles results in peptide-stabilized Ag nanoparticles that are stable between pH 4 and 12 and in 1 M solutions of NaCl. Peptide-stabilized Ag nanoparticles 8 nm in diameter can also be synthesized using a modified two-phase arrested precipitation method. These nanoparticles are also stable over a wide pH range (6–12) and in 1 M NaCl solutions.

8.3.3.6 Peptides as Capping Ligands for Fluorescent and Magnetic Nanoparticles

Similar approaches have been used successfully for the stabilization and functionalization of other types of nanomaterials. Weiss' group has used synthetic phytochelatin-related peptides as an organic coat on the surface of colloidal CdSe/

ZnS semiconductor nanocrystals [81]. The peptides are designed to bind to the nanocrystals through a C-terminal adhesive domain composed of multiple repeats of cysteine pairs flanked by hydrophobic 3-cyclohexylalanines. This adhesive domain is followed by a flexible hydrophilic linker domain to which various bio-affinity tags can be attached, resulting in water-soluble, monodisperse peptide-coated nanoparticles with high colloidal stability and ensemble photophysical properties similar to those of the original, TOPO-coated nanocrystals. PEG-modified peptides were used to improve the accessibility of bio-affinity tags (e.g., biotin). In a recent review focused on quantum dots in biology, the same authors discuss the possibilities offered by a *peptide toolkit* to control surface and photophysical properties [82]. These include switching the emission by using a quencher linked to the nanocrystal through an enzyme-cleavable peptide sequence.

Belcher and colleagues have reported phage display-selected peptides as a template to grow FePt magnetic nanoparticles [83]. The particles obtained are ferromagnetic at room temperature, possessing coercivities up to 1000 Oe and may have some applications in high-density memory devices. Fernig and colleagues have reported the first synthesis of peptide-capped water-soluble cobalt nanoparticles [84]. The peptides facilitated the formation of nanoparticles and partly protected the nanoparticles from oxidation.

8.3.4 Peptide Extensions to Introduce Functionalities

The introduction of specific recognition groups at the surface of gold nanoparticles is an important prerequisite for their use in bioanalytical assays. Peptides having extensions can be used to introduce functions on the nanoparticles surface. Using a peptide mixture containing a matrix peptide (e.g., CALNN) and one or more functional peptides (e.g., CALNN-XXX where XXX is or bears the functional group), particles having a wide range of functions can be prepared. In contrast to most previously reported approaches, the stabilization and the functionalization of particles in this system are independent, but, crucially, both are achieved preparatively in the same step. Therefore, the number of recognition functions present on each particle can be easily controlled and reduced to a single or very few moieties without compromising the stability of the particles [85]. Recently, particles presenting various chemical groups have been successfully prepared by this approach. These include peptide sequences consisting of natural amino acids as well as artificial amino acids and hybrid sequences consisting of amino acids and oligonucleotides.

8.3.4.1 Biotin and Strep-tag II

Nanoparticles functionalized with biotin and with a peptide analogue of biotin (Strep-tag II: WSHPQFEK) [86] have been obtained using a peptide mixture containing, on a molar basis, 90% CALNN and 10% CALNNGK(biotin)G or CALNNGGWSHPQFEK [79]. The nanoparticles were purified from excess peptides by size-exclusion chromatography and immobilized on a nitrocellulose mem-

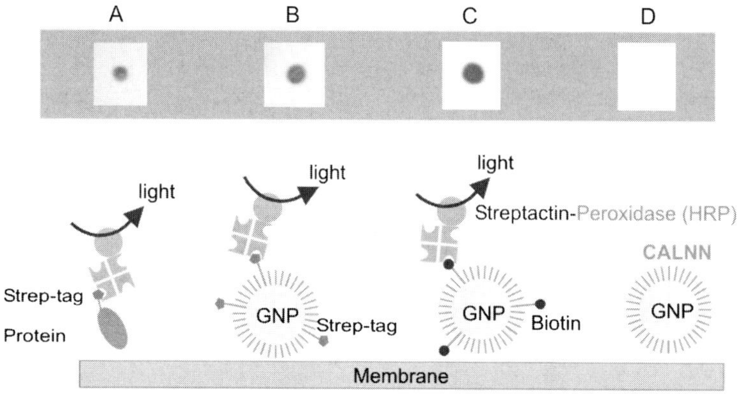

Fig. 8.9. Streptactin-peroxidase specific recognition of Strep-tag II and biotin on peptide-capped gold nanoparticles. (A) Engineered fibroblast growth factor receptor (FGFR) with a Strep-tag II sequence. (B) CALNN-capped nanoparticles decorated with Strep-tag II. (C) CALNN-capped nanoparticles decorated with biotin. (D) CALNN-capped nanoparticles. (Reprinted with permission from [79]. Copyright (2004) by ACS.)

brane. Streptactin-peroxidase was then used to detect the presence of biotin and of its peptide analogue on the membrane (Fig. 8.9). The results demonstrate the presence of functional groups as well as the absence of non-specific binding to the CALNN-capped nanoparticles by streptactin-peroxidase.

8.3.4.2 **Peptide-DNA Hybrids**

Gold nanoparticles stabilized by thiol-modified oligonucleotides have been used for the programmed self-assembly of nanostructures and for oligonucleotide detection. Wang and colleagues have shown that a peptide-DNA hybrid molecule, i.e., CALNN-*DNA*, provides a simple route to DNA functionalized particles. Moreover, the ratio of CALNN-*DNA* to CALNN in the preparation mixture directly controls the amount of DNA available on the nanoparticle surface. The particles retain the stability of the peptide-capped particles. Importantly, this work extends the peptide toolbox to DNA-based assays and DNA-based nanostructured materials. Thus, it is possible to prepare, in a one-pot synthesis, particles functionalized with DNA(s) and other recognition motifs (e.g., peptide recognition motif to inorganic materials). As proof of principle, particles bearing both DNA and biotin extensions have been prepared and detected in a microarray format (Fig. 8.10) [85].

8.3.4.3 **His-tag and Nickel Nitrilotriacetic Acid (Ni-NTA)**

Immobilized metal affinity chromatography (IMAC) is extensively used in biological research to purify engineered proteins having a histidine tag (generally composed of six consecutive histidines) [87, 88]. Nitrilotriacetic acid immobilized on a gel chelates nickel ions that interact specifically with the histidine tag. The relevant proteins are then eluted from the column using a competitor (imidazole) or a pH

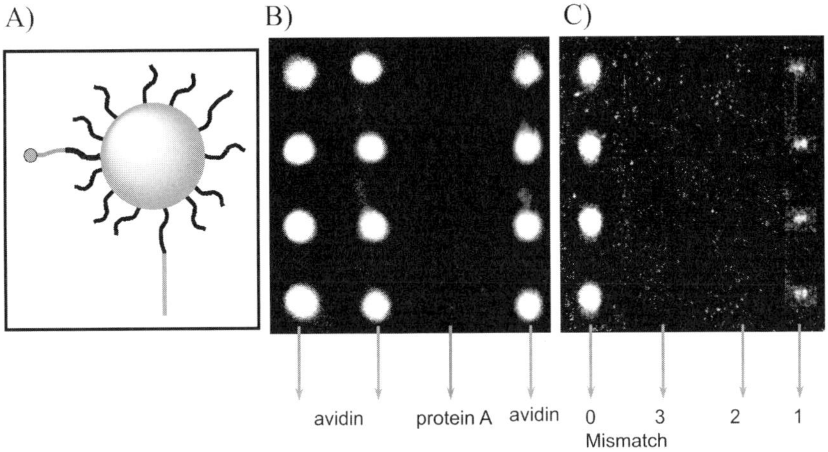

Fig. 8.10. Binding of bifunctional peptide-capped particles labeled both with biotin and DNA on microarrays. (A) Scheme of the bifunctional particles. (B) Dark field imaging of the protein microarray after binding of the particles and silver enhancing. (C) Dark field imaging of the DNA microarray after binding of the particles and silver enhancing. (Adapted from [85] with permission.)

change. A large variety of derived protocols based on this interaction have been developed, e.g., Ni-NTA magnetic beads and nanoparticles [89] for the separation of histidine tagged proteins, Ni-NTA gold clusters for their localization using electron microscopy [90] and Ni-NTA lipids for the 2D crystallization of histidine-tagged proteins [91].

Peptides having a histidine tag extension and peptides having a NTA extension could be obtained by standard peptide synthesis and coupling protocols. This will provide new tools to detect and follow histidine-tagged proteins. More importantly, as described in Section 8.3.5.2, it allows an unprecedented control of quantitative labeling through affinity chromatography and opens a new route to multistep synthesis of nanostructures.

8.3.5 Chromatography of Peptide-capped Nanoparticles

Protein chromatography techniques offer routes to separation based on size, charge, hydrophobicity and affinity. Chromatography media have been optimized to avoid unspecific interactions in the context of protein purification and, thus, are compatible with peptide-capped nanomaterials. This provides a range of protocols to obtain extremely well-defined and pure nanoparticles. Examples of size-exclusion and affinity chromatography are presented below to illustrate the possibilities these techniques offer. Ionic and hydrophobic exchange chromatographies have also been used in purifying peptide-capped nanoparticles.

8.3.5.1 Size-exclusion Chromatography

Size-exclusion chromatography on Sephadex G25 provides a rapid means of separating peptide-capped gold nanoparticles from small reagents, including free peptide resulting from the preparation [79]. This process can be scaled up easily for preparative and production purposes. By using a gel with a higher fractionation range, particles of different sizes can be separated (Fig. 8.11).

8.3.5.2 Affinity Chromatography

Achieving precise control over the number of functional groups per nanoparticle is an important challenge. Its resolution would open up new opportunities to probe the formation of biological complexes and be an important step towards the preparation of well-defined nanostructures. For DNA-labeled peptide-capped particles, Wang and colleagues have shown that the proportion of labeled peptide in the preparation mixture correlates directly with the amount of label at the nanoparticle surface [85]. Therefore, particles having a mean number of labels well below one can be prepared by using a very low percentage of the labeled peptides. In that case, simple combinatorial arguments show that the labeled particles will be mainly particles having a single label. The problem is then analogous to a simple protein purification problem (separation of labeled and unlabeled particles) and can be solved using IMAC (Fig. 8.12). Particles are loaded on a Ni-NTA column, and particles without a histidine tag do not bind, whereas particles having at least one histidine tag are immobilized and then eluted from the column [92].

8.3.6 Recognition of Materials

The peptide toolbox provides various molecular tools for the specific recognition of materials (Fig. 8.13, see p. 260). Phage display and cell-surface display are *in vivo* combinatorial biology protocols for identifying biological ligands. The power of such technologies relies on the size and diversity of the library used, combined with the efficiency of the molecular biology tools in allowing easy identification and amplification of the DNA encoding the selected peptide sequences. Libraries are generated by inserting randomized oligonucleotides within certain genes encoded on phage genomes or on bacterial plasmids, leading to the incorporation of a random polypeptide sequence within a protein residing on the surface of the organism (e.g., the coat protein of a phage or an outer membrane or flagellar protein of a cell). Following the pioneering work of Brown on genetically engineered binding of *E. coli* to iron oxide [93], these protocols have been used to select peptides that bind to various inorganic compounds [94]. Peptides with semiconductor binding specificity have been selected by phage display. Selective binding as a function of crystal composition (e.g., binding to GaAs but not to Si) and crystalline face [e.g., binding to (100) GaAs, but not to (111)B GaAs] was obtained [95]. A hexapeptide with specific binding to the surface of titanium was selected by phage display [96]. Gold binding sequences were selected by cell-surface display, and their folding

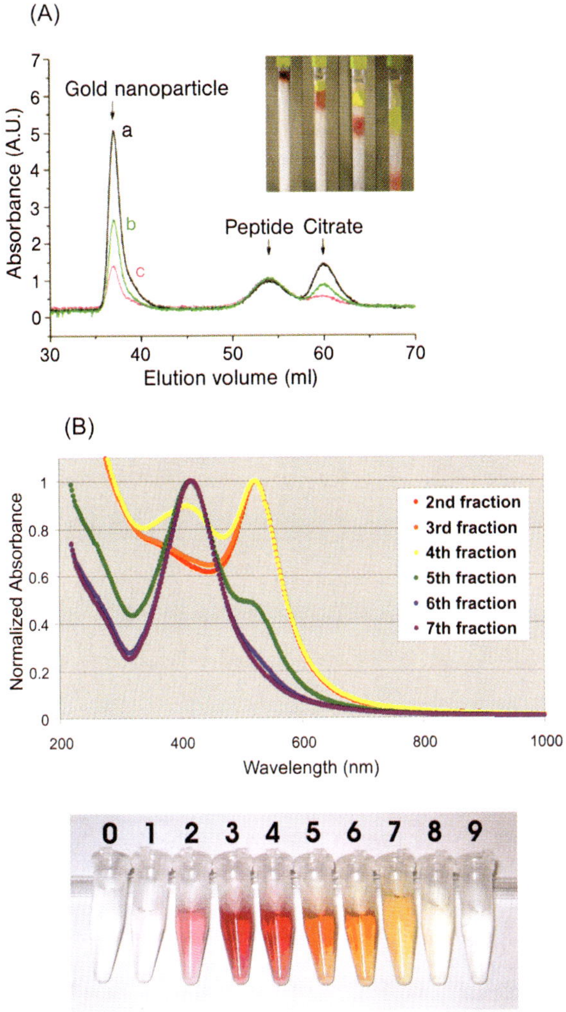

Fig. 8.11. Size-exclusion chromatography. (A) Separation of CALNN-capped gold nanoparticles from excess peptide and citrate using Sephadex G25. Inset: separation of CALNN-capped gold nanoparticles (red, diameter ~ 12 nm) from potassium dichromate. (Reprinted with permission from [79]. Copyright (2004) by ACS.) (B) Separation of CALNN-capped gold nanoparticles from 5 nm PEG-hydroxyl capped silver nanoparticles, (R.C. Doty, unpublished results). Top: absorbance spectra of collected fractions. Bottom: Photograph of collected fractions.

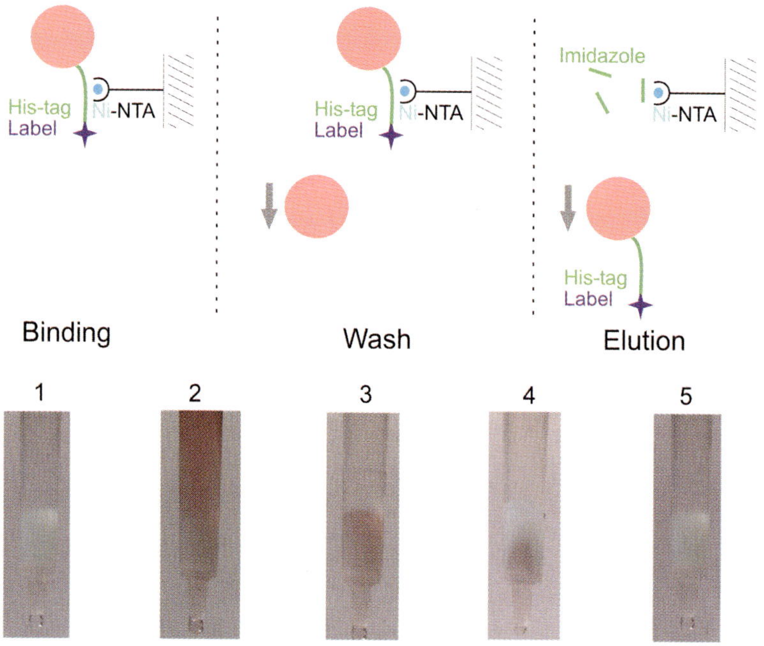

Fig. 8.12. Separation of labeled and unlabeled particles using IMAC (R. Lévy, unpublished results). Top: scheme of the main steps of affinity chromatography. Bottom: 1. Clean Ni-NTA gel. 2. Loading of the labeled and unlabeled particles. Only the labeled particles bind to the matrix. 3. Washing; the bound particles remain. 4. Elution with a competitor. 5. Clean Ni-NTA gel.

in the presence of crystalline gold has been investigated by computer modeling [94].

De novo design and molecular modeling, another strategy for obtaining affinity towards materials, has been applied successfully to the design of a peptide (nano-1) that binds and solubilizes carbon nanotubes [97, 98]. Nano-1 is designed to fold into an amphiphilic α-helix and coat carbon nanotubes. The hydrophobic face of the helix was intended to interact noncovalently with the aromatic surface of carbon nanotubes, and the hydrophilic face was designed to promote self-assembly through charged peptide–peptide interactions.

8.3.7
Peptide-based Linkers

The development of crosslinking systems based on noncovalent interactions facilitates the detection and purification of recombinant proteins [99]. Only a handful of these have been applied in the context of nanomaterials, and new affinity pairs are being developed. The capabilities and versatility of peptide-based linkers are illustrated below for peptide–peptide, peptide–DNA and peptide–synthetic organic molecule linkers.

8.3.7.1 A Peptide-Peptide Linker Based on Leucine-zipper Sequences

The peptide–peptide linker designed by Ryadnov and colleagues consists of three leucine-zipper sequences of *de novo* design: one peptide, "the belt", templates the co-assembly of the other two half-sized peptides, "the braces" [100]. When mixed, the three peptides reversibly formed a predominantly helical and stable 1:1:1 ternary complex. Surface plasmon resonance experiments demonstrated assembly of the complex on gold surfaces, while the ability of the system to bring together peptide-bound cargo was demonstrated using gold nanoparticles derivatized with the brace peptides before the addition of the belt.

8.3.7.2 A Peptide-DNA Linker Based on Metallopeptides

Metallopeptides of the form Cu(II) or Ni(II) Gly-Gly-His are implicated in nucleic acid recognition and reactivity phenomena. Recently, Fang and colleagues have studied the minor-groove recognition of A/T-rich DNA sites by Ni(II)-(L)-Arg-Gly-His and Ni(II)-(D)-Arg-Gly-His [101]. This study has important implications in understanding protein binding to DNA, but it could also form the basis of new assembly systems for DNA- and peptide-capped nanomaterials.

8.3.7.3 A Peptide-Texas Red Linker Obtained by Phage Display

A library of constrained peptides that form stable folded structures has been screened for aptamers that bind with high affinity to the fluorescent dye Texas red [102]. Two selected clones had binding constants to Texas red of 25 and 80 pM. Thus, minimal, constrained peptides can bind to organic fluorescent dyes in biological contexts, allowing *in vivo* imaging with highly sensitive dyes and some degree of genetic control. It also opens up new routes for the assembly of fluorophores and nanoparticles.

8.3.8 Biologically Active Peptides

Numerous biologically active peptides have been identified and their potential as biomarkers and drugs are under evaluation [103]. Moreover, phage-display technology provides novel peptides that bind protein targets with high affinity and specificity, offering many opportunities in drug discovery [104]. A review of natural and selected biologically active peptides is far beyond the aim of this chapter. The following example illustrates the benefits of conjugating some of these sequences to nanoparticles. The nanoparticles can play the role of geometrically defined support for the simultaneous presence of multiple sequences as well as the role of optical label for the real-time imaging of these conjugates. Tkachenko and colleagues have prepared peptide–BSA conjugated particles that carry both a receptor-mediated endocytosis peptide and a nuclear localization signal [105]. The particles' localization was monitored inside cells using a combination of video-enhanced color microscopy and differential interference contrast microscopy, revealing an effective targeting of the cell nucleus. Particles bearing only one of the two signal sequences did not target effectively the nucleus. Kanaras and colleagues have demonstrated the

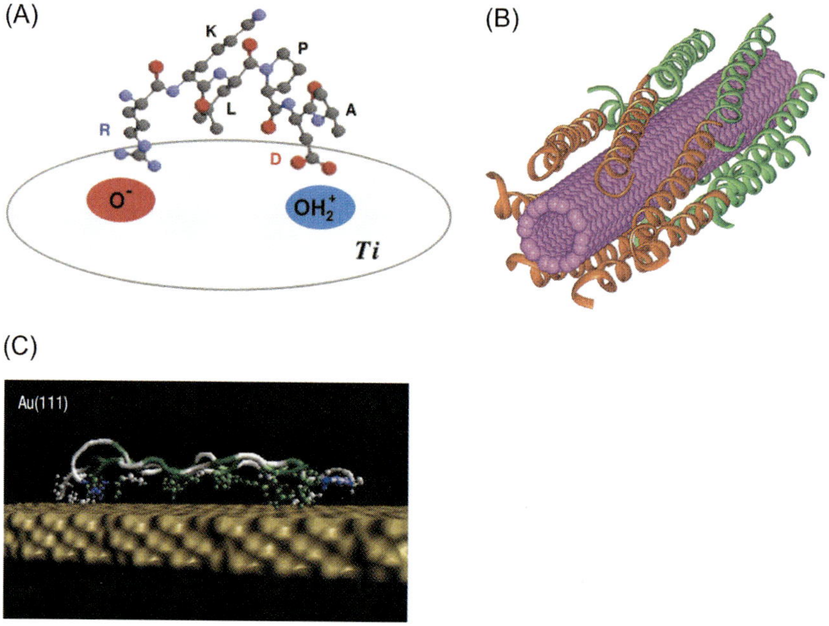

Fig. 8.13. Recognition of materials by selected or designed peptides. (A) Peptide selected by phage-display: model of the RKLPDA peptide binding to the surface of titanium. (B) Peptide designed through molecular modeling: model of the peptide Nano-1 wrapping around a carbon nanotube. (C) Peptide selected by cell-surface display: model of a gold binding peptide. (A) reprinted with permission from [96]. Copyright (2003) by ACS. (B) reprinted with permission from [97]. Copyright (2003)

use of DNA processing enzymes (restriction endonucleases, ligase) for multistep nanostructure synthesis using DNA-protected nanoparticles [106]. Similarly, nanoparticles conjugated with peptide sequences comprising enzyme recognition sites (e.g., proteases, kinases or phosphatases) will offer new perspectives for monitoring enzyme activity and for the controlled assembly of nanostructures.

8.3.9
Self-assembling Peptides

Recently, partly driven by the elucidation of the mechanisms of amyloid fibril formation, a series of articles have revealed the fascinating self-assembly properties of peptides into fibers, nanotubes, micelles, vesicles, and hydrogels (Fig. 8.14) [107–109]. These assemblies exploit various interactions and, eventually, mimic existing biological assemblies. Early work includes the development of biomimetic materials based on self-assembly of ionic self-complementary peptides [110].

8.3.9.1 Fibers and Nanotubes

Alzheimer's beta-amyloid diphenylalanine structural motif has been reported to self-assemble into discrete, stiff nanotubes. Reduction of ionic silver within the

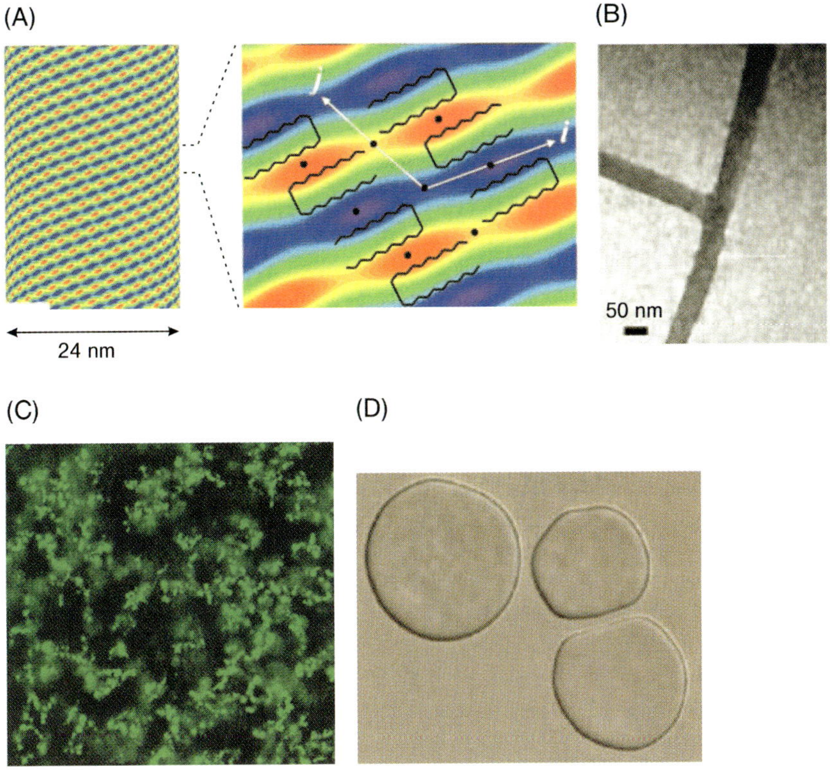

Fig. 8.14. Peptide self assemblies.
(A) Nanotubes: crystalline structure of the wall of Lanreotide nanotubes. Left: two-dimensional Patterson function, indicating the main electron density variations of the nanotubes wall. Right: Zoom of the unit cell, showing the beta-hairpin backbone of Lanreotide. The black circles indicate the 2-fold symmetry axes.
(B) Fibers: TEM image of a peptide fiber containing a proportion of a branch-promoting peptide. (C) Hydrogel: Laser scanning confocal microscopy image of hydrogel microstructure obtained by the assembly of a beta-hairpin designed peptide. Black regions are water-filled pores and channels. (D) Giant vesicles: DIC image of giant vesicles formed by the assembly of amphiphilic block copolypeptide. (A) reprinted with permission from [116]. Copyright (2003) by National Academy of Sciences of the USA. (B) reprinted with permission from [113]. (C) reprinted with permission from [118]. Copyright (2002) by the ACS. (D) reprinted with permission from [120]. Copyright (2002) by the NPG.

nanotubes, followed by enzymatic degradation of the peptide backbone, produced discrete nanowires with a length in the micron range and a diameter of around 100 nm [111].

Woolfson and colleagues have focused on fiber-forming peptides based on the alpha-helical coiled coil, which is a widespread and well-understood protein–protein interaction motif. These peptides form fibers that are over 10 μm long with diameters around 100 nm. Interestingly, a degree of control over their morphology was achieved with mutation-inducing kinks or branching [112–115].

Hierarchical self-assembly of a therapeutic octapeptide, namely Lanreotide, has been revealed at an atomic scale using a combination of characterization techniques (optical and electron microscopies, vibrational spectroscopies, and small and wide-angle X-ray scattering) [116]. This peptide forms hexagonal packing of nanotubes with a high degree of monodispersity in tube diameter (24 nm) and wall thickness ($\sim$1.8 nm). The diameter is tunable by suitable modifications of the molecular structure.

8.3.9.2 **Peptide-based Amphiphiles**

Amphiphilic molecules tend to form well-defined assemblies (e.g., micelles and bilayers) to minimize the contact between the hydrophobic moieties and the aqueous environment. Recent major developments in the design and the structures formed by amphiphilic peptides have been reviewed [117]. Selected papers illustrate the variety of structures formed: One of the attractive properties of these systems is the possibility of easily tuning assembly by external parameters such as the pH and temperature. Kretsinger and colleagues have presented a very elegant way to engineer a stimulus-dependant hydrogel [118]. They have designed a peptide with a pH-dependent intramolecular folding. When folded in a beta-hairpin, this peptide has a propensity to self-assemble into rigid hydrogels with shear-thinning properties and quick mechanical strength recovery. Cryo-transmission electron and laser scanning confocal microscopies revealed a water-filled porous scaffold on both the nano- and microscale. Larger block copolypeptides ($\sim$200 amino acids) have been studied by Deming and colleagues [119, 120]. In the first study, the authors used charged amino acids (polylysine and polyglutamate) as hydrophilic blocks. This resulted in hydrogels at very low concentration. In the second study, ethylene glycol-modified amino acid building blocks were used in the hydrophilic domain to give polypeptide segments with stable α-helical conformations, affording giant vesicles into which functionality could be incorporated.

8.4
Concluding Remarks

With the arrival of new detection systems for metallic nanoparticles, e.g., the photothermal method developed by Lounis and co-workers, restrictions on particle size have been greatly reduced. Previously, single-particle detection was limited to particles with diameters > 30 nm (by light scattering). However, now that particles with a diameter of < 5 nm can be detected photothermally, the emphasis for biological applications of nanotechnology has moved from particle stability to particle functionalization, where it belongs. Peptide capping ligands confer protein-like properties to nanoparticles in terms of water solubility, stability and molecular recognition properties. As a result of their protein-like behavior, functionalized particles can be separated easily from unfunctionalized particles by standard chromatographic techniques, i.e., ion-exchange or metal-ion affinity chromatography. Mixed peptide monolayers on nanoparticles might offer a route towards artificial proteins and enzymes. Peptides offer numerous possibilities in terms of self-assembly, molecular recognition, biological activity, etc., and peptide-capped nanoparticles offer a unique opportunity to integrate these properties into new and complex materials.

References

1 Frens, G., Controlled nucleation for regulation of particle-size in monodisperse gold suspensions. *Nat. Phys. Sci.* **1973**, *241*, 20–22.

2 Brown, K.R., Walter, D.G., Natan, M.J., Seeding of colloidal Au nanoparticle solutions. 2. Improved control of particle size and shape. *Chem. Mater.* **2000**, *12*, 306–313.

3 Jana, N.R., Gearheart, L., Murphy, C.J., Seeding growth for size control of 5–40 nm diameter gold nanoparticles. *Langmuir* **2001**, *17*, 6782–6786.

4 Nikoobakht, B., El-Sayed, M.A., Preparation and growth mechanism of gold nanrods (NRs) using seed-mediated growth method. *Chem. Mater.* **2003**, *15*, 1957–1962.

5 Sau, T.K., Murphy, C.J., Seeded high yield synthesis of short Au nanorods in aqueous solution. *Langmuir* **2004**, *20*, 6414–6420.

6 Sau, T.K., Murphy, C.J., Room temperature, high-yield synthesis of multiple shapes of gold nanoparticles in aqueous solution. *J. Am. Chem. Soc.* **2004**, *126*, 8648–8649.

7 Cao, Y., Jin, R., Mirkin, C.A., DNA-modified core-shell Ag/Au nanoparticles. *J. Am. Chem. Soc.* **2001**, *123*, 7961–7962.

8 Jana, N.R., Gearheart, L., Murphy, C.J., Wet chemical synthesis of silver nanorods and nanowires of controllable aspect ratio. *Chem. Commun.* **2001**, 617–618.

9 Jin, R., Cao, Y., Mirkin, C.A., Kelly, K.L., Schatz, G.C., Zheng, J.G., Photoinduced conversion of silver nanospheres to nanoprisms. *Science* **2001**, *294*, 1901–1903.

10 Chan, W.C.W., Nie, S.M., Quantum dot bioconjugates for ultrasensitive nonisotopic detection. *Science* **1998**, *281*, 2016–2018.

11 Mattoussi, H., Mauro, J.M., Goldman, E.R., Anderson, G.P., Sundar, V.C., Mikulec, F.V., Bawendi, M.G., Self-assembly of CdSe-ZnS quantum dot bioconjugates using an engineered recombinant protein. *J. Am. Chem. Soc.* **2000**, *122*, 12142–12150.

12 Kanaras, A.G., Kamounah, F.S., Schaumburg, K., Kiely, C.J., Brust, M., Thioalkylated tetraethylene glycol: A new ligand for water soluble monolayer protected gold clusters. *Chem. Commun.* **2002**, 2294–2295.

13 Gerion, D., Pinaud, F., Williams, S.C., Parak, W.J., Zanchet, D., Weiss, S., Alivisatos, A.P., Synthesis and properties of biocompatible water-soluble silica-coated CdSe/ZnS semiconductor quantum dots. *J. Phys. Chem. B* **2001**, *105*, 8861–8871.

14 Schroedter, A., Weller, H., Ligand design and bioconjugation of colloidal gold nanoparticles. *Angew. Chem. Int. Ed.* **2002**, *41*, 3218–3221.

15 Yguerabide, J., Yguerabide, E.E., Light-scattering submicroscopic particles as highly fluorescent analogs and their use as tracer labels in clinical and biological applications – I. Theory. *Anal. Biochem.* **1998**, *262*, 137–156.

16 Yguerabide, J., Yguerabide, E.E., Light-scattering submicroscopic particles as highly fluorescent analogs and their use as tracer labels in clinical and biological applications – II. Experimental characterization. *Anal. Biochem.* **1998**, *262*, 157–176.

17 Mie, G., Contributions to the optics of turbid media, especially colloidal metal solutions. *Ann. Physik* **1908**, *25*, 377–445.

18 Wilcoxon, J.P., Martin, J.E., Parsapour, F., Wiedenman, B., Kelley, D.F., Photoluminescence from

nanosize gold clusters. *J. Chem. Phys.* **1998**, *108*, 9137–9143.
19 Link, S., Beeby, A., FitzGerald, S., El-Sayed, M.A., Schaaff, T.G., Whetten, R.L., Visible to infrared luminescence from a 28-atom gold custer. *J. Phys. Chem. B* **2002**, *106*, 3410–3415.
20 Zheng, J., Petty, J.T., Dickson, R.M., High quantum yield blue emission from water-soluble Au_8 nanodots. *J. Am. Chem. Soc.* **2003**, *125*, 7780–7781.
21 Zheng, J., Zhang, C., Dickson, R.M., Highly fluorescent, water-soluble, size-tunable gold quantum dots. *Phys. Rev. Lett.* **2004**, *93*, 077402.
22 Zheng, J., Dickson, R.M., Individual water-soluble dendrimer-encapsulated silver nanodot fluorescence. *J. Am. Chem. Soc.* **2002**, *124*, 13982–13983.
23 Petty, J.T., Zheng, J., Hud, N.V., Dickson, R.M., DNA-templated Ag nanocluster formation. *J. Am. Chem. Soc.* **2004**, *126*, 5207–5212.
24 Boyer, D., Tamarat, P., Maali, A., Lounis, B., Orrit, M., Photothermal imaging of nanometer-sized metal particles among scatterers. *Science* **2002**, *297*, 1160–1163.
25 Cognet, L., Tardin, C., Boyer, D., Choquet, D., Tamarat, P., Lounis, B., Single metallic nanoparticle imaging for protein detection in cells. *Proc. Natl. Acad. Sci. U.S.A.* **2003**, *100*, 11350–11355.
26 Mirkin, C.A., Letsinger, R.L., Mucic, R.C., Storhoff, J.J., A DNA-based method for rationally assembling nanoparticles into macroscopic materials. *Nature* **1996**, *382*, 607–609.
27 Alivisatos, A.P., Johnsson, K.P., Peng, X., Wilson, T.E., Loweth, C.J., Bruchez, J., Marcel, P., Schultz, P.G., Organization of 'nanocrystal molecules' using DNA. *Nature* **1996**, *382*, 609–611.
28 Jin, R.C., Wu, G.S., Li, Z., Mirkin, C.A., Schatz, G.C., What controls the melting properties of DNA-linked gold nanoparticle assemblies? *J. Am. Chem. Soc.* **2003**, *125*, 1643–1654.
29 Elghanian, R., Storhoff, J.J., Mucic, R.C., Letsinger, R.L., Mirkin, C.A., Selective colorimetric detection of polynucleotides based on the distance-dependent optical properties of gold nanoparticles. *Science* **1997**, *277*, 1078–1081.
30 Storhoff, J.J., Lazarides, A.A., Mucic, R.C., Mirkin, C.A., Letsinger, R.L., Schatz, G.C., What controls the optical properties of DNA-linked gold nanoparticle assemblies? *J. Am. Chem. Soc.* **2000**, *122*, 4640–4650.
31 Taton, T.A., Mirkin, C.A., Letsinger, R.L., Scanometric DNA array detection with nanoparticle probes. *Science* **2000**, *289*, 1757–1760.
32 Taton, T.A., Lu, G., Mirkin, C.A., Two-color labeling of oligonucleotide arrays via size-selective scattering of nanoparticle probes. *J. Am. Chem. Soc.* **2001**, *123*, 5164–5165.
33 Park, S.J., Taton, T.A., Mirkin, C.A., Array-based electrical detection of DNA with nanoparticle probes. *Science* **2002**, *295*, 1503–1506.
34 Mucic, R.C., Storhoff, J.J., Mirkin, C.A., Letsinger, R.L., DNA-directed synthesis of binary nanoparticle network materials. *J. Am. Chem. Soc.* **1998**, *120*, 12674–12675.
35 Mitchell, G.P., Mirkin, C.A., Letsinger, R.L., Programmed assembly of DNA functionalized quantum dots. *J. Am. Chem. Soc.* **1999**, *121*, 8122–8123.
36 Fu, A., Micheel, C.M., Cha, J., Chang, H., Yang, H., Alivisatos, A.P., Discrete nanostructures of quantum dots/Au with DNA. *J. Am. Chem. Soc.* **2004**, *126*, 10832–10833.
37 Loweth, C.J., Caldwell, W.B., Peng, X., Alivisatos, A.P., Schultz, P.G., DNA-based assembly of gold nanocrystals. *Angew. Chem. Int. Ed.* **1999**, *38*, 1808–1812.
38 Zanchet, D., Micheel, C.M., Parak, W.J., Gerion, D., Alivisatos, A.P., Electrophoretic isolation of discrete Au nanocrystal/DNA conjugates. *Nano Lett.* **2001**, *1*, 32–35.
39 Zanchet, D., Micheel, C.M., Parak, W.J., Gerion, D., Williams, S.C., Alivisatos, A.P., Electrophoretic and structural studies of DNA-directed Au

nanoparticle groupings. *J. Phys. Chem. B* **2002**, *106*, 11758–11763.
40 Sung, K.-M., Mosley, D.W., Peelle, B.R., Zhang, S., Jacobson, J.M., Synthesis of monofunctionalized gold nanoparticles by Fmoc solid-phase reactions. *J. Am. Chem. Soc.* **2004**, *126*, 5064–5065.
41 Wilson, R., Chen, Y., Aveyard, J., One molecule per particle method for functionalising nanoparticles. *Chem. Commun.* **2004**, 1156–1157.
42 Shenton, W., Davis, S.A., Mann, S., Directed self-assembly of nanoparticles into macroscopic materials using antibody-antigen recognition. *Adv. Mater.* **1999**, *11*, 449–452.
43 Thanh, N.T.K., Rosenzweig, Z., Development of an aggregation-based immunoassay for anti-protein A using gold nanoparticles. *Anal. Chem.* **2002**, *74*, 1624–1628.
44 Hall, S.R., Shenton, W., Engelhardt, H., Mann, S., Site-specific organization of gold nanoparticles by biomolecular templating. *ChemPhysChem* **2001**, *2*, 184–186.
45 Bergkvist, M., Mark, S.S., Yang, X., Angert, E.R., Batt, C.A., Bionanofabrication of ordered nanoparticle arrays: Effect of particle properties and adsorption conditions. *J. Phys. Chem. B* **2004**, *108*, 8241–8248.
46 Pasquato, L., Pengo, P., Scrimin, P., Functional gold nanoparticles for recognition and catalysis. *J. Mater. Chem.* **2004**, *14*, 3481–3487.
47 Boal, A.K., Rotello, V.M., Fabrication and self-optimization of multivalent receptors on nanoparticle scaffolds. *J. Am. Chem. Soc.* **2000**, *122*, 734–735.
48 Pengo, P., Polizzi, S., Pasquato, L., Scrimin, P., Carboxylate-imidazole cooperativity in dipeptide-functionalized gold nanoparticles with esterase-like activity. *J. Am. Chem. Soc.* **2005**, *127*, 1616–1617.
49 Baltzer, L., Nilsson, H., Nilsson, J., De novo design of proteins – what are the rules? *Chem. Rev.* **2001**, *101*, 3153–3163.
50 Ventura, S., Serrano, L., Designing proteins from the inside out. *Proteins-Struct. Funct. Bioinformatics* **2004**, *56*, 1–10.
51 Venkatraman, J., Shankaramma, S.C., Balaram, P., Design of folded peptides. *Chem. Rev.* **2001**, *101*, 3131–3152.
52 Kaplan, J., DeGrado, W.F., De novo design of catalytic proteins. *Proc. Natl. Acad. Sci. USA* **2004**, *101*, 11566–11570.
53 Knez, M., Bittner, A.M., Boes, F., Wege, C., Jeske, H., Maiss, E., Kern, K., Biotemplate synthesis of 3-nm nickel and cobalt nanowires. *Nano Lett.* **2003**, *3*, 1079–1082.
54 Nam, K.T., Peelle, B.R., Lee, S.W., Belcher, A.M., Genetically driven assembly of nanorings based on the M13 virus. *Nano Lett.* **2004**, *4*, 23–27.
55 Goodsell, D.S., *Bionanotechnology: Lessons from Nature*, **2004**, Wiley-Liss.
56 Brust, M., Walker, M., Bethell, D., Schiffrin, D.J., Whyman, R., Synthesis of thiol-derivatized gold nanoparticles in a 2-phase liquid-liquid system. *J. Chem. Soc., Chem. Commun.* **1994**, 801–802.
57 Wilson, R., Haptenylated mercaptodextran-coated gold nanoparticles for biomolecular assays. *Chem. Commun.* **2003**, 108–109.
58 Zhang, J., Chi, Q., Nielsen, J.U., Friis, E.P., Andersen, J.E.T., Ulstrup, J., Two-dimensional cysteine and cystine cluster networks on Au(111) disclosed by voltammetry and in situ scanning tunneling microscopy. *Langmuir* **2000**, *16*, 7229–7237.
59 Mandal, S., Phadtare, S., Sastry, M., Interfacing biology with nanoparticles. *Curr. Appl. Phys.* **2005**, *5*, 118–127.
60 Mandal, S., Gole, A., Lala, N., Gonnade, R., Ganvir, V., Sastry, M., Studies on the reversible aggregation of cysteine-capped colloidal silver particles interconnected via hydrogen bonds. *Langmuir* **2001**, *17*, 6262–6268.
61 Selvakannan, P.R., Mandal, S., Phadtare, S., Pasricha, R., Sastry, M., Capping of gold nanoparticles by the amino acid lysine renders them water-dispersible. *Langmuir* **2003**, *19*, 3545–3549.

62 Selvakannan, P., Mandal, S., Phadtare, S., Gole, A., Pasricha, R., Adyanthaya, S.D., Sastry, M., Water-dispersible tryptophan-protected gold nanoparticles prepared by the spontaneous reduction of aqueous chloroaurate ions by the amino acid. *J. Colloid Interface Sci.* **2004**, *269*, 97–102.

63 Joshi, H., Shirude, P.S., Bansal, V., Ganesh, K.N., Sastry, M., Isothermal titration calorimetry studies on the binding of amino acids to gold nanoparticles. *J. Phys. Chem. B* **2004**, *108*, 11535–11540.

64 Xu, L., Guo, Y., Xie, R., Zhuang, J., Yang, W., Li, T., Three-dimensional assembly of Au nanoparticles using dipeptides. *Nanotechnology* **2002**, *13*, 725–728.

65 Zhong, Z.Y., Luo, J.Z., Ang, T.P., Highfield, J., Lin, J.Y., Gedanken, A., Controlled organization of Au colloids into linear assemblies. *J. Phys. Chem. B* **2004**, *108*, 18119–18123.

66 Pengo, P., Broxterman, Q.B., Kaptein, B., Pasquato, L., Scrimin, P., Synthesis of a stable helical peptide and grafting on gold nanoparticles. *Langmuir* **2003**, *19*, 2521–2524.

67 Zhang, F.X., Han, L., Israel, L.B., Daras, J.G., Maye, M.M., Ly, N.K., Zhong, C.J., Colorimetric detection of thiol-containing amino acids using gold nanoparticles. *Analyst* **2002**, *127*, 462–465.

68 Xie, H., Tkachenko, A.G., Glomm, W.R., Ryan, J.A., Brennaman, M.K., Papanikolas, J.M., Franzen, S., Feldheim, D.L., Critical flocculation concentrations, binding isotherms, and ligand exchange properties of peptide-modified gold nanoparticles studied by UV-visible, fluorescence, and time-correlated single photon counting spectroscopies. *Anal. Chem.* **2003**, *75*, 5797–5805.

69 Burt, J.L., Gutierrez-Wing, C., Miki-Yoshida, M., Jose-Yacaman, M., Noble-metal nanoparticles directly conjugated to globular proteins. *Langmuir* **2004**, *20*, 11778–11783.

70 Schaaff, T.G., Knight, G., Shafigullin, M.N., Borkman, R.F., Whetten, R.L., Isolation and selected properties of a 10.4 kDa gold: Glutathione cluster compound. *J. Phys. Chem. B* **1998**, *102*, 10643–10646.

71 Slocik, J.M., Moore, J.T., Wright, D.W., Monoclonal antibody recognition of histidine-rich peptide encapsulated nanoclusters. *Nano Lett.* **2002**, *2*, 169–173.

72 Slocik, J.M., Wright, D.W., Biomimetic mineralization of noble metal nanoclusters. *Biomacromolecules* **2003**, *4*, 1135–1141.

73 Djalali, R., Chen, Y., Matsui, H., Au nanowire fabrication from sequenced histidine-rich peptide. *J. Am. Chem. Soc.* **2002**, *124*, 13660–13661.

74 Djalali, R., Chen, Y.F., Matsui, H., Au nanocrystal growth on nanotubes controlled by conformations and charges of sequenced peptide templates. *J. Am. Chem. Soc.* **2003**, *125*, 5873–5879.

75 Yu, L.T., Banerjee, I.A., Matsui, H., Incorporation of sequenced peptides on nanotubes for Pt coating: Smart control of nucleation and morphology via activation of metal binding sites on amino acids. *J. Mater. Chem.* **2004**, *14*, 739–743.

76 McMillan, R.A., Howard, J., Zaluzec, N.J., Kagawa, H.K., Mogul, R., Li, Y.-F., Paavola, C.D., Trent, J.D., A self-assembling protein template for constrained synthesis and patterning of nanoparticle arrays. *J. Am. Chem. Soc.* **2005**, *127*, 2800–2801.

77 Naik, R.R., Jones, S.E., Murray, C.J., McAuliffe, J.C., Vaia, R.A., Stone, M.O., Peptide templates for nanoparticle synthesis derived from polymerase chain reaction-driven phage display. *Adv. Funct. Mater.* **2004**, *14*, 25–30.

78 Kramer, R.M., Li, C., Carter, D.C., Stone, M.O., Naik, R.R., Engineered protein cages for nanomaterial synthesis. *J. Am. Chem. Soc.* **2004**, *126*, 13282–13286.

79 Lévy, R., Thanh, N.T.K., Doty, R.C., Hussain, I., Nichols, R.J., Schiffrin, D.J., Brust, M., Fernig, D.G., Rational and combinatorial

design of peptide capping ligands for gold nanoparticles. *J. Am. Chem. Soc.* **2004**, *126*, 10076–10084.
80 Doty, R.C., Tshikhudo, T.R., Brust, M., Fernis, D.G., Extremely stable water-soluble Ag nanoparticles. Submitted to *Chem. Mater.* **2005**.
81 Pinaud, F., King, D., Moore, H.-P., Weiss, S., Bioactivation and cell targeting of semiconductor CdSe/ZnS nanocrystals with phytochelatin-related peptides. *J. Am. Chem. Soc.* **2004**, *126*, 6115–6123.
82 Michalet, X., Pinaud, F., Bentolila, L.A., Tsay, J.M., Doose, S., Li, J.J., Sundaresan, G., Wu, A.M., Gambhir, S.S., Weiss, S., Quantum dots for live cells, in vivo imaging, and diagnostics. *Science* **2005**, *307*, 538–544.
83 Reiss, B.D., Mao, C.B., Solis, D.J., Ryan, K.S., Thomson, T., Belcher, A.M., Biological routes to metal alloy ferromagnetic nanostructures. *Nano Lett.* **2004**, *4*, 1127–1132.
84 Thanh, N.T.K., Puntes, V.F., Tung, L.D., Fernig, D.G., Peptides as capping ligands for in situ synthesis of water soluble Co nanoparticles for bioapplications. *J. Phys. D – Appl. Phys.* **2005**, in the press.
85 Wang, Z., Lévy, R., Fernig, D.G., Brust, M., The peptide route to multifunctional gold nanoparticles. *Bioconjugate Chem.* **2005**, *16*, 457–500.
86 Skerra, A., Schmidt, T.G.M., Use of the strep-tag and streptavidin for detection and purification of recombinant proteins. In *Applications of Chimeric Genes and Hybrid Proteins, Pt A* (Vol. 326), **2000**, pp. 271–304.
87 Hochuli, E., Dobeli, H., Schacher, A., New metal chelate adsorbent selective for proteins and peptides containing neighbouring histidine residues. *J. Chromatogr.* **1987**, *411*, 177–184.
88 Gaberc-Porekar, V., Menart, V., Perspectives of immobilized-metal affinity chromatography. *J. Biochem. Biophys. Methods* **2001**, *49*, 335–360.
89 Xu, C.J., Xu, K.M., Gu, H.W., Zhong, X.F., Guo, Z.H., Zheng, R.K., Zhang, X.X., Xu, B., Nitrilotriacetic acid-modified magnetic nanoparticles as a general agent to bind histidine-tagged proteins. *J. Am. Chem. Soc.* **2004**, *126*, 3392–3393.
90 Hainfeld, J.F., Liu, W.Q., Halsey, C.M.R., Freimuth, P., Powell, R.D., Ni-NTA-gold clusters target His-tagged proteins. *J. Struct. Biol.* **1999**, *127*, 185–198.
91 Venien-Bryan, C., Balavoine, F., Toussaint, B., Mioskowski, C., Hewat, E.A., Helme, B., Vignais, P.M., Structural study of the response regulator HupR from Rhodobacter capsulatus. Electron microscopy of two-dimensional crystals on a nickel-chelating lipid. *J. Mol. Biol.* **1997**, *274*, 687–692.
92 Lévy, R., Unpublished results, **2005**.
93 Brown, S., Engineered iron oxide-adhesion mutants of the Escherichia-coli phage-lambda receptor. *Proc. Natl. Acad. Sci. U.S.A.* **1992**, *89*, 8651–8655.
94 Sarikaya, M., Tamerler, C., Jen, A.K.Y., Schulten, K., Baneyx, F., Molecular biomimetics: Nanotechnology through biology. *Nat. Mater.* **2003**, *2*, 577–585.
95 Whaley, S.R., English, D.S., Hu, E.L., Barbara, P.F., Belcher, A.M., Selection of peptides with semiconductor binding specificity for directed nanocrystal assembly. *Nature* **2000**, *405*, 665–668.
96 Sano, K.I., Shiba, K., A hexapeptide motif that electrostatically binds to the surface of titanium. *J. Am. Chem. Soc.* **2003**, *125*, 14234–14235.
97 Dieckmann, G.R., Dalton, A.B., Johnson, P.A., Razal, J., Chen, J., Giordano, G.M., Munoz, E., Musselman, I.H., Baughman, R.H., Draper, R.K., Controlled assembly of carbon nanotubes by designed amphiphilic peptide helices. *J. Am. Chem. Soc.* **2003**, *125*, 1770–1777.
98 Zorbas, V., Ortiz-Acevedo, A., Dalton, A.B., Yoshida, M.M., Dieckmann, G.R., Draper, R.K., Baughman, R.H., Jose-Yacaman, M., Musselman, I.H., Preparation and characterization of individual peptide-wrapped single-walled carbon

nanotubes. *J. Am. Chem. Soc.* **2004**, *126*, 7222–7227.

99 Terpe, K., Overview of tag protein fusions: From molecular and biochemical fundamentals to commercial systems. *Appl. Microbiol. Biotechnol.* **2003**, *60*, 523–533.

100 Ryadnov, M.G., Ceyhan, B., Niemeyer, C.M., Woolfson, D.N., "Belt and braces": A peptide-based linker system of de novo design. *J. Am. Chem. Soc.* **2003**, *125*, 9388–9394.

101 Fang, Y.Y., Ray, B.D., Claussen, C.A., Lipkowitz, K.B., Long, E.C., Ni(II)center dot Arg-Gly-His – DNA interactions: Investigation into the basis for minor-groove binding and recognition. *J. Am. Chem. Soc.* **2004**, *126*, 5403–5412.

102 Marks, K.M., Rosinov, M., Nolan, G.P., In vivo targeting of organic calcium sensors via genetically selected peptides. *Chem. Biol.* **2004**, *11*, 347–356.

103 Adermann, K., John, H., Standker, L., Forssmann, W.G., Exploiting natural peptide diversity: Novel research tools and drug leads. *Curr. Opin. Biotechnol.* **2004**, *15*, 599–606.

104 Kolonin, M., Pasqualini, R., Arap, W., Molecular addresses in blood vessels as targets for therapy. *Curr. Opin. Chem. Biol.* **2001**, *5*, 308–313.

105 Tkachenko, A.G., Xie, H., Coleman, D., Glomm, W., Ryan, J., Anderson, M.F., Franzen, S., Feldheim, D.L., Multifunctional gold nanoparticle-peptide complexes for nuclear targeting. *J. Am. Chem. Soc.* **2003**, *125*, 4700–4701.

106 Kanaras, A.G., Wang, Z.X., Bates, A.D., Cosstick, R., Brust, M., Towards multistep nanostructure synthesis: Programmed enzymatic self-assembly of DNA/gold systems. *Angew. Chem. Int. Ed.* **2003**, *42*, 191–194.

107 Wright, E.R., Conticello, V.P., Self-assembly of block copolymers derived from elastin-mimetic polypeptide sequences. *Adv. Drug Deliv. Rev.* **2002**, *54*, 1057–1073.

108 Zhang, S.G., Zhao, X.J., Design of molecular biological materials using peptide motifs. *J. Mater. Chem.* **2004**, *14*, 2082–2086.

109 MacPhee, C.E., Woolfson, D.N., Engineered and designed peptide-based fibrous biomaterials. *Curr. Opin. Solid State Mater. Sci.* **2004**, *8*, 141–149.

110 Zhang, S.G., Emerging biological materials through molecular self-assembly. *Biotechnol. Adv.* **2002**, *20*, 321–339.

111 Reches, M., Gazit, E., Casting metal nanowires within discrete self-assembled peptide nanotubes. *Science* **2003**, *300*, 625–627.

112 Ryadnov, M.G., Woolfson, D.N., Engineering the morphology of a self-assembling protein fibre. *Nat. Mater.* **2003**, *2*, 329–332.

113 Ryadnov, M.G., Woolfson, D.N., Introducing branches into a self-assembling peptide fiber. *Angew. Chem. Int. Ed.* **2003**, *42*, 3021–3023.

114 Ryadnov, M.G., Woolfson, D.N., Fiber recruiting peptides: Noncovalent decoration of an engineered protein scaffold. *J. Am. Chem. Soc.* **2004**, *126*, 7454–7455.

115 Smith, A.M., Acquah, S.F.A., Bone, N., Kroto, H.W., Ryadnov, M.G., Stevens, M.S.P., Walton, D.R.M., Woolfson, D.N., Polar assembly in a designed protein fiber. *Angew. Chem. Int. Ed.* **2005**, *44*, 325–328.

116 Valery, C., Paternostre, M., Robert, B., Gulik-Krzywicki, T., Narayanan, T., Dedieu, J.C., Keller, G., Torres, M.L., Cherif-Cheikh, R., Calvo, P., Artzner, F., Biomimetic organization: Octapeptide self-assembly into nanotubes of viral capsid-like dimension. *Proc. Natl. Acad. Sci. U.S.A.* **2003**, *100*, 10258–10262.

117 Lowik, D.W.P.M., van Hest, J.C.M., Peptide based amphiphiles. *Chem. Soc. Rev.* **2004**, *33*, 234–245.

118 Schneider, J.P., Pochan, D.J., Ozbas, B., Rajagopal, K., Pakstis, L., Kretsinger, J., Responsive hydrogels from the intramolecular folding and self-assembly of a designed peptide. *J. Am. Chem. Soc.* **2002**, *124*, 15030–15037.

119 Nowak, A.P., Breedveld, V., Pakstis,

L., Ozbas, B., Pine, D.J., Pochan, D., Deming, T.J., Rapidly recovering hydrogel scaffolds from self-assembling diblock copolypeptide amphiphiles. *Nature* **2002**, *417*, 424–428.

120 Bellomo, E.G., Wyrsta, M.D., Pakstis, L., Pochan, D.J., Deming, T.J., Stimuli-responsive polypeptide vesicles by conformation-specific assembly. *Nat. Mater.* **2004**, *3*, 244–248.

9
Folate-linked Lipid-based Nanoparticles for Tumor-targeted Gene Therapy

Yoshiyuki Hattori and Yoshie Maitani

9.1
Introduction

Cancer gene therapy has been intensively developed using non-viral vector [1]. Viral vectors such as retroviruses [2], adenoviruses [3], adeno-associated viruses [4] and several other viral types [5], are efficient in transfection, but pose risks to the host from the immunogenicity of viral proteins, a lack of desired tissue selectivity, the potential for oncogenesis due to chromosomal integration, and the generation of infectious viruses due to recombination, making non-viral vectors an attractive alternative. Synthetic vectors such as cationic polymers, liposomes and nanoparticles have been studied widely for DNA delivery due to their potential for tissue-specific targeting, their lack of immunogenicity, the relative safety, and relative ease of large-scale production. For targeted delivery to tumors, vitamin folic acid has been utilized for folate receptor (FR)-mediated drug delivery since the FR is frequently overexpressed on human tumors [6, 7]. Liposomes conjugated to folate ligand have been reported as carriers of chemotherapeutic agents to FR-bearing tumor cells *in vivo* [8–14]. While much has been published on folate-drug conjugates and folate-linked carriers, relatively little is known about the targeting of gene delivery. The use of a folate ligand as a targeting ligand to deliver DNA has also been reported *in vitro* [15–19], but has not been successful in *in vivo* gene therapy [20, 21]. Therefore, in this chapter, we describe the current understanding of tumor-targeting particle vectors and folate-linked lipid-based vectors such as liposomes and nanoparticles. Information pertaining to the formulation of folate-linked lipid-based nanoparticles, their transfection activity *in vitro* and *in vivo* in suicide gene therapy to treat prostate and nasopharyngeal tumors *in vivo* is also included.

9.2
Gene Delivery and Expression System

Plasmids for gene expression system contain a cDNA coding for either a full gene or minigene and several other genetic elements, including introns, polyadenylation

Nanotechnologies for the Life Sciences Vol. 1
Biofunctionalization of Nanomaterials. Edited by Challa S. S. R. Kumar

ISBN: 3-527-31381-8

sequences and transcript stabilizers to control transcription, translation, protein stability and secretion from the host cells [22]. The minimal transcription unit required for expression of a therapeutic protein consists of 5′ enhancer/promoter upstream of the gene encoding for the therapeutic protein (e.g., HSV-tk or cytosine deaminase, etc.) and a polyadenylation signal downstream of the gene. Several promoters originating from eukaryotic viruses, such as cytomegalovirus (CMV), similian virus 40 (SV40), Moloney murine leukemia virus (MoMLV), and Rous sarcoma virus (RSV) are widely used. Tumor-specific promoters (e.g., carcinoembryonic antigen (CEA) [23], alpha-fetoprotein (AFP) [24], midkine [25], prostate specific antigen (PSA) [26], etc.) for cancer gene therapy are also designed to interact with transcription factors or other nuclear proteins present in the desired target cells [27].

A major requirement for gene therapy is efficient transport of DNA through the cell membrane by processes that are not well defined. The mechanistic pathway for gene transfection includes the compaction of extended plasmid DNA chain. This process, also known as DNA condensation, has received considerable attention in recent years due to its biological importance in DNA packaging in the development of gene delivery [28, 29]. Multivalent cations such as polyamines (spermidine, spermine), positively charged polymers (polyethylenimine, PEI) and peptides (poly-L-lysine, PLL) provoke the condensation of DNA to nanoparticles [28, 30].

Non-viral particle systems generally entail complex/encapsulation of the gene of interest (present, along with appropriate promoters, etc., in a circular plasmid) with additional molecules, particularly various lipids. These generally display a positive charge and hence interact with the negatively charged DNA molecules. Inside the cytoplasm, endosomes are destabilized and release the plasmid DNA, although this is an inefficient process in many cases [31]. Once plasmid DNA is released into the cytoplasm, it may enter the nucleus. DNA is transported across the nuclear envelope through the nuclear pore. While smaller particles of 25 nm can freely diffuse through the nuclear pore, which is ~55 nm in diameter, larger molecules enter the nucleus through the nuclear pore complex [32, 33]. Finally, therapeutic protein is transcribed and translated from plasmid DNA. Genes introduced into cells using particle vectors are episomal and provide transient expression of transgenes.

9.3
Nanoparticles for Gene Delivery System

Systemic administration via intravenous injection rarely achieves meaningful cell transfection. This is most likely due to the high nuclease levels present in serum. Particle vectors can stabilize the DNA, protect it, e.g., from serum nuclease, and ideally interact with the biological system when particles modified with ligands, for example, help target the DNA to particular cells, leading to endocytosis. However, a major limitation of these systems is their inability to cross-intact endothelial barriers and leave general circulation. In general, particle carriers are phagocytosed by the macrophages of the mononuclear phagocytotic cells (MPS), thereby rapidly localizing predominantly in the liver and spleen [34]. However, sterically stabilized particle carriers such as polyethylene glycol (PEG)-coated nanoparticles have extended circulation times and can remain in the blood [35]. Such nanoparticles, known as long-circulating nanoparticles, tend to accumulate in tumors as a result of increased microvascular permeability and defective lymphatic drainage, a process also referred to as the enhanced permeability and retention (EPR) effect. This is a passive and non-specific process of extravasation that is statically improved by the prolonged residence time of nanoparticles in circulation and repeated passages through the tumor microvascular bed. These ideas have already been realized in liposomal products such as Doxil®.

Liposomes coated with the monoclonal antibodies (mAbs) (immunoliposomes) can provide target-specific binding to the cells [36]. The ligand can be coupled directly to the liposome surface; however, the PEG chains may provide steric hindrance to receptor binding. Alternatively, a bi-functional PEG linker can be used to couple liposomes to one end of PEG chains and ligands to the other end. Steric hindrance is not a problem in the latter approach. The primary focus of their use has been in the targeted delivery of anticancer agents. Hosokawa et al. [37] have reported efficacy of immunoliposomal doxorubicin on cancer models in a cell-surface-antigen-density-dependent manner.

Active targeting increases the affinity of the carrier system for the target site while passive targeting minimizes the non-specific interaction with non-targeted sites by the reticuloendothelial systems (RES). However, gene transfer activity after intravenous injection of a cationic liposome/plasmid DNA complex is most prevalent in the lung [38]. The challenge for tumor-specific targeting using particulate gene delivery systems is to decrease this non-specific gene transfer in the lung while simultaneously maintaining or increasing the level of gene transfer to the tumor tissues. Xu et al. [39] have reported that a cationic immunolipoplex system directed by a single-chain antibody variable region fragment (scFv) against the human transferrin receptor enhanced the transfection efficiency both *in vitro* and *in vivo*. Anti-Her-2 mAb [40], anti-transferrin receptor mAb [39], and growth factor, such as a transferrin, which is a high affinity ligand for the transferrin receptor [41, 42], have been used for tumor-targeting. Other ligands, such as sugar (galactose [43] and glucose [44]), folic acid [45], or RGD-peptide [46], which are associated with asialoglycoprotein receptor on the hepatocyte, folate receptor, and integrin, respectively, in actively growing cells and tumor, can be used.

9.4 Folate-linked Vectors

Folic acid as a targeting ligand offers many potential advantages: (a) a small targeting ligand, often leading to favorable pharmacokinetic properties of the folate conjugates and reduced probability of immunogenicity; (b) convenient availability and low cost; (c) relatively simple and defined conjugation chemistry; (d) high affinity for FR and lack of FR expression in normal tissue; (e) the receptor–ligand complex can be induced to internalize via endocytosis; and (f) high frequency of FR overexpression among human tumors. Therefore, folate-linked targeting systems show great potential for clinical and therapeutic application.

9.4.1 Folate Receptors

Folate receptor (FR) is overexpressed in a wide range of tumors, and is known as a high-affinity membrane folate-binding protein, which mediates uptake of the vitamin by receptor-mediated endocytosis. Therefore, it presents an attractive target for tumor-selective delivery. FR-targeting materials can continuously accumulate into cells due to receptor recycling. FR-targeting imaging agents arrived on the market in 2004. Three isoforms of FR have been identified and two, FR-α and -β, are attached to the cell by a glycosylphosphatidylinositol (GPI)-anchor, while FR-γ is secreted due to the lack of an efficient signal for GPI modification [7]. The role of FRs in the cellular transport of folate is not well understood, although a potocytosis (caveolin-coated endocytosis) model has been proposed [47]. FR-α was found to be clustered in a membrane region called caveolae or rafts [47]. While an elevated expression of FR has frequently been observed in various types of human tumors, the receptor is generally absent in normal tissues with the exception of the choroid plexus and placenta, with low levels in the lung, thyroid and kidney [48]. FR-α is frequently overexpressed in tumors, including ovarian, colorectal, breast, lung, renal cell carcinomas and brain metastases derived from epithelial cancers [6, 7]. FR-β is frequently overexpressed in tumors of non-epithelial cell lineages such as sarcomas and acute myeloid leukemia [49], and FR-γ is overexpressed in malignant hemopoietic cells [50]. The causes of FR overexpression in tumors are unclear, but high levels of FR may be associated with increased biological aggressiveness of carcinomas.

9.4.2 Folate Receptor-targeting Liposomes

Liposomes used in recent studies have been coated with folate-PEG-lipid to facilitate tumor-targeting by an active mechanism (via FR) and a passive mechanism (prevention/reduction of RES uptake) [20, 51]. PEGylated lipids can significantly reduce non-specific gene transfer activity in the lung, and conjugation of the targeting ligand, folate, to the PEG chain can restore this activity in FR-positive tumors *in vivo* [20]. For intravascular targeting to access tumor cells expressing FR, liposomes must cross the vascular endothelium and diffuse into the interstitial fluid (Fig. 9.1) [51]. The theoretical advantage of FR-targeting over non-targeting is related to a shift in the distribution of the liposomes to the tumor cell compartment and delivery of the genes. The disadvantage of a system targeting a cancer cell receptor such as FR is the difficulty that a large nano-size assembly has in penetrating a solid tumor mass. Many cell types, including most tumor cells, display a low endocytotic capacity. Since the intracellular mechanism of FR-targeted gene deliv-

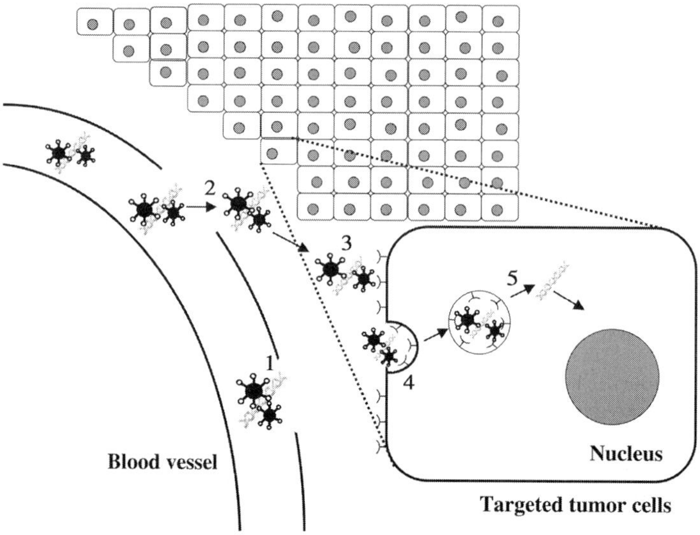

Fig. 9.1. Scheme illustrating the concept of using FR-targeting nanoparticles to deliver plasmid DNA to tumor cells. Dots and helixes on the nanoparticles represent the folate ligands and plasmid DNA, respectively. The various steps involved in the targeting process are numbered 1–5. Steps 1 and 2 are common to non-targeted and FR-targeting nanoparticles mixed with plasmid DNA (nanoplex). Steps 3–5 are specific to the FR-targeting vector. (1) long-circulating nanoplexes make more passages through the tumor microvasculature. (2) Increased vascular permeability in tumor tissue enables nanoplexes to extravasate and reach the tumor interstitial fluid. (3) FR-targeting nanoplexes bind to FR expressed on the tumor membrane via the folate ligand. (4) Nanoplexes are internalized by tumor cells via FR. (5) Internalized nanoplexes release their plasmid DNA in the cytoplasm.

ery with liposomes and nanoparticles is endocytosis, this is a serious limitation to the successful application of FR-targeted lipid-based particle delivery systems. The development of suitable delivery vectors for *in vivo* gene transfer is necessary for the clinical application of therapeutic genes.

Several cationic polymer–folate conjugates and/or cationic liposomes, and cationic nanoparticles incorporating folate-derivatives have been developed for FR-targeted gene delivery (Table 9.1). Folic acid retains its receptor-binding and endocytotic properties when covalently linked to a wide variety of molecules. Polyplexes are composed of charged complexes of plasmid DNA and a cationic polymer, such as poly-L-lysine (PLL), polyethylenimine (PEI) and polyamidoamine dendrimers. For FR-targeted gene delivery, PLL-folate [52–54], PLL-PEG-folate [55], PEI-folate [56], PEI-PEG-folate [56, 57], and poly(dimethylaminomethyl methacrylate) (pDMAEMA)-PEG-folate [58] have been synthesized (Fig. 9.2). These folate-conjugates facilitated efficient FR-targeted gene delivery without additional vector components *in vitro*. It appears that the incorporation of a long PEG spacer between folate and the cationic polymer is important for efficient FR-targeted gene delivery [54].

Tab. 9.1. FR-targeted nonviral vectors; all vectors were used in *in vitro* transfection.

Vector		*Description*	*In vivo*	*Ref.*
Polymer	Poly-L-Lys (PLL)	Polyplex prepared with PLL-folate or PLL-PEG_{3400}-folate	–	52–55
	Polyethylenimine (PEI)	Polyplex prepared with PEI-folate or PEI-PEG_{3350}-folate	–	56, 57
	Polydimethylamino methyl methacrylate (pDMAEMA)	Polyplex prepared with pDMAEMA-PEG_{3400}-folate	–	58
Liposome	Cationic	Incorporating 0.1 mol% folate-PEG_{3350}-DOPE, 5 mol% folate-DOPE, 0.5–5 mol% folate-PEG_{3400}-DSPE or 5 mol% folate-PEG_{4600}-cholesterol into liposome	i.v.	15, 17–20, 59
	LPDI type	Polyplex prepared from protamine was mixed with catonic liposome containing 0.03 mol% folate-PEG_{3400}-DSPE or 2 mol% folate-PEG_{5000}-DSPE	i.p. i.v.	21, 60
	LPDII type	Polyplex prepared from PLL or PEI was mixed with pH-sensitive anionic liposome containing 0.1 mol% folate-PEG_{3350}-DOPE or folate-PEG_{3350}-DSPE	–	16, 61
Nanoparticle		Polyplex prepared with cationic dithiol-detergent [$(C_{14}Corn)_2$] was mixed with 1 or 2 mol% folate-PEG_{3400}-DPPE	–	62
	NPI-F, NPII-F	Incorporating 2 mol% folate-PEG_{2000}-DSPE into cationic nanoparticle based DC-Chol	i.v. i.t.	63, 64, 73
	NPIII-F	Incorporating 1 mol% folate-PEG_{2000}-DSPE into cationic nanoparticle based OH-Chol	–	68

i.v.: intravenous injection, i.p.: intraperitoneal injection;
i.t.: intratumoral injection.

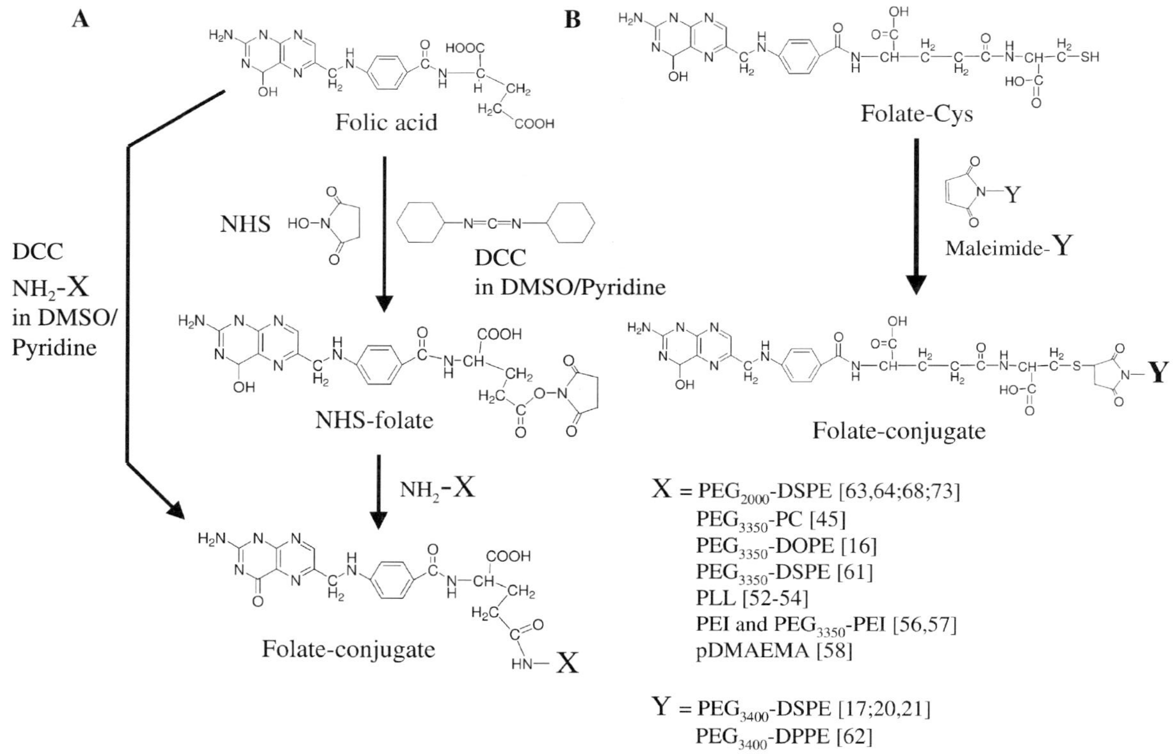

Fig. 9.2. Preparations of conjugation with folic acid. (A) *N*-Hydroxysuccinimidyl ester of folic acid (NHS-folate) is prepared by esterification of folic acid with *N*-hydroxysuccinimide (NHS) in the presence of 1,3-dicyclohexylcarbodiimide (DCC) and pyridine, and is then conjugated with amino-residues in targeted compounds (X). Alternatively, folic acid can be conjugated directly with compounds (X) in the presence of DCC and pyridine. (B) Folate-cysteine conjugate (Folate-Cys) is reacted with maleimide (MAL) conjugated with targeted compounds (Y).

Lipoplexes are composed of charge complexes of plasmid DNA and cationic liposome. Lipopolyplexes are composed of plasmid DNA attached to both polymers and lipids. Cationic liposomes are generally composed of a cationic lipid, such as dioleoyltrimethylammonium chloride (DOTMA), dioleoyltrimethylammonium propane (DOTAP), or 3-[*N*-(*N*,*N*′-dimethylaminoethanolamine)carbamoyl]cholesterol (DC-Chol), and a helper lipid, such as dioleoylphosphatidylethanolamine (DOPE) or cholesterol (Chol), which provides fusogenicity and stability to the lipoplex. Depending on the preparation, the lipoplex may not be a single aggregate, but an intricate structure in which the condensed DNA is surrounded by a lipid bilayer. FR-targeting cationic liposomes have been incorporated with folate-derivatives, folate-DOPE [59], folate-PEG-DOPE [15, 16], folate-PEG-DSPE [17–21, 60], folate-PEG-Chol [20], etc. (Fig. 9.2). Hofland et al. [20] have shown that both folate-PEG_{3400}-DSPE and folate-PEG_{4600}-Chol, when combined with a cationic lipid RPR209120 and DOPE, formed lipoplexes with greatly reduced normal tissue gene transfer and efficient *in vivo* tumor gene transfer.

LPDI-type lipoplexes (lipopolyplex) consist of a ternary complex of cationic liposomes, DNA-condensing polycation, and plasmid DNA. In a report by Reddy et al. [21], polyplexes prepared from protamine were mixed with cationic liposomes containing folate-PEG_{3400}-DSPE as a targeting ligand and DOPE as a helper lipid. This vector showed superior transfection activity in FR-positive M109 murine lung carcinoma cells as well as in ascitic cells derived from L1210A murine lymphocytic leukemia cells. LPDII-type lipoplexes (lipopolyplex) consist of a ternary complex of anionic liposomes, DNA-condensing polycation, and plasmid DNA. Lee et al. [16] have reported a formulation of LPDII-type vector, in which DNA was first attached to PLL and then mixed with pH-sensitive anionic liposomes composed of DOPE/CHEMS/folate-PEG_{3350}-DOPE. The pH-sensitive liposomes are fusogenic at acidic pH and thus can be used to facilitate endosomal disruption and subsequent release of plasmids in the cytoplasm. Shi et al. [61] have reported efficient gene delivery using an LPDII vector that incorporated PEI as a DNA-condensing agent and a cationic/anionic lipid pair, composed of dimethyldioctadecylammonium bromide (DDAB)/CHEMS/polyoxyethylene sorbitan monoolate (Tween80)/folate-PEG_{3350}-DSPE.

9.5 Folate-linked Lipid-based Nanoparticles

Preferential expression of a gene in tumor cells contributes to the safety and efficacy of gene therapy. For FR-targeted gene transfection, the concentrations of folic acid and linker in vectors are important.

9.5.1 Formulations

For drug delivery, folate-targeting liposomes contained 0.1–0.5 mol% folate PEG_{2000}-DSPE or folate-PEG_{3400}-DSPE for targeting, and about 4 mol% PEG_{2000}-

DSPE was used for PEG-coating [8–13]. For gene delivery, FR-targeting liposomes and nanoparticles contained 0.03–5 mol% folate-PEG-lipid. Reddy et al. [21] have reported that a cationic liposome formulated with less than 0.03 mol% of folate-PEG_{3400}-DSPE showed the greatest cell association. Folate moieties located at the distal end of the PEG spacers would likely not interact at concentrations lower than 0.03%. Bruckheimer et al. [60] have reported that 2 mol% folate-PEG_{3400}-DSPE conjugate increased the cellular association with tumor cells and transfection potency. FR-targeting cationic nanoparticles incorporating 2 mol% folate-PEG_{3400}-DPPE showed efficient FR-dependent cellular uptake and transfection [62], and cationic liposomes with 5 mol% folate-PEG_{4600}-Chol showed high gene transfer activity into a FR-positive cell line, M109 [20]. Xu et al. [59] have reported specific *in vivo* gene delivery to tumors with a liposome containing about 5 mol% folate-DOPE. Dauty et al. [62] have reported that an FR-targeting cationic nanoparticle incorporating folate-PEG_{3400}-DPPE and a cationic dithiol-detergent [dimerized tetradecyl-ornithinyl-cysteine, $(C14Corn)_2$] shows efficient FR-dependent cellular uptake and transfection.

As a linker of folate, PEG of M_r 2000–5000 has been used (Table 9.1). A certain distance between the folate moiety and the lipid particles is needed for FR-targeting, due to the need for folate to enter the binding pocket of FR on the cell surface. Lee et al. [45] first described the dependence of folate-liposome targeting on the distance between the folate and liposome, and reported that a PEG_{3400} linker was necessary for the targeting. Leamon et al. [17] optimized the targeting activity of the liposomes by modifying the length of the PEG-linker, and found that PEGs as small as M_r 1000 could function as effective linkers. Ward et al. [54] have reported that a folate-linked PEG_{800}-polymer-modified PLL/DNA complex did not lead to a significant increase in *in vitro* transgene expression. A PEG spacer with $M_r > 1000$ might be essential for FR-targeting.

Folate-linked microemulsions have been used composed of 0.24 mol% folate-lipid (F0/M), folate-PEG_{2000}-DSPE (F2/M) or folate-PEG_{5000}-DSPE (F5/M) for targeting, and 6.7 mol% PEG_{2000}-DSPE for PEG-coating and forming emulsion (Fig. 9.3) [14]. Selectivity of folate-linked microemulsions for delivery into KB cells was validated by flow cytometry (Fig. 9.4). The mean fluorescence intensities of F5/M

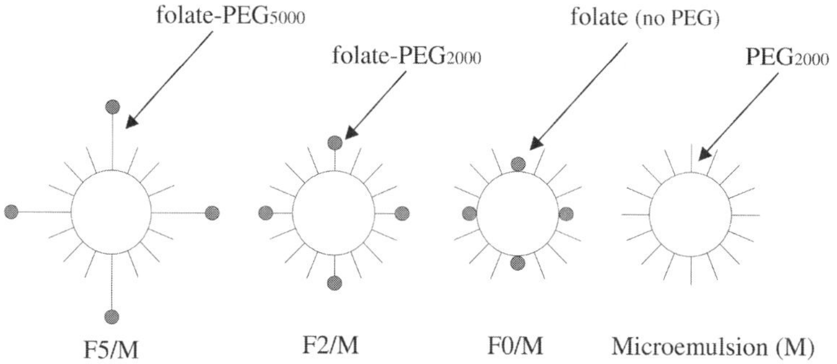

Fig. 9.3. Schematic diagrams of the microemulsion and the folate-linked microemulsions.

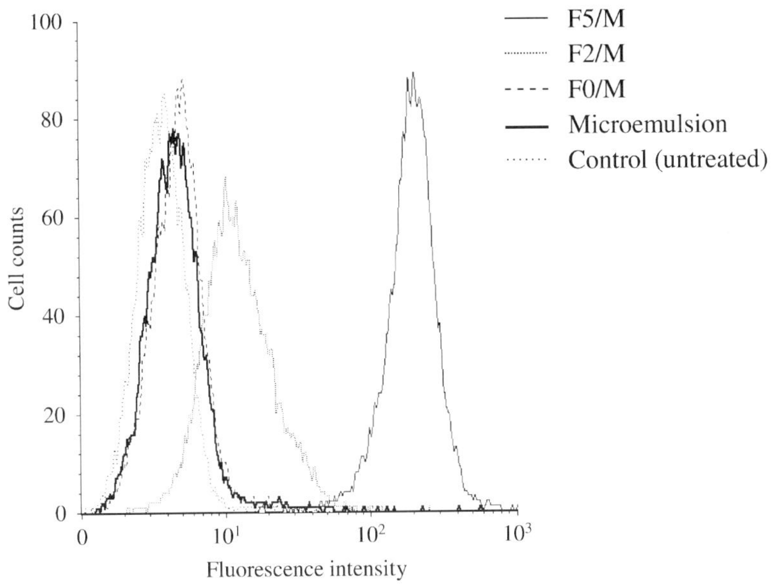

Fig. 9.4. Association of 1,1′-dioctadecyl-3,3,3′,3′-tetramethylindocarbocyanine perchlorate (DiI)-labeled F5/M, F2/M, F0/M and microemulsion with KB cells after 1 h incubation was analyzed by flow cytometry. [14]

and F2/M had ca. 200- and 4-fold greater association than non-folate microemulsion, respectively. In contrast, F0/M showed a similar curve to non-folate microemulsion. These results correspond well with the idea that conjugating folate to a shorter PEG polymer reduces folate exposure by interference with the ability of liposome to interact with FR [9]. Additionally, these increased associations of F5/M and F2/M could be blocked completely by adding 2 mM free folic acid to the medium [14]. Extending the PEG-chain length of the folate-PEG-lipid from 0 to M_r 2000, and M_r 2000–5000, dramatically improved the selective FR-mediated association and the cytotoxicity of folate-linked microemulsions loading anticancer drug *in vitro* [14].

Folate-linked nanoparticles (NPI), consisting of 1 mg mL^{-1} DC-Chol as a cationic lipid, 5 mol% conventional Tween 80 (about 50% pure), and 0–1 mol% folate-PEG_{2000}-DSPE (f-PEG_{2000}-DSPE) or folate-PEG_{5000}-DSPE (f-PEG_{5000}-DSPE), respectively, have been prepared by a modified ethanol injection method [63, 64]. All nanoparticles were about 100–200 nm in size, with an ζ-potential of about 50 mV. Here the definition of a lipid-based nanoparticle is a formula containing no bilayers like liposomes. Cholesterol derivatives are usually unable to form stable bilayers unless used in combination with DOPE or some other neutral lipid. Therefore, these particles may be nanoparticles. Figure 9.5 illustrates some folate linked nanoparticles.

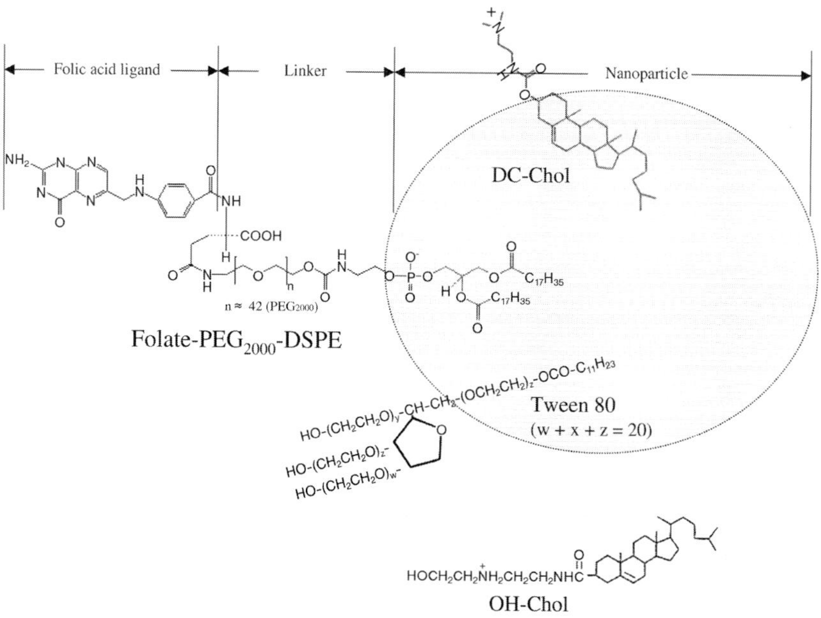

Fig. 9.5. Schematic structure of folate-linked nanoparticles composed of folate-PEG$_{2000}$-DSPE, DC-Chol, OH-Chol and Tween 80 (NPI-, NPII-, NPIII-F).

9.5.2
Nanoplex and Transfection Activity *In Vitro*

Nanoplexes are composed of charged complexes of plasmid DNA and cationic nanoparticles. The size of nanoplexes of NPI with 0.3 mol% f-PEG$_{2000}$-DSPE at a charge ratio (+/−) of cationic nanoparticle to DNA of 3:1 in the presence of 50% serum increased up to 940 nm. Nanoplexes of NPI with 1 mol% f-PEG$_{5000}$-DSPE did not increase greatly in size in serum-containing medium, but showed lower transfection activity than that with 1 mol% f-PEG$_{2000}$-DSPE [63].

Folate-linked nanoparticles (NPII) have been composed with the same composition as NPI with 1–3 mol% f-PEG$_{2000}$-DSPE except for the substitution of Tween 80 (purity 99%) for conventional Tween 80. Each NPII was, on average, ca. 100–200 nm [64] (Table 9.2). Three mol% of f-PEG$_{2000}$-DSPE may not be incorporated in NPII because no reduction in the ζ-potential of NPII was seen upon the addition of f-PEG$_{2000}$-DSPE (about 55 mV) [64]. The concentration of f-PEG$_{2000}$-DSPE in an ethanol–water mixture to prepare NPII-2F containing 2 mol% f-PEG$_{2000}$-DSPE, and NPII-3F containing 3 mol% f-PEG$_{2000}$-DSPE, was about 40 and 60 μM, respectively. f-PEG$_{2000}$-DSPE below the critical micelle concentration (c.m.c.) might lead to efficient incorporation into the particles. However, f-PEG$_{2000}$-DSPE above the c.m.c. may help to stabilize micellized f-PEG$_{2000}$-DSPE and lead to inefficient insertion into the particle. The c.m.c. of f-PEG$_{2000}$-DSPE may be between 40 and 60 μM

Tab. 9.2. Formulae, particle size and ζ-potential of folate-linked nanoparticles (NPII) and their nanoplexes [64].

Formulation	*Mol (%)*			*Nanoparticle*		*Nanoplex*[a]	
	DC-Chol	*Tween 80*	*folate-PEG_{2000}-DSPE (F)*	*Size (nm)*	*ζ-potential (mV)*	*Size (nm)*	*ζ-potential (mV)*
NPII	95	5	–	117.2 ± 2.0	53.1 ± 2.5	354.9 ± 8.8	39.0 ± 1.0
NPII-1F	94	5	1	146.1 ± 12.4	43.9 ± 1.7	515.2 ± 32.3	34.2 ± 1.6
NPII-2F (NPII-F)	93	5	2	165.3 ± 22.1	38.6 ± 1.5	233.7 ± 6.5	30.8 ± 1.9
NPII-3F	92	5	3	118.4 ± 4.3	54.8 ± 6.3	396.0 ± 7.8	35.1 ± 0.9

Nanoparticles prepared with lipids [e.g. DC-Chol/Tween 80/folate-PEG_{2000}-DSPE = 94/5/2, molar ratio = 10:1.3:1.3, weight (mg)] in 10 mL of water by a modified ethanol injection method. Nanoparticles consisted of 1 mg mL^{-1} DC-Chol and 5 mol% Tween 80 with 0, 1, 2 and 3 mol% folate-PEG_{2000}-DSPE (NPII, NPII-1F, NPII-2F and NPII-3F, respectively). The particle size and ζ-potential were measured after the nanoparticle and nanoplex were diluted with water. Charge ratio (+/−) of nanoparticle/DNA = 3:1. Each value represents the mean ± SD ($n = 3$).

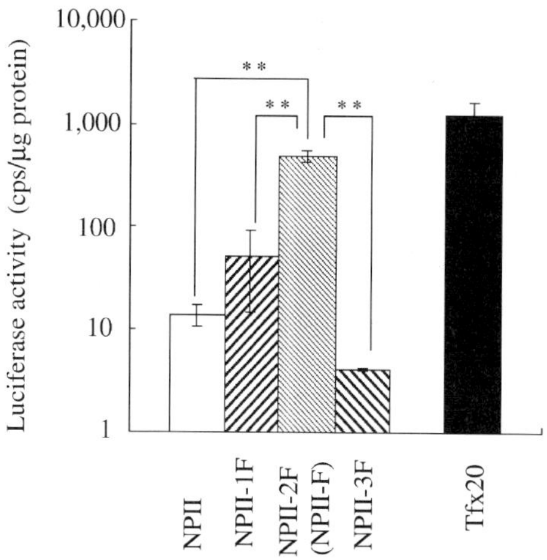

Fig. 9.6. Comparison of transfection efficiency in KB cells with luciferase expression between NPII nanoparticles and Tfx20. The NPII nanoplex and the lipoplex were prepared by mixing luciferase plasmid (2 μg) with the luciferase gene under the control of the cytomegalovirus (CMV) promoter, with nanoparticles and Tfx20, respectively. The luciferase assay was carried out 24 h after incubation of nanoplexes in the medium with 10% serum. Each column represents the mean ± S.D. ($n = 3$). $^{**}P < 0.01$, compared with NPII-F. NPII-F refers to the formulation in Table 9.2.

and might affect the incorporation of f-PEG_{2000}-DSPE in NPII-3F with 3 mol% f-PEG_{2000}-DSPE.

In the presence of 10% and 50% serum, NPII-2F with 2 mol% f-PEG_{2000}-DSPE (NPII-F) formed injectable-sized nanoplexes (Table 9.2), which showed the highest transfection efficiency among NPII with 0–3 mol% f-PEG_{2000}-DSPE, at the optimal charge ratio (+/−) of 3:1 in nasopharyngeal cancer KB cells, being comparable to Tfx20, a commercially available DNA transfection reagent (Fig. 9.6) [64].

9.5.3
Selectivity of Folate-linked Nanoparticle

NPII-F showed greater transfection efficiency in human prostate cancer LNCaP cells, human prostate adenocarcinoma PC-3 cells, and human cervix carcinoma HeLa cells, than in KB cells, in the comparison with Tfx20 (Fig. 9.7A). There were three FR isoforms, α, β and γ, each with a distinctive tissue distribution. FR-α mRNA was expressed strongly in KB and HeLa cells, but not in either LNCaP or PC-3 cells (Fig. 9.7B). FR-β and -γ mRNAs were not detected in any of the cell lines using the RT-PCR method. Reduced folate carrier (RFC), a carrier-mediated folate transporter, was weakly expressed in all cell lines examined (Fig. 9.7B). Cellular uptake of NPII-F in HeLa and KB cells was mediated via FR-α, following the induction of transfection activity. The selectivity of NPII-F to carry genes into KB cells

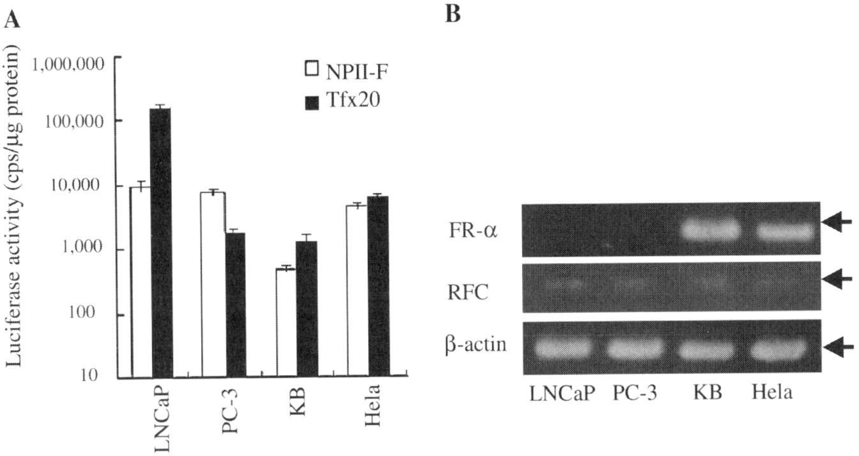

Fig. 9.7. Comparison of transfection efficiency between NPII-F and Tfx20 in the NPII-F nanoplexes and Tfx20 lipoplex delivered with the luciferase plasmid into various cell lines (A). Each column represents the mean ± S.D. ($n = 3$). FR-α, RFC and β-actin mRNA expression were detected in various cell lines by RT-PCR (B). NPII-F refers to the formulation in Table 9.2.

was validated using FITC-oligodeoxynucleotide (FITC-ODN) from the result of a competitive experiment in the presence of folic acid by flow cytometry [64].

In LNCaP and PC-3 cells, FR mRNAs were not often observed. In the human prostate, a high-affinity folate binding protein has been characterized [65] and folic acid binds to the membrane fraction that cross-reacts with the anti-prostate-specific membrane antigen (PSMA) antibody. PSMA is a transmembrane protein with a pattern of overexpression restricted to malignant human prostate tissue and LNCaP cells [66]. The physiological role of PSMA in prostate cancer remains unknown, but PSMA shows hydrolase enzymatic activity with a folate substrate [66] and is internalized via an endocytic mechanism [67]. If PSMA functions as a receptor mediating the internalization of a putative ligand similar to folic acid, this suggests that the folate-linked nanoparticle binds to PMSA and is then taken up via an endocytic mechanism by LNCaP cells as we reported [63].

In PC-3 cells, our study using RT-PCR confirmed the presence of RFC mRNA, but found no FR or PSMA mRNA [64]. A FITC-labeled folate-BSA conjugate was taken up by PC-3 cells and the cellular association was significantly decreased in the presence of 1 mM folic acid [64]. Xu et al. [59] also reported that a folate-cationic liposome system could mediate gene therapy with p53 antisense DNA in prostate cancer (DU145 cells). We found that NPII-F is a useful vector for transfection in prostate androgen-dependent and -independent cancer cells as well as KB cells.

Nanoparticles composed of cholesteryl-3β-carboxyamidoethylene-*N*-hydroxylamine (OH-Chol) instead of DC-Chol (NPIII) could incorporate up to 5 mol% f-PEG$_{2000}$-DSPE (Fig. 9.5). For FR-targeted vectors, NPIII-1F (NPIII-F), -2F and -5F

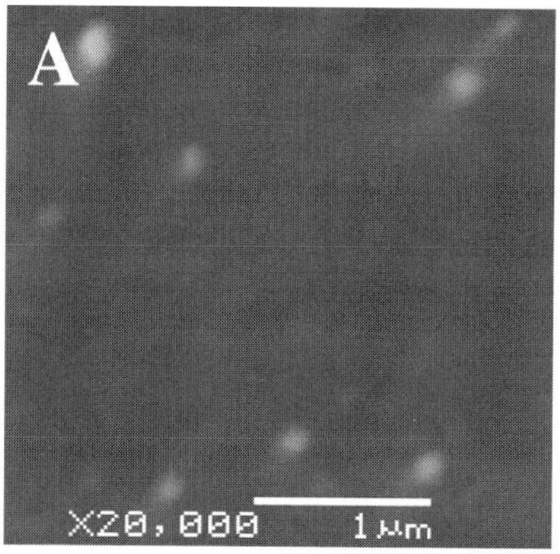

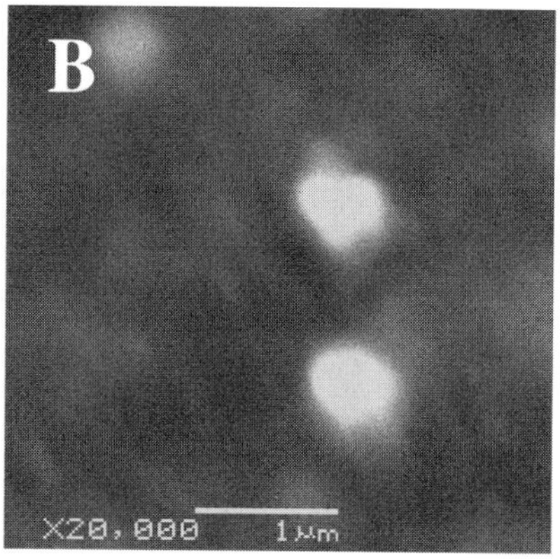

Fig. 9.8. Scanning electron micrographs of NPIII-F nanoparticles (A) and NPIII-F nanoplexes (B). In (B), NPIII-F nanoparticles, NPIII with 1 mol% folate-PEG_{2000}-DSPE, were mixed for 10 min at a charge ratio (+/−) of 3:1 with plasmid DNA in water. The method used to visualize the nanoparticles and nanoplexes was adapted [44]. Briefly, aliquots of 10 μL prepared samples were placed on the copper platform and dried. The nanoparticle and nanoplex layers on the copper platform were coated with platinum and observed with a scanning electron microscope (SEM).

consisted of NPIII with 1, 2 and 5 mol% f-PEG_{2000}-DSPE, respectively. The average size of each nanoparticle was 100–200 nm (Fig. 9.8A) [68]. When the NPIII nanoparticles were mixed with DNA at a charge ratio (+/−) of 3:1 in water, each NPIII nanoplex increased from 250 to 300 nm (Fig. 9.8B) [68]. When the amount of f-PEG_{2000}-DSPE in NPIII was increased, association of plasmid DNA with nanoparticles was inhibited significantly (Fig. 9.9) and a reduction in luciferase activity was observed [68]. A large amount of f-PEG_{2000}-DSPE in nanoparticles might prevent enough DNA being carried into the cells, and/or reduce the cellular association with the nanoplex as reported in PEG-lipid [69]. The NPIII-F based on OH-Chol exhibited about 40× higher transfection efficiency than the NPII-F based on DC-Chol in KB cells [64, 68]. The hydroxyl group of OH-Chol reportedly reduced the stability of the lipoplex, and enhanced transfection efficiency by facilitating the process by which DNA was liberated from the endosome [70].

It is reported that a negatively charged folic acid forms a charge-mediated complex with positively charged particles through its carboxyl groups and has an effect on transfection efficiency [71]. We prepared nanoplexes in water at a charge ratio (+/−) of 1:1 to protect to form complex for co-incubation of the positively charged NPIII with folic acid in the medium, and then incubated them with KB cells. Cellular association of FR-targeting NPIIIs occurred via FR and the interaction of 1 mol% f-PEG_{2000}-DSPE in the NPIII with FR was higher than that of 2 and 5 mol% ones (Fig. 9.10). NPIII-F with 1 mol% f-PEG_{2000}-DSPE nanoplexes at a charge ratio (+/−) of NP-F to DNA of 1:1 exhibited higher selectivity to FR, but lower transfection activity relative to that at a charge ratio (+/−) of 3:1 *in vitro*

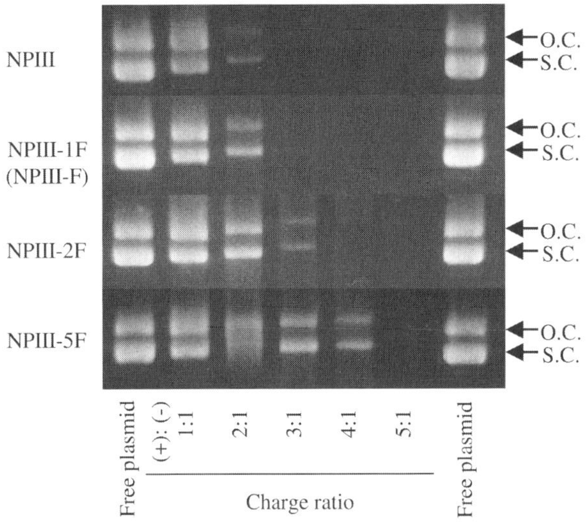

Fig. 9.9. Association of plasmid DNA with NPIII nanoplexes formed in water at various charge ratios (+/−), analyzed using agarose gel electrophoresis. One microgram of Plasmid DNA was mixed with aliquots of NPIII at various charge ratios in water. After a 10 min-incubation, the nanoplexes were analyzed by 1.5% agarose gel electrophoresis. Charge ratios (+/−) of nanoparticle:plasmid DNA = 1:1, 2:1, 3:1, 4:1 and 5:1. O.C. indicates open circular plasmid; S.C. indicates supercoiled plasmid. NPIII refers to the formulation in Table 9.2, substituting OH-Chol for DC-Chol. NPIII-F contains NPIII with 1 mol% folate-PEG_{2000}-DSPE.

[68]. From a competitive experiment of luciferase assay in the presence of free folic acid in the medium, gene expression of the NPIII-F with 1 mol% f-PEG_{2000}-DSPE nanoplexes was reduced [68]. For selectivity and transfection activity in FR-targeted gene delivery, the charge ratio of folate-linked lipid-based nanoparticles to DNA needs to be optimized.

9.5.4
Transfection Activity *In Vivo*

Both systemic and local administration offers several biological opportunities for gene therapy. The systemic route allows non-invasive access to many target cells that are not accessible otherwise by direct administration. Folate-linked liposomes showed efficient FR-dependent cellular uptake and transfection *in vitro*. However, the use of a folate ligand as a targeting ligand to deliver DNA has not been successful in *in vivo* gene therapy [20, 21]. The major limitation of *in vivo* gene therapy using liposomes is the low transfection efficiency. Several factors can adversely affect FR-targeted gene transfer *in vivo*. The first is the presence of endogenous folate in the systemic circulation, which potentially can block FR-binding. Plasma folic acid may interfere with the binding of FR. The human serum folic acid con-

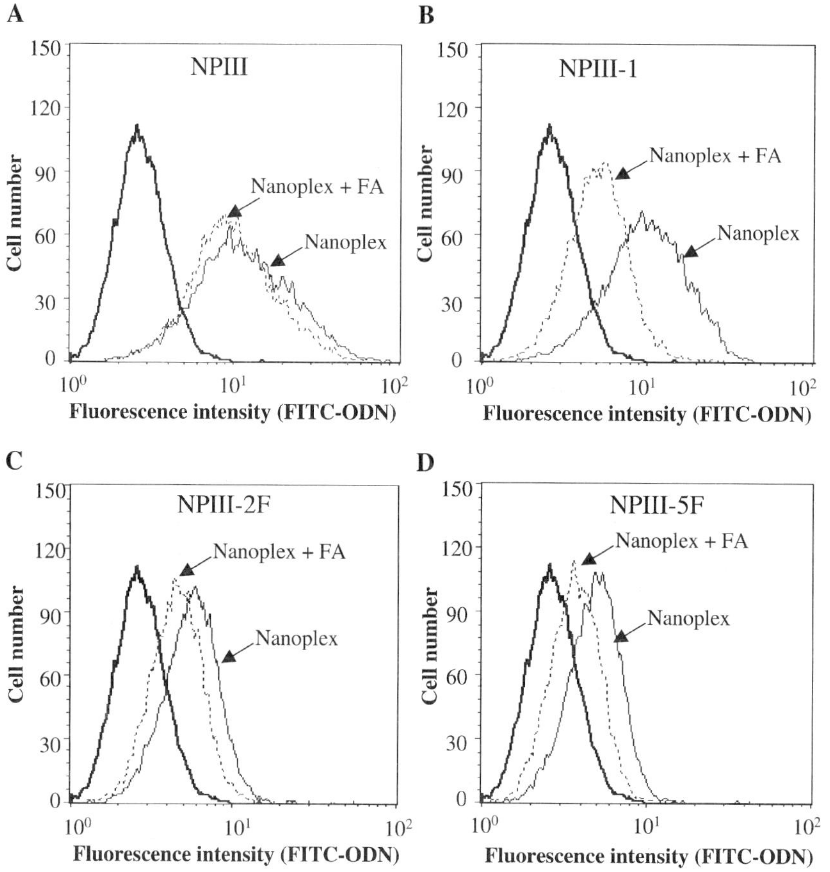

Fig. 9.10. Association of FITC-labeled NPIII nanoplex formed in water with KB cells 3 h after transfection in the absence or presence of free folic acid. Each NPIII nanoparticle was mixed with 2 μg of FITC-ODN at a charge ratio (+/−) of 1:1. Association was determined based on FITC-fluorescence by flow cytometry. Flow cytometry of cells exposed to the nanoplex (continuous line). Dotted line, plus 1 mM folic acid (FA); Bold line, autofluorescence of the cells. NPIII refers to the formulation in Table 9.2, substituting OH-Chol for DC-Chol. NPIII-F contains NPIII with 1 mol% folate-PEG_{2000}-DSPE.

centration, following FDA-mandated dietary supplementation, is ~42 nM [72]. Earlier reports [45] indicated that serum folic acid at this concentration should not inhibit significantly the binding of FR mediated by liposomes. Our recent study [64] showed that mice on a folate-deficient were actually able to maintain a plasma folate level within the physiologic range of humans diet. In contrast, mice on a normal diet maintained a much higher serum concentration of folic acid. Therefore, mice on a folate-deficient diet should be considered relevant to humans with respect to serum folate levels. A second concern is that the size of gene transfer vectors, escaping the vasculature and intratumoral diffusion, could be limiting to targeted delivery. To address this issue, formulation parameters can potentially be optimized to improve the pharmacokinetic properties of the vectors. For example, the vector can be PEGylated to reduce plasma protein binding and RES uptake, resulting in an extended systemic circulation time [35]. In addition, the vector should be kept under 300 nm since this is the approximate limit for efficient tumor extravasation. Non-specific cell uptake by the RES (e.g., Kupffer cells in the liver) is expected to be reduced by incorporating PEGylated lipid within the lipid–DNA complex.

When the NPII-F nanoplex was injected via a tail vein, DNA in the blood was still detectable 4 h later by PCR [73]. Free DNA has an extremely short $T_{1/2}$ in blood (0.5–1 h), depending on the DNA dose [38, 74]. The NPII-F seemed to keep the DNA stable in circulation by forming a nanoplex. NPII-F induced greater gene expression in liver and kidney than NP (unpublished data). FR is on the brush borders of proximal renal tubes and provides for the reabsorption of folate. Recently, Paulos et al. discovered that activated liver-derived macrophages (Kupffer cells) in mice do express the FR [75]. Kupffer cells in the liver and the tubular cells in kidneys of mice may be responsible for capturing NPII-F by FR. Therefore, FR-targeted delivery of therapeutic genes damages normal cells in organs such as the liver and kidney and may subsequently cause death [13]. For cancer gene therapy, using a tumor-specific promoter to regulate expression transcriptionally in target cancer cells has promise. It will be essential to use a strong and tissue-specific promoter region if a therapeutic gene is to be selectively expressed in the cancer cells.

Intraperitoneal and intratumoral injections of lipoplex and nanoplex have been applied in mice bearing tumors. Reddy et al. [21] have reported that maximum *in vivo* transfection activity of reporter gene (luciferase) occurred with intraperitoneally administered folate-liposome using a disseminated intraperitoneal L1210A tumor model. When the NPII-F nanoplexes of the luciferase plasmid were injected directly into the nasopharyngeal tumor, KB, xenografts, NPII-F showed about 100-fold more luciferase activity than Tfx20, suggesting that the NPII-F nanoplex remained small enough to migrate into the tumorous tissue [64].

9.6
Application of Suicide Gene Therapy

Cancer gene therapy has become an increasingly important strategy for treating various human diseases [1]. Currently, cancer gene therapy is being researched, especially in the field of cancer treatment [76]. Suicide gene therapy is a strategy whereby a gene is introduced into cancer cells, making them sensitive to a drug that is normally non-toxic. The suicide genes used often encode enzymes that metabolize non-toxic prodrugs into toxic metabolites. One of the most frequently used suicide genes is the herpes simplex virus thymidine kinase (HSV-tk) gene [77], which phosphorylates a prodrug, ganciclovir (GCV), into a toxic form (GCV triphosphate, GCV-PPP). GCV, an acyclic analog of natural nucleoside 2′-deoxyguanosine, is an antiviral agent used against human cytomegalovirus, herpes simplex

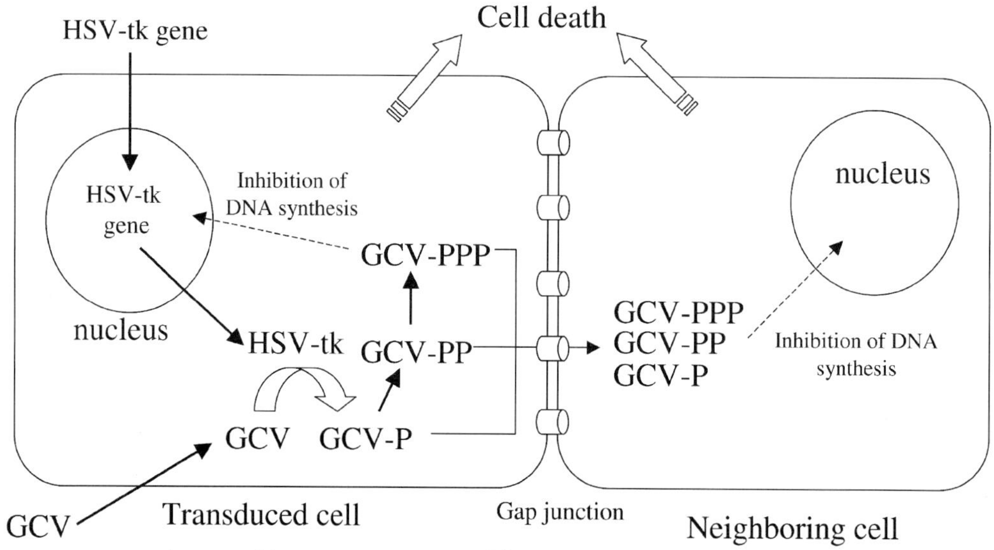

Fig. 9.11. Schematic representation of the HSV-tk/GCV system's mode of action and the bystander effect. In HSV-tk-transduced cells, GCV is intracellularly phosphorylated and converted into the triphosphate derivative (GCV-PPP), which acts as a competitive inhibitor of deoxyguanosine triphosphate. The production of GCV monophosphate (GCV-P) appears to be catalyzed by HSV-tk in the transduced cells. Subsequent formation of the diphosphate and triphosphate GCV derivatives (GCV-PP and -PPP) is catalyzed by cellular guanylate kinase. After incorporation of GCV-PPP into DNA, the synthesis of DNA is immediately inhibited in the cells and this leads to cell death. Cell to cell transfer of HSV-tk-activated GCV between HSV-tk-transduced tumor cells and neighboring cells via gap junctions is a major mechanism of the widespread tumor-cell death (bystander effect).

virus type 1 and 2, varicella zoster virus and Epstein-Barr virus [78]. The effect appears when GCV is intracellularly phosphorylated and converted into the triphosphate derivative GCV triphosphate, which acts as a competitive inhibitor of deoxyguanosine triphosphate (Fig. 9.11) [77]. GCV monophosphate (GCV-P) production appears to be catalyzed in the cells transfected with HSV-tk gene. Subsequent formation of the diphosphate and triphosphate GCV derivatives (GCV-PP and -PPP) is catalyzed by cellular guanylate kinase. GCV-PPP, due to its analogy with the purinic nucleotide 2′-deoxyguanosine triphosphate, becomes substrate for DNA polymerase. Once bound to DNA polymerase, GCV-PPP is either incorporated into DNA or inhibits the polymerase. Consequently, chain termination immediately occurs after GCV incorporation into DNA, and leads to cell death [79].

A powerful characteristic of HSV-tk/GCV therapy is that the transduction of a small fraction of tumor cells with the suicide gene can result in widespread tumor-cell death (bystander effect) (Fig. 9.11). The cell to cell transfer of HSV-tk-activated GCV between HSV-tk-transduced tumor cells and neighboring unmodified cells via gap junctions is a major mechanism of the bystander effect [80, 81]. Gap junctions are composed of connexin subunits and connect the cytoplasmic domains of contacting cells, allowing ionic and metabolic exchange between them [82]. However, many cancer cell lines are deficient in gap junctions [83]. Such a deficiency, which is also found in human tumors [84], can limit the extent of the bystander effect in suicide gene therapy. The bystander effect has been reported to be enhanced by introducing a connexin gene with the HSV-tk gene *in vitro* [81]. In the normal human prostate, the cells communicate via gap junctions, whereas in poorly differentiated prostate cancer the expression of connexin 43 (Cx43) decreased and gap junctional intracellular communication failed [83, 84]. Transfection of the Cx43 gene into a Cx43-deficient prostate cancer cells may enhance the bystander effect, and also has been reported to inhibit cell growth, retard tumorigenicity and induce differentiation [85].

The use of a folate ligand as a targeting ligand to deliver DNA has not been successful in *in vivo* gene therapy [20, 21]. In prostate cancer, suicide gene therapy by local injection using adenoviral vectors has been reported as an alternative treatment [86, 87]. The use of non-viral vectors is a novel approach. A NPII-F nanoplex of HSV-tk was transiently transfected into KB, LNCaP and PC-3 cells. The first evidence of transfection was that GCV-PPP, the most abundant triphosphate produced, was clearly detected in LNCaP cells transfected with the HSV-tk gene after incubation with GCV by HPLC [73]. These findings were also made in KB and PC-3 cancer cells [64]. Further evidence was that HSV-tk plasmid-transfected LNCaP cells showed significantly greater sensitivity to GCV than the controls (IC_{50} 9.4 μg mL^{-1}) (Fig. 9.12A). Cx43 plasmid-transfected cells showed significantly higher sensitivity to GCV (IC_{50} 62.4 μg mL^{-1}) than the controls. Cells co-transfected with HSV-tk and Cx43 plasmids exhibited increased sensitivity to GCV (IC_{50} 7.9 μg mL^{-1}). This result suggests that HSV-tk and Cx43, individually, induced a cytotoxic effect by GCV in the transfected cells, and that the combination of HSV-tk plus Cx43 genes may display a bystander effect. HSV-tk plasmid-transfected PC-3 cells showed significant sensitivity to GCV (IC_{50} 6.6 μg mL^{-1}) compared with the controls, but Cx43 plasmid-transfected cells did not (Fig. 9.12B) [64]. Sensitivity to GCV was not enhanced in cells transfected with HSV-tk plus Cx43 plasmids. This result suggests that Cx43 plasmid did not display a bystander effect in PC-3 cells.

The *in vivo* anti-tumor effect of the NPII-F nanoplex with the HSV-tk gene has been evaluated. First, we determined the anti-tumor effect by direct injection into KB tumor xenografts with the NPII-F nanoplex of HSV-tk. When KB cells were transiently transfected with the NPII-F nanoplex using various plasmids, HSV-tk, Cx43 plasmid and combinations thereof, the HSV-tk-transfected cells showed significant sensitivity to GCV compared with the control, but did not with cells co-transfected with HSV-tk and Cx43 plasmids (unpublished data). Therefore, HSV-tk plasmid was used as a therapeutic gene for KB xenograft. When the NPII-F nanoplex of the HSV-tk plasmid was injected directly into the tumor, the growth of KB nasopharyngeal tumors was inhibited significantly in mice treated with the plasmid on day 13 (Fig. 9.13A). A comparison of tumor weight and appearance after excision also demonstrated that the tumor growth was attenuated in mice treated with the plasmid (Fig. 9.13B and C) [64].

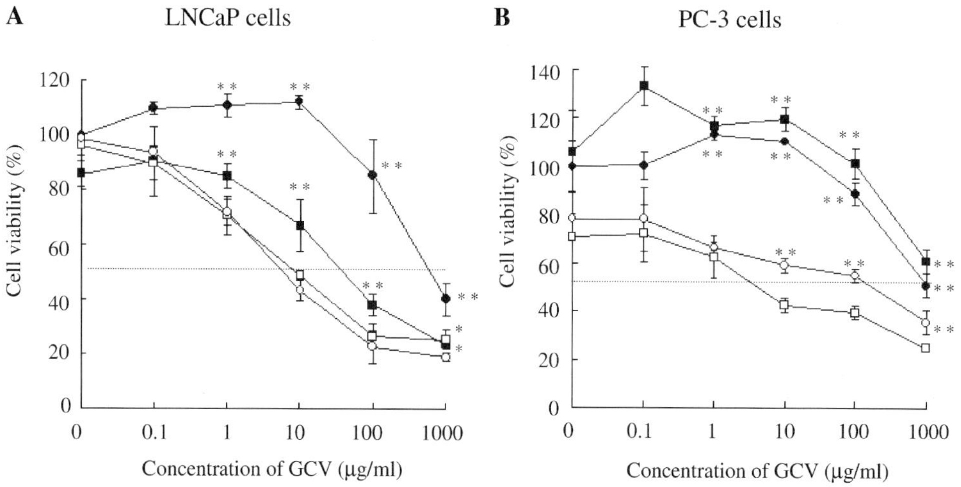

	IC_{50} (μg/ml)
Control	804.3
Cx43 plasmid	62.4
HSV-tk plasmid	9.4
Cx43 + HSV-tk plasmids	7.9

	IC_{50} (μg/ml)
Control	> 1000.0
Cx43 plasmid	> 1000.0
HSV-tk plasmid	6.6
Cx43 + HSV-tk plasmids	334.9

Fig. 9.12. Sensitivity of LNCaP (A) and PC-3 (B) cells to GCV. Cells were transfected with various plasmids using NPII-F. After 12 h incubation, the culture medium was replaced with one containing a concentration of GCV ranging from 0.1 to 1000 μg mL^{-1}. Plasmids used were: control plasmid (●), HSV-tk (□), Cx43 (■), and HSV-tk plus Cx43 plasmids (○). The number of surviving cells was determined with a WST-8 assay after 4 days exposure to the GCV. Data points indicate the mean ± S.D. ($n = 3$). *$p < 0.05$ and **$p < 0.01$, compared with HSV-tk and Cx43 plasmids in (A). **$p < 0.01$, compared with HSV-tk plasmid in B [64].

We then evaluated the anti-tumor effect by direct injection into LNCaP tumor xenografts with the NPII-F nanoplex of HSV-tk plus Cx43 plasmid (Fig. 9.14), because this nanoplex was the most effective in *in vitro* experiments with LNCaP cells (Fig. 9.12A). Tumor growth was suppressed in mice treated with the NPII-F nanoplex of HSV-tk plus Cx43 plasmids, but not in the control mice. The mean survival times of the control mice and the mice treated with the nanoplex of HSV-tk plus Cx43 plasmids were 21.5 and 33 days, respectively [64]. The observed reduction in tumor size may not be wholly due to the direct effect of the phosphorylated GCV on the transduced tumor cells. An indirect mechanism (the bystander effect) might be contributing to the antitumor activity. It is reported that a 1–5% *in vivo* transfection efficiency could generate a significant anti-tumoral effect in suicide gene therapy [88]. However, a deficiency of gap junctions is found in human prostate tumors [83, 84], which may limit the extent of the bystander effect in suicide gene therapy. Therefore, to examine the *in vivo* anti-tumor effects of direct injection into LNCaP prostate xenografts, the nanoplex of HSV-tk plus Cx43 plasmids was used, with the result that the tumor growth was suppressed [64] (Fig. 9.14).

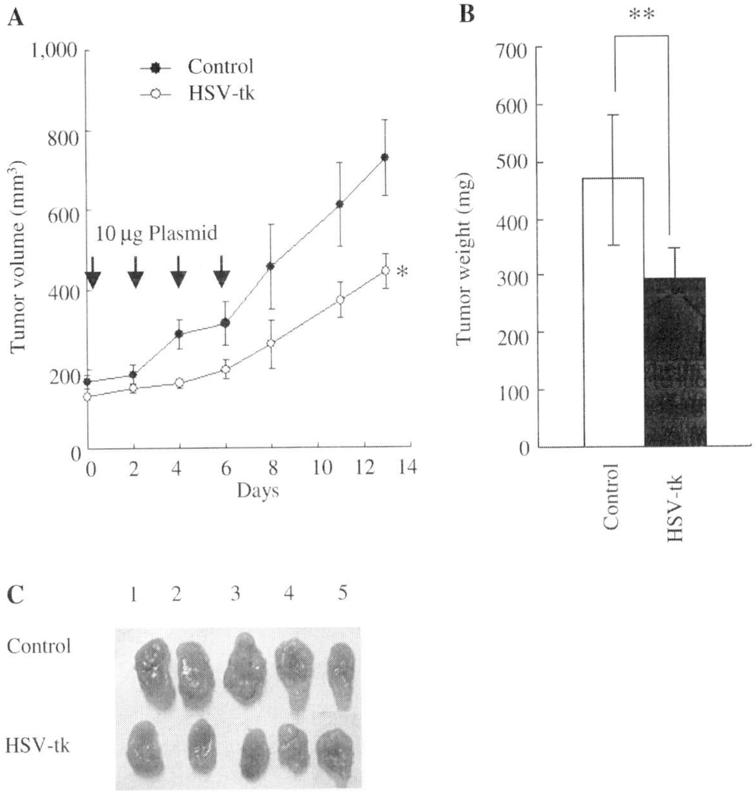

Fig. 9.13. *In vivo* suicide gene therapy for KB tumor xenografts with GCV in mice. Mice were divided into two groups: group I, control plasmid (10 μg); group II, HSV-tk plasmid (10 μg). NPII-F nanoplexes of the plasmids were injected directly into the tumor four times (day 0, 2, 4, and 6). GCV (25 mg kg^{-1}) was administered i.p. at 24 and 36 h after the injections. Tumor volume (A), excised tumor weight (B) and macroscopic tumor appearance (C) when all the mice in Fig. 9.13(A) were sacrificed at day 14. The results are indicated in (A) and (B) as the mean volume and weight ± S.E. or S.D., respectively ($n = 5$). $*P < 0.05$ and $**P < 0.01$, compared with control [64].

9.7 Conclusions

We have shown that folate-linked lipid-based nanoparticles can deliver DNA with high transfection efficiency and selectivity, inhibiting tumor growth following intratumoral injection into human nasopharyngeal and prostate cancer using an HSV-tk/GCV therapy system. These findings indicate that folate-linked lipid-based nanoparticles have potential as a clinically effective vector in cancer suicide gene therapy. However, several factors have the potential to adversely affect FR-targeted gene transfer *in vivo*. The size of gene transfer vectors, escaping the vasculature and intratumoral diffusion, could be limiting to targeted delivery. They should be

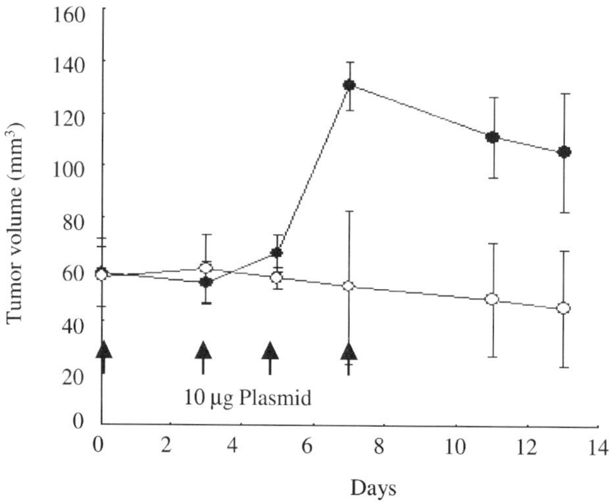

Fig. 9.14. Suicide gene therapy for LNCaP tumor xenografts with GCV in mice. Mice were divided into two groups: group I, control plasmid (●); group II, HSV-tk plus Cx43 plasmids (○). NPII-F nanoplexes of the plasmids indicated were injected directly into the tumor four times (day 1, 3, 5, and 7). GCV (25 mg kg^{-1}) was administered i.p. at 24 and 36 h after the injections. The results are indicated as the mean volume ± S.E. ($n = 6$) [64].

kept under 300 nm since this is the approximate limit for long circulation and efficient tumor extravasation. In addition, PEGylated vectors can reduce plasma protein binding and RES uptake, resulting in an extended systemic circulation time. Non-specific cell uptake by the RES (e.g., Kupffer cells in the liver) is expected to be reduced by incorporating PEGylated lipid within the particle/DNA complex. However, PEGylated particles may prevent enough DNA being carried into cells by inhibition of association of plasmid DNA with particles. For gene therapy, a balance of long-circulating vectors and FR-targeting vectors will be key to using folate-PEG-lipid. Further efforts aimed at optimizing FR-targeting vector formulations from a systemic approach should lead to the clinical evaluation of these vectors for cancer gene therapy.

List of Abbreviations

CHEMS	Cholesteryl hemisuccinate
Chol	Cholesterol
DC-Chol	3-[*N*-(*N′*,*N′*-dimethylaminoethane)carbamoyl]cholesterol
DOPE	Dioleoylphosphatidylethanolamine
DPPE	Dipalmitoyl phosphatidylethanolamine
DSPE	Distearoyl phosphatidylethanolamine
FR	Folate receptor

GCV	Ganciclovir
HSV-tk	Herpes simplex virus thymidine kinase
OH-Chol	Cholesteryl-3β-carboxyamidoethylene-*N*-hydroxylamine
ODN	Oligodeoxynucleotide
PEG	Poly(ethylene glycol)
PEI	Polyethylenimine
PLL	Poly-L-lysine
PEG-DSPE	Poly(ethylene glycol)-distearoylphosphatidylethanolamine
PSMA	Prostate specific membrane antigen
RES	Reticuloendothelial systems
RFC	Reduced folate carrier

References

1 Dass, C. R., Burton, M. A. Lipoplexes and tumours. A review. *J. Pharm. Pharmacol.*, **1999**, *51*, 755–770.

2 Rosenberg, S. A., Aebersold, P., Cornetta, K., Kasid, A., Morgan, R. A., Moen, R., Karson, E. M., Lotze, M. T., Yang, J. C., Topalian, S. L. Gene transfer into humans – immunotherapy of patients with advanced melanoma, using tumor-infiltrating lymphocytes modified by retroviral gene transduction. *N. Engl. J. Med.*, **1990**, *323*, 570–578.

3 Hoffman, M. New vector delivers genes to lung cells. *Science*, **1991**, *252*, 374.

4 Flotte, T. R., Solow, R., Owens, R. A., Afione, S., Zeitlin, P. L., Carter, B. J. Gene expression from adeno-associated virus vectors in airway epithelial cells. *Am. J. Respir. Cell Mol. Biol.*, **1992**, *7*, 349–356.

5 Dachs, G. U., Dougherty, G. J., Stratford, I. J., Chaplin, D. J. Targeting gene therapy to cancer: a review. *Oncol. Res.*, **1997**, *9*, 313–325.

6 Wu, M., Gunning, W., Ratnam, M. Expression of folate receptor type alpha in relation to cell type, malignancy, and differentiation in ovary, uterus, and cervix. *Cancer Epidemiol. Biomarkers Prev.*, **1999**, *8*, 775–782.

7 Antony, A. C. Folate receptors. *Annu. Rev. Nutr.*, **1996**, *16*, 501–521.

8 Lee, R. J., Low, P. S. Folate-mediated tumor cell targeting of liposome-entrapped doxorubicin *in vitro*. *Biochim. Biophys. Acta*, **1995**, *1233*, 134–144.

9 Gabizon, A., Horowitz, A. T., Goren, D., Tzemach, D., Mandelbaum-Shavit, F., Qazen, M. M., Zalipsky, S. Targeting folate receptor with folate linked to extremities of poly(ethylene glycol)-grafted liposomes: *in vitro* studies. *Bioconjug. Chem.*, **1999**, *10*, 289–298.

10 Goren, D., Horowitz, A. T., Tzemach, D., Tarshish, M., Zalipsky, S., Gabizon, A. Nuclear delivery of doxorubicin via folate-targeted liposomes with bypass of multidrug-resistance efflux pump. *Clin. Cancer Res.*, **2000**, *6*, 1949–1957.

11 Pan, X. Q., Zheng, X., Shi, G., Wang, H., Ratnam, M., Lee, R. J. Strategy for the treatment of acute myelogenous leukemia based on folate receptor beta-targeted liposomal doxorubicin combined with receptor induction using all-trans retinoic acid. *Blood*, **2002**, *100*, 594–602.

12 Pan, X. Q., Wang, H., Lee, R. J. Antitumor activity of folate receptor-targeted liposomal doxorubicin in a KB oral carcinoma murine xenograft model. *Pharm. Res.*, **2003**, *20*, 417–422.

13 Gabizon, A., Horowitz, A. T., Goren, D., Tzemach, D., Shmeeda, H., Zalipsky, S. *In vivo* fate of folate-

targeted polyethylene-glycol liposomes in tumor-bearing mice. *Clin. Cancer Res.*, **2003**, *9*, 6551–6559.

14 Shiokawa, T., Hattori, Y., Kawano, K., Ohguchi, Y., Kawakami, H., Toma, K., Maitani, Y. Effect of the polyethylene glycol linker chain length of folate-linked microemulsions loading aclacinomycin A on targeting ability and antitumor effect *in vitro* and *in vivo*. *Clin. Cancer Res.*, **2005**, *11*, 2018–2025.

15 Reddy, J. A., Dean, D., Kennedy, M. D., Low, P. S. Optimization of folate-conjugated liposomal vectors for folate receptor-mediated gene therapy. *J. Pharm. Sci.*, **1999**, *88*, 1112–1118.

16 Lee, R. J., Huang, L. Folate-targeted, anionic liposome-entrapped polylysine-condensed DNA for tumor cell-specific gene transfer. *J. Biol. Chem.*, **1996**, *271*, 8481–8487.

17 Leamon, C. P., Cooper, S. R., Hardee, G. E. Folate-liposome-mediated antisense oligodeoxy-nucleotide targeting to cancer cells: evaluation *in vitro* and *in vivo*. *Bioconjug. Chem.*, **2003**, *14*, 738–747.

18 Yang, L., Li, J., Zhou, W., Yuan, X., Li, S. Targeted delivery of antisense oligodeoxynucleotides to folate receptor-overexpressing tumor cells. *J. Controlled Release*, **2004**, *95*, 321–331.

19 Wang, S., Lee, R. J., Cauchon, G., Gorenstein, D. G., Low, P. S. Delivery of antisense oligodeoxyribo-nucleotides against the human epidermal growth factor receptor into cultured KB cells with liposomes conjugated to folate via polyethylene glycol. *Proc. Natl. Acad. Sci. U.S.A.*, **1995**, *92*, 3318–3322.

20 Hofland, H. E., Masson, C., Iginla, S., Osetinsky, I., Reddy, J. A., Leamon, C. P., Scherman, D., Bessodes, M., Wils, P. Folate-targeted gene transfer *in vivo*. *Mol. Ther.*, **2002**, *5*, 739–744.

21 Reddy, J. A., Abburi, C., Hofland, H., Howard, S. J., Vlahov, I., Wils, P., Leamon, C. P. Folate-targeted, cationic liposome-mediated gene transfer into disseminated peritoneal tumors. *Gene Ther.*, **2002**, *9*, 1542–1550.

22 Papadakis, E. D., Nicklin, S. A., Baker, A. H., White, S. J. Promoters and control elements: designing expression cassettes for gene therapy. *Curr. Gene Ther.*, **2004**, *4*, 89–113.

23 Humphreys, M. J., Ghaneh, P., Greenhalf, W., Campbell, F., Clayton, T. M., Everett, P., Huber, B. E., Richards, C. A., Ford, M. J., Neoptolemos, J. P. Hepatic intra-arterial delivery of a retroviral vector expressing the cytosine deaminase gene, controlled by the CEA promoter and intraperitoneal treatment with 5-fluorocytosine suppresses growth of colorectal liver metastases. *Gene Ther.*, **2001**, *8*, 1241–1247.

24 Ido, A., Nakata, K., Kato, Y., Nakao, K., Murata, K., Fujita, M., Ishii, N., Tamaoki, T., Shiku, H., Nagataki, S. Gene therapy for hepatoma cells using a retrovirus vector carrying herpes simplex virus thymidine kinase gene under the control of human alpha-fetoprotein gene promoter. *Cancer Res.*, **1995**, *55*, 3105–3109.

25 Yoshida, Y., Tomizawa, M., Bahar, R., Miyauchi, M., Yamaguchi, T., Saisho, H., Kadomatsu, K., Muramatsu, T., Matsubara, S., Sakiyama, S., Tagawa, M. A promoter region of midkine gene can activate transcription of an exogenous suicide gene in human pancreatic cancer. *Anticancer Res.*, **2002**, *22*, 117–120.

26 Suzuki, S., Tadakuma, T., Kunitomi, M., Takayama, E., Sato, M., Asano, T., Nakamura, H., Hayakawa, M. Liposome-mediated gene therapy using HSV-TK/ganciclovir under the control of human PSA promoter in prostate cancer cells. *Urol. Int.*, **2001**, *67*, 216–223.

27 Saukkonen, K., Hemminki, A. Tissue-specific promoters for cancer gene therapy. *Expert Opin. Biol. Ther.*, **2004**, *4*, 683–696.

28 Vijayanathan, V., Thomas, T., Thomas, T. J. DNA nanoparticles and development of DNA delivery vehicles for gene therapy. *Biochemistry*, **2002**, *41*, 14085–14094.

29 Bloomfield, V. A. DNA condensation. *Curr. Opin. Struct. Biol.*, **1996**, *6*, 334–341.

30 De Smedt, S. C., Demeester, J., Hennink, W. E. Cationic polymer based gene delivery systems. *Pharm. Res.*, **2000**, *17*, 113–126.

31 Kamiya, H., Fujimura, Y., Matsuoka, I., Harashima, H. Visualization of intracellular trafficking of exogenous DNA delivered by cationic liposomes. *Biochem. Biophys. Res. Commun.*, **2002**, *298*, 591–597.

32 Nigg, E. A. Nucleocytoplasmic transport: signals, mechanisms and regulation. *Nature*, **1997**, *386*, 779–787.

33 Gorlich, D. Nuclear protein import. *Curr. Opin. Cell Biol.*, **1997**, *9*, 412–419.

34 Allen, T. M., Hansen, C., Rutledge, J. Liposomes with prolonged circulation times: factors affecting uptake by reticuloendothelial and other tissues. *Biochim. Biophys. Acta*, **1989**, *981*, 27–35.

35 Klibanov, A. L., Maruyama, K., Beckerleg, A. M., Torchilin, V. P., Huang, L. Activity of amphipathic poly(ethylene glycol) 5000 to prolong the circulation time of liposomes depends on the liposome size and is unfavorable for immunoliposome binding to target. *Biochim. Biophys. Acta*, **1991**, *1062*, 142–148.

36 Park, J. W., Hong, K., Kirpotin, D. B., Papahadjopoulos, D., Benz, C. C. Immunoliposomes for cancer treatment. *Adv. Pharmacol.*, **1997**, *40*, 399–435.

37 Hosokawa, S., Tagawa, T., Niki, H., Hirakawa, Y., Nohga, K., Nagaike, K. Efficacy of immunoliposomes on cancer models in a cell-surface-antigen-density-dependent manner. *Br. J. Cancer*, **2003**, *89*, 1545–1551.

38 Mahato, R. I., Kawabata, K., Takakura, Y., Hashida, M. *In vivo* disposition characteristics of plasmid DNA complexed with cationic liposomes. *J. Drug Target*, **1995**, *3*, 149–157.

39 Xu, L., Huang, C. C., Huang, W., Tang, W. H., Rait, A., Yin, Y. Z., Cruz, I., Xiang, L. M., Pirollo, K. F., Chang, E. H. Systemic tumor-targeted gene delivery by anti-transferrin receptor scFv-immunoliposomes. *Mol. Cancer Ther.*, **2002**, *1*, 337–346.

40 Lee, C. H., Hsiao, M., Tseng, Y. L., Chang, F. H. Enhanced gene delivery to HER-2-overexpressing breast cancer cells by modified immunolipoplexes conjugated with the anti-HER-2 antibody. *J. Biomed. Sci.*, **2003**, *10*, 337–344.

41 Joo, S. Y., Kim, J. S. Enhancement of gene transfer to cervical cancer cells using transferrin-conjugated liposome. *Drug Dev. Ind. Pharm.*, **2002**, *28*, 1023–1031.

42 Kakudo, T., Chaki, S., Futaki, S., Nakase, I., Akaji, K., Kawakami, T., Maruyama, K., Kamiya, H., Harashima, H. Transferrin-modified liposomes equipped with a pH-sensitive fusogenic peptide: an artificial viral-like delivery system. *Biochemistry*, **2004**, *43*, 5618–5628.

43 Nishikawa, M., Kawakami, S., Yamashita, F., Hashida, M. Glycosylated cationic liposomes for carbohydrate receptor-mediated gene transfer. *Methods Enzymol.*, **2003**, *373*, 384–399.

44 Hwang, S. H., Hayashi, K., Takayama, K., Maitani, Y. Liver-targeted gene transfer into a human hepatoblastoma cell line and *in vivo* by sterylglucoside-containing cationic liposomes. *Gene Ther.*, **2001**, *8*, 1276–1280.

45 Lee, R. J., Low, P. S. Delivery of liposomes into cultured KB cells via folate receptor-mediated endocytosis. *J. Biol. Chem.*, **1994**, *269*, 3198–3204.

46 Harbottle, R. P., Cooper, R. G., Hart, S. L., Ladhoff, A., McKay, T., Knight, A. M., Wagner, E., Miller, A. D., Coutelle, C. An RGD-oligolysine peptide: a prototype construct for integrin-mediated gene delivery. *Hum. Gene Ther.*, **1998**, *9*, 1037–1047.

47 Sabharanjak, S., Mayor, S. Folate receptor endocytosis and trafficking. *Adv. Drug Deliv. Rev.*, **2004**, *56*, 1099–1109.

48 Weitman, S. D., Lark, R. H., Coney, L. R., Fort, D. W., Frasca, V., Zurawski, V. R., Jr., Kamen, B. A. Distribution of the folate receptor GP38 in normal and malignant cell lines and tissues. *Cancer Res.*, **1992**, *52*, 3396–3401.

49 Shen, F., Ross, J. F., Wang, X., Ratnam, M. Identification of a novel folate receptor, a truncated receptor, and receptor type beta in hematopoietic cells: cDNA cloning, expression, immunoreactivity, and tissue specificity. *Biochemistry*, **1994**, *33*, 1209–1215.

50 Shen, F., Wu, M., Ross, J. F., Miller, D., Ratnam, M. Folate receptor type gamma is primarily a secretory protein due to lack of an efficient signal for glycosylphosphatidylinositol modification: protein characterization and cell type specificity. *Biochemistry*, **1995**, *34*, 5660–5665.

51 Gabizon, A., Shmeeda, H., Horowitz, A. T., Zalipsky, S. Tumor cell targeting of liposome-entrapped drugs with phospholipid-anchored folic acid-PEG conjugates. *Adv. Drug Deliv. Rev.*, **2004**, *56*, 1177–1192.

52 Gottschalk, S., Cristiano, R. J., Smith, L. C., Woo, S. L. Folate receptor mediated DNA delivery into tumor cells: potosomal disruption results in enhanced gene expression. *Gene Ther.*, **1994**, *1*, 185–191.

53 Mislick, K. A., Baldeschwieler, J. D., Kayyem, J. F., Meade, T. J. Transfection of folate-polylysine DNA complexes: evidence for lysosomal delivery. *Bioconjug. Chem.*, **1995**, *6*, 512–515.

54 Ward, C. M., Pechar, M., Oupicky, D., Ulbrich, K., Seymour, L. W. Modification of pLL/DNA complexes with a multivalent hydrophilic polymer permits folate-mediated targeting *in vitro* and prolonged plasma circulation *in vivo*. *J. Gene Med.*, **2002**, *4*, 536–547.

55 Leamon, C. P., Weigl, D., Hendren, R. W. Folate copolymer-mediated transfection of cultured cells. *Bioconj. Chem.*, **1999**, *10*, 947–957.

56 Guo, W., Lee, R. L. Receptor-targeted gene delivery via folate-conjugated polyethylenimine. *AAPS. PharmSci.*, **1999**, *1*, E19.

57 Benns, J. M., Mahato, R. I., Kim, S. W. Optimization of factors influencing the transfection efficiency of folate-PEG-folate-graft-polyethylenimine. *J. Controlled Release*, **2002**, *79*, 255–269.

58 van Steenis, J. H., van Maarseveen, E. M., Verbaan, F. J., Verrijk, R., Crommelin, D. J., Storm, G., Hennink, W. E. Preparation and characterization of folate-targeted pEG-coated pDMAEMA-based polyplexes. *J. Controlled Release*, **2003**, *87*, 167–176.

59 Xu, L., Pirollo, K. F., Chang, E. H. Tumor-targeted p53-gene therapy enhances the efficacy of conventional chemo/radiotherapy. *J. Controlled Release*, **2001**, *74*, 115–128.

60 Bruckheimer, E., Harvie, P., Orthel, J., Dutzar, B., Furstoss, K., Mebel, E., Anklesaria, P., Paul, R. *In vivo* efficacy of folate-targeted lipid-protamine-DNA (LPD-PEG-Folate) complexes in an immunocompetent syngeneic model for breast adenocarcinoma. *Cancer Gene Ther.*, **2004**, *11*, 128–134.

61 Shi, G., Guo, W., Stephenson, S. M., Lee, R. J. Efficient intracellular drug and gene delivery using folate receptor-targeted pH-sensitive liposomes composed of cationic/anionic lipid combinations. *J. Controlled Release*, **2002**, *80*, 309–319.

62 Dauty, E., Remy, J. S., Zuber, G., Behr, J. P. Intracellular delivery of nanometric DNA particles via the folate receptor. *Bioconjug. Chem.*, **2002**, *13*, 831–839.

63 Hattori, Y., Maitani, Y. Enhanced *in vitro* DNA transfection efficiency by novel folate-linked nanoparticles in human prostate cancer and oral cancer. *J. Controlled Release*, **2004**, *97*, 173–183.

64 Hattori, Y., Maitani, Y. Folate-linked nanoparticle-mediated suicide gene therapy in human prostate cancer and

nasopharyngeal cancer with herpes simplex virus thymidine kinase. *Cancer Gene Ther.*, **2005**, in press.

65 Holm, J., Hansen, S. I., Hoier-Madsen, M. High-affinity folate binding in human prostate. *Biosci. Rep.*, **1993**, *13*, 99–105.

66 Pinto, J. T., Suffoletto, B. P., Berzin, T. M., Qiao, C. H., Lin, S., Tong, W. P., May, F., Mukherjee, B., Heston, W. D. Prostate-specific membrane antigen: a novel folate hydrolase in human prostatic carcinoma cells. *Clin. Cancer Res.*, **1996**, *2*, 1445–1451.

67 Rajasekaran, S. A., Anilkumar, G., Oshima, E., Bowie, J. U., Liu, H., Heston, W., Bander, N. H., Rajasekaran, A. K. A novel cytoplasmic tail MXXXL motif mediates the internalization of prostate-specific membrane antigen. *Mol. Biol. Cell*, **2003**, *14*, 4835–4845.

68 Hattori, Y., Kubo, H., Higashiyama, K., Maitani, Y. Folate-linked nanoparticles formed with DNA complexes in sodium chloride solution enhance transfection efficiency. *J. Boimed. Nanotechnol.*, **2005**, in press.

69 Song, L. Y., Ahkong, Q. F., Rong, Q., Wang, Z., Ansell, S., Hope, M. J., Mui, B. Characterization of the inhibitory effect of PEG-lipid conjugates on the intracellular delivery of plasmid and antisense DNA mediated by cationic lipid liposomes. *Biochim. Biophys. Acta*, **2002**, *1558*, 1–13.

70 Hasegawa, S., Hirashima, N., Nakanishi, M. Comparative study of transfection efficiency of cationic cholesterols mediated by liposomes-based gene delivery. *Bioorg. Med. Chem. Lett.*, **2002**, *12*, 1299–1302.

71 Guo, W., Lee, R. J. Efficient gene delivery via non-covalent complexes of folic acid and polyethylenimine. *J. Controlled Release*, **2001**, *77*, 131–138.

72 Lawrence, J. M., Petitti, D. B., Watkins, M., Umekubo, M. A. Trends in serum folate after food fortification. *Lancet*, **1999**, *354*, 915–916.

73 Hattori, Y., Maitani, Y. Folate-linked lipid-based nanoparticle for targeted gene delivery. *Curr. Drug Delivery*, **2005**, *2*, 243–252.

74 Mahato, R. I., Kawabata, K., Nomura, T., Takakura, Y., Hashida, M. Physicochemical and pharmacokinetic characteristics of plasmid DNA/cationic liposome complexes. *J. Pharm. Sci.*, **1995**, *84*, 1267–1271.

75 Paulos, C. M., Turk, M. J., Breur, G. J., Low, P. S. Folate receptor-mediated targeting of therapeutic and imaging agents to activated macrophages in rheumatoid arthritis. *Adv. Drug Deliv. Rev.*, **2004**, *56*, 1205–1217.

76 El Aneed, A. An overview of current delivery systems in cancer gene therapy. *J. Controlled Release*, **2004**, *94*, 1–14.

77 Fillat, C., Carrio, M., Cascante, A., Sangro, B. Suicide gene therapy mediated by the Herpes Simplex virus thymidine kinase gene/Ganciclovir system: fifteen years of application. *Curr. Gene Ther.*, **2003**, *3*, 13–26.

78 Faulds, D., Heel, R. C. Ganciclovir. A review of its antiviral activity, pharmacokinetic properties and therapeutic efficacy in cytomegalovirus infections. *Drugs*, **1990**, *39*, 597–638.

79 Ilsley, D. D., Lee, S. H., Miller, W. H., Kuchta, R. D. Acyclic guanosine analogs inhibit DNA polymerases alpha, delta, and epsilon with very different potencies and have unique mechanisms of action. *Biochemistry*, **1995**, *34*, 2504–2510.

80 Hamel, W., Magnelli, L., Chiarugi, V. P., Israel, M. A. Herpes simplex virus thymidine kinase/ganciclovir-mediated apoptotic death of bystander cells. *Cancer Res.*, **1996**, *56*, 2697–2702.

81 Mesnil, M., Piccoli, C., Tiraby, G., Willecke, K., Yamasaki, H. Bystander killing of cancer cells by herpes simplex virus thymidine kinase gene is mediated by connexins. *Proc. Natl. Acad. Sci. U.S.A.*, **1996**, *93*, 1831–1835.

82 Lampe, P. D., Lau, A. F. Regulation of gap junctions by phosphorylation of connexins. *Arch. Biochem. Biophys.*, **2000**, *384*, 205–215.

83 Tsai, H., Werber, J., Davia, M. O., Edelman, M., Tanaka, K. E., Melman, A., Christ, G. J., Geliebter, J. Reduced connexin 43 expression in high grade, human prostatic adenocarcinoma cells. *Biochem. Biophys. Res. Commun.*, **1996**, *227*, 64–69.

84 Habermann, H., Ray, V., Habermann, W., Prins, G. S. Alterations in gap junction protein expression in human benign prostatic hyperplasia and prostate cancer. *J. Urol.*, **2002**, *167*, 655–660.

85 Mehta, P. P., Perez-Stable, C., Nadji, M., Mian, M., Asotra, K., Roos, B. A. Suppression of human prostate cancer cell growth by forced expression of connexin genes. *Dev. Genet.*, **1999**, *24*, 91–110.

86 Cheon, J., Kim, H. K., Moon, D. G., Yoon, D. K., Cho, J. H., Koh, S. K. Adenovirus-mediated suicide-gene therapy using the herpes simplex virus thymidine kinase gene in cell and animal models of human prostate cancer: changes in tumour cell proliferative activity. *BJU Int.*, **2000**, *85*, 759–766.

87 Shalev, M., Miles, B. J., Thompson, T. C., Ayala, G., Butler, E. B., Aguilar-Cordova, E., Kadmon, D. Suicide gene therapy for prostate cancer using a replication-deficient adenovirus containing the herpesvirus thymidine kinase gene. *World J. Urol.*, **2000**, *18*, 125–129.

88 Huber, B. E., Austin, E. A., Richards, C. A., Davis, S. T., Good, S. S. Metabolism of 5-fluorocytosine to 5-fluorouracil in human colorectal tumor cells transduced with the cytosine deaminase gene: significant antitumor effects when only a small percentage of tumor cells express cytosine deaminase. *Proc. Natl. Acad. Sci. U.S.A.*, **1994**, *91*, 8302–8306.

10
Magnetic Core Conducting Polymer Shell Nanocomposites for DNA Attachment and Hybridization

Jean-Paul Lellouche

10.1
Introduction

Micro- and nanosized magnetically responsive particles or particulates have become an important class of micro-/nanomaterials that have found numerous applications in electronics (data storage technology), catalysis, and biotechnology [1–5]. Generally, these nanoparticulate materials display a range of magnetic, electrical, optical, and chemical properties that clearly differ from that of their bulk materials, thus making them very attractive for property-based applications. The main applications of nanosized magnetic particles in biomedical research are magnetism-driven separations of small biological components and cells; magnetic detoxification of undesirable molecules and antigens; magnetic field-guided delivery of drugs (targeting) and genes; relaxation and contrast enhancement in non-invasive magnetic resonance imaging (MRI) of tissues; piezoelectric immunosensors; and magnetic fluid hyperthermia for cancer therapy [6–13].

To exploit the full potential of corresponding magnetic nanoparticles and related nanocomposites, some key general issues need to be consistently addressed regarding their synthesis and further subsequent use. Accordingly, controlling the shape, size, and size distribution of nanoparticles toward spherical or non-spherical anisotropic materials is one significant issue. In addition, magnetic nanoparticles need to be stabilized sterically or by using charge repulsion against aggregation in both organic and/or aqueous media. The versatility of chemical modifications that can be introduced onto particle/composite surfaces is another key question that requires careful investigation. Finally, for *in vivo* use of nanoparticles/related nanocomposites, their biocompatibility profiles and systemic toxicity properties need to be examined in depth.

Related to this field, magnetically responsive core–shell iron oxide-conducting polymer (CP) [14–21] nanosized composites form a relatively recent class of magnetic nanocomposites (NCs) [22, 23]. They display thin outer layers of insoluble CPs, such as doped polypyrrole, that have been oxidatively deposited around nanosized magnetite/magnetite silica cores. Armes and co workers, in particular, have

Nanotechnologies for the Life Sciences Vol. 1
Biofunctionalization of Nanomaterials. Edited by Challa S. S. R. Kumar

ISBN: 3-527-31381-8

reported the fabrication of colloidal stable core–shell magnetite-silica-polypyrrole NCs with diameters in the range 100–520 nm that are superparamagnetic [24, 25]. Both aqueous oxidants $H_2O_2/Fe^{3+}/HCl$ and $(NH_4)_2S_2O_8$ have been used to chemically oxidize *non-functional* pyrrole around inorganic hybrid magnetite-silica cores (5–20 nm diameter). Nanosized ferromagnetic Fe_3O_4-crosslinked polyaniline NCs have recently been described by the Peng's group using aniline (monomer) and $(NH_4)_2S_2O_8$ (oxidant) [26]. Related conducting NCs were found polydispersed, 20–30 nm in diameter, and of a core–shell morphology. Consequently, both maghemite (γ-Fe_2O_3) and magnetite (Fe_3O_4) nanoparticles should be considered as attractive inorganic magnetic cores toward related magnetic CPs-based NCs. These readily prepared iron oxide nanoparticles are prone to minimal oxidation, are of low systemic toxicity, and present a high magnetic susceptibility, in the range of 76–81 and 90–98 emu g^{-1}, respectively.

Notably, in this related framework, various non-magnetic organic and inorganic cores have been engaged as micro-/nanosized supports to polymerize oxidatively *non-functional* and *functional* CPs monomers in their presence. For example, to develop color visual immunodiagnostic assays, core–shell micrometer-sized polystyrene latex-CPs [27–30] and colloidal nanosized silica-CPs [31–37] composites have been produced by oxidative deposition of insoluble CPs around corresponding cores. Tin(IV) oxide-polypyrrole colloidal NCs have been similarly fabricated by the same group for solid-state conductivity studies [38]. The main CPs studied include polypyrrole, polyaniline, poly(3,4-ethylenedioxythiophene), poly(3-pyrrol-1-yl-propionic acid), poly(3-(1*H*-pyrrol-3-yl)-propionic acid), poly(*N*-succinimidyl ester of 3-pyrrol-1-yl-propionic acid), and related copolymers. Interestingly, the last reported example [37] demonstrated that amine-sensitive *N*-succinimidyl ester of pyrrolyl-3-acetic acid survived the aqueous acidic medium that developed during monomer polymerization onto silica core nanoparticles. The resulting NCs were able to covalently attach proteins without the need for any additional post-polymerization activation step. Gold nanoparticles in a 5–200 nm diameter range have been also used as templating metallic cores to polymerize pyrrole and *N*-methylpyrrole monomers around them [39, 40]. Following core gold etching, hollow nanosized polymeric polypyrrolic capsules were synthesized as useful vehicles for drug physical entrapment and targeted delivery.

This chapter describes our most recent progress in the field of magnetically responsive new core–shell iron oxide-CPs NCs. It consists of four main sections, dealing with (a) the modular chemical design and synthesis of oxidizable dipyrrole- (DPyr) and dicarbazole- (DCbz) containing monomers to introduce molecular diversity at the monomer level (Sections 10.2 and 10.3); (b) the fabrication of magnetic NCs (chemical polymerization around magnetite cores) and their thorough characterization by means of modern spectral and analytical methods (Section 10.4); and (c) the investigation of covalent/quasi-covalent DNA attachments and hybridizations at NCs surfaces (Section 10.5). Additionally, Section 10.6 contains robust and reliable typical experimental procedures that relate to each separate step.

10.2
Chemical Design of DPyr- and DCbz-containing Monomers: Introduction of Molecular Diversity

Based on the literature considerations cited above, the full potential of magnetically responsive CPs-maghemite/magnetite nanocomposites (NCs) has still to be developed regarding novel (electro-)chemically oxidizable monomers that possess (a) heterocycles different from nonfunctional pyrrole, as well as (b) appropriate functionalities that can be appended by biological species after polymerizing over nanoparticles, e.g., grafting COOH functions that can be readily amidated using well-known amide chemistry. Considering the above points, four generic chemical structures (Fig. 10.1) of mono/dicarboxylate DPyr- and DCbz-containing monomers **1–2a** (index **a** specific for the DPyr-series) and **1–2b** (index **b** specific for the DCbz-series) readily emerged from the indicated planned innovative chemical design. These generic structures have been designed to be modular and clearly accentuated the key roles played by L- or D-amino acid building blocks and appropriate linkers of variable lengths, in order to introduce chirality and molecular diversity [41–43] at the monomer level. C_2-Symmetrization operations used have been included based on generally high-yielding, stable amide connections between monocarboxylated or monoaminated Pyr- and Cbz-containing building blocks and diaminated or dicarboxylated linkers, respectively. More precisely, molecular diversity at the monomer level should arise from (a) both types of heterocyclic DPyr- and DCbz-units; (b) the existing number of COOH functions (one or two); (c) absolute (*S*) or (*R*) chiralities of asymmetric centers (from L- or D-amino acid building blocks); and, finally, (d) linkers of different chemical types and lengths.

Another notable aspect is that, in these *bis*-heterocyclic generic structures, both pyrrole and carbazole heterocycles of suitable monomers would be simultaneously engaged in polymer chain propagation at positions 2,5 and 5,5′, respectively,

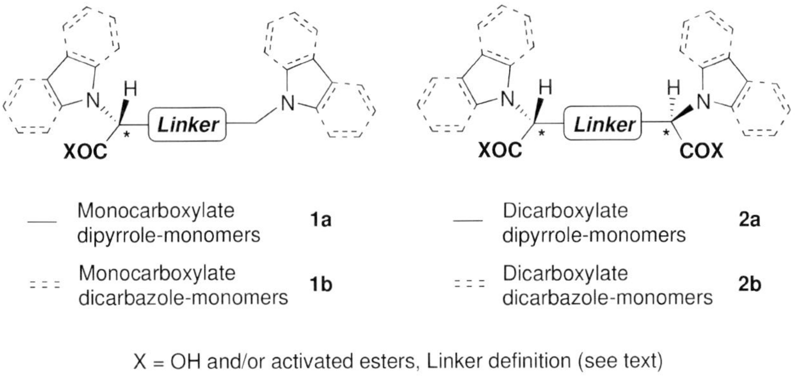

Fig. 10.1. Generic structures **1a/2a** and **1b/2b** of optically active mono- and dicarboxylate DPyr- and DCbz-containing oxidizable monomers.

through C–C bond formation, leading to reticulated and more stable polymers. Literature data more particularly emphasized the lack of stability of polycarbazole polymers in the carbazole series of oxidizable monomers. Accordingly, tentative electrosyntheses of polycarbazole films from N-substituted *mono*carbazole monomers resulted chiefly in short tetramers that are soluble in the electrochemical medium [44, 45]. In contrast, our laboratory has overcame this limitation. Electrochemically stable poly(DCbz)-films containing amine-sensitive pentafluorophenol esters have been formed using the electropolymerization of innovative DCbz-monomers synthesized according to the bis-podant bis-heterocyclic design cited above [46]. An example potential applications of these functional polyDCbz-films is the successful covalent attachment of polyphenol and glucose oxidases onto them as a step towards biosensor constructs [47–49].

10.3
Synthetic Approaches for Mono- and Dicarboxylated DPyr-/DCbz-based Monomers

According to synthetic approaches described below in Schemes 10.1–10.4, a range of *thirteen* enantiomerically pure mono-/dicarboxylated DPyr- and DCbz-monomers has been routinely prepared and used for the fabrication of targeted polyDPyr- and polyDCbz-magnetite NCs. Several key synthetic steps deserve some comments so as to best grasp the power and maneuverability of our planned chemical design for monomers. First, the well-known Clauson-Kaas reaction, a one-step acid-catalyzed transformation of an aromatic or alkyl NH_2 function into a pyrrole heterocycle unit using 2,5-dimethoxytetrahydrofuran (DMT, **4**) (Scheme 10.1) [50], has been modified to moderate reaction conditions (less acidic, salt buffered, solvent diluted, lower temperatures/shorter reaction times) [46]. Similar preparation of carbazole-based monomers generally required higher temperatures for a while

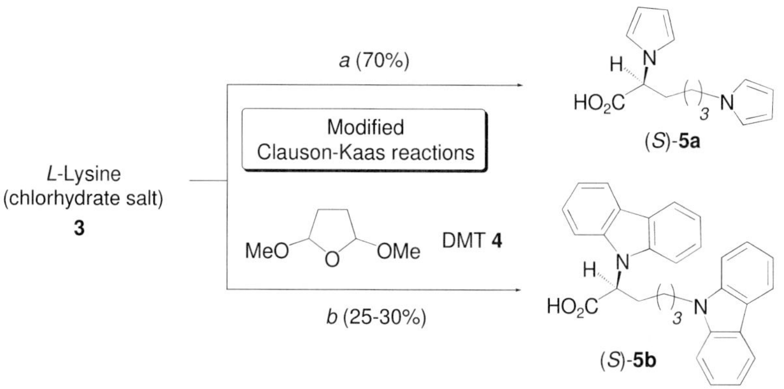

Scheme 10.1. Reagents and conditions: (a) 2,5-Dimethoxytetrahydrofuran (DMT, **4**), NaOAc, H_2O, AcOH–1,2-dichloroethane, 1 h, 76 °C; (b) DMT (**4**), AcOH–dioxane, 3 h at reflux then overnight at 20 °C.

and longer reaction times. Thus, two separate sets of experimental conditions allowed the synthesis of both DPyr- and DCbz-containing monocarboxylated monomers **5a–b**, as well as of intermediates **7a–b**, and **14–17a–b** from enantiomerically pure L-lysine, L-aspartic, and L-glutamic acid derivatives. However, contrary to what was usually observed under harsher conditions, racemization of existing asymmetric centers was nonexistent (*ee* 97–99%, Schemes 10.1–10.4, steps a and b) [46].

A stability issue has been encountered during the preparation of aminated Pyr-based intermediate **7a**, which readily cyclizes intramolecularly to the corresponding seven-membered lactam **8** (**7a**:**8** = 4:1 assayed by high-field ^{1}H NMR for a quasi-quantitative 91% recovery yield after separation from reaction mixture) during chromatographic purifications on silica gel columns. This intramolecular amidation did not, however, occur for the sterically more hindered Cbz-based precursor **7b**, therefore allowing its corresponding C_2-symmetrization, as described later (Scheme 10.2).

Intermediates and monomer yields were consistently higher in the modified Clauson-Kaas pyrrole synthesis than for the synthesis of carbazoles (70–80% and 25–40%, respectively). In addition, C_2-symmetrization operations toward bis-heterocyclic oxidizable monomers have been operated straightforwardly, using powerful amide connecting chemistries that do not racemize existing asymmetric centers, e.g., the use of highly reactive diacid dichlorides and of a dicyclohexylcarbodiimide (DCC)/1-hydroxybenzotriazole (HOBt) system in the

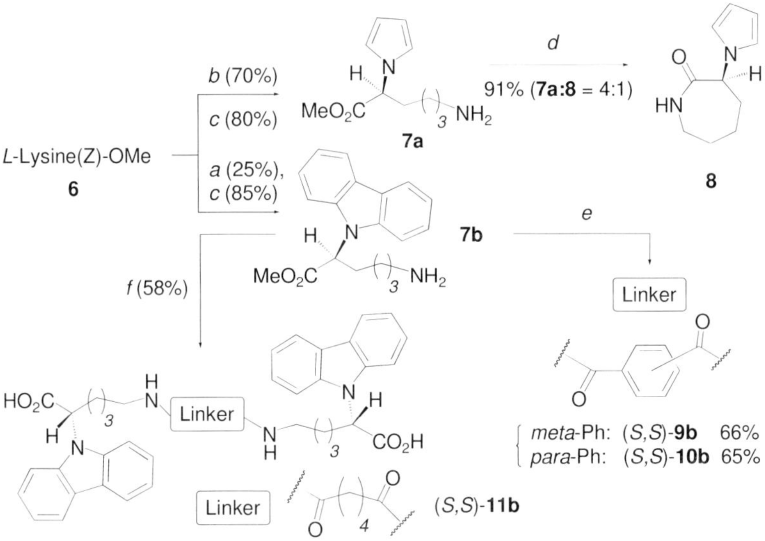

Scheme 10.2. Reagents and conditions: (a) and (b) same as Scheme 10.1; (c) cyclohexene, MeOH, 10% Pd/C, reflux, 0.5 h; (d) spontaneous cyclization during purification on silica gel column, **7a**:**8a** = 4:1 by ^{1}H NMR, 91% recovery; (e) (i) $CHCl_3$–Et_3N, terephthaloyl or isophthaloyl chloride, 2 h, 20 °C, (ii) 1.0 M KOH, 1/1 v/v MeOH–$PhCH_3$, reflux, 4 h then 0.1 M HCl; (f) (i) CH_2Cl_2–Et_3N, adipoyl chloride, 2 h, 20 °C, (ii) 1.0 M KOH, 1/1 v/v MeOH–$PhCH_3$, reflux, 4 h then 0.1 M HCl.

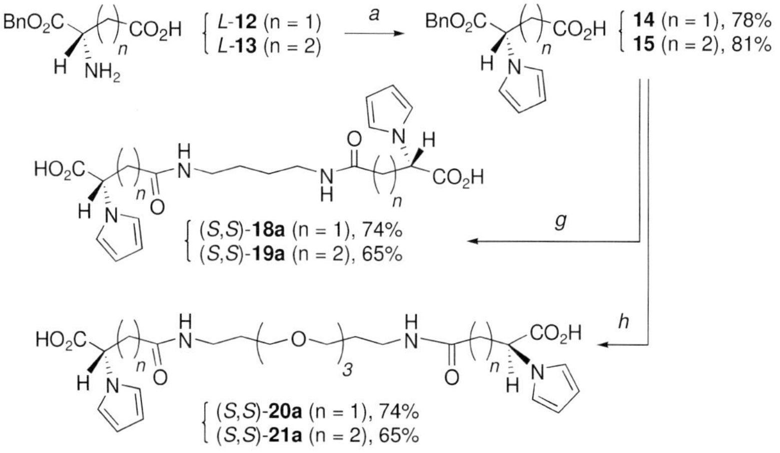

Scheme 10.3. Reagents and conditions: (a)–(f): same as Schemes 10.1 and 10.2; (g) (i) Dicyclohexylcarbodiimide (DCC), 1-hydroxybenzotriazole (HOBt), CH_2Cl_2, *N*-methylmorpholine, 1,4-diaminobutane, 3 h, 20 °C, (ii) 1:4 v/v cyclohexene–2-propanol, 10% Pd/carbon, 1.5 h, 20 °C; (h) same conditions as for step g but using a different 1,ω-diamine, e.g., 4,7,10-trioxatridecane-1,13-diamine.

presence of *N*-methylmorpholine (Schemes 10.2–10.4, Steps e–h). Appropriate monoPyr-/monoCbz-intermediates **7a–b** and **14–17** ($n = 1$ or 2) prepared from L-lysine(Z)-OMe **6** (Z: benzyloxycarbonyl) and monobenzyl esters of L-aspartic/L-glutamic acids **12–13** ($n = 1$ or 2) presented free NH_2 and COOH groups for C_2-symmetrical amide coupling. Diacids as well as diamide linkers variable in length and lipophilicity/hydrophilicity characteristics included aromatic terephthaloyl/isophthaloyl and alkyl adipoyl chlorides, the alkyl 1,4-diaminobutane, and, finally, the more hydrophilic polyoxyethylenyl 1,ω-diamine 4,7,10-trioxa-1,13-tridecanediamine.

Consequently, these synthetic efforts facilitated routine preparation of five DPyr- and eight DCbz mono-/dicarboxylated homochiral based monomers in a 0.5–1.0 g weight range. From commercially available L-amino acid derivatives, and apart from monocarboxylated monomers (*S*)-**5a**/(*S*)-**5b** (Scheme 10.1, *one* synthetic step from **3**, 70 and 25–30% yields), only *three* to *four* synthetic steps were necessary to obtain the entire range of dicarboxylated oxidizable monomers (*S*,*S*)-**18–21a**, (*S*,*S*)-**9–11b**, and (*S*,*S*)-**18–21b** in global 53–58%, 12–14%, and 19–27% yields, respectively (Schemes 10.1–10.4).

All these monomers have been fully characterized, their chemical structures confirmed and their purities checked before fabrication of the corresponding NCs by appropriate analytical means (thin-layer and high-performance liquid chromatographies, optical rotations) and spectroscopic analyses (FT-IR, 1D/2D-high-field $^1H/^{13}C$ NMR, low- and high-resolution FAB-MS). Additionally, and only after completion of synthetic amidations by starting block C_2-symmetrization, 1D high-field $^1H/^{13}C$ NMR techniques allowed us to again check that optical purities of resulting

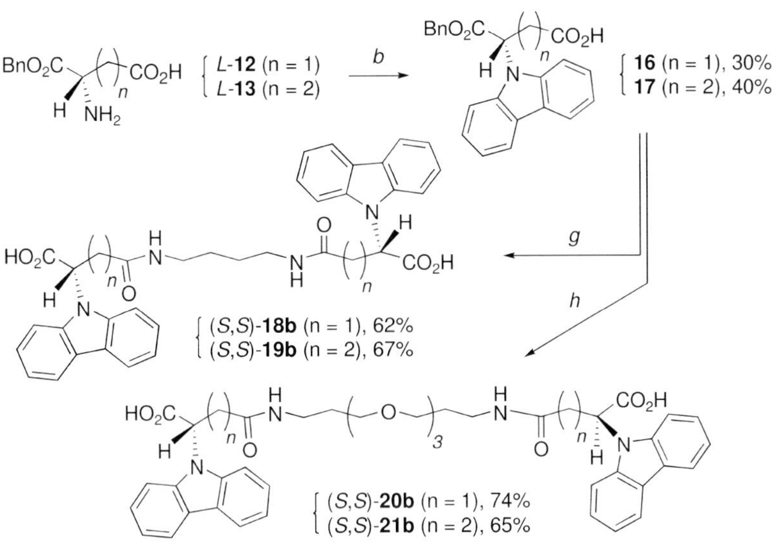

Scheme 10.4. Same reagents and conditions as in Schemes 10.1 and 10.3.

monomers were in a 97–98% range, based on the non-detection of meso diastereoisomers arising from asymmetric center racemization.

10.4 Oxidative Polymerization of DPyr-/DCbz-based Monomers around Magnetite Nanoparticles

10.4.1 General Considerations

The availability of DPyr- and DCbz-based monomers allowed us to test various oxidative polymerization conditions in the presence of nanosized magnetite particles (Fig. 10.2) towards corresponding magnetic NCs. Numerous methods and related modifications have been reported for the preparation of magnetite nanoparticles, and, significantly, dealing with stabilization against aggregation of the particles [1–4]. With this goal in mind, we modified slightly the original Sugimoto method, and, accordingly, the oxidative hydrolysis of iron(II) sulfate heptahydrate (Fe_2SO_4 $7H_2O$) by KNO_3 in an alkaline KOH medium under nitrogen [51, 52] (see optimized protocols for NC fabrication in Section 10.6.1) that afforded magnetite sheet-like nanoparticles (mean particle size of 20–40 nm by TEM analysis) as a free-flowing, brilliant black water suspension that can be used immediately or stored under nitrogen if necessary. FT-IR peaks characteristics of pure magnetite (Fe_3O_4, $\nu = 410, 510\ cm^{-1}$) confirmed its nature, and, in particular, the absence of contaminating maghemite (γ-Fe_2O_3) [51, 52].

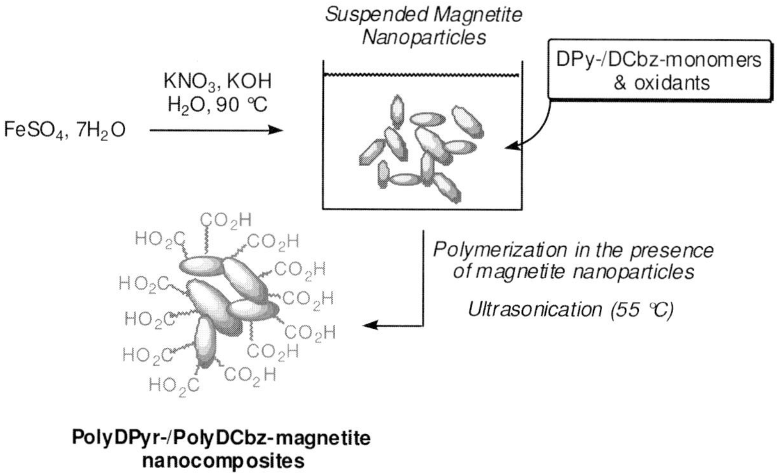

Fig. 10.2. Oxidative polymerization of DPyr-/DCbz-based monomers in the presence of magnetite nanoparticles.

Regarding oxidative polymerization of DPyr-/DCbz-based monomers in the presence of nanosized magnetite particles toward corresponding magnetic NCs (Fig. 10.2), several experimental parameters were considered important and, subsequently, examined carefully during extensive screening, keeping in mind the best practicality, reliability, and robustness of NC fabrication protocols. Polymerization parameters examined included different (a) polymerization times; (b) mono- or bi-electronic chemical oxidants; (c) molar/weight ratios of DPyr- and DCbz-monomers/magnetite nanoparticles; (d) polymerization solvents (low-molecular weight alcohols, acetone, acetonitrile, dimethylformamide, and their respective mixtures with water, chloroform, hexane); (e) medium temperatures [25–55 °C when using or not ultrasonic irradiation (ultrasonic cleaner Bransonic at full 42 kHz power)]; and finally (f) magnetite concentrations (0.5–5% w/v range at constant experiment volume).

Two main problems arose that were successfully solved during this selection process, ending with the delivery of optimized protocols for NC fabrication [53]. First, both DPyr- and DCbz-based oxidizable monomers must be minimally soluble in water, since magnetite nanoparticles had an irreversible strong tendency to aggregate in non-aqueous media. For example, the dicarboxylate DCbz-containing (*S*,*S*)-**18b** (Scheme 10.4) could not be solubilized in any water-miscible organic solvent mixture and, therefore, could not be polymerized around magnetite nanoparticles. Due to the heterocycle type, DCbz-based monomers are consistently more hydrophobic, or less water-soluble than DPyr-related monomers. Therefore, two different polymerization media have been specifically adapted for monomers of both DPyr- and DCbz-type (water–methanol mixtures and acetone, respectively; see typical procedures for NC fabrication in Section 10.6.1). Secondly, DCbz-based monomers that were expected to polymerize with difficultly under usual chemical oxidative conditions polymerized efficiently when using the *only* oxidizing Ce(IV) salt CAN [$(NH_4)_2Ce(NO_3)_6$] among a range of currently tested oxidants [$FeCl_3$, $Fe(NO_3)_3$, $Fe(ClO_4)_3$, $H_2O_2/FeCl_3/0.1$ M HCl, $CuCl_2$, $K_2Cr_2O_7$, $K_2S_2O_8$, $(NH_4)_2S_2O_8$, I_2, PbO_2, etc.] [53].

Conversely, DPyr-based monomers readily polymerize when using $FeCl_3$ and ammonium peroxodisulfate, $(NH_4)_2S_2O_8$, with the latter oxidant being preferred since it affords much cleaner polyDPyr-magnetite NCs (absence of shorter, water-bleachable, dark colored DPyr-oligomers). Interestingly, the resulting carboxylated polyDPyr-/polyDCbz-magnetite nanocomposites did not always show colloidal stability for the entire range of parameter combinations and during storage (at 4 °C in a neutral PBS phosphate buffer). In fact, preliminary TGA (Thermogravimetric Analysis) analyses over 200–750 °C, together with FT-IR spectroscopic analyses, helped to confirm successful monomer polymerizations. This large screening towards optimized polymerization parameters rapidly disclosed two separate optimal sets of polymerization conditions specific for each DPyr- and DCbz-series of monomers in the presence of nanosized magnetite. Beyond the use of oxidizers specific to each monomer series, the main protocol differences related to (a) optimal polymerization media, e.g., a 45/55 v/v H_2O–CH_3OH mixture for DPyr-based monomers and pure CH_3COCH_3 for more hydrophobic DCbz-based ones, and (b) optimal ultrasound-assisted polymerization times, e.g., 1 h for DPyr-based monomers versus 5 h for DCbz-based ones. Typical preparations of magnetically responsive polyDPyr- and polyDCbz-magnetite NCs are reported in Section 10.6.1.

10.4.2
Characterization of Magnetically Responsive PolyDPyr- and PolyDCbz-Magnetite Nanocomposites

Magnetically responsive polyDPyr- and polyDCbz-magnetite NCs have been characterized using a range of analytical and spectroscopic methods that included FT-IR and ^{57}Fe Mössbauer spectroscopies, C,H,N elemental and TGA analyses, magnetism measurements, and low- and high-resolution TEM microscopies with Energy-Dispersive X-Ray Microanalysis (EDAX). Additionally, as discussed in Section 10.5, a DNA-based biological parallel screening system has also been developed to characterize the fabricated NCs. In fact, NCs have been systematically tested for (a) DNA attachment using both covalent amide and noncovalent streptavidin/biotin linkages, and (b) NC surface-confined DNA hybridizations using an amplifying colored HRP-based enzymatic system (HRP: Horse Radish Peroxidase) towards detection and quantification of optically read signal outputs.

In a first step, carboxylated polyDPyr-/polyDCbz-magnetite NCs have been characterized by TGA analysis (TGA-Mettler apparatus, TG-50 DSS50 model, executed temperature profile: 25–130 °C at 20 °C min^{-1}, 130 °C for 15 min, and then 130–800 °C at 15 °C min^{-1} under nitrogen) and high-resolution FT-IR spectroscopy (Bomen-Hartmann & Braun instrument, KBr pellets, 4 cm^{-1} resolution) to check the formation of polyDPyr-/polyDCbz-polymers in the presence of nanosized magnetite nanoparticles. TGA curves showed quite similar two-step profiles, which

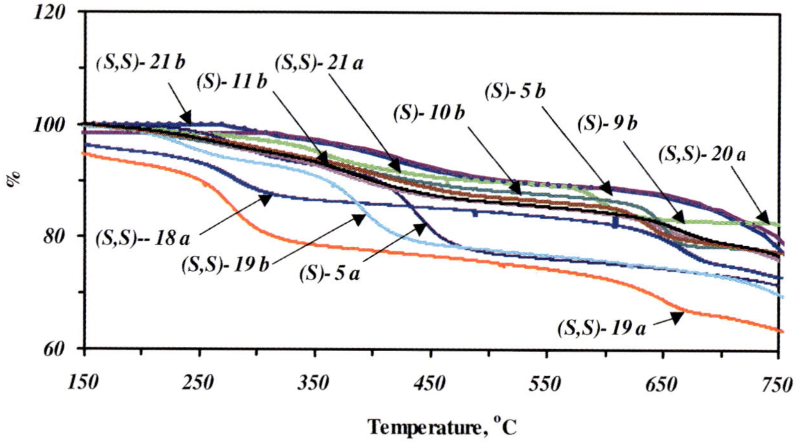

Fig. 10.3. TGA curves of magnetically responsive polyDPyr-/polyDCbz-magnetite NCs.

were more or less pronounced depending on NCs over a 200–750 °C temperature range (Fig. 10.3 and Table 10.1). Observed weight losses match up, most likely, to the evaporation of shorter, more volatile polymeric chains followed by final polymer burning. Interestingly, C,H,N elemental analyses (EA 1110/CHNS-O CE instrument) data, corrected for oxygen (Table 10.1), matched with TGA NC composition data and, therefore, allowed us to check for data homogeneity. Both DPyr- and DCbz-based monomers afforded NCs of similar polymer compositions with polymer deposits in a w/w range of 18–30% and 20–32%, respectively. FT-IR spectra

Tab. 10.1. NC compositions from gravimetric measurements (TGA graphs) and from C, H, N elemental analyses.

Nanocomposite poly(monomer)-magnetite	*Elemental analysis[a] (%)*			*NC Composition (% w/w)[a]*	*TGA weight loss (% w/w)*
	C	*H*	*N*		
5a	18.63	2.01	3.20	27	28
18a	15.40	1.71	3.50	25	27
19a	19.37	1.76	2.91	28	30
20a	11.39	1.39	2.11	19	19
21a	13.33	1.65	2.35	22	18
5b	19.52	1.40	2.01	25	24
9b	20.87	1.78	2.41	32	31
10b	21.18	1.67	2.32	30	29
11b	14.11	1.62	1.67	20	23
19b	19.34	1.65	2.48	27	30
21b	13.96	1.39	1.38	20	21

[a] Values corrected for oxygen content.

of NCs showed quite similar absorption peaks. They included mixed absorption peaks characteristic of both freshly prepared non-oxidized magnetite ($\nu = 1083$–1099, 1017–1024, and 568–585 cm^{-1}) and of polyDPyr- and polyDCbz-polymeric systems [$\nu = 2850$–2922 and 2958–2964 ($\delta_{Csp3\text{-}H}$), 1650–1750 ($\nu_{C=O}$, carboxyl), 1454–1558 ($\nu_{Csp2\text{-}Csp2}$, polypyrrole and polycarbazole aromatics), 1258–1264 ($\nu_{(C=O)\text{-}O}$, acid), 800–808 ($\delta_{Csp2\text{-}H}$, out of plane stretching) cm^{-1}].

Bulk magnetization versus applied magnetic field experiments (Oxford VSM system Magnetometer equipped with an Aerosonic VSM 3001 controller) have been conducted at 300 K on all magnetically responsive, carefully dried NCs. Saturation magnetizations M_s have been observed in a range of 32–55 emu g^{-1}, with coercivity factors H_c of 35–132 Oe (Fig. 10.4 and Table 10.2). Subsequently, these materials cannot be strictly considered as superparamagnetic materials since they presented a low- to medium-range hysteresis. This resulted most likely from the partial oxidation of the former magnetite Fe_3O_4 core during the oxidative processes used for monomer polymerizations. In fact, inorganic magnetic cores were formed of nonstoichiometric magnetite, $Fe_{3-x}O_4$ ($0 \leq x \leq 0.33$), or of γ-Fe_2O_3 (maghemite)–magnetite mixtures as determined by ^{57}Fe Mössbauer analysis at 300 K (two superposed magnetic subspectra compatible with Fe^{3+} and $Fe^{2.5+}$ atoms located in tetrahedral and octahedral sites, respectively, with different relative intensities were obtained). For example, polyDCbz(**9b**)- and polyDCbz(**10b**)-magnetite NCs were analyzed and found to contain 30% and 60% maghemite, respectively.

Interestingly, DCbz-containing monomers, which were more difficult to polymerize oxidatively around magnetite particles, mainly afforded NCs of lower M_s and higher H_c than similarly prepared polyDPyr-based NCs (Table 10.2). These data are likely to be related to higher contents of less magnetic maghemite/nonstoichiometric magnetite ($Fe_{3-x}O_4$) within corresponding NCs, while magnetic spin blocking effects could arise from formation of oxidized magnetite/polymer interfacial domains.

In a second series of analyses, all these NCs were systematically examined by low- and high-resolution transmission electron microscopies TEM (JEOL-1200EX) and HR-TEM (JEOL-JEM 2010 of Oxford Instruments, 200 kV accelerating voltage, Gatan CCD video camera for microphotograph digitization). Even using ultrasonic irradiation, NC fabrication processes were not found to alter the sheet-like morphology of starting magnetite nanoparticles nor the average particle size (20–40 nm). More interestingly, mixed structures of the discrete polyDPyr-/polyDCbz-particulates–magnetite nanoparticle type could not be detected, clearly emphasizing polymerization processes, during which deposition of insoluble polymer chains occurred around magnetite nanoparticles. These observations are consistent with the relatively low quantities of polymers deposited onto magnetite nanoparticles independent of starting DPyr-/DCbz-monomers (~18–32% w/w).

Since polymer–magnetite NC morphology remained a central issue, unambiguous confirmation of the core–shell nature for *all* the fabricated NCs came from HR-TEM analysis combined with EDAX. For illustration, HR-TEM microphoto graphs of poly(**5a**)-, poly(**10b**)- and poly(**21a**)-magnetite NCs belonging to both poly-

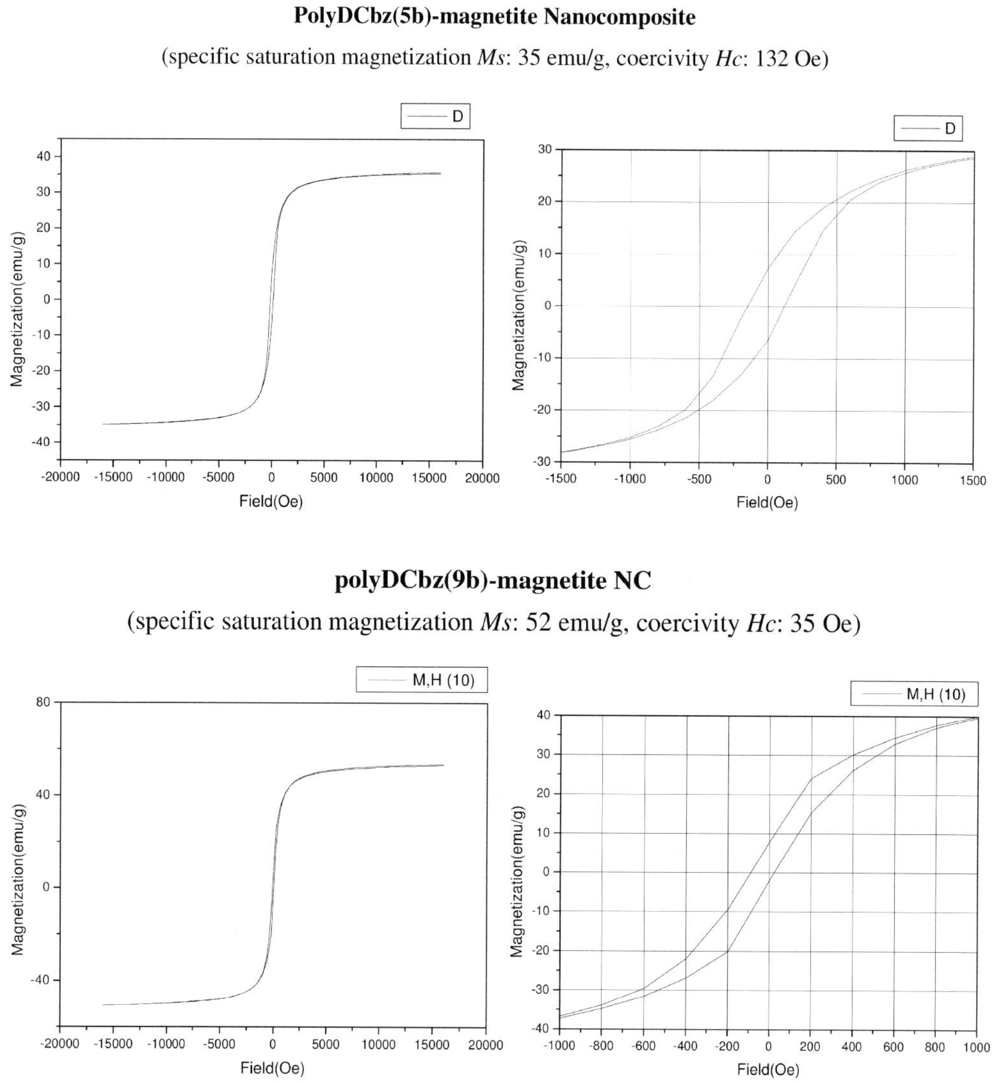

Fig. 10.4. Magnetism measurements/graphs for polyDCbz(**5b**)- and polyDCbz(**9b**)-magnetite NCs.

DPyr- and polyDCbz-series of NCs have been reported that showed clearly amorphous 5.0–7.5 nm thick polyDPyr-/polyDCbz-deposits decorating highly ordered magnetite/maghemite crystals (Fig. 10.5, samples prepared on 400 mesh Au grids free of carbon-containing pollutants). Corresponding elemental compositions have been determined by EDAX microanalysis using an Oxford Instruments X-ray detector and INCA software with electron beams focused at both 15 and 30 nm diameters, depending on the samples. All chemical elements have been analyzed, nor-

Tab. 10.2. Saturation magnetizations M_s and coercivities H_c of polyDPyr-/polyDCbz-magnetite NCs.

Nanocomposite poly(monomer)-magnetite	*Saturation magnetization M_s (emu g^{-1})*	*Coercivity H_c (Oe)*
5a	50	55
18a	52	55
19a	55	55
20a	50	40
21a	55	50
5b	35	132
9b	52	35
10b	51	55
11b	35	130
19b	32	130
21b	35	130

malized, and their results obtained in weight percentages. Examples of such EDAX microanalyses are shown for poly(**5a**)- and poly(**21a**)-magnetite NCs in Fig. 10.5, wherein crystal edges have been found to be systematically carbon-rich and iron-poor, while crystal centers appear to be carbon-poor and iron-rich, arguing for the presence of organic polymer deposits around magnetite nanoparticles [poly(**5a**)-magnetite NC, spectrum 1: 55.2 and 18.0% for C and Fe versus spectrum 2: 1.9 and 63.4%; poly(**21a**)-magnetite NC: spectrum 9: 39.6 and 44.1% for C and Fe versus spectrum 6: 1.7 and 48.8%].

10.5 Development of a DNA-based Biological System for Nanocomposite Parallel Screening

Among the critical steps identified for screening the properties and optimization of fabricated polyDPyr-/polyDCbz-magnetite NCs, realization of a reliable highly-parallel (use of 96-well microtiter plates), low cost, less laborious and robust biological screening system were quite essential. Accordingly, a natural choice was to turn to a DNA-based hybridization system, supported on these novel nanosized magnetic NCs, because of the extreme relevance of DNA-based diagnostics using magnetically responsive nanomaterials [54, 55]. Although numerous examples of DNA hybridizations onto various non-planar solid phases have been reported, they are mainly concerned with micrometer-sized beads that generally did not suffer from critical aggregation and non-specific binding (NSB) issues often encountered with nanosized materials [56, 57].

During our studies involving polyDPyr-/polyDCbz-magnetite NCs, two different modes of DNA probe attachments were tested – covalent (via amide bonds) and

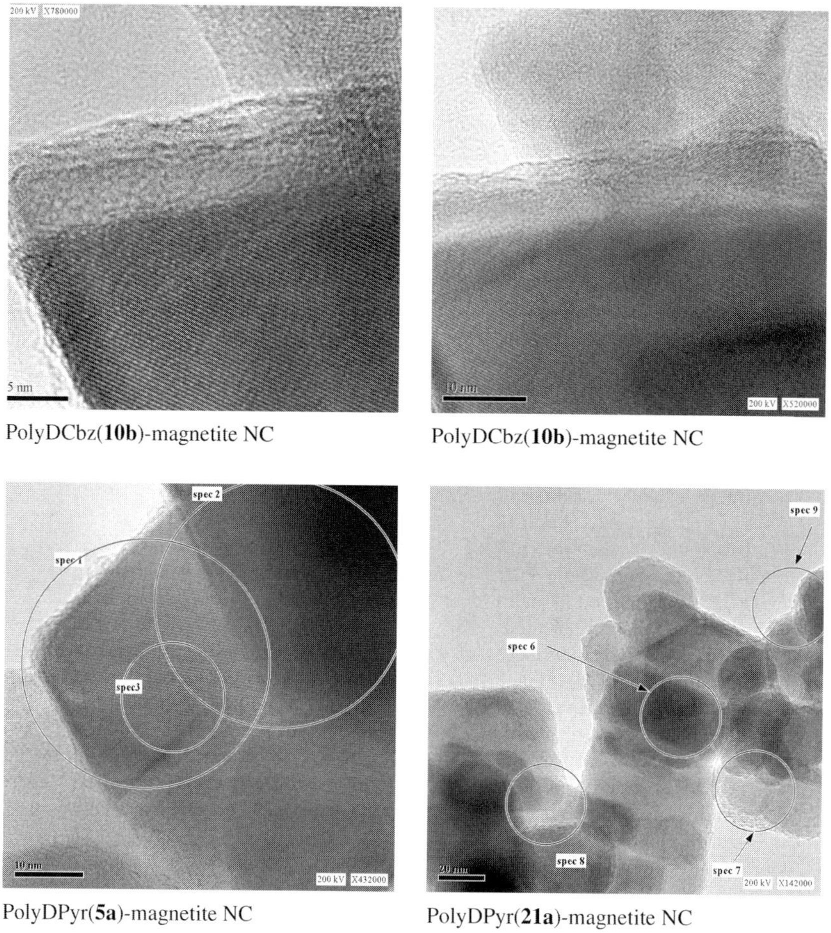

Fig. 10.5. High-resolution TEM microphotographs of selected polyDPyr-/polyDCbz-magnetite NCs.

quasi-covalent (via streptavidin–biotin interactions [58–60]). These brought out the great versatility of the chemistry of surface COOH groups of NCs set up by polycarboxylated polyDPyr-/polyDCbz-deposits. After simple chemical activation of COOH groups by water-soluble carbodiimides [61–63], the addition of an NH_2-$^{5'}$-modified DNA sequence as a model molecular DNA probe resulted in covalent attachment of DNA through stable amide bonds. Alternatively, second-generation streptavidin-modified magnetic NCs could be fabricated using a similar activation protocol of polymeric COOH groups followed by incubation with streptavidin. Covalent attachment of streptavidin occurs via amidation of ε-NH_2 groups of surface lysines of the protein. Then, the same, albeit biotin-$^{5'}$-modified, DNA sequence will be quasi-covalently (via streptavidin–biotin interactions) attached to modified NCs upon incubation, resulting in the testing and comparison of DNA-decorated

NCs using both probe attachment methodologies. The streptavidin/avidin-biotin system has many advantages [58–60]. Noncovalent streptavidin–biotin supramolecular interactions are very strong ($K_d \sim 10^{-15}$ M) and, furthermore, the system is more biocompatible, and is therefore less denaturing for DNA/protein molecular probe attachments. Additionally, its great versatility makes it particularly attractive for a wide range of biological and non-biological probes (sugars, peptides, proteins/antibodies, DNA/RNA sequences, and catalysts, small ligands, fluorescent dyes, quantum dots and nanoparticles/clusters).

10.5.1
Covalent Attachment of an NH_2-$^{5'}$-modified 20-mer DNA Probe onto NCs towards DNA-Biofunctionalized NCs. Covalent Amide Bond Chemistry and Resulting NC-Supported DNA Hybridizations

The simple but powerful DNA-based test described in Fig. 10.6 constitutes the basic biological screening system used to investigate the properties of fabricated polyDPyr-/polyDCbz-magnetite NCs in parallel mode [53]. Whether the covalent (amide bond chemistry) or quasi-covalent (streptavidin–biotin system) DNA probe attachments were used in NC functionalization, DNA hybridizations on NC surfaces were characterized and quantified using a blue color-emitting, HRP-based enzymatic amplifying system (HRP: Horse Radish Peroxidase). Resulting hybridization signal outputs were processed in parallel, using 96-well plastic microtiter plates optically read in an Elisa Plate Reader Anthos ht II at 620 nm.

Practically, the amine-modified 20-mer oligonucleotide DNA_1 H_2N-$(CH_2)_{12}$-$^{5'}$GCACTGGGAGCATTGAGGCT that characterized the 20210 mutation in the Human Factor II gene (G → A single oligonucleotide mutation at position 20210) [64, 65] was chosen as a model DNA probe and, through incubation, has been covalently attached to a full range of fabricated NCs after carboxylate activation in

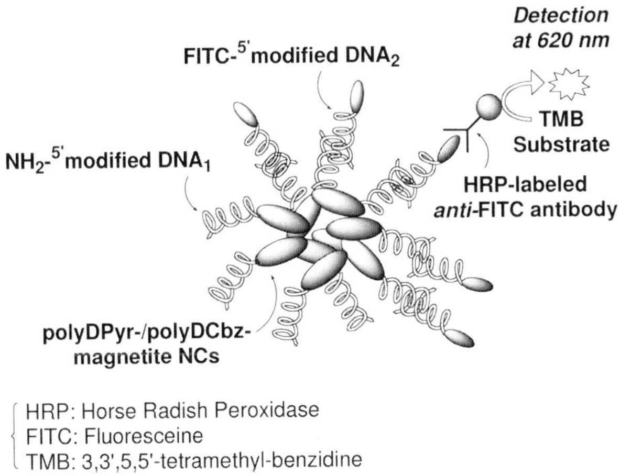

Fig. 10.6. DNA covalent attachment onto polyDPyr-/polyDCbz-magnetite NCs and hybridization.

a 0.4 M MES buffer (pH 5.0) by the water-soluble carbodiimide EDC [63] [EDC: N'-(3-dimethylamino-propyl)-N-ethylcarbodiimide hydrochloride, 0.4 M MES buffer, 2 h incubation at 20 °C]. NC-supported DNA hybridizations have been performed with the fluoresceine-labeled *anti*-sense 20-mer oligonucleotide FITC-DNA_2 (fluoresceine-$^{5'}$AGCCTCAATGCTCCCAGTGC, 60 min, 60 °C). After addition of an *anti*-FITC HRP-labeled mouse monoclonal antibody and incubation (20 min, 20 °C), the HRP substrate TMB (3,3′,5,5′-tetramethylbenzidine) was added and reacted with the NC-immobilized amplifying enzymatic construct for 1.5 min at the same temperature before visible signal reading at 620 nm (Elisa Plate Reader Anthos ht II). Accordingly, the resulting optical reading data (OD_{Total}) allowed the characterization of all the tested DNA-functionalized NCs. These were systematically averaged for six to ten similar parallel experiments for each separate NC, providing minimal signal output variations in a 5–8% range.

Additionally, and for better characterization of DNA-decorated NCs, Non-specific binding (NSB) data were systematically collected during similar averaged parallel experiments, where the complementary FITC-labeled DNA_2 probe was omitted. NSB data allowed us to estimate the affinity of tested DNA-decorated polyDPyr-/polyDCbz-magnetite NCs to physically adsorb the reporter *anti*-FITC HRP-labeled antibody. Furthermore, micrometer-sized COOH-Dynabeads® M-270 (∅ 2.8 µm, Dynal AS, Oslo, Norway) [66] that are routinely used for magnetism-driven suspension assays were also included in those experiments as an internal standard for comparison.

In a first series of experiments for screening of NC-supported DNA hybridizations, the concentrations of FITC-5′ labeled complementary probe FITC-DNA_2 and tested NCs were 10^{-7} M and at 50 µg (1.0% w/v), respectively, per microtiter plate well (Fig. 10.7). From patterns of optical signal outputs (OD_{Total}) and specific binding (SB = OD_{Total} − NSB)/NSB ratios, the three polyDCbz-magnetite NCs, e.g., polyDCbz(**9b**)-, polyDCbz(**10b**)-, and polyDCbz(**19b**)-magnetite NCs, were as efficient as the COOH-Dynabeads tested under similar conditions. Calculated SB/NSB averaged ratios of 19.0–22.8 were in a high range. In contrast, polyDPyr-magnetite NCs were less efficient than standard COOH-Dynabeads with SB/NSB data in a low to medium (4.2–16.3) range. Here, polyDPyr(**19a**) was the most efficient NC in the polyDPyr-based series of NCs (SB/NSB = 16.3 vs. 22.2 for COOH-Dynabeads).

Interestingly, both couples of NCs polyDPyr(**19a**)/polyDCbz(**19b**)- and polyDPyr(**21a**)/polyDCbz(**21b**)-magnetite fabricated from DPyr-/DCbz-monomers **19/21a–b**, possessing an hydrophobic 1,4-diaminobutane and an hydrophilic 4,7,10-trioxa-1,13-tridecaneamine linker, were related. Among the tested NCs, they exhibited the higher and the lower efficiencies, respectively. Confirming this specific trend, the polyDPyr(**20a**)-magnetite NC built on the same hydrophilic 4,7,10-trioxa-1,13-tridecaneamine linker showed the lowest efficiency of all the tested NCs (SB/NSB = 4.2). Additionally, both polyDPyr(**5a**)- and polyDCbz(**5b**)-magnetite NCs arising from the same monocarboxylated L-lysine-based precursor exhibited similar efficiencies (13.2 and 15.4, respectively).

Subsequently, while keeping other assay parameters constant (see the typical

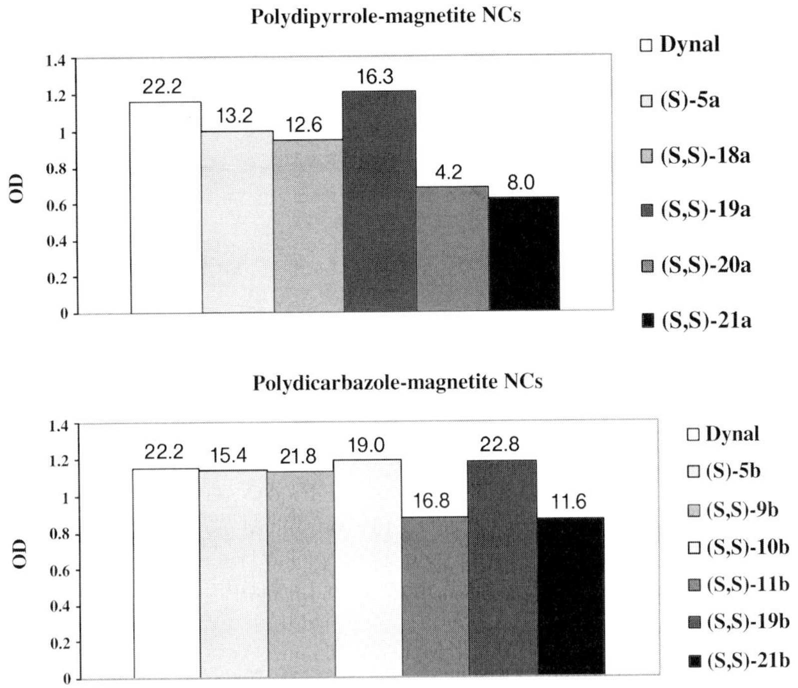

Fig. 10.7. Screening of polyDPyr-/polyDCbz-magnetite NCs at a 10^{-7} M DNA_2 concentration and related specific binding/non-specific binding (SB/NSB) ratios.

procedure reported below), a second larger parallel screening of NC properties was performed to find a minimum assay sensitivity limit to detect the model analyte FITC-labeled DNA_2 (Fig. 10.8). For this purpose, a concentration range of 10^{-7}–10^{-14} M of FITC-labeled DNA_2 was investigated. In this concentration range, NSB averaged data were uniformly observed in a low 0.05–0.09 range for all tested NCs, except for the polyDPyr(**20a**)-magnetite NC fabricated from the hydrophilic 4,7,10-trioxa-1,13-tridecanediamine (averaged NSB = 0.11). The previously observed trend of being the least efficient system for the SB/NSB ratio was consistent and reproducible for all tested concentrations of FITC-labeled DNA_2. These data precluded its further use as a sensitive detection of this model analyte. In contrast, three polyDPyr- and three polyDCbz-magnetite NCs were disclosed as the most sensitive NCs, able to achieve reproducible SB/NSB ratios in the range 1.6–2.7, at very low 10^{-12}–10^{-14} M concentrations of FITC-labeled DNA_2. These NCs were polyDPyr(**5a**)-, polyDPyr(**18a**)-, and polyDPyr(**19a**)-magnetite in the polyDPyr-series and, in the polyDCbz-series, were polyDCbz(**5b**)-, polyDCbz(**9b**)-, and polyDCbz(**10b**)-magnetite. COOH-Dynabeads, tested in parallel under identical concentration range and conditions, were quite inefficient. This emphasized the potential of these novel nanosized magnetic NCs for highly sensitive DNA detec-

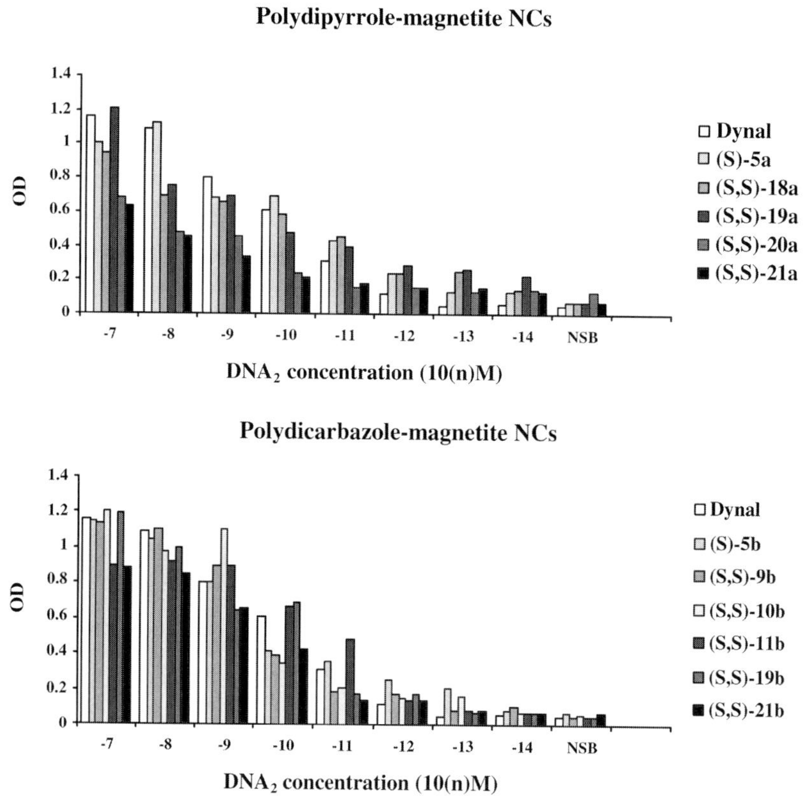

Fig. 10.8. Sensitivity patterns of PolyDPyr-/polyDCbz-magnetite NCs at decreasing FITC-labeled DNA_2 concentrations.

tion. Interestingly, and among all tested polyDPyr-/polyDCbz-NCs, the unique polyDPyr(**19a**)-magnetite NC was the most sensitive (SB/NSB = 2.7 at 10^{-14} M), while both polyDCbz(**5b**)- and polyDCbz-(**10b**)-magnetite NCs were just an order less sensitive for similar SB/NSB ratios (SB/NSB = 2.0 and 1.6, respectively, at 10^{-13} M).

Importantly, these low-range detection levels were consistently achieved without employing any additional passivating step (Egg albumin, BSA, PEG_{1000} or Triton X surfactants, dextran) commonly used in the diagnostic field.

Concentrating on both typical polyDPyr(**5a**)- and polyDCbz(**5b**)-magnetite NCs, sensitivity issues were further examined by investigating the influence of two additional parameters, i.e. minimal amounts of (a) capture NH_2-modified DNA_1 probe covalently attached onto NCs and (b) NCs used per microtiter plate well to afford reliably quantifiable optical outputs with SB/NSB ratios in a 1.0–1.5 range (Fig. 10.9). First, concentrations of the capture NH_2-$^{5'}$-modified DNA_1 probe for the covalent functionalization of both NCs were varied in a 10^{-5}–10^{-16} M range. Other

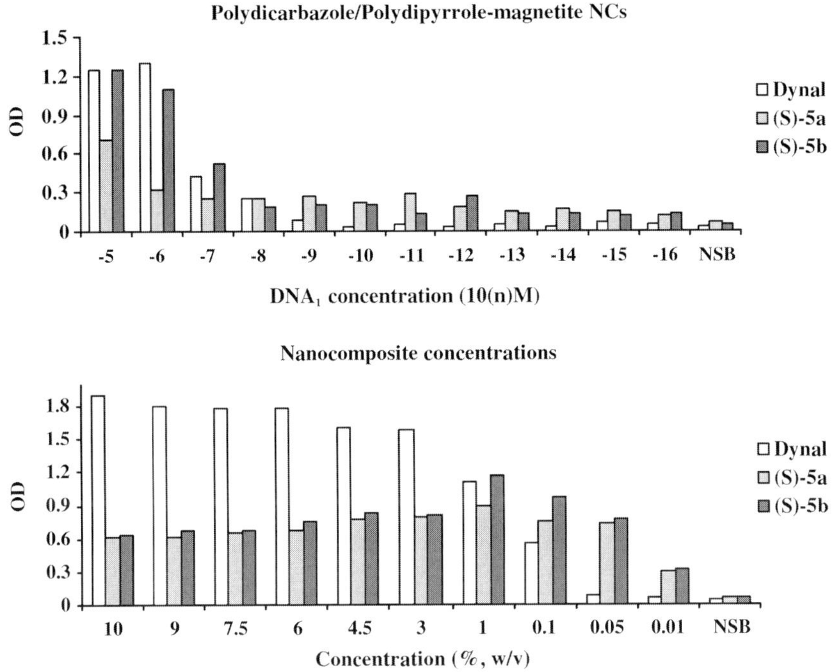

Fig. 10.9. Sensitivities of polyDPyr(**5a**)- and polyDCbz(**5b**)-magnetite NCs for decreasing DNA_1 and NC concentrations (the value 1% w/v corresponds to 50 μg of NC per microtiter plate well).

protocol parameters were identical to values used in the typical experimental protocol described in Section 10.6.2. For comparison, a DNA_1 concentration of 10^{-7} M for probe attachment onto NCs was used (standardized experimental protocol). Second, variable NC amounts per microtiter plate well were investigated in a 10–10^{-2}% w/v range (500.0–0.5 μg) when the same standardized experimental protocol made use of a 1% w/v NC concentration, e.g., use of 50.0 μg of NC per well. The resulting data (Fig. 10.9) led to some interesting conclusions.

A rather wide range of concentrations in NH_2-$^{5'}$-modified DNA_1 probe, from 10^{-9} to the very low 10^{-16} M, afforded reliable SB/NSB ratios in a 0.9–4.0 range, depending on NCs and DNA_1 concentrations. In contrast, standard COOH-Dynabeads treated under similar conditions were totally unresponsive. Both polyDPyr(**5a**)- and polyDCbz(**5b**)-magnetite NCs were effective even at the lowest tested DNA_1 concentration (10^{-16} M, SB/NSB = 0.9 and 1.4, respectively). Regarding usable NC concentration per microtiter plate well, only limited decreases in signal outputs were registered when using NC amounts per well as low as 5.0 [0.1% w/v; polyDPyr(**5a**)- and polyDCbz(**5b**)-magnetite NCs: SB/NSB = 14.0 and 18.6, respectively] and 0.5 μg [0.01% w/v; polyDPyr(**5a**) and polyDCbz(**5b**)-magnetite NCs: SB/NSB = 13.6 and 14.4, respectively]. In parallel, COOH-Dynabeads afforded lower or background-level SB/NSB ratios for both NC concentrations (0.1% w/v: SB/NSB = 13.0; 0.01% w/v: SB/NSB = 0.8).

10.5.2 Attachment of a Biotin-$^{5'}$-modified 20-mer DNA Probe to DNA-biofunctionalized NCs. Quasi-covalent Linkage Using the Streptavidin–Biotin System and the Resulting NC-supported DNA Hybridizations

A second methodology for DNA probe attachment onto polyDPyr(**5a**)-/polyDCbz(**5b**)-magnetite NCs has been investigated that exploited the strong quasi-covalent streptavidin–biotin interactions. In the first step, two previously fabricated magnetic polycarboxylated polyDPyr(**5a**)-/polyDCbz(**5b**)-magnetite NCs were chemically activated at room temperature by the same water-soluble carbodiimide EDC (COOH activation) in a mixture of neutral PBS and 0.4 M MES (pH 5.0) buffers. This activation step is immediately followed by covalent grafting of a high purity commercial recombinant streptavidin (Roche Inc.), leading to second-generation streptavidin-modified polyDPyr(**5a**)-/polyDCbz(**5b**)-magnetite NCs. As usually performed, excess chemical reagents and biological components/buffers were readily eliminated or exchanged by magnetic decantation and appropriate washings before DNA hybridizations (see the typical experimental procedure given below).

In the second step, streptavidin-modified NC-supported DNA hybridizations were similarly tracked using the blue-emitting HRP-based enzymatic amplifying system mentioned previously (Fig. 10.6), providing the use of a biotinylated DNA_1 capture probe biotin–(triethylene glycol) linker-$^{5'}DNA_1$. Notably, in this particular case, NSB data were attributed to the noncovalent binding affinity of streptavidin-modified NCs (e.g., of protein-decorated, instead of polycarboxylated DNA-decorated, NCs) to physically adsorb the reporter *anti*-FITC HRP-labeled antibody.

Interestingly, efficiency comparisons of both covalent (amide chemistry) and quasi-covalent (streptavidin–biotin system) modes of DNA_1 probe attachment showed a particularly strong dependency on NC concentration (NC weight/Elisa plate well) (Fig. 10.10). For example, at a 1% NC concentration (50.0 μg of NC/Elisa plate well), SB/NSB ratios for streptavidin-modified NCs were in a low to medium range (5.3–10.1), with the streptavidin-modified polyDCbz(**5b**)-magnetite NC being the most efficient system (SB/NSB = 10.1). Streptavidin-modified micrometer-sized Dynabeads, prepared in the same way, were as efficient, with a SB/NSB ratio of 11.0. Though, while in covalent NH_2-$^{5'}$-linked DNA_1 probe attachment mode, both polyDPyr(**5a**)-/polyDCbz(**5b**)-magnetite NCs always exhibited a greater efficiency (SB/NSB = 13.2 and 15.4 respectively), they were not comparable to micrometer-sized DNA_1-decorated Dynabeads, which performed better as the most efficient support (SB/NSB = 22.2).

Conversely, lowering NC concentration to 0.25% w/v (12.5 μg of NC/Elisa plate well) strongly diminished the previous, detrimentally high NSB, resulting in marked differences. Whatever the covalent or streptavidin/biotin modes of DNA_1 probe attachment, the polyDPyr(**5a**)-/polyDCbz(**5b**)-magnetite NCs systematically afforded more efficient responses than that of carboxylated Dynal microbeads

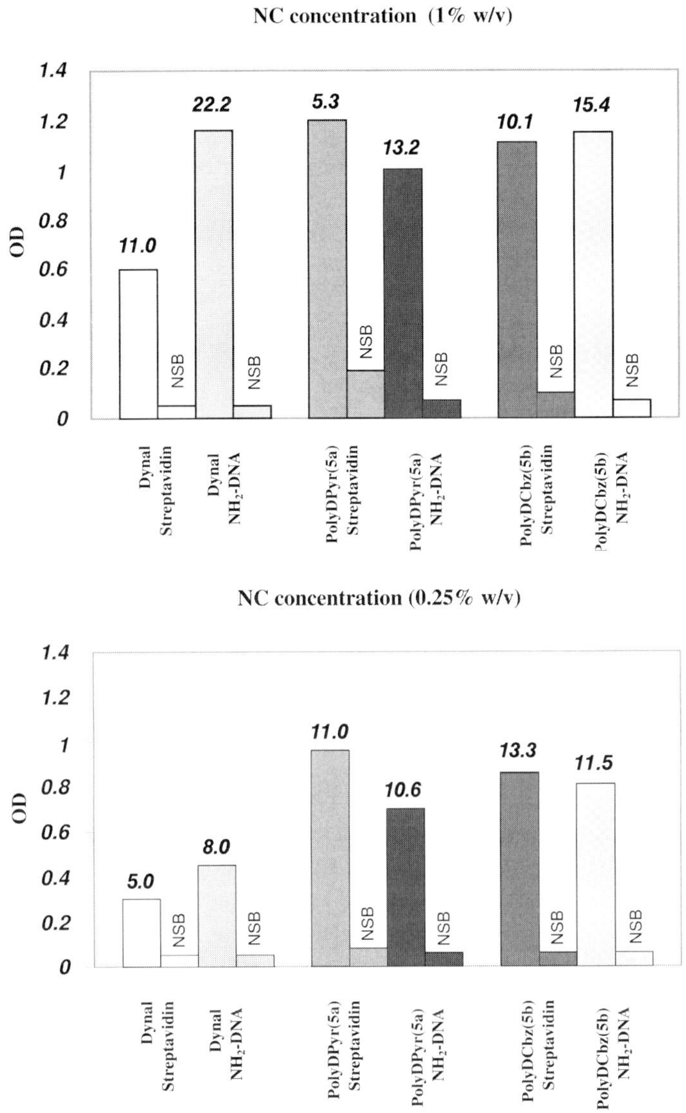

Fig. 10.10. Covalent (amide chemistry) and quasi-covalent (streptavidin–biotin system) attachment modes of both NH_2- and biotin-$^{5'}$-modified DNA_1 probes onto polyDPyr(**5a**)- and polyDCbz(**5b**)-magnetite NCs.

(SB/NSB = 10.6–13.3 vs. 5.0–8.0, respectively). Interestingly for this low NC concentration, both streptavidin-modified polyDPyr(**5a**)-/polyDCbz(**5b**)-magnetite NCs displayed better efficiencies than did carboxylated covalently modified ones (SB/NSB = 11.0 and 13.3 vs. 10.6 and 11.5, respectively). These preliminary data featured the important disclosure that optimized conditions dealing with polyDPyr-/polyDCbz-magnetite NCs should be investigated when testing both types of covalent (amide chemistry) and noncovalent (streptavidin–biotin system) DNA probe attachments.

10.5.3
Storage: Medium-term Stability of Some PolyDPyr-/PolyDCbz-Magnetite NCs

The colloidal stability of some of these novel polyDPyr-/polyDCbz-magnetite NCs was also examined during storage in a neutral PBS buffer (1% w/v NC concentration) at 4 °C. For this investigation, three freshly prepared polyDPyr- and polyDCbz-magnetite NCs, polyDPyr(**5a**)-, polyDPyr(**19a**)-, polyDPyr(**21a**)-, and polyDCbz-(**5b**)-, polyDCbz(**10b**)-, and polyDCbz(**19b**)-magnetite NCs, and COOH-Dynabeads for reference were stored in the above-described neutral PBS buffer. Regular controls (quadruplicate parallel experiments) were performed on aliquots from these stored NCs on a fifteen day-basis over a period of seven and a half months, using our powerful DNA-based biological screening test. This test was operated using standard conditions of concentrations for DNA_1, the complementary FITC-labeled DNA_2 and NC components (typical experimental procedure given in Section 10.6.2), for which NSB data were always in a low 0.04–0.05 range.

Importantly, during this period the HRP-based amplifying enzymatic system revealed a slow but regular time-dependent decrease in detection efficiency, probably because of component ageing. This ageing phenomenon, most likely, is due to the natural thermodynamic instabilities of both the HRP-labeled *anti*-FITC antibody (antibody and HRP components), and of the FITC label/epitope of the complementary FITC-labeled DNA_2 (light-induced degradation). Consequently, NC stability data were calculated and presented graphically as ratios of SB data of NCs/SB data of reference COOH-Dynabeads® M-270 treated in a similar time-dependent manner. Figure 10.11 depicts the resulting characteristic time-dependent ratio evolutions for each separate NC. More specifically, the three NCs polyDPyr(**5a**)-, polyDPyr(**19a**)- and polyDCbz(**10b**)-magnetite NCs underwent quite noticeable decreases in efficiency (11, 11, and 27%, respectively), most likely due to slow time-dependent NC aggregation. In contrast, the other three NCs belonging to both polyDPyr- and polyDCbz-series displayed reasonable time-dependent stabilities for the examined period and for these specific storage conditions.

10.6
Typical Experimental Procedures for NC Fabrication and NC-Supported DNA Hybridizations

10.6.1
Typical Optimized Procedures for NC Fabrication Including Magnetite Preparation

10.6.1.1 Magnetite Preparation Using the Oxidative Hydrolysis of Iron(II) Sulfate in an Alkaline KOH Medium [51, 52]

A solution of iron(II) sulfate heptahydrate ($FeSO_4$, $7H_2O$) (17.71 g, 60.0 mmol) in high-purity nitrogen-deoxygenated water (200 mL) was heated at 90 °C in a 1 L

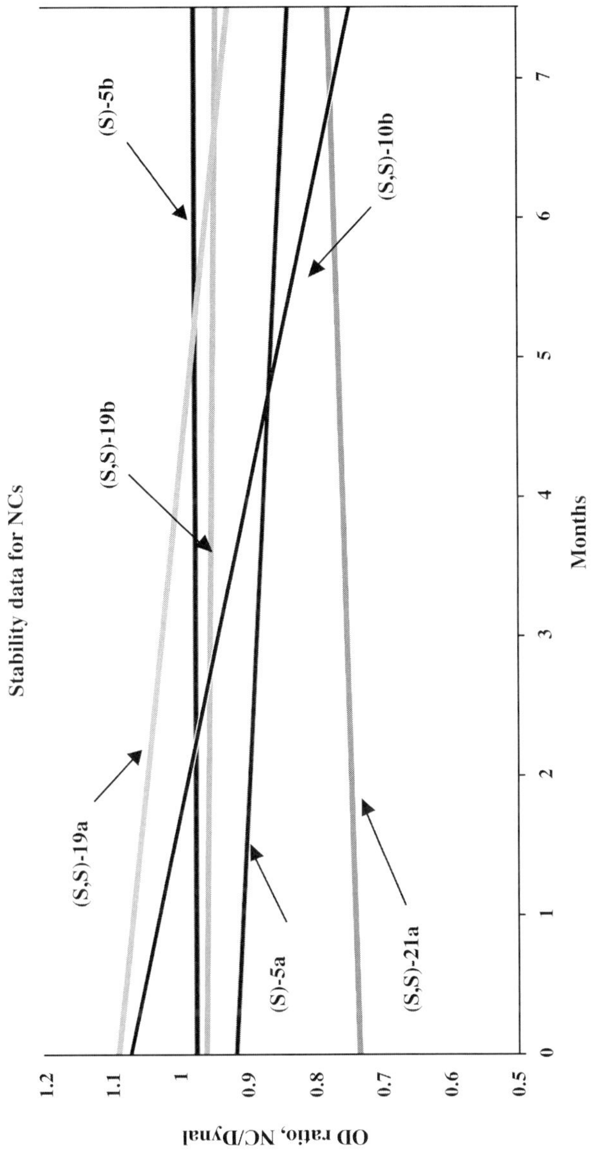

Fig. 10.11. Stability data for polyDPyr-/polyDCbz-magnetite NCs during medium-term storage using a DNA-hybridization screening system.

round-bottomed flask while stirring with an overhead stirrer. In parallel, deoxygenated aqueous solutions of KNO_3 (10.11 g, 100.0 mmol, 100 mL of H_2O) and of KOH (13.81 g, 250.0 mmol, 50 mL of H_2O) were prepared and then mixed under nitrogen until complete dissolution of the salts. The resulting basic salt mixture was then slowly added to the $FeSO_4$ solution at 90 °C under a constant flow of nitrogen. The oxidative hydrolysis lasted 2 h at 90 °C, affording a brilliant black precipitate of magnetite nanoparticles. After cooling to room temperature (1 h), the black Fe_3O_4 nanoparticle suspension was washed twice with H_2O (2 × 2 L), with 1 M HNO_3 (2 L), and twice again with H_2O (2 × 2 L). These washings were repeated if necessary until a visually clear and neutral supernatant aqueous phase was obtained. The suspension volume of precipitated magnetite nanoparticles was adjusted to 1 L with deoxygenated H_2O and kept in a polyethylene storage bottle at 4 °C (stock suspension of magnetite nanoparticles). Preferably, magnetite nanoparticles should be used immediately for polyPyr-/polyCbz-magnetite NC fabrication [final storage concentration of Fe_3O_4 nanoparticles: 46 mg (mL of suspension)$^{-1}$].

10.6.1.2 **PolyDPyr-Magnetite Nanocomposites**

Freshly prepared magnetite nanoparticles (100.0 mg, 2.3 mL of a 3.5% w/v water suspension of magnetite nanoparticles as prepared above) were added with the mono- or dicarboxylated DPyr-monomer (*S*)-**5a** or (*S*,*S*)-**18–21a** dissolved in MeOH (0.41 mmol, 3.0 mL of MeOH) and sonicated for 1 min (ultrasonic cleaner Bransonic at full 42 kHz power). Thereafter, the oxidizer (ammonium peroxodisulfate, $(NH_4)_2S_2O_8$, 98% purity from Riedel-de-Haën, 436.0 mg, 2.05 mmol, 5.0 equiv.) was added in one portion to the sonicated methanolic suspension of magnetite. The resultant fine black suspension (magnetite concentration of 2.0% at constant experiment volume) was then ultrasonicated for 1 h, during which time the medium temperature increased to 55 °C (ultrasound-mediated constant stirring). The resulting brown-black polyDPyr-magnetite NC was magnetically decanted with the help of a powerful external magnet. It was serially washed by 4 × 10 mL of each of the indicated deoxygenated solvents/buffers, CH_3COCH_3, 0.4 M MES buffer (pH 5.0), neutral PBS buffer, TNET buffer (pH 7.5), and, finally, again with neutral PBS buffer to eliminate soluble by-products (inorganic salts, excess oxidants, unreacted monomers, and short, colored monomer-related oligomers). (The preparation of these particular buffers is described in a corresponding typical experimental procedure given in Section 10.6.2.). Colorless supernatants must be obtained at each last separate washing. The resulting magnetically responsive carboxylated polyDPyr-magnetite NCs were suspended in a deoxygenated neutral PBS buffer at a 1% w/v concentration and stored at 4 °C. These colloidal suspensions were stable for at least 2–3 months under these storage conditions.

10.6.1.3 **PolyDCbz-Magnetite Nanocomposites [53]**

The protocol cited above was modified slightly to take into account the fact that mono- or dicarboxylated DCbz-containing monomers are much more hydrophobic than DPyr-based ones. Magnetite nanoparticles (same quantity as above) were first magnetically decanted, washed with CH_3COCH_3 (3 × 2.0 mL), and immediately added with the DCbz-based monomer (*S*)-**5b**, (*S*,*S*)-**9–11b**, or (*S*,*S*)-**18–21b** solubilized in CH_3COCH_3 (0.22 mmol, 2.0 mL of CH_3COCH_3, magnetite concentration of 2.5% at constant experiment volume). After medium sonication for 1 min for best mixing, the ammonium cerium(IV) nitrate oxidizer [CAN: $(NH_4)_2Ce(NO_3)_6$] dissolved in CH_3COCH_3 (CAN, 99% purity, Fluka, 0.18 mmol, 100.0 mg, 2.0 mL of CH_3COCH_3) was added under sonication in one portion. The resultant fine black suspension was ultrasonicated for 5 h at 55 °C (ultrasound-mediated constant stirring). Work-up procedures and storage conditions of the resulting poly-DCbz-magnetite NCs were strictly identical to those of the former polymerization protocol.

10.6.2
Covalent Attachment of an Aminated NH_2-$^{5'}$-modified DNA Probe. Hybridization Experiments onto PolyDPyr-/PolyDCbz-Magnetite NCs. Typical Experimental Procedures

An appropriate polyDPyr-/polyDCbz-magnetite NC suspension (1% w/v suspension in a neutral PBS buffer, 100 μL, 1.0 mg) was washed by (a) the same PBS neutral buffer (3 × 100 μL) and by (b) a 0.4 M MES buffer (pH 5.0, 100 μL). After magnetically-driven decantation, the supernatant was removed and (a) EDC (0.52 M EDC in 0.4 M MES buffer, 30 μL, 3.0 mg) and (b) the 20-mer amine-modified oligonucleotide DNA_1 NH_2-$(CH_2)_{12}$-$^{5'}$GCACTGGGAGCATTGAGGCT (0.4 M MES buffer at pH 5.0, 70 μL, 1.68×10^{-5} M; Danyiel Biotech Ltd, Israel, chemical purity ≥ 98%) were added successively at 20 °C. The so-obtained mixture was then incubated at room temperature for 2 h (smooth vortex agitation) for carboxylate activation.

Upon completion, polyDPyr-/polyDCbz-magnetite NCs were washed with 4 × 100 μL of PBS buffer to remove excess DNA_1. DNA-coated nanocomposites can be stored for weeks at 4 °C at a 1% w/v NC concentration in this same neutral PBS buffer, but containing NaN_3 (0.02% w/v), without noticeable degradation.

DNA-linked NCs (1.0 mg) were washed in a TNET buffer (100 μL, pH 7.5) and distributed as 5.0 μL (50.0 μg) portions to the wells of a thermowell polycarbonate non-sterile 96-well microtiter plate, which was then connected to a Dynal MPC® magnetic particle concentrator to separate magnetically the nanocomposites. Each well was added with the FITC-labeled *anti*-sense oligonucleotide DNA_2 FITC-$^{5'}$AGCCTCAATGCTCCCAGTGC dissolved in a pH 7.5 TNET buffer (50 μL, 10^{-7} M; Danyiel Biotech Ltd, Israel, chemical purity ≥ 98%) and the microtiter plate was incubated for 60 min at 60 °C for hybridization. Hybridized polyDPyr-/polyDCbz-magnetite NCs were washed by a TNET buffer (4 × 100 μL, pH 7.5) and by 50 μL of a commercially available Assay Solution® (Savyon Diagnostics Ltd, Israel) before incubation with the reporter *anti*-FITC HRP-labeled mouse monoclonal antibody (commercially available from Hoffman la Roche Inc., 0.1 μg mL^{-1}, 20 min at 20 °C, 50 μL of an Assay® Solution). After magnetically-driven decantation and plate washings (4 × 100 μL of a washing solution), the TMB substrate (0.05% w/w TMB solution in de-ionized water, 50 μL, Savyon Diagnostics Ltd) was added for color development for 1.5 min.

Following decantation, supernatants were removed and 80 μL fractions for each well were transferred to a second PS 96-well microplate for optical reading at 620 nm, using an Elisa plate reader Anthos ht II.

10.6.2.1 Specific Reagents, Buffers and Washing/Assay Solutions

PBS buffer (pH 7.0) prepared from Dubelcco's Phosphate Buffered Saline (Sigma); 0.4 M MES (pH 5.0): prepared using 2-morpholinoethanesulfonic acid hydrate 99%, adjusted to pH 5.0 by addition of 10 M NaOH and stored at 4 °C; TNET buffer (pH 7.5): prepared from a mixture of 10 mM Tris-HCl, 0.5 M NaCl, 1 mM EDTA and 0.02% Tween-20; washing solution: prepared from a mixture of 3 M NaCl and 2 M Tris-HCl (pH 7.5). Assay solution: prepared from a mixture of 154 m NaCl, 50 mM Tris-HCl (pH 7.8), 0.5% BSA, and 0.1% Tween 20; EDC: *N*′-(3-dimethylaminopropyl)-*N*-ethylcarbodiimide hydrochloride, >98% purity (Aldrich).

10.6.3
Quasi-covalent Attachment of a Biotin-5′-modified DNA Probe and DNA Hybridization Experiments onto Streptavidin-modified PolyDPyr-(5a)/PolyDCbz(5b)-magnetite NCs. Typical Experimental Procedures

Previously prepared polyDPyr(**5a**)-/polyDCbz(**5b**)-magnetite NCs (1% w/v suspension in a neutral PBS buffer, 200 μL, 2.0 mg) were first washed by the same neutral PBS buffer (3 × 200 μL), and then gently suspended in a freshly prepared cold 0.4 M MES buffer solution of the activating carbodiimide EDC (100.0 mg EDC/1.0 mL of a 0.4 M MES buffer at pH 5.0, 60 μL, 0–4 °C). After 5 min of gentle mixing for carboxylate activation, the commercially available, highly purified recombinant streptavidin dissolved in the same 0.4 M MES buffer [0.5 (mg of protein) mL^{-1} of a 0.4 M MES buffer at pH 5.0, 140 μL, 0–4 °C, Roche Inc.] was injected for a 1 h of incubation at room temperature (gentle NC mixing/vortexing). The resulting streptavidin-modified NCs were decanted magnetically, washed by a PBS neutral buffer (4 × 200 μL), and finally suspended in the same PBS neutral buffer (200 μL) to obtain a 1% w/v suspension of modified NCs ready for use. If necessary, they can be stored at 4 °C for several days without noticeable degradation.

DNA hybridizations operated on streptavidin-modified polyDPyr(**5a**)-/polyDCbz(**5b**)-magnetite NCs made use of the 20-mer biotinylated oligonucleotide DNA_1 biotin–(triethylene glycol) linker-$^{5'}$GCACTGGGAGCATTGAGGCT (1.2 nmol, 0.4 M MES buffer at pH 5.0; Danyiel Biotech Ltd, Israel, chemical purity ≥ 98% as checked by HPLC analysis, incubation time 2.0 h). DNA hybridizations onto NC surfaces were probed and optically quantified using the same (a) complementary FITC-$^{5'}$-labeled DNA_2 and (b) HRP-based amplifying enzymatic system, according to the formerly described protocol (covalent amide chemistry). Again, specific (SB) and non-specific binding (NSB) data were averaged values of three to six parallel experiments so as to minimize dispersion of optical output data.

10.7
Conclusions and Research Outlook

Novel chemically oxidizable COOH-DPyr- and DCbz-monomers have been synthesized using a general modular synthetic route (C_2-symmetrization of NH_2-/COOH-amino acid-related building blocks) towards a vast range of functionalized polycarboxylated polyDPyr-/polyDCbz-magnetite NCs. A combination of updated analytical and spectroscopic means has established – without ambiguity – that these magnetically responsive NCs possess a core–shell morphology (sheet-like nanoparticles 20–40 nm in size). This core–shell morphology basically results from chemical oxidative deposition of insoluble polyDPyr-/polyDCbz-polymers from the corresponding DPyr-/DCbz-monomers around magnetite nanoparticles. As a result of NC functionalization [introduction of COOH groups by poly(DPyr)-poly(DCbz)-polymers], DNA attachments and hybridizations have been successfully operated on them under various conditions and attachment formats (covalent and noncovalent) for DNA capture probes. These studies have emphasized their interesting potential for DNA-based diagnostic applications. Additionally, this research clearly offers an original way to combinatorially engineer polyDPyr-/polyDCbz-polymeric shell coverages of these novel magnetic NCs for the optimization of any desired application (NC functionalization by proteins/antibodies/enzymes, small peptides/oligosaccharides, locked nucleic acids, small chemical ligands/receptors). The novel materials, processes, and knowledge produced during this research could also have major applications in materials science and/or sensing technologies. For example, the fabrication of (a) polyDPyr-/polyDCbz-nanorods/nanotubules by template-oxidative polymerization of appropriate monomers within nanosized pores of template membranes, (b) new carbon nanotube–polyDPyr-/polyDCbz NCs, and (c) arrays of nanoporous polyDPyr-/polyDCbz-covered nanoelectrodes for biosensing applications are currently being developed in our laboratory.

Acknowledgments

This work has been funded under both Vth/VIth Framework European CHEMAG (n° GRD2-2000-30122) and NACBO (n° NMP3-2004-500802-2) projects. J.P.L. warmly acknowledges his close collaborators, Drs. Nurit Perlman, Senthil Govindaraji, Ludmila Buzhanski, and Augustine Joseph for investment in terms of much effort and many ideas during their research period at Bar-Ilan University (Israel). Professor Ian Bruce (Universities of Greenwich, England and of Urbino, Italy), and his main collaborator Dr. M. J. Davies (University of Greenwich, England) contributed much to the success of this research and are particularly thanked. Many Israeli collaborators/colleagues also supported various aspects of this program, which included specific nanotechnology-related analyses as well as stimulating scientific discussions/support. More particularly, the technical/scientific assistance of Professor Shlomo Margel, Dr. Ishai Bruckental (Departments of Chemistry and Physics, Bar-Ilan University, Israel), and Dr. Erika Rivka Bauminger (Racah Institute of Physics, Hebrew University of Jerusalem, Israel) has been highly appreciated. Drs. Aline Yakir, Nir Navot and Jacob Schlessinger (Savyon Diagnostics Ltd, Ashdod, Israel) are particularly commended for having sensitized us to DNA-based biological techniques.

References

1 R. Arshady, D. Pouliquen, A. Halbreich, J. Roger, J. N. Pons, J. C. Bacri, M. Da Silva, U. Häfeli, Magnetic nanospheres and nanocomposites in *Microspheres, Microcapsules & Liposomes* (Ed.: R. Arshady), Citrus Books, **2002**, Vol. 5, 283–329.

2 T. Hyeon, Chemical synthesis of magnetic nanoparticles. *Chem. Commun.* **2003**, 927–934.

3 M. Hilgendorff, M. Giersig, Synthesis of colloidal magnetic nanoparticles: Properties and applications in the *NATO Science Series, II: Mathematics, Physics and Chemistry*, Springer, **2003**, Vol. 91, 151–161.

4 M. A. Willard, L. K. Kurihara, E. E. Carpenter, S. Calvin, V. G. Harris, Chemically prepared magnetic nanoparticles in the *Encyclopedia of Nanoscience and Nanotechnology* (Ed.: J. A. Schwarz, C. Contescu, K. Putyera), Marcel Dekker, **2004**, Vol. 1, 815–848.

5 T. Pellegrino, S. Kudera, T. Liedl, A. M. Javier, L. Manna, W. J. Parak, On the development of colloidal nanoparticles towards multifunctional structures and their possible use for biological applications. *Small* **2005**, *1*, 48–63.

6 *Scientific and Clinical Applications of Magnetic Carriers*, (Eds.: U. Häfeli, W. Schütt, J. Teller, M. Zborowski), Plenum Press, New York, **1997**.

7 I. Safarik, M. Safarikova, Magnetic nanoparticles and biosciences. *Monatsh. Chem.* **2002**, *133*, 737–759.

8 R. Hergt, R. Hiergeist, I. Hilger, W. Kaiser, Magnetic nanoparticles for thermoablation in *Recent Res. Develop. Mater. Sc.* **2002**, *3*, 723–742.

9 C. C. Berry, A. S. G. Curtis, Functionalisation of magnetic nanoparticles for applications in biomedicine. *J. Phys. D: Appl. Phys.* **2003**, *36*, R198–R206.

10 K. K. Jain, Nanodiagnostics: application of nanotechnology in molecular diagnostics. *Expert Rev. Mol. Diagn.* **2003**, *3*, 153–161.

11 Q. A. Pankhurst, J. Connolly, S. K. Jones, J. Dobson, Applications of magnetic nanoparticles in biomedicine. *J. Phys. D: Appl. Phys.* **2003**, *36*, R167–R181.

12 S. Mornet, S. Vasseur, F. Grasset, E. Duguet, Magnetic nanoparticle design for medical diagnosis and therapy. *J. Mater. Chem.* **2004**, *14*, 2161–2175.

13 A. G. Payne, Using immunomagnetic technology and other means to facilitate stem cell homing. *Med. Hypotheses* **2004**, *62*, 718–720.

14 G. Bidan, Electroconducting conjugated polymers: new sensitive matrices to build-up chemical or electrochemical sensors. A review. *Sens. Actuators, B* **1992**, *6*, 45–56.

15 A. Deronzier, J. C. Moutet, Functionalized polypyrroles as versatile molecular materials for

electrode modification. A review. *Curr. Top. Electrochem.* **1994**, *3*, 159–200.

16 S. Cosnier, Biosensors based on immobilization of biomolecules by electrogenerated polymer films new perspectives. *Appl. Biochem. Biotechnol.* **2000**, *89*, 127–138.

17 A. Malinauskas, Chemical deposition of conducting polymers. *Polymer* **2001**, *42*, 3957–3972.

18 R. Gangopadhyay, A. De, Conducting polymer nanocomposite in the *Handbook of Organic-Inorganic Hybrid Materials and Nanocomposites* (Ed.: H. S. Nalwa), American Scientific Publishers: Calcutta, India, **2003**, Vol. 2, 217–263.

19 J. F. Rubinson, From biology to engineering: The present status of conducting polymers. *ACS Symp. Ser.* **2003**, *832*, 2–15.

20 R. Gangopadhyay, Conducting polymer nanostructures in the *Encyclopedia of Nanoscience and Nanotechnology* (Ed.: J. A. Schwarz, C. Contescu, K. Putyera), Marcel Dekker, Sapporo, Japan, **2004**, Vol. 2, 105–131.

21 G. G. Wallace, P. C. Innis, L. A. P. Kane-Maguire, Inherently conducting polymer nanostructures in the *Encyclopedia of Nanoscience and Nanotechnology* (Ed.: J. A. Schwarz, C. Contescu, K. Putyera), Marcel Dekker, Wollogong, Australia, **2004**, Vol. 4, 113–130.

22 S. P. Armes, Conducting polymer colloids. *Curr. Opin. Colloid Interface Sci.* **1996**, *1*, 214–220.

23 R. Gangopadhyay, A. De, Conducting polymer nanocomposites: A brief overview. *Chem. Mater.* **2000**, *12*, 608–622.

24 M. D. Butterworth, S. P. Armes, Poly(pyrrole)-silica-magnetite composite colloids. *Polym. Mater.: Sci. Eng.* **1995**, *72*, 300–301.

25 M. D. Butterworth, S. A. Bell, S. P. Armes, A. W. Simpson, Synthesis and characterization of polypyrrole-magnetite-silica particles. *J. Colloid Interface Sci.* **1996**, *183*, 91–99.

26 J. Deng, X. Ding, W. Zhang, Y. Peng, J. Wang, X. Long, P. Li, A. S. C. Chan, Magnetic and conducting Fe_3O_4-cross-linked polyaniline nanoparticles with core-shell structure. *Polymer* **2002**, *43*, 2179–2184.

27 S. F. Lascelles, S. P. Armes, Synthesis and characterization of micrometer-sized, polypyrrole-coated polystyrene latexes. *J. Mater. Chem.* **1997**, *7*, 1339–1347.

28 C. Barthet, S. P. Armes, S. F. Lascelles, S. Y. Luk, H. M. E. Stanley, Synthesis and characterization of micrometer-sized, polyaniline-coated polystyrene latexes. *Langmuir* **1998**, *14*, 2032–2041.

29 D. B. Cairns, S. P. Armes, L. G. B. Bremer, Synthesis and characterization of submicrometer-sized polypyrrole-polystyrene composite particles. *Langmuir* **1999**, *15*, 8052–8058.

30 M. A. Khan, S. P. Armes, Synthesis and characterization of micrometer-sized poly(3,4-ethylenedioxythiophene)-coated polystyrene latexes. *Langmuir* **1999**, *15*, 3469–3475.

31 S. Maeda, S. P. Armes, Preparation of novel polypyrrole-silica colloidal nanocomposites. *J. Colloid Interface Sci.* **1993**, *159*, 257–259.

32 S. Maeda, S. P. Armes, Preparation and characterization of novel polypyrrole-silica colloidal nanocomposites. *J. Mater. Chem.* **1994**, *4*, 935–942.

33 S. Maeda, R. Corradi, S. P. Armes, Synthesis and characterization of carboxylic acid-functionalized polypyrrole-silica microparticles. *Macromolecules* **1995**, *28*, 2905–2911.

34 M. R. Pope, S. P. Armes, P. J. Tarcha, Specific activity of polypyrrole nanoparticulate immunoreagents: Comparison of surface chemistry and immobilization options. *Bioconj. Chem.* **1996**, *7*, 436–444.

35 G. P. McCarthy, S. P. Armes, S. J. Greaves, J. F. Watts, Synthesis and characterization of carboxylic acid-functionalized polypyrrole-silica microparticles using a 3-substituted pyrrole comonomer. *Langmuir* **1997**, *13*, 3686–3692.

36 H. M. Han, S. P. Armes, Synthesis of

poly(3,4-ethylenedioxythiophene)/silica colloidal nanocomposites. *Langmuir* **2003**, *19*, 4523–4526.
37 A. Azioune, A. Ben Slimane, L. A. Hamou, A. Pleuvy, M. M. Chehimi, C. Perruchot, S. P. Armes, Synthesis and characterization of active ester-functionalized polypyrrole-silica nanoparticles: application to the covalent attachment of proteins. *Langmuir* **2004**, *20*, 3350–3356.
38 S. Maeda, S. P. Armes, Polypyrrole-tin(IV) oxide colloidal nanocomposites. *Synth. Met.* **1995**, *69*, 499–500.
39 S. M. Marinakos, J. P. Novak, L. C. III Brousseau, A. B. House, E. M. Edeki, J. C. Feldhaus, D. L. Feldheim, Gold particles as templates for the synthesis of hollow polymer capsules. Control of capsule dimensions and guest encapsulation. *J. Am. Chem. Soc.* **1999**, *121*, 8518–8522.
40 S. M. Marinakos, D. A. Shultz, D. L. Feldheim, Gold nanoparticles as templates for the synthesis of hollow nanometer-sized conductive polymer capsules. *Adv. Mater.* **1999**, *11*, 34–37.
41 H. V. Meyers, Chemical and biological approaches to molecular diversity: Applications to drug discovery in the *Biology-Chemistry Interface* (Ed.: K. Nakanishi, R. Cooper, J. K. Snyder III), Marcel Dekker: Framingham, USA, **1999**, 271–287.
42 L. Weber, Molecular diversity analysis and combinatorial library design in *Methods and Principles in Medicinal Chemistry* (Ed.: D. E. Clark), Wiley-VCH: Weinheim, Germany, **2000**, Vol. 8, 137–157.
43 D. L. Wright, R. S. Oruganty, C. V. Robotham, The role of organic synthesis in the generation of molecular diversity in *Organic Synthesis: Theory and Applications* (Ed.: T. Hudlicky), JAI Press, **2001**, Vol. 5, 197–254.
44 G. Helary, C. Chevrot, G. Sauvet, A. Slove, Electroactive poly(3,6-carbazolediyl) with lateral amino-alkyldisiloxane groups. *Polym. Bull.* **1991**, *26*, 131–138.
45 A. Desbene-Monvernay, P. C. Lacaze, M. Delamar, A quantitative study of cross-linking in electro-deposited carbazole films using tetrabutylammonium tribromide bromination and XPS analysis. *J. Electroanal. Chem.* **1992**, *354*, 241–246.
46 K. Périé, R. S. Marks, S. Szumerits, S. Cosnier, J.-P. Lellouche, Novel electro-oxidizable chiral *N*-substituted dicarbazoles and resulting electro-active films for covalent attachment of proteins. *Tetrahedron Lett.* **2000**, *41*, 3725–3729.
47 S. Cosnier, R. S. Marks, J.-P. Lellouche, K. Périé, D. Fologea, S. Szumerits, Electrogenerated poly(chiral dicarbazole) films for the reagentless grafting of enzymes. *Electroanalysis* **2000**, *12*, 1107–1112.
48 S. Cosnier, S. Szunerits, R. S. Marks, J.-P. Lellouche, K. Périé, Mediated electrochemical detection of catechol by tyrosinase-based poly(dicarbazole) electrodes. *J. Biochem. Biophys. Methods* **2001**, *50*, 65–77.
49 S. Cosnier, A. Le Pellec, R. S. Marks, K. Périé, J.-P. Lellouche, A permselective biotinylated polydicarbazole film for the fabrication of amperometric enzyme electrodes. *Electrochem. Commun.* **2003**, *5*, 973–977.
50 N. Elming, N. Clauson-Kaas, The preparation of pyrroles from furans. *Acta Chim. Scand.* **1952**, 867–874.
51 T. Sugimoto, E. Matijevic, Formation of uniform spherical magnetite particles by crystallization from ferrous hydroxide gels. *J. Colloid Interface Sci.* **1980**, *74*, 227–243.
52 J. I. Taylor, C. D. Hurst, M. J. Davies, N. Sachsinger, I. J. Bruce, Application of magnetite and silica-magnetite composites to the isolation of genomic DNA. *J. Chromatogr., A* **2000**, *890*, 159–166.
53 J.-P. Lellouche, N. Perlman, A. Joseph, S. Govindaraji, L. Buzhansky, A. Yakir, I. Bruce, New magnetically responsive polydicarbazole-magnetite nano-

particles. *Chem. Commun.* **2004**, 560–561.

54 L. Josephson, J. M. Perez, R. Weissleder, Magnetic nanosensors for the detection of oligonucleotide sequences. *Angew. Chem., Int. Ed.* **2001**, *40*, 3204–3206.

55 K. Abdel-Nasser, J. Wang, Amplified electrical transduction of DNA hybridization based on polymeric beads loaded with multiple gold nanoparticle tags. *Electroanalysis* **2004**, *16*, 101–107.

56 D. A. Vignali, Multiplexed particle-based flow cytometric assays. *J. Immunol. Methods* **2000**, *243*, 243–255.

57 J. Wang, A. Erdem, An overview to magnetic beads used in electrochemical DNA biosensors in the *NATO Science Series, II: Mathematics, Physics and Chemistry*, Springer: Heidelberg, **2003**, Vol. 102, 297–303.

58 E. P. Diamandis, T. K. Christopoulos, The biotin-(strept)avidin system: principles and applications in biotechnology. *Clin. Chem.* **1991**, *37*, 625–636.

59 M. Wilchek, E. A. Bayer, Avidin-biotin immobilization systems in *Immobilised Macromolecules: Application Potentials* (Ed.: U. B. Sleytr, U. Bernd), Springer: Heidelberg, **1993**, 51–60.

60 E. A. Bayer, M. Wilchek, The avidin-biotin system. *Immunoassay* **1996**, 237–267.

61 J. V. Staros, *N*-Hydroxysulfosuccinimide active esters: bis(*N*-hydroxysulfosuccinimide) esters of two dicarboxylic acids are hydrophilic, membrane-impermeant, protein cross-linkers. *Biochemistry* **1982**, *21*, 3950–3955.

62 F. S. Gibson, M. S. Park, H. Rapoport, Bis[[4-(2,2-dimethyl-1,3-dioxolyl)]methyl]-carbodiimide (BDDC) and its application to residue-free esterifications, peptide couplings, and dehydrations. *J. Org. Chem.* **1994**, *59*, 7503–7507.

63 I. Grayson, Water-soluble carbodiimide – an efficient coupling agent for synthesis. *Speciality Chem.* **2000**, *20*, 86–88.

64 S. R. Poort, F. R. Rosendaal, P. H. Reitsma, R. M. Bertina, A common genetic variation in the 3′-untranslated region of the prothrombin gene is associated with elevated plasma prothrombin levels and an increase in venous thrombosis. *Blood* **1996**, *88*, 3698–3703.

65 V. Vicente, R. Gonzalez-Conejero, J. Rivera, J. Corral, The prothrombin gene variant 20210A in venous and arterial thromboembolism. *Haematologica* **1999**, *84*, 356–362.

66 Dynabeads® M-270 (carboxylic acid form, 2.8 μm diameter, 2–5 $m^2\ g^{-1}$ specific area) are superparamagnetic beads composed of highly cross-linked polystyrene with a magnetic iron oxide material precipitated and trapped in evenly distributed pores. A hydrophilic outer layer of glycidyl ether provides functional carboxylate groups (150 μmol per g beads). The iron content of the beads is 15% w/w for a magnetic mass susceptibility in a 88–126 × $10^{-6}\ m^3\ g^{-1}$ range.

11
Gelatin Nanoparticles and Their Biofunctionalization

Sushma Kommareddy, Dinesh B. Shenoy, and Mansoor M. Amiji

11.1
Introduction

Progress in nanotechnology and medicine has led to an expansion of novel dosage forms for the delivery of drugs to diseased areas while minimizing toxicity to healthy tissues. Popular nanocarriers include polymeric micelles, dendrimers, micro-nano-emulsions, liposomes, niosomes, supramolecular complexes, nanosuspensions and nanoparticles [1–10]. Most of these can be generally classified as colloidal drug delivery systems (by virtue of their size and physico-chemical properties), each having their own merits and demerits. Nanoparticles, especially those prepared from polymeric materials, enjoy tremendous popularity due to ease of preparation, ease of tuning physico-chemical properties (through an array of polymeric materials), possibility of surface modification, excellent stability and scalability to industrial production. Since their conception in the mid-1970s, nanoparticles have found applicability in almost every section of medicine and biology (besides a host of other fields) in general, in particular for controlled/targeted delivery of drugs and genetic materials [11–21].

Nanoparticles can be categorized as colloidal carrier systems of submicron size that are made from synthetic or natural polymers. Based on the method used for their formation, they could be either nanospheres (or nanoparticles), which are essentially monolithic systems having a solid matrix or nanocapsules that have hollow interior that is filled with the compound of interest and are surrounded by a polymeric shell [16]. Drug-loaded nanoparticles have been developed for almost every route of administration – nasal, ocular, mucosal, inhalation, oral, transdermal and parenteral. Clinically, they have found applications for diagnosing and treating a wide range of pathological conditions.

Polymers used to prepare nanoparticles may be biodegradable or non-biodegradable. An ideal polymer should be biocompatible, biodegradable with minimum toxicity, sterile and non-pyrogenic, and must have a high capacity to accommodate drugs and protect them from degradation. Nanoparticles have been prepared using both natural and synthetic biopolymers. Poly(D,L-lactide-*co*-

Nanotechnologies for the Life Sciences Vol. 1
Biofunctionalization of Nanomaterials. Edited by Challa S. S. R. Kumar

ISBN: 3-527-31381-8

glycolide), poly(ε-caprolactone), polyalkylcyanoacrylates, poly(styrene-*co*-maleic anhydride), poly(divinylether-*co*-maleic anhydride), poly(vinyl alcohol), and poly-(ethylene glycol) are some of the synthetic, non-immunogenic polymers used extensively for the preparation of nanoparticles [1, 14, 19, 22–25]. Similarly, poly-(amino acids), hyaluronic acid, albumin, dextran, chitosan and gelatin are a few of the natural biodegradable polymers [26–32]. While each polymer has its own advantages, nanoparticles can be synthesized with a high degree of reproducibility from most of them; natural polymers, due to their natural origin, are preferred considering non-toxicity and biodegradability. The striking advantage of synthetic polymers is the possibility of synthesizing them reproducibly with well-defined physico-chemical properties. Advances in biotechnology are helping natural polymers overcome this drawback and we can expect a surge in delivery systems based on them. In the sections that follow, the properties of gelatin, its chemical modification, synthesis of nanoparticles using gelatin and its derivatives, characterization of the formed nanoparticles, loading and release of the payload from the nanoparticles and the biocompatibility of gelatin nanoparticles and their conjugates are discussed. Further, the use of these nanoparticles in various drug delivery applications is elaborated.

11.2 Gelatin and Gelatin Derivatives

Gelatin, one of the most versatile, naturally occurring biopolymers, is widely used in food products and pharmaceutical dosage forms. It is a proteinaceous hydrocolloid obtained by partial hydrolysis of collagen. Natural gelatins or recombinant gelatins have been tailored to enhance product performance – thus expanding their applicability in biology and medicine. The following sub-sections give an overview of such gelatins.

11.2.1 Gelatin

Gelatin is a heterogeneous mixture of single or multi-stranded polypeptides, each with extended left-handed proline helix conformations and containing between 300 and 4000 amino acids. Figure 11.1 depicts the composition of gelatin in terms of amino acids. The triple helix of type I collagen extracted from skin and bones consists of alpha and beta helical strands together with their oligomers and breakdown (and other) polypeptides and has a molecular mass of ~95 kDa, is ~1.5 nm wide and ~0.3 mm long. It is obtained commercially by acidic or basic cleavage of the intermolecular and intramolecular covalent bonds that stabilize porcine or bovine collagen. Figure 11.2 shows the basic structure of gelatin. Based on the process used for its manufacture, gelatin is obtained either as Type-A or -B. Type-A gelatin is obtained by acidic treatment of collagen and has an isoelectric point (pI) between

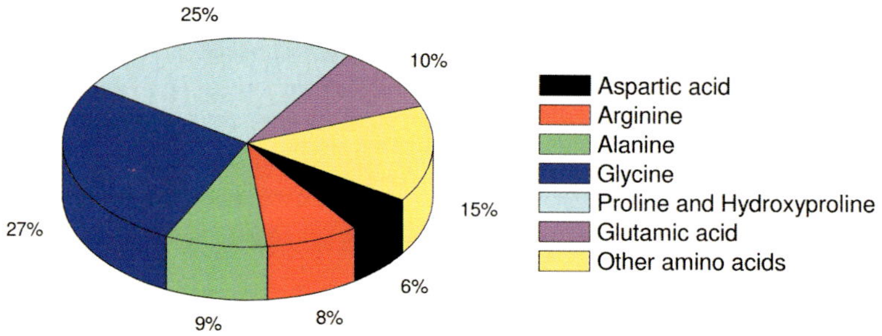

Fig. 11.1. Amino acid composition of gelatin.

7.0 and 9.0. Type-B gelatin, however, is obtained by alkaline hydrolysis of collagen and has a pI between 4.8 and 5.0. [33–35].

Gelatin is a polyampholyte that gels below 35–40 °C. The heterogeneous nature of the molecular weight profile of this biopolymer is affected by pH and temperature, which in turn affects the noncovalent interactions and phase behavior of gelatin in solution [35]. The numerous pendant functional groups throughout the polymeric chain present many opportunities for a pharmaceutical chemist to induce novel functionality via chemical derivatization. The purpose could be as simple as crosslinking and/or hardening or could be as complex as ligand-mediated active targeting at the cellular level.

11.2.2
Chemical Modification of Gelatin

Different modifications of polymer gelatin are carried out to control the biofunctional properties: biodistribution, targetability and stability of the formulations prepared from the modified polymer [36]. Poly(ethylene glycol) (PEG) conjugation (PEGylation), thiolation and conjugation with other synthetic block copolymers and antibodies are some of the currently studied modifications of gelatin.

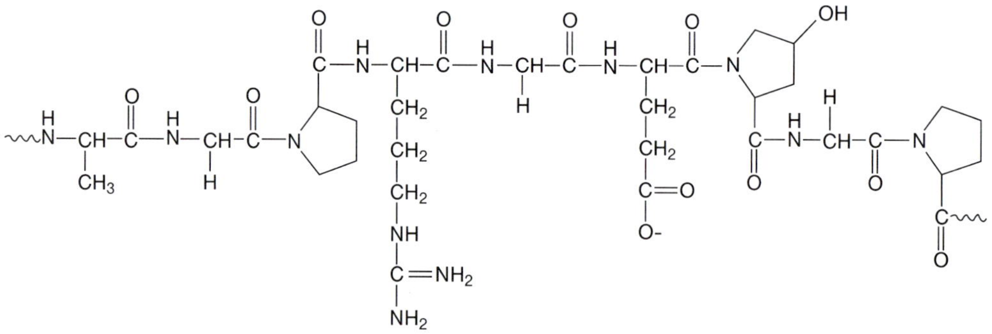

Fig. 11.2. Basic chemical structure of gelatin.

11.2.2.1 PEGylation

PEGylation is the simplest and most popular methodology employed to increase the systemic circulation time of colloidal carriers like liposomes, micelles and nanoparticles [37–41]. It is the most widely accepted and commercially utilized technique to improve drug performance by optimizing pharmacokinetics, increasing bioavailability, decreasing immunogenicity and dosing frequency [42–47]. The basic strategy of PEGylation is to hydrophilize the surface and to induce a steric barrier by anchoring long, mobile PEG chains – thus preventing opsonin recognition in the reticuloendothelial system (RES) based blood clearance pathway. Based on the properties of colloids, the stability can be increased by limiting the mutual interactions (hydrophobic, van der Waal's, electrostatic etc.) by usage of hydrophilic and chemically inert polymers that form a protective layer around each particle, resulting in steric stabilization [48]. The major outcome of PEGylation is the significantly increased circulation time, the advantages of which include maintenance of optimal therapeutic concentration of drug in the blood after single administration of the drug carrier, increased probability of extravasation and retention of the colloidal carrier in areas of fenestrated vasculature and enhancement of active targeting ability to areas of diminished blood supply by using a ligand [11]. Besides PEG, polymers such as poly(vinyl alcohol), poly(acryl amide), poly(vinyl pyrrolidone) are also used to modify the physico-chemical properties of colloidal carriers [36].

PEG is a linear or branched polymer with terminal hydroxyl groups and is synthesized by anionic ring-opening polymerization of ethylene oxide initiated by nucleophilic attack of hydroxide ion on epoxide ring. Monomethoxy PEG (mPEG) is another widely used modification where polymerization is initiated by methoxide ion. To conjugate PEG to molecules such as polypeptides, polysaccharides, polynucleotides or other polymers, a derivative of PEG is generally prepared by functionalizing one or both the hydroxyl end groups and then coupled to the reactive amino, hydroxyl or carboxyl groups present on the molecules of interest [42]. The protective action (Stealth® property) of PEG is mainly due to the formation of a dense, hydrophilic cloud of long polyethylene chains on the surface of the molecule/colloidal particle. The tethered/chemically anchored PEG chains can undergo spatial conformations, thus preventing the opsonization of particles by the RES of the liver and spleen and hence improving the circulation time of molecules/particles in the blood. In addition, excellent biocompatibility and lack of toxicity/immunogenicity make PEG the polymer of choice for chemically modifying molecule/particles of interest to induce Stealth® properties [49–51]. The best known commercial success that employs the PEGylation technology to increase the circulation half-life of an intravenously injected formulation is the Stealth® liposomal formulation of doxorubicin (Doxil®) [39].

We have prepared PEG-modified gelatin for drug delivery applications by reacting Type-B gelatin with PEG-epoxide according to the scheme depicted in Fig. 11.3 [52]. Carboxylated mPEG can also be prepared, and subsequently coupled to the amine groups of gelatin by the dichlorohexylcarbodiimide method [53]. FTIR and NMR analysis confirmed the carboxylation and coupling reactions, and by estimat-

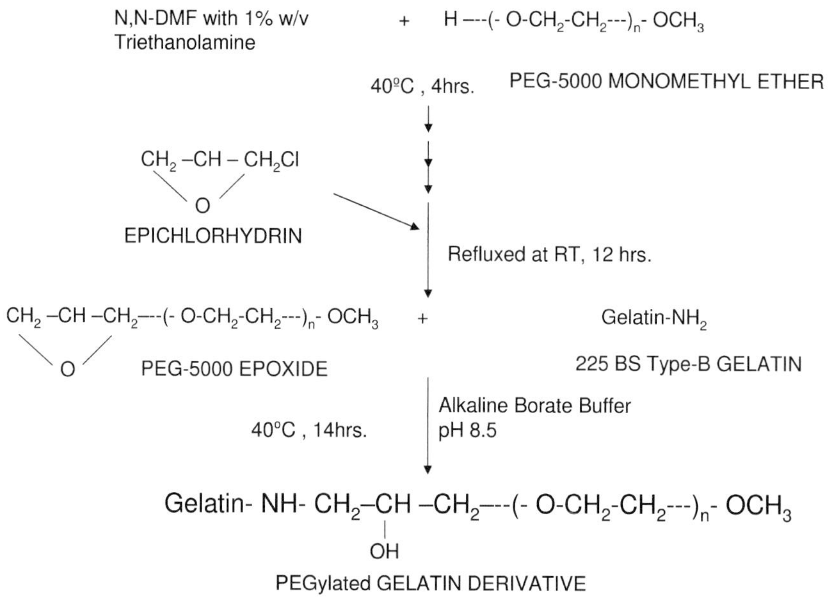

Fig. 11.3. Scheme of poly(ethylene glycol) (PEG) conjugation with Type-B gelatin.

ing the unreacted mPEG it was determined that each molecule of gelatin was coupled to 205 molecules of mPEG. In another study, an ester-activated PEG (mPEG) was coupled to the amino group of gelatin to prepare PEG-grafted gelatin (PEG-gelatin). This PEG-gelatin formed a micellar structure with PEG chains positioned on the outer surface of the micelle [54].

When hydrated in an aqueous medium, the chain-like PEG molecule is swiftly hydrated and set in rapid motion. This extended, quick motion causes the PEG to sweep out a large volume around it, preventing the approach and interference of other molecules/particles. As a result, when attached to a drug or a particle, PEG chains can influence not only inter-molecular/particulate interactions but also protect the underlying core from immune response and other clearance mechanisms, thus sustaining drug bioavailability. The size, molecular weight and shape of the PEG fraction and the linkage used to connect it to the entity of interest determine the consequences of PEGylation in relation to protein adsorption and pharmacokinetics (like volume of distribution, circulation time and renal clearance). When formulated into colloidal particles, the PEG density on the colloidal surface can be changed by using a PEG of appropriate molecular weight (hence length of poly (ethylene glycol) chains) and molar ratio (hence the grafting efficiency) between gelatin and PEG. Longer PEG chains offer greater steric influence around the colloidal entity – similar to increased grafting density with shorter PEG chains. Longer PEG chains may also collapse onto the nanoparticle surface, thus providing a hydrophilic shield.

11.2.2.2 **Thiolation**

Thiolated derivatives of gelatin have been prepared by different methods to create disulfide crosslinked hydrogels that can act as substrates for cell growth, improve the mucoadhesive properties of the nanoparticulate material and to functionalize the gelatin for conjugation with other molecules like antibodies or drugs. Thiolated gelatin can be synthesized by carbodiimide-mediated reaction of the carboxyl groups of gelatin with disulfide-containing dithiobis(propionic hydrazide) (DTP) followed by reduction with dithiothreitol (DTT) (Fig. 11.4) [55]. As this chemical reaction is based on the modification of carboxyl groups of gelatin, the carboxyl rich Type-B gelatin is preferred to Type-A. The reaction is carried out at pH 4.7 to obtain gelatin-DTPH after reduction with DTT [55]. Other thiolation reactions that involve modification of carboxyl residues are activation of carboxyl groups using carbodiimide followed by covalent reaction of a sulfhydryl group containing substrate, like cystaminium dichloride [56].

The ε-amino groups of the proteins can also be modified to introduce a free thiol group. Traut's reagent (2-iminothiolane) undergoes a ring-opening reaction with amino groups to expose the sulfhydryl group. Reagents like succinimidyl 3-(2-pyridyldithio) propionate (SPDP), succinimidyl 4-(*p*-maleimidophenyl) butyrate (SMPB), *N*-succinimidyl[4-iodoacetyl] aminobenzoate (SIAB), succinimidyl 4-[*N*-maleimidomethyl] cyclohexane-1-carboxylate (SMCC) are also used as bifunctional crosslinkers that react with amino groups of proteins to produce a free sulfhydryl group on the surface. Alternatively, gelatin nanoparticles can be thiolated after crosslinking with glutaraldehyde (post-modification). In such cases, aldehyde groups are quenched with cysteine, which generates free sulfhydryl groups on the surface of gelatin nanoparticles [57]. The disulfide content or the free thiol groups can be determined by Ellman's assay or by ^{1}H NMR [56].

Thiolated gelatin obtained by utilizing any of the above-mentioned reactions can be further modified by conjugation with moieties like avidin, which is complexed with biotinylated peptide nucleic acids or biotinylated antibodies [58, 59]. Hyaluronan–gelatin hydrogels have been prepared by disulfide crosslinking of thiol derivatives of hyaluronan and gelatin that were synthesized separately. Such disulfide crosslinked hydrogels have been used as a substrate for cell growth [60].

11.2.2.3 **Other Conjugates of Gelatin**

Gelatin has been conjugated with chitosan by the enzymatic action of tyrosinase on gelatin [61]. The enzyme tyrosinase is an oxidative enzyme that converts phenols into O-quinones – hence it reacts with tyrosyl groups present on the telopeptide region of gelatin to convert them into O-quinones that react with nucleophilic amino groups of chitosan non-enzymatically. Chemical conjugation of gelatin to chitosan was confirmed by UV/Visible, IR and ^{1}H NMR spectroscopy. Viscosity measurements carried out at different reaction conditions also indicated the conjugation of gelatin with chitosan, as it has thermal behavior compared with gels formed by cooling gelatin. These studies indicate that the mechanical properties of tyrosinase-mediated conjugates of gelatin can be further explored for medical and industrial applications [61].

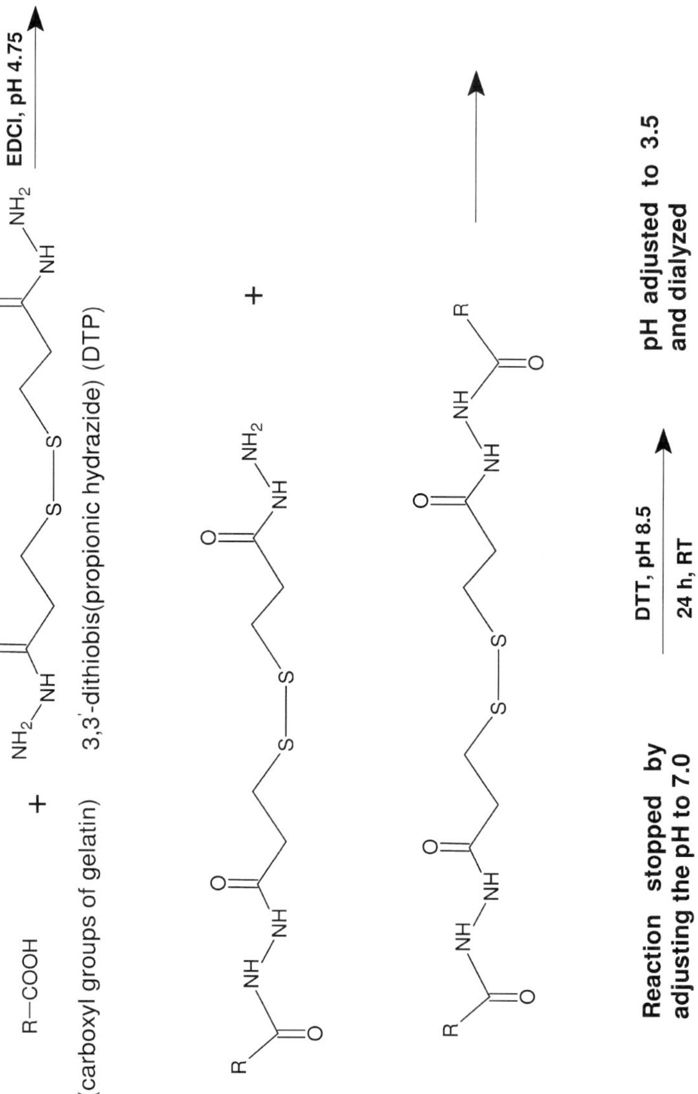

Fig. 11.4. Scheme of thiolation of carboxyl groups of gelatin with disulfide-containing dithiobis(propionic hydrazide) (DTP) mediated by carbodiimide.

Semi-synthetic, biodegradable, amphiphilic copolymers of poly(D,L-lactide) grafted gelatins have been prepared by ring-opening polymerization of D,L-lactide onto gelatin and a trimethylsilyl derivative of gelatin in the presence of a catalyst, tin(II) bis(2-ethylhexanoate), at 80 °C [62]. The solution polymerization was carried out in DMSO and the copolymers formed were characterized by elemental and thermal analysis, and IR and ^{1}H NMR spectroscopy. Molecular weights of the copolymers were calculated and were found to increase with increasing ratio of D,L-lactide to gelatin, indicating the possibility of fabricating polymers with required properties for tissue engineering [62].

Gelatin nanoparticles have recently been conjugated to antibodies by avidin–biotin complex formation [63, 64]. Following crosslinking, some of the reactive amino groups on the gelatin surface were activated with 2-iminothiolane to introduce reactive sulfhydryl groups. The thiolated nanoparticles were coupled to NeutrAvidin™ (NAv) previously activated by a hetero-bifunctional crosslinker. The NAv-modified nanoparticles were then used for the binding of biotinylated antibodies by avidin–biotin complex formation. The biotinylated antibody attached may be an anti-CD3 antibody that is used for specific drug targeting to T-lymphocytes or trastuzumab (Herceptin), which could be used for targeting HER2 overexpressing tumor cells [63, 64].

11.3 Nanoparticulate Carriers of Gelatin and Gelatin Derivatives

Preparation of nanoparticles from a pre-formed polymer is, in general, relatively straightforward, having high degree of reproducibility. However, the physicochemical properties of gelatin, especially its heterogeneity in molecular weight distribution, make it a challenging polymer with which to produce stable nanoparticles. Nonetheless, many groups have successfully prepared nanoparticles, from gelatin and its derivatives, that have been evaluated for a range of biomedical applications [65–70]. Desolvation is the most popular technique for preparing gelatin nanoparticles, followed by techniques such as coacervation and water-in-oil emulsification.

11.3.1 Desolvation

Desolvation is the process in which solvents of different polarity and hydrogen bonding, when added to solution of proteins, bring about rolling up or controlled precipitation of proteins due to the displacement of water molecules from the surface of proteins [71]. In solution, the gelatin molecules are well stretched and upon addition of (non-)solvents, such as ethanol, acetone or isopropanol, the solubility of gelatin molecules decreases (as the high hydrogen-bonding capacity of these solvents displaces water molecules), resulting in phase separation of the rolled-up gelatin molecules. These molecules have a size range of 100–200 nm and are further hardened by crosslinking with aldehydes such as formaldehyde or glutaraldehyde. The pH and stirring conditions affect the size range and yield of these particles [15, 35].

11.3.1.1 Desolvation Using Ethanol

The folding of gelatin in solution is determined by noncovalent interactions with the water molecules and the presence of solvents such as ethanol, which in turn affect these interactions. Marty et al. first observed that the complex phase behavior of gelatin was affected by temperature and other experimental conditions [13]. Farrugia et al. have investigated the affect of temperature, pH and ethanol concentration on the molecular weight distribution profile of gelatin in solution in order to develop a robust method for preparing gelatin nanoparticles [35]. The molecular weight profile of gelatin remained unchanged at pH 5.0 to 7.0. However, at pH < 6.0, the gelatin particles lacked a net charge, resulting in aggregation. At pH > 7.5, the increased charge on the particles contributed to increased resistance to dehydration. In addition, the turbidity of the solution during nanoparticles preparation was constant at all temperatures within the pH range, and the percentage of molecular weight fractions precipitated was optimum at ethanol concentrations ranging from 62.5 to 75% w/w [35].

We have standardized preparation procedures for gelatin and PEGylated gelatin nanoparticles using the solvent displacement (based on principles of desolvation) process [52, 72]. Typically, ethanol is used as the non-solvent for gelatin. A 1% w/v solution of gelatin is prepared at 37 °C and the pH adjusted to 7.0 with 0.2 M sodium hydroxide. Nanoparticles are formed when the solvent composition is changed from 100% water to 65% (by volume) hydro-alcoholic solution under continuous stirring. The nanoparticles are further crosslinked with a 40% v/v aqueous solution of glyoxal for the desired time and any unreacted aldehyde is quenched with 12% w/v sodium metabisulfite. Particles so-obtained have a size range of 200–500 nm.

11.3.1.2 Two-step Desolvation

Nanoparticles can be prepared from both Type-A and -B gelatins using this method. In the first step gelatin molecules of low molecular weight are separated (through a first-stage desolvation process) and discarded. The sediment obtained is rich in high-molecular weight gelatin fractions and is resolvated (redissolved in suitable aqueous medium) to carry out a second-stage desolvation process. Gelatin nanoparticles obtained by the two-step desolvation process have high stability (predominantly by virtue of high molecular weight) and do not show any aggregation or flocculation [73–75].

11.3.2 Coacervation

Coacervation is a process of spontaneous phase separation in the presence of two oppositely charged polyelectrolytes in solution. Electrostatic interaction between the electrolytes and the macromolecules results in the separation of a polymer-rich phase, the coacervate, and a polymer-poor phase, the supernatant [76]. This concept of coacervation or phase separation can be used for preparing nanoparticles to encapsulate proteins and drugs.

Leong et al. [68, 76, 77] have synthesized gelatin nanoparticles as vehicles for gene delivery, by coacervation brought about by desolvation of water molecules using polyelectrolytes. Gelatin nanoparticles so-obtained form at gelatin concentrations ranging from 1.5 to 5% w/v and sodium sulfate from 0.2 to 1.2% w/v. The conditions of coacervation also depend to a great extent on the mixing conditions and presence or absence of electrolytes in solution. When plasmid DNA was co-encapsulated with endolysolytic agents such as chloroquine the required sodium sulfate concentration was reduced by 10–20% w/v. The uncrosslinked nanoparticles formed were relatively stable in acidic pH; however, as they dissociate at high ionic strength and neutral pH, the formed nanoparticles were separated by centrifugation and crosslinked using 0.1 mg mL^{-1} (1-ethyl-3-[3-dimethylaminopropyl]-carbodiimide hydrochloride) (EDC); the excess was quenched using glycine at a concentration of 0.2 M in the final solution.

In other instances, the concept of coacervation was used in combination with phase separation, in which a 1% w/v solution of gelatin containing surfactant (polysorbate 20, at 0.5% w/v) was mixed with sodium sulfate (at 20% w/v) to bring about coacervation followed by phase separation using isopropanol under continuous stirring. The nanoparticles formed were stabilized by crosslinking with glutaraldehyde; the excess aldehyde groups were quenched with sodium metabisulfite. The nanoparticles formed were stabilized by crosslinking with glutaraldehyde; the excess was quenched using sodium metabisulfite. Nanoparticles with an average size of 200 nm were separated from the salts by gel-chromatography using Sephadex G-50 [69, 70, 78].

11.3.3
Nano-encapsulation by Water-in-oil Emulsion Method

Nanoencapsulation involves wrapping small amounts of material in individual coatings or sheaths in discrete, sub-micron sized particles. Materials such as proteins or conventional drugs can be encapsulated, wherein the coatings aid in protecting the encapsulated material and in achieving prolonged or controlled release. Gelatin nanoparticles can be prepared by using the emulsifier-free water-in-oil (W/O) emulsion method either by solvent evaporation [67] or homogenization [79]. The gelling property of gelatin enables the separation of the hydrogel particles that are formed in the emulsion, which can be further stabilized/hardened by glutaraldehyde crosslinking [67]. Typically, a W/O emulsion is prepared with a gelatin solution as the internal aqueous phase and a vegetable oil as the external phase. The payload is incorporated in the internal aqueous phase itself and the two phases are emulsified under high-speed. The emulsion is then cooled to below the gelling point of gelatin to facilitate formation of payload-entrapped hydrogel particles. These are then collected by filtration, the oil phase is washed off with a suitable solvent and the hydrogel particles are then freeze-dried to obtain free flowing gelatin nanoparticles with an average size range of 840 nm [79].

The size distribution of these particles was affected by the nanoencapsulation process – mainly by the time and speed of homogenization and the viscosity of the gelatin solution. The size of these nanocapsules decreased with increasing time and speed of homogenization. However, prolonged homogenization resulted in flocculation of the droplets. The particle size was also increased with increasing viscosity, with a 1–3% w/w gelatin solution having optimum viscosity. The nanoencapsulation process was simple, with mild reaction conditions in the absence of emulsifiers and surfactants that might have harmful effects on the protein and peptide drugs co-encapsulated. The gelatin nanoparticulate system thus produced could be used for controlled delivery of protein and peptide drugs by intravenous, subcutaneous or intramuscular injection [79].

In the method involving solvent evaporation, the external phase is an organic solvent mixture (e.g., a 1:1 mixture of chloroform and toluene) containing a stabilizer [such as poly(methyl methacrylate) (PMMA)] and the internal aqueous phase is gelatin in phosphate-buffered saline (PBS). After high-speed homogenization of the mixture, the internal phase is evaporated under controlled conditions of temperature and pressure to obtain nanoparticles. The particles can then be crosslinked with an aldehyde if necessary. The nanoparticles are collected by centrifugation, washed with toluene to remove any excess of polymer and freeze-dried to obtain a free flowing product with a size range of 100–200 nm. The major advantage of this method is the use of PMMA in the oil phase, which prevents coagulation of the gelatin nanoparticles before and after crosslinking [67].

11.4 Characterization of Gelatin and Modified Gelatin Nanoparticles

Gelatin nanoparticles prepared by different methods are generally characterized for size, morphology, surface charge and water content. The mean particle size and size distribution of the gelatin nanoparticles can be measured by photon correlation spectroscopy (PCS) or any suitable technique that is sensitive to detecting particles in the nanometric range. Particle size analysis also helps in ensuring batch-to-batch reproducibility of the nanoparticles and hence can be used as a major quality control tool. Most nanoparticles prepared by the above methods have reported mean sizes ranging from 200 to 400 nm. Colloidal stability, drug encapsulation efficiency, loading capacity, drug release and biodistribution profile, cell internalization kinetics etc. are strongly influenced by the particle size.

Scanning electron microscopy (SEM) is widely used to study the morphology and size of nanoparticles. Nanoparticles separated from suspension either by centrifugation or filtration are dried by lyophilization. Cryoprotectants (such as mannitol, trehalose etc.) can be used if necessary to promote stability of the particle during reconstitution. The dried nanoparticles are mounted on an aluminum sample mount, sputter coated with gold–palladium and observed by SEM. SEM images reveal the morphology of these nanoparticles and their actual diameter when compared with the hydrodynamic diameter obtained by PCS. Hence, nanoparticles

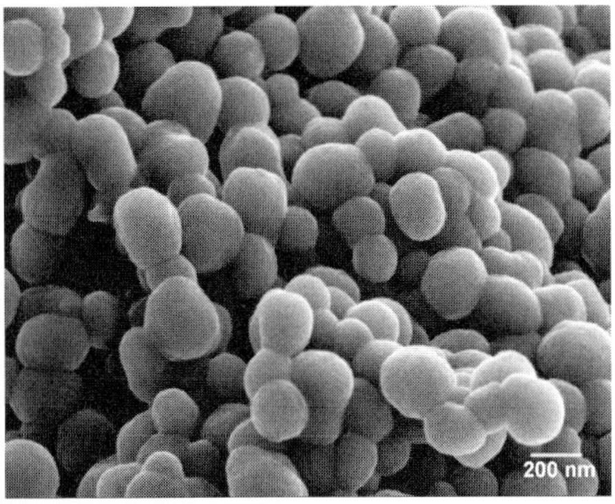

Fig. 11.5. Scanning electron microscopy image of non-crosslinked gelatin nanoparticles prepared by desolvation using ethanol.

sized by SEM would be relatively smaller than when determined by PCS [13, 52, 72, 73, 80]. Figure 11.5 shows the SEM image of non-crosslinked gelatin nanoparticles prepared by desolvation using ethanol.

The surface charge on the gelatin nanoparticles is measured by the zeta potential (the electrical potential due to the charged particles on the thin film of liquid bound to the surface of nanoparticles). Measurement of the zeta potential is one of the most important parameters in characterizing colloids, denoting their stability. Colloids with high zeta potentials ($>\pm 30$ mV) are very stable due to electrostatic repulsions, when the zeta potential is close to zero coagulation and sedimentation of the colloidal particles is faster. The gelatin nanoparticles are dispersed in deionized water (or suitable buffer if necessary) and the zeta potential measured at the default parameters of dielectric constant, refractive index and viscosity of water [81].

Measurement of water content is important for any drug delivery system containing a moisture-sensitive compound like proteins. Gelatin nanoparticles are a kind of nano-hydrogel system that consists of a network of polymer with water molecules incorporated and the polymer crosslinked to enhance stability. The high water content in these systems plays a significant role in their biocompatibility, mechanical strength and drug release. Diffusion of water molecules into the hydrophilic matrix and formation of a gel barrier affects the release of drug from the system [82]. Water molecules can be associated with the hydrophilic polymer gels in three ways: freezing or bound water, freezing interfacial or intermediate water and free water [83]. Each molecule of associated water can exert its influence on the stability and reactivity of the polymeric carrier system in different ways.

Li et al. have determined the water content of hydrogel particles of gelatin prepared by the W/O emulsion method [79]. In this method the nanoparticles were suspended in deionized water and left in a water bath at different temperatures overnight; each sample was then vacuum filtered using a nylon filter membrane and the weight of swollen gelatin nanoparticles was compared with the dry weight of gelatin nanoparticles to calculate the percentage water content at each temperature. The water content of gelatin was linearly dependent on the temperature, taking up about 51.6% water at 15 °C and 71.4% at 42 °C. NMR spectroscopy and differential scanning calorimetry (DSC) are also widely used to determine the water content of gelatin nanoparticles. In addition, NMR spectroscopy is used to study the structure mobility and hydration properties of the polymers [82].

The nano-structured surfaces of the nanoparticles of gelatin and its derivatives can be characterized by electron spectroscopy for chemical analysis (ESCA) – a surface analysis technique that exploits the photoelectric effect to obtain information about elemental composition and identify the functional groups present within a few nanometers-thick surface layers. This method involves irradiating the sample with photons (mainly low energy X-rays) that interact with the surface of the material and eject electrons, which are then analyzed by a spectrophotometer to identify the elements they come from. We have analyzed gelatin and PEG-modified gelatin nanoparticles prepared in our laboratory by ESCA to provide evidence for the presence of surface PEG chains on the nanoparticles. The results showed surface functional groups identified by high-resolution peak analysis of carbon-1S (C_{1S}), oxygen-1S (O_{1S}) and nitrogen-1S (N_{1S}) envelopes that indicate the presence of ethylene oxide residues of PEG on the surface of modified gelatin [52].

11.5 Loading and Release of Payload from Gelatin Nanoparticles

The payload of drugs or other substances such as proteins or plasmid DNA may be distributed throughout the matrix, or encapsulated in the cavity enclosed by the polymer, or adsorbed on the surface of the nanoparticles. Interaction of gelatin with these substances may be through chemical conjugation, ionic interaction or physical entrapment. The extent of drug loading and encapsulation efficiency of the gelatin nanoparticles depends on the molecular weight and also on the nature of the substance incorporated. Studies by Truong-Le et al. have shown that the encapsulation efficiency of gelatin nanoparticles increases with increasing molecular weight, with some exceptions where charge interactions have a profound affect [68].

The amount of substance incorporated into the gelatin nanoparticles is generally estimated either by assaying the supernatant for the free drug or by determining the amount of drug encapsulated in the particles by subjecting them to enzymatic hydrolysis. We have used tetramethylrhodamine-labeled dextran (TMR-dextran) as a model to represent a hydrophilic macromolecular drug. The TMR-dextran was added to the gelatin solution during nanoparticle preparation, the free drug was separated by centrifugation and the drug-loaded nanoparticles were dissolved in protease (0.2 mg mL^{-1}) containing PBS. The florescence intensity of the resulting solution was measured to account for the amount of drug loaded in the gelatin nanoparticles, and the loading efficiency was found to be 51% [52]. In certain cases the loading of conventional drugs like doxorubicin and proteins like bovine serum albumin (BSA) was estimated by UV/Visible spectrophotometry and that of plasmid DNA by picogreen assay or by radiolabeling the DNA and accounting for its activity [68, 69, 72, 79].

Drug release from the gelatin nanoparticles may be due to leaching, erosion, rupture or degradation of the particulate material. Generally, it is suggested that the release of the payload is via diffusion and bioerosion for the gelatin nanoparticles [52, 72]. The hydrolysis/biodegradation process is accelerated in presence of enzymes (such as hydrolases or proteases). When the drug is distributed throughout the matrix, slow erosion or degradation can lead to prolonged drug release [15].

In vitro release studies of drugs from gelatin nanoparticles is generally carried out in a known amount of PBS, with constant shaking in the presence or absence of protease. Samples are removed at predetermined time intervals to analyze the amount of payload released. Sink conditions are maintained throughout the release study by replenishing the released medium with fresh PBS, and the drug released is calculated as a function of time [52].

Leo et al. have studied the release of doxorubicin from gelatin nanoparticles by dynamic dialysis [78]. The release study was carried out in 0.9% w/v NaCl in both the absence and presence of trypsin in the donor compartment separated by dialysis membrane with a cut-off size of 3.5 kDa. About 9 to 13% of the drug was released in the absence of the enzyme compared with 12.6 to 23.5% in the presence of trypsin [78]. The drug release rate from the gelatin nanoparticles was affected by the degree of crosslinking. This indicated the possibility of achieving controlled release by manipulating the degree of crosslinking. Gel electrophoresis indicated that the crosslinking had no effect on the structure and electrophoretic mobility of the encapsulated DNA [68].

11.6 Biocompatibility Studies

Gelatin has several unique properties that support its usability in medicine and biology. However, its animal origin and protein nature make it a material with safety risks, too, especially when intended for medical applications. These safety risks are related to the presence of prions and other infectious contaminations. Currently, there are commercial suppliers that produce gelatin by recombinant DNA technology (refer to the websites of companies like FibroGen, Fuji-Tilburg, etc.).

To evaluate cellular biocompatibility, cytotoxicity assays have been carried out to determine the affect of gelatin and modified gelatin nanoparticles on the viability of the cells in culture. Lactate dehydrogenase (LDH), the enzyme present in the cytosol of the cells, is a marker of membrane integrity of the living cells, and the LDH released by the rupture of the membrane of the dead cells is estimated to determine the affect of nanoparticles on the viability of the cells. Brzoska et al. have compared the cytotoxicity of gelatin nanoparticles with that of human serum albumin (HSA) and poly(hexylcyanoacrylate) nanoparticles by incubating them at concentrations of 0–50 μg mL^{-1} for 6 h with pulmonary epithelial cells, monitoring the levels of LDH up to 96 h after replacing the supernatant. LDH levels of the cells incubated with gelatin nanoparticles were constant and were comparable with that of negative control. The same group has also looked into the ability of gelatin nanoparticles to initiate the expression of interleukin-8 (IL-8) by the pulmonary epithelial cells. ELISA was used to estimate the concentration of IL-8 in the supernatant after 24 h incubation of nanoparticles. Notably, gelatin nanoparticles did not initiate any expression of IL-8 even at concentrations as high as 100 $\mu g\ mL^{-1}$ [75].

One of the most popular methods of estimating cytotoxicity is the MTS assay (commercially available as CellTiter 96® AQ_{ueous} Non-Radioactive Cell Proliferation Assay from Promega). It is based on the principle that when a novel tetrazolium compound [3-(4,5-dimethylthiazol-2-yl)-5-(3-carboxymethoxyphenyl)-2-(4-sulfophenyl)-2*H*-tetrazolium, inner salt or MTS] is incubated with cells, the metabolically active cell population converts MTS into purple formazan that is soluble in the culture medium (unlike the MTT assay, wherein the formazan salt is not soluble). Mitochondrial dehydrogenase enzymes present in the viable cells cleave the yellow tetrazolium compound to a purple formazan salt that is estimated by calorimetry. We have evaluated the cellular toxicity of gelatin and modified gelatins (PEGylated form) in comparison with polyethyleneimine and lipofectin. Cells incubated with gelatin remained 100% viable even at concentrations up to 200 $\mu g\ mL^{-1}$ [52]. These studies indicate that gelatin is biocompatible and non-toxic, and hence is safe and could be used as a vehicle for drug delivery applications.

11.7 Applications of Gelatin and Modified Gelatin Nanoparticles

Gelatin has been widely used for various industrial applications, primarily in food, pharmaceuticals and medicine. It is used extensively in the food industry – confectionary, dairy, meat, desserts, in bakery products as thickening agents, stabilizer and emulsifier. Gelatin is an inexpensive, non-toxic, biocompatible and biodegradable polymer that can be easily formulated – the most popular conventional pharmaceutical dosage form being soft and hard gelatin capsules. Hydrogels, films, micro- and nanoparticles based on gelatin represent a few of the novel formulations, which are being explored widely for pharmaceutical and drug delivery applications.

Gelatin nanoparticles have been used as a carrier for gene delivery applications [84]. Cellular uptake of these nanoparticles is mainly attributed to endocytosis, wherein the cells engulf the nanoparticles, forming a vesicular structure (endosome) that fuses with the lysosomes within the cytoplasmic space. Upon acidification of the endo-lysosomal complex, the nanoparticles degrade and the contents are released into the cytoplasm to exert pharmacological action. Gelatin nanoparticles have several advantages as a non-viral gene delivery vector. They can be conjugated to moieties that stimulate receptor-mediated endocytosis, multiple plasmids or bioactive agents can be encapsulated and the bioactivity of the encapsulated DNA could be improved by preventing digestion by nucleases and by using long-circulating nanoparticles that are modified by PEG [76]. In other instances the DNA is adsorbed onto the surface of the gelatin nanoparticles by modifying the surface of gelatin with cholamine (a quaternary amine) to increase ionic interactions [81].

Gelatin nanoparticles can be crosslinked with dialdehydes (glutaraldehyde, glyoxal etc.) and those aldehyde groups can then be used as chemical handles for further modification. Crosslinking also helps to control the degradation kinetics of the nanoparticles. One limitation of using crosslinked gelatin nanoparticles is that the nature of transfectability of the nanoparticles is reduced due to the reduction in release rate of the DNA from the nanospheres [68, 77].

Nanoparticulate carriers of gelatin have been used for efficient intracellular delivery of the encapsulated payload. Our laboratory is engaged in exploring gelatin and modified gelatin-based nanoparticles for drug delivery. We have carried out cell trafficking studies using gelatin and PEGylated gelatin nanoparticles loaded with TMR-dextran as a model hydrophilic drug in BT-20 cells. We observed the localization of TMR-dextran loaded nanoparticles in the perinuclear region of the cells. The particles were mainly taken up by endocytosis, which later escaped the endosomal system and were found around the perinuclear area in the cytoplasm [52, 72]. In addition, we have reported the gene delivery efficiency of nanoparticles prepared from gelatin and PEGylated gelatin [85]. Most of the administered gelatin and PEGylated gelatin nanoparticles were internalized in NIH-3T3 fibroblast cells within the first 6 h of incubation. A large fraction of the administered nanoparticles was concentrated in the perinuclear region of the cells after 12 h. Green fluorescent protein expression was observed after 12 h of nanoparticle incubation and remained stable for up to 96 h. Flow cytometry results showed that the DNA transfection efficiency with gelatin and PEGylated gelatin nanoparticles was 43% and 61%, respectively, after 96 h. This study illustrates that PEGylated gelatin nanoparticles were rapidly internalized by the cells through nonspecific endocytosis and remained intact in the cytosol for up to 12 h [85]. A similar study was carried out using non-crosslinked gelatin nanoparticles loaded with plasmid DNA; confocal images in Fig. 11.6 show the florescence observed at 24 and 96 h post-transfection.

Kushibiki et al. have proven the long-circulation property of PEGylated gelatin by using ^{125}I-labeled gelatin [54]. The grafted polymer was obtained by incubating succinimidyl succinate methoxy-PEG with gelatin followed by radio-iodination by the chloramine-T method. Nanoparticulates with an average size of 100 nm were prepared by micellization of gelatin and PEGylated gelatin solutions at concentrations ranging from 0.04 to 10 mg mL^{-1} in the presence of 5 mM *N*-pheny-1-naphthylamine (PNA) in methanol. Results of the biodistribution studies indicated a parallel increase in area under the curve (AUC) with an increase in molecular weight of the grafted PEG at the same degree of PEGylation, [54].

We have prepared nanoparticles from gelatin (Type-B) and PEGylated gelatin, radiolabeled with ^{125}I for *in vivo* biodistribution studies after intravenous (i.v.) administration in mice bearing Lewis lung carcinoma [58]. From the radioactivity in

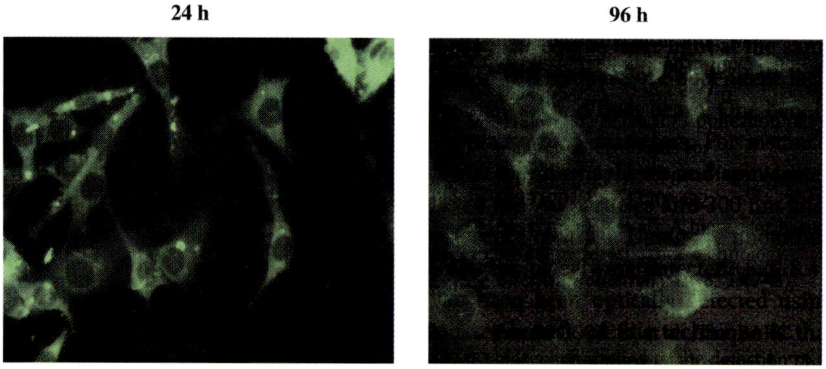

Fig. 11.6. Fluorescence confocal microscopy images of NIH-3T3 murine fibroblast cells transfected with enhanced green fluorescent protein plasmid DNA (EGFP-N1)-loaded gelatin nanoparticles after 24 and 96 h post-transfection.

plasma and various organs collected, most PEGylated nanoparticles were evidently present either in the blood pool or taken up by the tumor mass and liver. For instance, after 3 h, the concentrations of PEGylated gelatin nanoparticles were almost two-fold higher in the blood pool than the control gelatin nanoparticles. PEGylated gelatin nanoparticles remained in the blood pool for a longer due to the steric repulsion effect of the PEG chains as compared with the gelatin nanoparticles. In addition, ca. 4–5% of the recovered dose of PEGylated gelatin nanoparticles was present in the tumor mass for up to 12 h. Plasma and the tumor half-lives, mean residence time, and the AUC of the PEGylated gelatin nanoparticles were significantly higher than those for the gelatin nanoparticles. These results showed that PEGylated gelatin nanoparticles possess long-circulating properties and can preferentially distribute in the tumor mass after systemic delivery.

Leong et al. have studied the *in vivo* transfection efficiency of gelatin nanoparticles containing the LacZ plasmid in the tibialis anterior muscle of 6-week-old BALB/c mice; the muscle was isolated and homogenized 3 weeks after injection to assay the expression of β-galactosidase. The gelatin nanoparticles exhibited a more profound and sustained gene expression than the naked plasmid DNA and lipofectamine complexes [76].

Research carried out by Farrugia et al. has indicated the antitumor activity of empty gelatin nanoparticles, which effectively inhibited the formation of melanoma tumors by binding to the fibronectin surfaces that interfere with tumor growth [80]. This property can allow gelatin nanoparticles to be used as a possible alternative to Bacillus Calmette-Guerin vaccine in the treatment of melanoma [80]. In yet another study, nanoparticles of gelatin and PEGylated gelatin, ranging in size from 100–1000 nm, have been prepared via a self-assembly process. These nanoparticles were degraded by collagenase IV within 1 min and the degraded fragments had a molecular weight of 2000 and below, which is smaller than the cut-off molecular size for the kidney membrane. This indicates the possibility of using these complexes for anticancer therapy wherein the payload is released by the action of matrix metalloproteases (MMPs) at the cancer site. all-*trans*-Retinoic acid has been used as a model drug, and the loading efficiency was found to be about 92% when loaded at 1% weight of polymer. Release studies of the drug-loaded PEGylated gelatin nanoparticles revealed an accelerated release profile in the presence of collagenase IV – an enzyme present in high concentrations in tumor tissues [53].

Gelatin-based nanoparticulate systems have also been used to deliver protein and peptide drugs. Macromolecules such as proteins are degraded in the gastrointestinal tract when administered orally and these drugs require multiple injections to achieve the desired therapeutic effect if administered via the parenteral route. Li et al. have studied gelatin nanoparticles to overcome these hurdles for the delivery of a model protein (BSA) [59, 79].

Gelatin nanoparticles have been explored to encapsulate antitumor drugs, which resulted in increased efficiency, controlled release, and targeting of drugs to the affected area. Paclitaxel-loaded gelatin nanoparticles were used to enhance the solubility of the drug and its partitioning across biological membranes that are sensitive to Cremophor EL, a constituent used to solubilize paclitaxel in commercial formulations. X-Ray diffraction analysis indicated an amorphous state of the entrapped drug, thus confirming its enhanced solubility. These paclitaxel-loaded gelatin nanoparticles were used to treat dogs with intravesical bladder carcinoma and a 2.6× higher drug concentration was achieved in tumors compared with control dogs treated with Cremophor EL containing a commercial paclitaxel injection [86]. Studies have been conducted by injecting doxorubicin-loaded glutaraldehyde-crosslinked gelatin nanoparticles into rats by intraperitoneal injection [69]. The animals were monitored for side effects by electrocardiogram and body weight and the results indicated that control nanoparticles (without any drug) did not show any toxicity. Although the efficiency of the anticancer drug was enhanced, upon repeated administration the formulation (doxorubicin-loaded gelatin nanoparticles) showed high cardiotoxicity. This was attributed to covalent attachment of the drug to the carrier and the toxicity of the degradation products of these drug-peptide conjugates [69, 78]. Michaelis et al. also observed similar results, by conjugating diethylenetriamine pentaacetic acid (DTPA – an extracellular chelator) to gelatin. The attachment to gelatin enhanced cellular uptake and increased the cytotoxic and antiviral activity of DTPA by five- to eight-fold [74].

11.8 Conclusions

The unique physical, chemical and biological properties of gelatin and its modified derivatives make it a best possible alternative for drug delivery and therapeutic applications. The safety of traditional gelatins, especially in terms of immunogenicity, presence of biological impurities and other drawbacks associated with tissue-derived material are some of the reasons why researchers have developed a complete set of new recombinant gelatins. Advances in biotechnology have provided gelatins with well-defined molecular weights, pI, guaranteed lot-to-lot reproducibility, and the ability to tailor the molecule to match a specific application. They are also biodegradable, non-immunogenic, have excellent cell binding properties, and can be delivered with a purity of >99.9%. Thus the new generation recombinant gelatins are the most appropriate materials for a range of medical and pharmaceutical applications, including hydro-gels for controlled release functions, tissue engineering scaffolds, and stabilizing additives of vaccines or bio-pharmaceuticals. It is also evident that gelatin is useful in maintaining the therapeutic activity of biotechnological products such as proteins, peptides and oligonucleotides, in reducing the toxicity of cytotoxic compounds such as doxorubicin and help in improving the targeting ability of various drugs to the diseased site. The examples cited in this chapter show a broad potential for a wide range of clinical and therapeutic applications using gelatin, and ongoing studies should help to improve therapeutic approaches for the effective use of this natural polymer.

References

1 Soppimath, K. S., Aminabhavi, T. M., Kulkarni, A. R., Rudzinski, W. E., Biodegradable polymeric nanoparticles as drug delivery devices. *J. Controlled Release* **2001**, *70* (1–2), 1–20.

2 Adams, M. L., Lavasanifar, A., Kwon, G. S., Amphiphilic block copolymers for drug delivery. *J. Pharm. Sci.* **2003**, *92* (7), 1343–1355.

3 Kataoka, K., Harada, A., Nagasaki, Y., Block copolymer micelles for drug delivery: design, characterization and biological significance. *Adv. Drug Deliv. Rev.* **2001**, *47* (1), 113–131.

4 Rao, G. C., Kumar, M. S., Mathivanan, N., Rao, M. E., Nanosuspensions as the most promising approach in nanoparticulate drug delivery systems. *Pharmazie* **2004**, *59* (1), 5–9.

5 Uchegbu, I. F., Vyas, S. P., Non-ionic surfactant based vesicles (niosomes) in drug delivery. *Int. J. Pharm.* **1998**, *172* (1–2), 33–70.

6 De Miguel, I., Ioualalen, K., Bonnefous, M., Peyrot, M., Nguyen, F., Cervilla, M., Soulet, N., Dirson, R., Rieumajou, V., Imbertie, L., et al., Synthesis and characterization of supramolecular biovector (SMBV) specifically designed for the entrapment of ionic molecules. *Biochim. Biophys. Acta* **1995**, *1237* (1), 49–58.

7 Rabinow, B. E., Nanosuspensions in drug delivery. *Nat. Rev. Drug Discov.* **2004**, *3* (9), 785–796.

8 Boas, U., Heegaard, P. M., Dendrimers in drug research. *Chem. Soc. Rev.* **2004**, *33* (1), 43–63.

9 Sonneville-Aubrun, O., Simonnet, J. T., L'Alloret, F., Nanoemulsions: a new vehicle for skincare products. *Adv. Colloid Interface Sci.* **2004**, *108–109*, 145–149.

10 Tenjarla, S., Microemulsions: an overview and pharmaceutical applications. *Crit. Rev. Ther. Drug Carrier Syst.* **1999**, *16* (5), 461–521.

11 Torchilin, V. P., Drug targeting. *Eur. J. Pharm. Sci.* **2000**, *11* (Suppl 2), S81–91.

12 Kreuter, J., Nanoparticles and nanocapsules – new dosage forms in the nanometer size range. *Pharm. Acta Helv.* **1978**, *53* (2), 33–39.

13 Marty, J. J., Oppenheim, R. C., Speiser, P., Nanoparticles – a new colloidal drug-delivery system. *Pharm. Acta Helv.* **1978**, *53*, 17–23.

14 Douglas, S. J., Davis, S. S., Illum, L., Nanoparticles in drug delivery. *Crit. Rev. Ther. Drug Carrier Syst.* **1987**, *3* (3), 233–261.

15 Kreuter, J., Drug targeting with nanoparticles. *Eur. J. Drug Metab. Pharmacokinet.* **1994**, *19* (3), 253–256.

16 Couvreur, P., Dubernet, C., Puisiex, F., Controlled drug delivery with nanoparticles: current possibilities and future trends. *Eur. J. Pharm. Biopharm.* **1995**, *41* (1), 2–13.

17 Ravi Kumar, M., Hellermann, G., Lockey, R. F., Mohapatra, S. S., Nanoparticle-mediated gene delivery: state of the art. *Expert Opin Biol Ther.* **2004**, *4* (8), 1213–1224.

18 Muller, R. H., Radtke, M., Wissing, S. A., Solid lipid nanoparticles (SLN) and nanostructured lipid carriers (NLC) in cosmetic and dermatological preparations. *Adv. Drug Del. Rev.* **2002**, *54* (Suppl 1), S131–155.

19 Moghimi, S. M., Hunter, A. C., Murray, J. C., Long-circulating and target-specific nanoparticles: theory to practice. *Pharmacol. Rev.* **2001**, *53* (2), 283–318.

20 Alonso, M. J., Polymeric nanoparticles: new systems for improving ocular bioavailability of drugs. *Arch. Soc. Esp. Oftalmol.* **2001**, *76* (8), 453–454.

21 Kreuter, J., Nanoparticles and microparticles for drug and vaccine delivery. *J. Anat.* **1996**, *189* (3), 503–505.

22 Panyam, J., Labhasetwar, V., Biodegradable nanoparticles for drug and gene delivery to cells and tissue. *Adv. Drug Del. Rev.* **2003**, *55* (3), 329–347.

23 Barratt, G., Colloidal drug carriers: achievements and perspectives. *Cell. Mol. Life Sci.* **2003**, *60* (1), 21–37.

24 Brigger, I., Dubernet, C., Couvreur, P., Nanoparticles in cancer therapy and diagnosis. *Adv. Drug Del. Rev.* **2002**, *54* (5), 631–651.

25 Speiser, P. P., Nanoparticles and liposomes: a state of the art. *Methods Find. Exp. Clin. Pharmacol.* **1991**, *13* (5), 337–342.

26 Lavasanifar, A., Samuel, J., Kwon, G. S., Poly(ethylene oxide)-block-poly(L-amino acid) micelles for drug delivery. *Adv. Drug Del. Rev.* **2002**, *54* (2), 169–190.

27 Goa, K. L., Benfield, P., Hyaluronic acid. A review of its pharmacology and use as a surgical aid in ophthalmology, and its therapeutic potential in joint disease and wound healing. *Drugs* **1994**, *47* (3), 536–566.

28 Chuang, V. T., Kragh-Hansen, U., Otagiri, M., Pharmaceutical strategies utilizing recombinant human serum albumin. *Pharm. Res.* **2002**, *19* (5), 569–577.

29 Cascone, M. G., Barbani, N., Cristallini, C., Giusti, P., Ciardelli, G., Lazzeri, L., Bioartificial polymeric materials based on polysaccharides. *J. Biomater. Sci. Polym. Ed.* **2001**, *12* (3), 267–281.

30 Mehvar, R., Dextrans for targeted and sustained delivery of therapeutic and imaging agents. *J. Controlled Release* **2000**, *69* (1), 1–25.

31 Suh, J. K., Matthew, H. W., Application of chitosan-based polysaccharide biomaterials in cartilage tissue engineering: a review. *Biomaterials* **2000**, *21* (24), 2589–2598.

32 Djagny, V. B., Wang, Z., Xu, S., Gelatin: a valuable protein for food and pharmaceutical industries: review. *Crit. Rev. Food Sci. Nutr.* **2001**, *41* (6), 481–492.

33 Courts, A., The N-terminal amino acid residues of gelatin 2. Thermal degradation. *Biochem. J.* **1954**, *58* (1), 74–79.

34 Flory, P. J., Weaver, E. S., Helix–coil transitions in dilute aqueous collagen solutions. *J. Am. Chem. Soc.* **1960**, *82*, 4518–4525.

35 Farrugia, C. A., Groves, M. J., Gelatin behaviour in dilute aqueous solution: designing a nanoparticulate formulation. *J. Pharm. Pharmacol.* **1999**, *51* (6), 643–649.

36 Torchilin, V. P., How do polymers prolong circulation time of liposomes? *J. Liposome Res.* **1996**, *6* (1), 99–116.

37 Torchilin, V. P., PEG-based micelles as carriers of contrast agents for

different imaging modalities. *Adv. Drug Del. Rev.* **2002**, *54* (2), 235–252.
38 Gref, R., Domb, A. J., Quellec, P., Blunk, T., Müller, R. H., Verbavatz, J. M., Langer, R., The controlled intravenous delivery of drugs using PEG-coated sterically stabilized nanospheres. *Adv. Drug Del. Rev.* **1995**, *16* (2–3), 215–233.
39 Lewanski, C. R., Stewart, S., Pegylated liposomal adriamycin: a review of current and future applications. *Pharm. Sci. Technol. Today* **1999**, *2* (12), 473–477.
40 Reddy, K. R., Controlled-release, pegylation, liposomal formulations: new mechanisms in the delivery of injectable drugs. *Ann. Pharmacother.* **2000**, *34* (7–8), 915–923.
41 Otsuka, H., Nagasaki, Y., Kataoka, K., PEGylated nanoparticles for biological and pharmaceutical applications. *Adv. Drug Del. Rev.* **2003**, *55* (3), 403–419.
42 Roberts, M. J., Bentley, M. D., Harris, J. M., Chemistry for peptide and protein PEGylation. *Adv. Drug Del. Rev.* **2002**, *54* (4), 459–476.
43 Bhadra, D., Bhadra, S., Jain, P., Jain, N. K., Pegnology: a review of PEG-ylated systems. *Pharmazie* **2002**, *57* (1), 5–29.
44 Yowell, S. L., Blackwell, S., Novel effects with polyethylene glycol modified pharmaceuticals. *Cancer Treat. Rev.* **2002**, *28* (Suppl A), 3–6.
45 Crawford, J., Clinical uses of pegylated pharmaceuticals in oncology. *Cancer Treat. Rev.* **2002**, *28* (Suppl A), 7–11.
46 Harris, J. M., Martin, N. E., Modi, M., Pegylation: a novel process for modifying pharmacokinetics. *Clin. Pharmacokinet.* **2001**, *40* (7), 539–551.
47 Francis, G. E., Delgado, C., Fisher, D., Malik, F., Agrawal, A. K., Polyethylene glycol modification: relevance of improved methodology to tumour targeting. *J. Drug Target.* **1996**, *3* (5), 321–340.
48 Naper, D. H., *Polymeric Stabilization of Colloidal Dispersions.* ed., Academic Press, New York, **1983**.
49 Torchilin, V. P., Polymer-coated long-circulating microparticulate pharmaceuticals. *J. Microencapsul.* **1998**, *15* (1), 1–19.
50 Torchilin, V. P., Papisov, M. I., Why do polyethylene glycol-coated liposomes circulate so long? *J. Liposome Res.* **1994**, *4* (1), 725–739.
51 Zalipsky, S., Functionalized poly(ethylene glycol) for preparation of biologically revalant conjugates. *Bioconj. Chem.* **1995**, *6*, 150–165.
52 Kaul, G., Amiji, M., Long-circulating poly(ethylene glycol)-modified gelatin nanoparticles for intracellular delivery. *Pharm. Res.* **2002**, *19* (7), 1062–1068.
53 Kim, K. J., Byun, Y., Preparation and characterizations of self-assembled PEGylated gelatin nanoparticles. *Biotechnol. Bioprocess Eng.* **1999**, *4*, 210–214.
54 Kushibiki, T., Matsuoka, H., Tabata, Y., Synthesis and physical characterization of poly(ethylene glycol)-gelatin conjugates. *Biomacromolecules* **2004**, *5* (1), 202–208.
55 Shu, X. Z., Liu, Y., Luo, Y., Roberts, M. C., Prestwich, G. D., Disulfide crosslinked hyaluronan hydrogels. *Biomacromolecules* **2002**, *3*, 1304–1311.
56 Weber, C., Reiss, S., Langer, K., Preparation of surface modified protein nanoparticles by introduction of sulfhydryl groups. *Int. J. Pharm.* **2000**, *211* (1–2), 67–78.
57 Coester, C., Kreuter, J., von Briesen, H., Langer, K., Preparation of avidin-labelled gelatin nanoparticles as carriers for biotinylated peptide nucleic acid (PNA). *Int. J. Pharm.* **2000**, *196* (2), 147–149.
58 Kaul, G., Amiji, M., Biodistribution and targeting potential of poly(ethylene glycol)-modified gelatin nanoparticles in subcutaneous murine tumor model. *J. Drug Target.* **2004**, *12* (9–10), 585–591.
59 Li, J. K., Wang, N., Wu, X. S., A novel biodegradable system based on gelatin nanoparticles and poly(lactic-co-glycolic acid) microspheres for protein and peptide drug delivery. *J. Pharm. Sci.* **1997**, *86* (8), 891–895.
60 Shu, X. Z., Liu, Y., Palumbo, F., Prestwich, G. D., Disulfide-

crosslinked hyaluronan-gelatin hydrogel films: a covalent mimic of the extracellular matrix for in vitro cell growth. *Biomaterials* **2003**, *24* (21), 3825–3834.
61 Chen, T., Embree, H. D., Wu, L. Q., Payne, G. F., In vitro protein-polysaccharide conjugation: tyrosinase-catalyzed conjugation of gelatin and chitosan. *Biopolymers* **2002**, *64* (6), 292–302.
62 Ma, J., Cao, H., Li, Y., Li, Y., Synthesis and characterization of poly(DL-lactide)-grafted gelatins as bioabsorbable amphiphilic polymers. *J. Biomater. Sci. Polymer Ed.* **2002**, *13* (1), 67–80.
63 Balthasar, S., Michaelis, K., Dinauer, N., von Briesen, H., Kreuter, J., Langer, K., Preparation and characterisation of antibody modified gelatin nanoparticles as drug carrier system for uptake in lymphocytes. *Biomaterials* **2005**, *26* (15), 2723–2732.
64 Wartlick, H., Michaelis, K., Balthasar, S., Strebhardt, K., Kreuter, J., Langer, K., Highly specific HER2-mediated cellular uptake of antibody-modified nanoparticles in tumour cells. *J. Drug Target.* **2004**, *12* (7), 461–471.
65 Gupta, A. K., Gupta, M., Yarwood, S. J., Curtis, A. S., Effect of cellular uptake of gelatin nanoparticles on adhesion, morphology and cytoskeleton organisation of human fibroblasts. *J. Controlled Release* **2004**, *95* (2), 197–207.
66 Vandervoort, J., Ludwig, A., Preparation and evaluation of drug-loaded gelatin nanoparticles for topical ophthalmic use. *Eur. J. Pharm. Biopharm.* **2004**, *57* (2), 251–261.
67 Cascone, M. G., Lazzeri, L., Carmignani, C., Zhu, Z., Gelatin nanoparticles produced by a simple W/O emulsion as delivery system for methotrexate. *J. Mater. Sci. Mater. Med.* **2002**, *13* (5), 523–526.
68 Truong-Le, V. L., August, J. T., Leong, K. W., Controlled gene delivery by DNA-gelatin nanospheres. *Hum. Gene Ther.* **1998**, *9* (12), 1709–1717.
69 Leo, E., Arletti, R., Forni, F., Cameroni, R., General and cardiac toxicity of doxorubicin-loaded gelatin nanoparticles. *Farmaco* **1997**, *52* (6–7), 385–388.
70 Oppheneium, R. C., Nanoparticulate drug delivery systems based on gelatin and albumin. In: *Polymeric Nanoparticles and Microspheres*, Ed. Guiot, P., Couvreur, P., CRC Press, Boca Raton, FL, **1986**, pp. 1–25.
71 Weber, C., Coester, C., Kreuter, J., Langer, K., Desolvation process and surface characterisation of protein nanoparticles. *Int. J. Pharm.* **2000**, *194* (1), 91–102.
72 Kaul, G., Lee-Parsons, C., Amiji, M., Poly(ethylene glycol)-modified gelatin nanoparticles for intracellular delivery. *Pharm. Eng.* **2003**, *23* (5), 1–5.
73 Coester, C. J., Langer, K., Briesen, H. V., Kreuter, J., Gelatin nanoparticles by two step desolvation–a new preparation method, surface modifications and cell uptake. *J. Microencapsul.* **2000**, *17* (2), 187–193.
74 Michaelis, M., Langer, K., Arnold, S., Doerr, H. W., Kreuter, J., Cinatl, J., Jr., Pharmacological activity of DTPA linked to protein-based drug carrier systems. *Biochem. Biophys. Res. Commun.* **2004**, *323* (4), 1236–1240.
75 Brzoska, M., Langer, K., Coester, C., Loitsch, S., Wagner, T. O., Mallinckrodt, C., Incorporation of biodegradable nanoparticles into human airway epithelium cells – in vitro study of the suitability as a vehicle for drug or gene delivery in pulmonary diseases. *Biochem. Biophys. Res. Commun.* **2004**, *318* (2), 562–570.
76 Leong, K. W., Mao, H. Q., Truong-Le, V. L., Roy, K., Walsh, S. M., August, J. T., DNA-polycation nanospheres as non-viral gene delivery vehicles. *J. Controlled Release* **1998**, *53*, 183–193.
77 Truong-Le, V. L., Walsh, S. M., Schweibert, E., Mao, H. Q., Guggino, W. B., August, J. T.,

Leong, K. W., Gene transfer by DNA-gelatin nanospheres. *Arch. Biochem. Biophys.* **1999**, *361* (1), 47–56.

78 Leo, E., Cameroni, R., Forni, F., Dynamic dialysis for the drug release evaluation from doxorubicin-gelatin nanoparticle conjugates. *Int. J. Pharm.* **1999**, *180*, 23–30.

79 Li, J. K., Wang, N., Wu, X. S., Gelatin nanocapsulation of protein/peptide drugs using an emulsifier-free emulsion method. *J. Microencapsul.* **1998**, *15* (2), 163–172.

80 Farrugia, C. A., Groves, M. J., The activity of unloaded gelatin nanoparticles on murine melanoma B16-F0 growth in vivo. *Anticancer Res.* **1999**, *19* (2A), 1027–1031.

81 Zwiorek, K., Kloeckner, J., Wagner, E., Coester, C., *In Vitro Gene Transfection with Surface Modified Gelatin Nanoparticles*, 2004 International conference on MEMS and NANO and smart systems, Banff, Alberta, Canada, August 25–27, **2004**, pp. 60–63.

82 Baumgartner, S., Lahajnar, G., Sepe, A., Kristl, J., Investigation of the state and dynamic of water in hydrogels of cellulose ethers by ^{1}H NMR spectroscopy. *AAPS Pharm. Sci. Tech.* **2003**, *3* (4).

83 Hatekeyama, H., Hatekeyama, T., Interaction between water and hydrophillic polymers. *Thermochim. Acta* **1998**, *308*, 3–22.

84 Kaul, G., Amiji, M., Protein nanoparticles for gene delivery. In: *Polymeric Gene Delivery: Principles and Applications*, Ed. Amiji, M., CRC Press LLC, Boca Raton, FL, **2005**, pp. 429–447.

85 Kaul, G., Amiji, M., Cellular interactions and in vitro DNA transfection studies with poly(ethylene glycol)-modified gelatin nanoparticles. *J. Pharm. Sci.* **2004**, *94* (1), 184–198.

86 Lu, Z., Yeh, T. K., Tsai, M., Au, J. L., Wientjes, M. G., Paclitaxel-loaded gelatin nanoparticles for intravesical bladder cancer therapy. *Clin. Cancer Res.* **2004**, *10* (22), 7677–7684.

Index

Nanotechnologies for the Life Sciences Vol. 1
Biofunctionalization of Nanomaterials. Edited by Challa S. S. R. Kumar

ISBN: 3-527-31381-8